MANUAL OF CLINICAL PROBLEMS
IN CARDIOLOGY
WITH ANNOTATED KEY REFERENCES

MANUAL OF CLINICAL PROBLEMS IN CARDIOLOGY
WITH ANNOTATED KEY REFERENCES

SECOND EDITION

L. DAVID HILLIS, M.D.

Associate Professor of Internal Medicine, The University of Texas Southwestern Medical School at Dallas; Director, Cardiac Catheterization Laboratory, Parkland Memorial Hospital, Dallas

BRIAN G. FIRTH, M.D., D. Phil.

Assistant Professor of Internal Medicine, The University of Texas Southwestern Medical School at Dallas; Associate Director, Cardiac Catheterization Laboratory, Parkland Memorial Hospital, Dallas

JAMES T. WILLERSON, M.D.

Professor of Internal Medicine and Chief, Cardiovascular Division, The University of Texas Southwestern Medical School at Dallas; Chief, Cardiology Division, Parkland Memorial Hospital, Dallas

LITTLE, BROWN AND COMPANY   BOSTON/TORONTO

CONTENTS

PREFACE

In this second edition of *Manual of Clinical Problems in Cardiology* we have attempted to achieve several goals. First, we have increased the number of topics from 91 to 114 so that we could introduce for discussion new areas of interest in cardiology. These include thrombolytic therapy of acute myocardial infarction, percutaneous transluminal coronary angioplasty, anthracycline-induced cardiomyopathy, systemic arterial hypertension, the digoxin-quinidine interaction, and the newest of the antiarrhythmic agents. Second, we have updated the discussions of those subjects that were covered in the first edition and, when appropriate, have lengthened them somewhat to add new information. Finally, we have extensively updated the references at the end of each discussion, and, as a result, a substantial number of them are from 1980–1983. At the same time, however, we have not deleted older references that are still worthy of note. In short, we have attempted to provide a maximal amount of up-to-date factual data and worthy reference material within the context of a manual rather than an exhaustive textbook.

We want to express our sincere thanks to several people who labored for many hours and whose help was immeasurable: Ms. Juanita Alexander and Ms. Laurie Christian for secretarial help; Ms. Sarah Hawkins for proofreading, photocopying, and helping to review the many references; and Ms. Kay Fulton for verifying the accuracy of the references.

L. D. H.
B. G. F.
J. T. W.

MANUAL OF CLINICAL PROBLEMS
IN CARDIOLOGY
WITH ANNOTATED KEY REFERENCES

RHYTHM AND CONDUCTION DISTURBANCES

SINUS TACHYCARDIA, SINUS BRADYCARDIA, AND SINUS ARRHYTHMIA

Sinus tachycardia is a rhythm in which each cardiac impulse arises normally from the sinoatrial node and in which the rate exceeds 100 beats per minute. The P–R interval is usually shortened but may be unchanged or even lengthened. With rates of 100 to 130 per minute, the P waves are easily identifiable before each QRS complex. When the rate approaches 150 per minute, the P waves may be superimposed on the preceding T waves, rendering P wave identification difficult or impossible. At this rate, sinus tachycardia is often difficult to differentiate from paroxysmal supraventricular tachycardia or atrial flutter with 2:1 conduction. If such differentiation is difficult, carotid sinus massage may help to clarify which tachyarrhythmia is present. In response to this maneuver, sinus tachycardia gradually slows and then gradually accelerates after massage is discontinued. In contrast, with paroxysmal supraventricular tachycardia, carotid massage induces either no change or an abrupt reversion to normal sinus rhythm. With atrial flutter and 2:1 conduction, such massage usually acutely increases the magnitude of AV block, thus slowing the ventricular response.

Sinus tachycardia represents a response to several pathologic or physiologic phenomena, including intravascular volume depletion, fever, hypermetabolism, anxiety, and physical exertion. It can occur as a manifestation of an increased intravascular catecholamine concentration, such as occurs in pheochromocytoma. Alcohol and caffeine-containing beverages, as well as certain drugs (e.g., epinephrine and atropine), often cause sinus tachycardia. Finally, sinus tachycardia is present in about one-third of patients with acute myocardial infarction, which may signify extensive pump damage with a resultant low cardiac output.

The therapy of sinus tachycardia is directed at its underlying cause. For instance, if it is due to intravascular volume depletion, the patient should receive adequate fluid replacement. If it is due to fever, the patient's body temperature should be lowered by cooling or with antipyretic medications. No therapy should be aimed at the tachycardia itself, since it is simply a reflection of disordered homeostasis. Especially in the setting of acute myocardial infarction, the underlying cause of sinus tachycardia should be determined and corrected quickly, since persistent tachycardia augments the extent of myocardial ischemic injury.

Sinus bradycardia is a rhythm in which each cardiac impulse arises normally from the sinoatrial node and in which the rate is less than 50 to 60 per minute. In about 25 percent of healthy young men, the sinus rate is between 50 and 60 beats per minute, leading some authors to suggest that 50 per minute be used as the lower limit of normal sinus rhythm. The P waves recur regularly, and each is followed by a QRS complex. The P–R interval is often prolonged.

Sinus bradycardia is a normal occurrence in some people, especially in well-trained athletes, who may have resting heart rates as low as 40 beats per minute. It can result from vagal stimulation by any of several mechanisms, including carotid sinus pressure, the Valsalva maneuver, vomiting, and facial immersion in cold water. Increased intracranial pressure may be accompanied by sinus bradycardia. Many pharmacologic agents can induce it, including the beta-adrenergic blocking agents, verapamil, digitalis, reserpine, guanethidine, methyldopa, various pressor amines, and occasionally quinidine, procainamide, and lidocaine. Certain electrolyte imbalances, such as hyperkalemia, and both hypothermia and hypothyroidism can cause sinus bradycardia. Finally, sinus bradycardia occurs in 10 to 15 percent of patients in the setting of acute myocardial infarction. However, its incidence in the very early phase of infarction (i.e., within 1–3 hr) is even higher, especially when the infarction involves the inferior portion of the left ventricle.

Although most patients with sinus bradycardia are asymptomatic, it can occasionally cause dizziness or even syncope, angina pectoris, or symptoms of biventricular congestive heart failure. If these symptoms appear, treatment should be initiated. First, any of the drugs known to cause sinus bradycardia should be discontinued. Second, atropine sulfate, 0.5 to 1.0 mg, should be administered intravenously and repeated 2 to 3 times if necessary. Third, if symptomatic sinus bradycardia persists, temporary and then permanent pacing should be instituted.

Sinus arrhythmia is a rhythm in which each cardiac impulse arises normally from the sinoatrial node but in which the rhythmicity of the beats varies, so that the P–P interval varies by more than 0.16 seconds. Most commonly, this change in sinus rate is related to respiration: the heart rate increases gradually during inspiration and decreases with expiration. These fluctuations in vagal tone are caused by reflex changes in the pulmonary and systemic vascular systems. Sinus arrhythmia is most common in patients with a resting bradycardia, presumably because baseline vagal influences are prominent. In these patients, the rhythm usually becomes regular when the rate is increased with exercise or atropine.

Sinus arrhythmia occurs most often in children and in the elderly. It may be seen following digitalis administration, during convalescence from various infectious diseases, and as a cardiovascular sign of increased intracranial pressure. It is common after an acute inferior myocardial infarction. In almost all patients with sinus arrhythmia, no symptoms can be attributed to the rhythm. At times, sinus arrhythmia can be difficult to distinguish from sinoatrial block or an ectopic atrial rhythm.

Since sinus arrhythmia is usually of no clinical importance, it requires no treatment. However, if severe bradycardia is also present, dizziness or syncope can occur, and intravenous atropine is the appropriate therapeutic agent, with transvenous temporary pacing held in reserve.

Sinus Tachycardia

1. Gifford RW Jr, Kvale WF, Maher FT, Roth GM, Priestley JT. Clinical features, diagnosis, and treatment of pheochromocytoma: a review of 76 cases. Mayo Clin Proc 1964; 39:281–302.
   Of these 76 patients with pheochromocytoma, 47 (62%) complained of palpitations.
2. DeSanctis RW, Block P, Hutter AM Jr. Tachyarrhythmias in myocardial infarction. Circulation 1972; 45:681–702.
   About one-third of patients with infarction demonstrate sinus tachycardia; most common causes are pump failure, fever, anxiety, pericarditis, and cardioaccelerator drugs.
3. Lown B, Klein MD, Hershberg PI. Coronary and precoronary care. Am J Med 1969; 46:705–24.
   In the setting of myocardial infarction, sinus tachycardia is often associated with pump failure; as a result, it carries a substantial mortality (34% in this study).
4. Julian DG, Valentine PA, Miller GG. Disturbances of rate, rhythm, and conduction in acute myocardial infarction. Am J Med 1964; 37:915–27.
   Of 100 consecutive patients with acute infarction, 43 had sinus tachycardia. Except for ventricular premature beats, this was the most frequent arrhythmia.
5. Redwood DR, Smith ER, Epstein SE. Coronary artery occlusion in the conscious dog: effects of alterations in heart rate and arterial pressure on the degree of myocardial ischemia. Circulation 1972; 46:323–32.
   In the dog with coronary artery occlusion, tachycardia worsens the severity of myocardial ischemic injury.

Sinus Bradycardia

6. Rotman M, Wagner GS, Wallace AG. Bradyarrhythmias in acute myocardial infarction. Circulation 1972; 45:703–22.
   The incidence of sinus bradycardia in monitored patients with acute myocardial infarction ranges from 10% to 30%, with an average incidence of about 15%.
7. Haden RF, Langsjoen PH, Rapoport MI, McNerney JJ. The significance of sinus bradycardia in acute myocardial infarction. Dis Chest 1963; 44:168–73.
   In this study, sinus bradycardia appeared to be a prelude to cardiac standstill or ventricular fibrillation.
8. Agruss NS, Rosin EY, Adolph RJ, Fowler NO. Significance of chronic sinus bradycardia in elderly people. Circulation 1972; 46:924–30.
   A heart rate below 50 beats/minute in elderly people (ages 67–79) does not indicate depressed cardiac performance.
9. Hiss RG, Lamb LE, Allen MF. Electrocardiographic findings in 67,375 asymptomatic subjects. X. Normal values. Am J Cardiol 1960; 6:200–31.
   In patients less than 25 years of age, 25–30% had a resting heart rate less than 60 beats/minute.
10. Hiss RG, Lamb LE. Electrocardiographic findings in 122,043 individuals. Circulation 1962; 25:947–61.
    Sinus tachycardia, sinus bradycardia, and sinus arrhythmia all occur most commonly in young (less than 25 years old) individuals.
11. Eraut D, Shaw DB. Sinus bradycardia. Br Heart J 1971; 33:742–9.
    In this group of 46 patients with persistent sinus bradycardia, sick sinus syndrome was eventually diagnosed in almost all.
12. Jose AD, Collison D. The normal range and determinants of the intrinsic heart rate in man. Cardiovasc Res 1970; 4:160–7.
    Normal standards are provided for resting heart rate from among 432 healthy adults, ages 16 to 70.
13. Dighton DH. Sinus bradycardia: Autonomic influences and clinical assessment. Br Heart J 1974; 36:791–7.
    Some patients with sinus bradycardia have poor autonomic responses, whereas in others the bradycardia is simply a marked physiologic phenomenon.

PREMATURE BEATS

Premature beats, or extrasystoles, are cardiac contractions of ectopic origin that occur earlier than expected in the usual rhythm. They are the most common of the cardiac arrhythmias. The activating impulse may be located in the atria, AV junction, or ventricles.

Atrial premature beats (APBs) are extremely common, even in individuals without organic heart disease. They occur with even greater frequency in persons who abuse alcohol or cigarettes, in persons with excessive fatigue or anxiety, and in persons with a variety of infectious diseases. Finally, their incidence is increased in patients with atrial disease or atrial enlargement of any kind, including mitral valve disease and cor pulmonale. Their occurrence is not increased in individuals with coronary artery disease. Although the patient may note "skipped beats" or "fluttering" of the heart, he is usually asymptomatic. On physical examination, palpation of the peripheral pulse reveals an occasional early beat.

Since the premature impulse originates from an ectopic focus in the atria, the normal sequence of atrial activation is altered, so that the P wave not only appears early but is also abnormal in configuration. It may or may not be conducted to the ventricles, depending on the degree of prematurity. The P–R interval of the premature beat may remain unchanged, become shorter, or lengthen. The QRS complex following an APB is usually morphologically normal, since the course of the impulse through the ventricular conduction system is normal. However, if the APB occurs at a time when the ventricular conduction system is partially refractory, the QRS complex may demonstrate various degrees of aberration; in fact, it may be so altered as to resemble a ventricular premature beat. The degree of aberration of ventricular activation is related to the degree of prematurity of the APB: an extremely early APB is usually conducted with a great deal of aberration, whereas a later APB is likely to be conducted normally. As the ectopic atrial impulse propagates and depolarizes the sinoatrial node, it resets the sinus cycle; as a result, the cycle length after the APB is similar to the basic cycle length. In contrast to ventricular premature beats, therefore, the pause following an APB is usually not fully compensatory.

Atrial premature beats usually require no therapy. If suppression is desired, quinidine or propranolol is usually efficacious.

Like APBs, *AV nodal or junctional premature beats* usually cause no symptoms. Since the premature beat originates in the AV node and follows the normal pathway of ventricular activation, the QRS complex usually is morphologically normal. The P wave may appear abnormal in position and configuration, representing either retrograde activation of the atria by the nodal impulse or normal sinus activation of the atria in close temporal proximity to the activation of the ventricles by the junctional depolarization. In the former circumstance, the P wave is morphologically abnormal and may appear before, simultaneously with, or after the QRS complex; in the latter instance, the P wave is normal in appearance and is positioned before, within, or immediately after the QRS complex.

In most instances, AV junctional premature beats function as an "escape" rhythm in patients with sinus arrhythmia, sinus bradycardia, sinus arrest, or high-degree AV block. Occasionally, they may occur following the pause after cessation of a supraventricular tachyarrhythmia or an atrial or ventricular premature beat. Thus, AV junctional escape beats are usually a secondary phenomenon, and they carry the same clinical implications as those of the underlying primary rhythm disturbance. For example, drugs, such as digitalis or propranolol, that suppress the sinoatrial node or impair AV conduction may be accompanied by AV junctional escape beats.

Ventricular premature beats (VPBs) arise from an ectopic ventricular focus and occur earlier than the prevailing sinus beat. Infrequent VPBs occur even in young and apparently healthy persons, in which case they are often the result of fatigue, anxiety, or overindulgence in tobacco, coffee, tea, or alcohol. In these healthy individuals, the frequency of VPBs may increase or decrease in response to exercise. More frequently, the appearance of VPBs is associated with several disease entities. Various electrolyte disturbances, such as hypokalemia or hypercalcemia, are associated with VPBs. Digitalis intoxication commonly is heralded by their appearance. They occur frequently in patients who have received sympathomimetic agents, such as dextroamphetamine or isoproterenol. They can appear in patients with many kinds of organic heart disease, including valvular and primary myocardial dysfunction. Finally, they are especially common and worrisome in those with ischemic heart disease.

The patient with an occasional VPB may complain of palpitations, and rarely the patient may actually note chest discomfort induced by a VPB. On physical examination, the VPB occurs earlier than the expected sinus beat and is usually followed by a long pause, the so-called compensatory pause. On the ECG, the VPB has a wide, bizarre QRS morphology that differs strikingly from normal, since the ectopic impulse takes an abnormal and longer course through the ventricles. The QRS complex is usually of high voltage, is somewhat slurred, and is widened to at least 0.13 second. The T wave is oriented in a direction opposite to its QRS complex. Those VPBs that arise from the same focus have a constant coupling interval; that is, the interval between the VPB and the preceding beat of the basic rhythm is reproducible. In most instances, the VPB is followed by the abnormally long compensatory pause. The P wave and QRS complex of the beat following a VPB are morphologically normal, but the T wave of that beat may be abnormal.

The prognostic significance of VPBs depends mainly on the patient population in which they occur. In those without demonstrable underlying heart disease, VPBs do not adversely influence mortality. In contrast, VPBs are associated with an increased risk of sudden death in individuals with any kind of organic heart disease, especially those ischemic in origin. Both in the setting of acute myocardial infarction and in the postinfarction period, frequent or complex VPBs are accompanied by a greatly enhanced likelihood of ventricular tachycardia and fibrillation. In these patients, therefore, antiarrhythmic medications should be administered in an attempt to suppress ventricular ectopic activity. Those VPBs that are especially ominous include (1) those that occur frequently (more than 5–10/min), (2) those that occur close to the T wave of the preceding sinus beat, (3) those that occur in pairs, and (4) those that originate from more than one focus within the ventricles.

Those VPBs that fulfill any of these criteria should be treated aggressively. Disturbances in serum electrolytes and acid-base balance should be corrected. Acutely, intravenous lidocaine is usually effective in abolishing VPBs: a bolus of 50 to 100 mg is followed by a continuous infusion of 1 to 4 mg per minute. If lidocaine is unsuccessful, intravenous procainamide or bretylium can be used in an attempt to suppress them. Chronically, VPB suppression can be accomplished with oral quinidine, procainamide, propranolol, or any of several new antiarrhythmics, including tocainide, amiodarone, and disopyramide.

It is often advantageous to differentiate VPBs from ventricular parasystole, since they differ substantially both in pathophysiology and prognosis. Although VPBs are often a manifestation of digitalis intoxication, parasystole does not occur in this setting. VPBs should be treated aggressively in the setting of myocardial ischemia or infarction, since they are often the precursor of ventricular tachycardia or fibrillation. In contrast, ventricular parasystole is a more benign rhythm, even in the setting of ischemic injury.

In ventricular parasystole, there is an ectopic ventricular pacemaker that activates the ventricles independently of the basic rhythm. As a result, the coupling intervals vary, and the longer interectopic intervals are whole-number multiples of the shortest one. Finally, since a parasystolic focus is independent of the basic cardiac rhythm, it can discharge its impulse at approximately the same time that the basic rhythm impulse arrives at the ventricles. Therefore, the ventricles are depolarized by two activation fronts, resulting in a fusion beat. Although such fusion beats are not unique to ventricular parasystole, they are most commonly seen in association with it.

Ventricular parasystole is relatively uncommon. It can occur in patients with or without underlying organic heart disease. Since it does not portend the same ominous prognosis as VPBs, it does not require as aggressive a therapeutic approach.

Atrial Premature Beats

1. Hinkle LE, Carver ST, Stevens M. The frequency of asymptomatic disturbances of cardiac rhythm and conduction in middle-aged men. Am J Cardiol 1969; 24:629–50.

Of 301 adult men (mean age, 55 years old), APBs occurred in 229 (76%), VPBs in 187 (62%).

Ventricular Premature Beats

2. Chiang BN, Perlman LV, Ostrander LD, Epstein FH. Relationship of premature systoles to coronary heart disease and sudden death in the Tecumseh epidemiologic study. Ann Intern Med 1969; 70:1159–66.
   In patients with coronary artery disease, the presence of VPBs increases the risk of sudden death.

3. Jelinek MV, Lown B. Exercise stress testing for exposure of cardiac arrhythmias. Prog Cardiovasc Dis 1974; 16:497–522.
   Exercise testing constitutes a safe and effective method for exposing arrhythmias that are infrequently seen at rest.

4. McHenry PL, Morris SN, Kavalier M, Jordan JW. Comparative study of exercise-induced ventricular arrhythmias in normal subjects and patients with documented coronary artery disease. Am J Cardiol 1976; 37:609–16.
   During moderate exercise, fewer than 10% of individuals without heart disease develop VPBs, whereas 27% of those with documented coronary artery disease develop ventricular ectopy.

5. Romhilt DW, Bloomfield SS, Chou T, Fowler NO. Unreliability of conventional electrocardiographic monitoring for arrhythmia detection in coronary care units. Am J Cardiol 1973; 31:457–61.
   In the setting of acute myocardial infarction, virtually all patients demonstrate ventricular ectopy.

6. Bigger JT, Dresdale RJ, Heissenbuttel RH, Weld FM, Wit AL. Ventricular arrhythmias in ischemic heart disease: mechanism, prevalence, significance, and management. Prog Cardiovasc Dis 1977; 19:255–300.
   A complete and very thorough review of ischemia and infarction-related ventricular ectopic activity.

7. Ambos HD, Roberts R, Oliver GC, Cox JR Jr, Sobel BE. Infarct size: a determinant of persistence of severe ventricular dysrhythmia. Am J Cardiol 1976; 37:116.
   In patients with acute myocardial infarction, the complexity of ventricular ectopy is closely linked to the quantity of damaged myocardium.

8. Devereux RB, Perloff JK, Reichek N, Josephson ME. Mitral valve prolapse. Circulation 1976; 54:3–14.
   About one-third of patients with prolapse have VPBs on routine ECGs. A much larger fraction has VPBs during ambulatory electrocardiographic monitoring.

9. Winkle RA, Lopes MG, Fitzgerald JW, Goodman DJ, Schroeder JS, Harrison DC. Arrhythmias in patients with mitral valve prolapse. Circulation 1975; 52:73–81.
   Of 24 unselected patients with mitral valve prolapse, 12 (50%) had frequent VPBs, and another 6 (25%) had infrequent VPBs. Five of the 24 had runs of ventricular tachycardia.

10. Engel TR, Meister SG, Frankl WS. The "R on T" phenomenon: an update and critical review. Ann Intern Med 1978; 88:221–5.
    Although early observations suggested that R-on-T was likely to initiate sustained ventricular tachyarrhythmias, more recent evidence suggests that R-on-T is not a critical determinant of primary ventricular fibrillation and sudden death.

11. Kennedy HL, Underhill SJ. Frequent or complex ventricular ectopy in apparently healthy subjects. Am J Cardiol 1976; 38:141–8.
    Exercise caused ventricular ectopy to disappear in almost all of 25 apparently healthy subjects with ventricular ectopy.

12. Lown B, Calvert AF, Armington R, Ryan M. Monitoring for serious arrhythmias and high risk of sudden death. Circulation 1975; 51, 52 (Suppl 3):189–198.
    A classification of VPBs based on their frequency, multiformity, repetitive pattern, and degree of prematurity appears to be helpful in identifying patients at high risk of sudden death.

13. Ruberman W, Weinblatt E, Frank CW, Goldberg JD, Shapiro S, Feldman CL. Ventricular premature beats and mortality of men with coronary heart disease. Circulation 1975; 51, 52 (Suppl 3):199–203.
    Among a large group of men with coronary disease, mortality was higher in those with VPBs than those without such ectopy.

14. Moss AJ, DeCamilla J, Mietlowski W, Greene WA, Goldstein S, Locksley R. Prognostic grading and significance of ventricular premature beats after recovery from myocardial infarction. Circulation 1975; 51, 52 (Suppl 3):204–10.
   In postinfarction patients, multiform and frequent VPBs portend a poor prognosis.
15. Ruberman W, Weinblatt E, Goldberg JD, Frank CW, Shapiro S, Chaudhary BS. Ventricular premature complexes in prognosis of angina. Circulation 1980; 61:1172–8.
   The risk of sudden death among patients with coronary artery disease is increased by the occurrence of ventricular ectopic activity not only among those who have had a myocardial infarction but also among those with angina only.
16. Krone RJ, Miller JP, Kleiger RE, Clark KW, Oliver GC. The effectiveness of antiarrhythmic agents on early-cycle premature ventricular complexes. Circulation 1981; 63:664–9.
   In patients with frequent VPBs, both quinidine and procainamide reduced the number of VPBs with short coupling intervals (less than 400 milliseconds) even though neither agent diminished their overall frequency.
17. Ruberman W, Weinblatt E, Goldberg JD, Frank CW, Shapiro S. Ventricular premature beats and mortality after myocardial infarction. N Engl J Med 1977; 297:750–7.
   In a group of 1,739 men with prior myocardial infarction, VPBs were associated with a three-fold increase in sudden death.
18. Hammermeister KE, DeRouen TA, Dodge HT. Variables predictive of survival in patients with coronary disease: selection by univariate and multivariate analyses from the clinical, electrocardiographic, exercise, arteriographic, and quantitative angiographic evaluations. Circulation 1979; 59:421–30.
   In patients with coronary artery disease treated either medically or surgically, the presence or absence of VPBs on a resting ECG was predictive of prognosis.
19. Kostis JB, McCrone K, Moreyra AE, Gotzoyannis S, Aglitz NM, Natarajan N, Kuo PT. Premature ventricular complexes in the absence of identifiable heart disease. Circulation 1981; 63:1351–6.
   Of 101 subjects without organic heart disease, only 4 had more than 100 VPBs/24 hours; in addition, 4 had multiform VPBs.
20. Velebit V, Podrid P, Lown B, Cohen BH, Graboys TB. Aggravation and provocation of ventricular arrhythmias by antiarrhythmic drugs. Circulation 1982; 65:886–94.
   In a retrospective analysis, a worsening of arrhythmia was observed in 11% of patients receiving therapy for ventricular tachyarrhythmias.
21. Kotler MN, Tabatznik B, Mower MM, Tominaga S. Prognostic significance of ventricular ectopic beats with respect to sudden death in the late postinfarction period. Circulation 1973; 47:959–66.
   All complex ventricular ectopy was associated with an excess risk of sudden cardiac death in patients at least 3 months post myocardial infarction.

Ventricular Parasystole
22. Myburgh DP, Lewis BS. Ventricular parasystole in healthy hearts. Am Heart J 1971; 82:307–11.
   Of 81 apparently normal individuals with ectopic beats, parasystole was present in 37.
23. Chung EKY. Parasystole. Prog Cardiovasc Dis 1968; 11:64–81.
   A concise yet thorough review of the electrocardiographic and clinical features of parasystole.
24. Moe GK, Jalife J, Mueller WJ, Moe B. A mathematical model of parasystole and its application to clinical arrhythmias. Circulation 1977; 56:968–79.
   Many electrocardiographic patterns attributed to a reentrant "extrasystolic" rhythm may actually represent the modulated activity of a parasystolic focus.

PAROXYSMAL SUPRAVENTRICULAR TACHYCARDIA

Paroxysmal supraventricular tachycardia (PSVT) occurs in persons of all ages, including infants, children, and adults. It is often seen in otherwise healthy young adults, but it also occurs in patients with rheumatic, atherosclerotic, hypertensive, or thyrotoxic heart disease. It has been described in 2 to 8 percent of patients with acute myocardial infarction. It is the most common tachyarrhythmia in individuals with the Wolff-Parkinson-White syndrome. In some patients, PSVT appears in relation to emotional stress, mental or physical fatigue, or excessive use of tobacco, coffee, or alcoholic beverages. Other precipitating factors include deep inspiration, hyperventilation, physical exertion, changes in position, and swallowing.

Episodes of PSVT usually have a sudden onset and termination. In persons with otherwise normal hearts, symptoms are usually mild and include palpitations or an uneasy feeling in the chest. Some patients describe precordial pain, weakness, dizziness, nausea, vomiting, and even syncope. In patients with atherosclerotic heart disease, episodes of PSVT may be accompanied by angina or even myocardial infarction. In those with rheumatic or hypertensive heart disease, symptoms of pulmonary and peripheral venous congestion may arise, and an occasional patient may develop evidence of vascular collapse during a sustained episode. Such collapse is especially likely to occur when the heart rate exceeds 200 beats per minute.

Electrocardiographically, PSVT has the following characteristics. First, the P waves are morphologically different from the sinus P waves. In most instances, they are small and difficult to identify, since they are often superimposed on the preceding T waves. Second, the atrial rate is between 150 and 250 per minute, with an average of 180 to 200 per minute. Third, a QRS complex follows each P wave; although it usually resembles that of the sinus beats, it may appear different because of aberrant ventricular conduction. Fourth, PSVT is a regular rhythm, although one sometimes observes a gradual increase in rate at the beginning of an episode (the so-called warm-up period). Finally, as with sinus tachycardia, S–T segment depression and T wave alterations may occur during episodes of PSVT, and they may persist for hours or even days after its conversion to sinus rhythm.

Paroxysmal supraventricular tachycardia can have one of four electrophysiologic mechanisms. Most commonly, it is due to a reentry circuit within the AV node utilizing dual AV nodal pathways. Such AV nodal reentry accounts for 60 percent of cases of PSVT. Second, PSVT can occur by a reentry mechanism in which the normal AV pathway is used for antegrade conduction and an AV bypass tract is employed for retrograde conduction. This electrophysiologic mechanism is responsible for about 30 percent of cases of PSVT. Lastly, PSVT can be produced by reentry within (1) the sinoatrial node or (2) intra-atrial tissues, together accounting for less than 10 percent of cases.

The conversion of PSVT to sinus rhythm can be accomplished in several ways. A number of so-called vagal maneuvers are designed to stimulate the vagus nerve, thereby inducing a reversion to sinus rhythm, including carotid sinus massage, the Valsalva maneuver, direct pressure on the eyeballs, and the so-called diving reflex (facial immersion in cold water for 5–10 sec). If these maneuvers are unsuccessful in causing a reversion, pharmacologic conversion is usually accomplished with intravenous verapamil, 5 to 10 mg by bolus injection, which is successful in converting approximately 90 percent of PSVTs to sinus rhythm. If intravenous verapamil is not available, one of the following pharmacologic agents can be administered: propranolol (1 mg intravenously every 3–5 min to a total dose of 0.1 mg/kg of body weight), digoxin (0.5–1.0 mg by bolus injection), edrophonium (10 mg by bolus injection), or lidocaine (50–100 mg by bolus injection).

If pharmacologic conversion is unsuccessful, electrical means can be employed. Rapid atrial pacing is used in a manner similar to that described under

Atrial Flutter (see p. 13). If this is unsuccessful, DC countershock, 50 to 200 watt-sec, usually accomplishes a reversion to sinus rhythm.

For the patient with frequent and recurrent PSVT episodes, several medications appear efficacious in maintaining sinus rhythm during chronic, long-term therapy. Digoxin or propranolol is effective in some patients with recurrent PSVT. More recently, chronic administration of oral verapamil, 240 to 480 mg per day, has been shown to reduce the frequency of PSVT episodes in patients whose PSVT is recurrent. Finally, an occasional patient whose PSVT utilizes an AV bypass tract for retrograde conduction may require surgical or catheter-electrode ablation of the tract to control episodes of PSVT.

Etiology and Precipitating Causes

1. Kissane RW, Brooks R, Clark T. Relation of supraventricular paroxysmal tachycardia to heart disease and the basal metabolism rate. Circulation 1950; 1:950–1.
   Of a group of patients with PSVT, 34% had underlying rheumatic heart disease. There was no relationship between PSVT and thyroid dysfunction.
2. Julian DG, Valentine PA, Miller GG. Disturbances of rate, rhythm, and conduction in acute myocardial infarction. Am J Med 1964; 37:915–27.
   In 100 consecutive patients with acute myocardial infarction, PSVT occurred in 4.
3. DeSanctis RW, Block P, Hutter AM Jr. Tachyarrhythmias in myocardial infarction. Circulation 1972; 45:681–702.
   In the setting of acute myocardial infarction, PSVT occurs in from 1 to 7½% of patients.
4. Berry K. Paroxysmal auricular tachycardia related to phases of respiration. Am Heart J 1959; 57:782–5.
   A patient whose PSVT occurred only during the inspiratory phase of the respiratory cycle is described.
5. Wildenthal K, Fuller DS, Shapiro W. Paroxysmal atrial arrhythmias induced by hyperventilation. Am J Cardiol 1968; 21:436–41.
   A case report of a 29-year-old man who consistently developed PSVT while hyperventilating.

Electrophysiologic Mechanisms

6. Gillette PC, Garson A. Electrophysiologic and pharmacologic characteristics of automatic ectopic atrial tachycardia. Circulation 1977; 56:571–5.
   Automatic ectopic atrial tachycardia is rare in adults but often occurs in children. It is typically extremely difficult to manage, even when drugs such as digoxin and propranolol are administered in combination.
7. Josephson ME, Kastor JA. Supraventricular tachycardia: mechanisms and management. Ann Intern Med 1977; 87:346–58.
   A superb review of the electrophysiologic mechanisms of all kinds of PSVT.
8. Wu D, Denes P, Amat-y-Leon F, Dhingra R, Wyndham CRC, Bauernfiend R, Latif P, Rosen KM. Clinical, electrocardiographic, and electrophysiologic observations in patients with paroxysmal supraventricular tachycardia. Am J Cardiol 1978; 41:1045–51.
   In about 90% of patients with PSVT, the arrhythmia can be induced by electrophysiologic stimulation, allowing delineation of its mechanism.
9. Holmes DR Jr, Hartzler GO, Maloney JD. Concealed retrograde bypass tracts and enhanced atrioventricular nodal conduction: an unusual subset of patients with refractory paroyxsmal supraventricular tachycardia. Am J Cardiol 1980; 45:1053–60.
   This report describes 8 patients with unusually rapid and medically refractory PSVT. The tachycardia resulted from antegrade enhanced AV nodal conduction combined with retrograde conduction by a concealed left atrial–left ventricular accessory pathway.
10. Brugada P, Ross D, Bär FWHM, Vanagt EJ, Dassen WRM, Wellens HJJ. Observations on spontaneous termination of atrioventricular nodal reentrant tachycardia. Am J Cardiol 1981; 47:703–7.
    In 2 patients with AV nodal reentrant tachycardia, the mechanism of termination was based on the use of a reentrant pathway other than the one used during tachycardia.

11. Goldreyer BN, Bigger JT Jr. Site of reentry in paroxysmal supraventricular tachycardia in man. Circulation 1971; 43:15–26.
    His bundle recordings during spontaneous and induced episodes of PSVT have shown that the site of reentry responsible for PSVT is the AV node.

Therapy

12. Wildenthal K, Atkins JM, Leshin SJ, Skelton CL. The diving reflex used to treat paroxysmal atrial tachycardia. Lancet 1975; 1:12–14.
    Immersion of the face in cold water while the breath is held is a powerful vagal stimulant; in this report, it reverted 7 of 7 episodes of PSVT to sinus rhythm.
13. Josephson ME, Seides SE, Batsford WB, Caracta AR, Damato AN, Kastor JA. The effects of carotid sinus pressure in reentrant paroxysmal supraventricular tachycardia. Am Heart J 1974; 88:694–7.
    In 12 of 13 patients in whom carotid sinus pressure terminated PSVT, gradual slowing occurred prior to conversion to sinus rhythm.
14. Waxman MB, Wald RW, Sharma AD, Huerta F, Cameron DA. Vagal techniques for termination of paroxysmal supraventricular tachycardia. Am J Cardiol 1980; 46:655–64.
    Of 68 consecutive episodes of PSVT, 57 were terminated with carotid massage alone or after pretreatment with edrophonium; 5 ended with Valsalva; and 6 were terminated by phenylephrine. In most patients, PSVT can be rapidly, safely, and consistently terminated by maneuvers that directly or reflexly increase vagal tone.
15. Waxman MB, Bonet JF, Finley JP, Wald RW. Effects of respiration and posture on paroxysmal supraventricular tachycardia. Circulation 1980; 62:1011–20.
    In many patients, a deep inspiration or assumption of a dependent position dramatically raised arterial blood pressure and terminated episodes of PSVT by reflexly increasing vagal tone.
16. Schamroth L, Krikler DM, Garrett C. Immediate effects of intravenous verapamil in cardiac arrhythmias. Brit Med J 1972; 1:660–2.
    Twenty consecutive patients with PSVT were treated with intravenous verapamil, 10 mg administered in 15–30 seconds. All reverted to sinus rhythm.
17. Krikler DM, Spurrell RAJ. Verapamil in the treatment of paroxysmal supraventricular tachycardia. Postgrad Med J 1974; 50:447–53.
    Of 60 consecutive patients with PSVT, intravenous verapamil induced a conversion to sinus rhythm in 57 (95%).
18. Waxman HL, Myerburg RJ, Appel R, Sung RJ. Verapamil for control of ventricular rate in paroxysmal supraventricular tachycardia and atrial fibrillation or flutter. Ann Intern Med 1981; 94:1–6.
    Of 29 individuals with PSVT, intravenous verapamil, 5 mg in 1 minute, caused conversion to sinus rhythm in 23 (79%).
19. Mauritson DR, Winniford MD, Walker WS, Rude RE, Cary JR, Hillis LD. Oral verapamil for paroxysmal supraventricular tachycardia: a long-term, double-blind, randomized trial. Ann Intern Med 1982; 96:409–12.
    In patients with frequent episodes of PSVT, oral verapamil reduces their number and duration.
20. Klein HO, Hoffman BF. Cessation of paroxysmal supraventricular tachycardias by parasympathomimetic interventions. Ann Intern Med 1974; 81:48–50.
    In 39 episodes of PSVT reverted to sinus rhythm by various parasympathomimetic interventions, a definite slowing of the rate of the supraventricular tachycardia was observed before the actual cessation of the tachyarrhythmia.
21. Cantwell JD, Dawson JE, Fletcher GF. Supraventricular tachyarrhythmias—treatment with edrophonium. Arch Intern Med 1972; 130:221–4.
    Twelve of 16 (75%) episodes of PSVT were terminated abruptly with intravenous edrophonium, 5–20 mg.
22. Lister JW, Cohen LS, Bernstein WH, Samet P. Treatment of supraventricular tachycardias by rapid atrial stimulation. Circulation 1968; 38:1044–59.
    In many patients with PSVT, rapid atrial stimulation causes a reversion to sinus rhythm.
23. Kitchen JG III, Goldreyer BN. Demand pacemaker for refractory paroxysmal supraventricular tachycardia. N Engl J Med 1972; 287:596–9.

A patient with PSVT refractory to conventional drug therapy is described. Competitive ventricular pacing was used to terminate episodes.

24. Gallagher JJ, Svenson RH, Kasell JH, German LD, Bardy GH, Broughton A, Critelli G. Catheter technique for closed-chest ablation of the atrioventricular conduction system. A therapeutic alternative for the treatment of refractory supraventricular tachycardia. N Engl J Med 1982; 306:194–200.
    A catheter technique for ablating the His bundle and its application in 9 patients with refractory supraventricular tachycardia are described.

25. Harrison L, Gallagher JJ, Kasell J, Anderson RH, Mikat E, Hackel DB, Wallace AG. Cryosurgical ablation of the AV node–His bundle. A new method for producing A-V block. Circulation 1977; 55:463–70.
    A cryosurgical technique was used to ablate AV conduction in 20 dogs and 3 patients with drug resistant and life-threatening supraventricular tachycardia.

26. Sealy WC, Anderson RH, Gallagher JJ. Surgical treatment of supraventricular tachyarrhythmias. J Thorac Cardiovasc Surg 1977; 73:511–22.
    A review of the first episode of supraventricular tachyarrhythmia with the direct surgical treatment.

27. Klein GJ, Sealy WC, Pritchett ELC, Harrison L, Hackel DB, Davis D, Kasell J, Wallace AG, Gallagher JJ. Cryosurgical ablation of the atrioventricular node–His bundle: long-term follow-up and properties of the junctional pacemaker. Circulation 1980; 61:8–15.
    A cryosurgical technique was used to ablate the AV node–His bundle in 22 patients with disabling supraventricular tachycardia unresponsive to medical therapy; it was successful in 17.

28. Lie KI, Duren DR, Cats VM, David GK, Durrer D. Long-term efficacy of verapamil in the treatment of paroxysmal supraventricular tachycardias. Am Heart J 1983; 105:688.
    These preliminary data suggest that oral, long-term verapamil is an effective agent in many patients with recurrent PSVT.

29. Sakurai M, Yasuda H, Kato N, Nomura A, Fujita M, Nishino T, Fujita K, Koike Y, Saito H. Acute and chronic effects of verapamil in patients with paroxysmal supraventricular tachycardia. Am Heart J 1983; 105:619–28.
    In 15 patients with frequent episodes of PSVT, oral verapamil was efficacious as prophylactic therapy. It appeared to be more effective in those with AV nodal reentry than in those in whom an accessory pathway was operative.

30. Wu D, Kou HC, Yeh SJ, Lin FC, Hung JS. Effects of oral verapamil in patients with atrioventricular reentrant tachycardia incorporating an accessory pathway. Circulation 1983; 67:426–33.
    Electrophysiologic testing 5–6 hours after verapamil can be used to predict clinical responses in patients with atrioventricular reentrant tachycardia.

31. Betriu A, Chaitman BR, Bourassa MG, Brevers G, Scholl JM, Bruneau P, Gagne P, Chabot M. Beneficial effect of intravenous diltiazem in the acute management of paroxysmal supraventricular tachyarrhythmias. Circulation 1983; 67:88–94.
    Of 15 patients with paroxysmal supraventricular tachycardia treated with intravenous diltiazem, conversion to sinus rhythm occurred in 13 (87%).

ATRIAL FLUTTER

Atrial flutter is a supraventricular tachycardia with an atrial rate of 250 to 350 per minute; in most patients, it is close to 300 per minute. In an occasional elderly patient or a patient who is taking quinidine or procainamide, the atrial rate may be slower than 250 per minute (i.e., 220–240/min). In most patients, atrial flutter is associated with second degree AV block, usually 2:1, 3:1, or 4:1; thus, with an atrial rate of 300 per minute, the ventricular rate is usually 75 to 150 per minute. Most patients with atrial flutter have underlying organic heart disease, most commonly mitral valve disease, primary myocardial disease, coronary artery disease, or pericardial disease. In addition, atrial flutter occasionally occurs in the setting of acute myocardial infarction. It can occur in toxic or metabolic conditions that affect the heart, such as thyrotoxicosis, alcoholism, or beriberi. As a general rule, it does not occur as a manifestation of digitalis intoxication.

The patient with atrial flutter may complain of palpitations. Because of a reduced cardiac output, the patient may note fatigue, weakness, coolness of the skin, and dizziness. He may have symptoms of left ventricular failure (dyspnea, orthopnea, and paroxysmal nocturnal dyspnea), inadequate coronary perfusion (angina pectoris or myocardial infarction), or inadequate cerebral perfusion (dizziness, syncope, or focal neurologic symptoms and signs if there is underlying cerebrovascular disease). On physical examination, the peripheral and precordial pulses correspond to the ventricular rate. The jugular venous pulse may demonstrate regular flutter waves at 250 to 350 per minute. Otherwise, the general physical examination reveals the findings of whatever underlying cardiac disease is present.

On the ECG, atrial flutter waves may appear regularly at 250 to 350 per minute. As a result, the baseline of the standard ECG often assumes a sawtooth pattern. The P waves are usually oriented negatively in the inferior leads (II, III, and aVF). The P–R interval is often slightly prolonged (but may be difficult to measure). Alternatively, it may be impossible to identify atrial activity on the ECG. The QRS complexes are usually normal in duration and configuration, occurring at a rate of 75 to 150 per minute.

In untreated cases of atrial flutter, the most common mode of AV conduction is 2:1, resulting in a regular ventricular rhythm of 150 beats per minute. A higher degree of AV block (e.g., 3:1, 4:1) is usually the result of digitalis, propranolol, or verapamil therapy. Alternatively, such high-degree AV block in the absence of these pharmacologic agents may indicate intrinsic conduction system disease.

Atrial flutter with 1:1 conduction is very uncommon. When it occurs, it is usually precipitated by emotional excitement, strenuous exercise, induction of anesthesia, or certain drugs, including atropine, quinidine, and procainamide. In most instances, 1:1 AV conduction leads rapidly to hemodynamic deterioration, and as a result, it usually constitutes a serious medical emergency.

When vagal stimulation is applied to the patient with atrial flutter, an increase in the degree of AV block may occur, resulting in the appearance of several flutter waves in succession without a QRS complex. As vagal stimulation is withdrawn, the degree of AV block lessens, and the ECG returns to its previous appearance. Such vagal stimulation is often helpful in differentiating atrial flutter from sinus tachycardia and paroxysmal supraventricular tachycardia. Carotid sinus massage in the setting of sinus tachycardia typically induces a gradual decline in heart rate, which returns to its previous level when massage is discontinued. In the patient with paroxysmal supraventricular tachycardia, vagal stimulation causes either no change or an abrupt reversion to normal sinus rhythm.

Some patients with atrial flutter suffer no hemodynamic embarrassment from it. Over a course of days to weeks, atrial flutter usually reverts spontaneously to either atrial fibrillation or sinus rhythm. If conversion of atrial flutter is desired but not emergent, it can be attempted pharmacologically. Digitalis alone ordinarily does little to convert atrial flutter to sinus rhythm, but it usually allows control of the ventricular rate. Such rate control can also be achieved with propranolol or verapamil. Once the ventricular response is adequately controlled with digitalis, propranolol, or verapamil, quinidine or procainamide can be administered in an attempt to induce a reversion to sinus rhythm.

If atrial flutter cannot be converted pharmacologically, it can be treated electrically. Rapid atrial pacing appears to be a safe and effective method of converting atrial flutter. A pacing catheter is placed in the right atrium, and pacing is initiated at a rate faster than the flutter rate (i.e., 400–450 beats/min). After pacing at this rate for 10 to 15 seconds, the pacing rate is slowed steadily over several seconds. In many patients, reversion to sinus rhythm or atrial fibrillation occurs. Rapid atrial pacing is especially advantageous in the patient with possible digitalis excess (in whom DC countershock is dangerous) and in the patient with an underlying disease in whom a mild anesthetic represents a risk (e.g., one with severe pulmonary disease). In addition, rapid atrial pacing can be used repetitively without cumulative effects.

If appropriate drugs and rapid atrial pacing do not convert the atrial flutter to sinus rhythm, DC countershock can be employed. The current usually required to convert atrial flutter to sinus rhythm is small (i.e., 5 to 25 watt-sec). Rarely are more than 50 watt-sec required. Electrical cardioversion should be performed while the patient is taking quinidine, propranolol, or procainamide, since these medications will help the patient to remain in sinus rhythm once reversion occurs.

Etiology

1. Fosmoe RJ, Averill KH, Lamb LE. Electrocardiographic findings in 67,375 asymptomatic subjects. II. Supraventricular arrhythmias. Am J Cardiol 1960; 6:84–95.
   Atrial flutter is rarely seen in normal subjects. It was found only once in this very large group of healthy individuals.
2. Julian DG, Valentine PA, Miller GG. Disturbances of rate, rhythm, and conduction in acute myocardial infarction. Am J Med 1964; 37:915–27.
   In 100 consecutive patients with acute myocardial infarction, 2 had atrial flutter.
3. Meltzer LE, Kitchell JB. The incidence of arrhythmias associated with acute myocardial infarction. Prog Cardiovasc Dis 1966; 9:50–63.
   Atrial flutter occurs uncommonly in the setting of acute myocardial infarction; when it occurs, it is almost always in the setting of congestive heart failure.
4. Delman AJ, Stein E. Atrial flutter secondary to digitalis toxicity. Circulation 1964; 29:593–7.
   Atrial flutter rarely occurs as a manifestation of digitalis intoxication.
5. Friedberg CK, Donoso E. Arrhythmias and conduction disturbances due to digitalis. Prog Cardiovasc Dis 1960; 2:408–31.
   Atrial flutter is only rarely a manifestation of digitalis intoxication.

Electrophysiologic Mechanisms

6. Watson RM, Josephson ME. Atrial flutter. I. Electrophysiologic substrates and modes of initiation and termination. Am J Cardiol 1980; 45:732–41.
   In patients with atrial flutter, intraatrial reentry appears to be the underlying electrophysiologic mechanism.
7. Inoue H, Matsuo H, Takayanagi K, Murao S. Clinical and experimental studies of the effects of atrial extrastimulation and rapid pacing on atrial flutter cycle. Evidence of macro-reentry with an excitable gap. Am J Cardiol 1981; 48:623–31.
   Again, intraatrial reentry appears to be the operative mechanism in patients with atrial flutter.

Therapy

8. Schamroth L, Krikler DM, Garrett C. Immediate effects of intravenous verapamil in cardiac arrhythmias. Brit Med J 1972; 1:660–2.
   Of 15 patients with atrial flutter, intravenous verapamil caused a reversion to sinus rhythm in 4 (27%). In the other 11, it slowed the ventricular response.
9. Aronow WS, Landa D, Plasencia G, Wong R, Karlsberg RP, Ferlinz J. Verapamil in

atrial fibrillation and atrial flutter. Clin Pharmacol Ther 1979; 26:578–83.
In most patients with flutter, verapamil slows the ventricular response. In 10–20% of patients it induces a reversion to sinus rhythm.

10. Hagemeijer F. Verapamil in the management of supraventricular tachyarrhythmias occurring after a recent myocardial infarction. Circulation 1978; 57:751–5.
In patients with atrial flutter in the setting of acute myocardial infarction, intravenous verapamil caused a reversion to sinus rhythm in 87%, a surprisingly high percentage.

11. Wolfson S, Herman MV, Sullivan JM, Gorlin R. Conversion of atrial fibrillation and flutter by propranolol. Br Heart J 1967; 29:305–9.
In several patients with atrial flutter in whom digitalis, quinidine, and direct current countershock did not induce a reversion to sinus rhythm, propranolol was successful.

12. Wellens HJJ, Bär FW, Gorgels AP, Muncharaz JF. Electrical management of arrhythmias with emphasis on the tachycardias. Am J Cardiol 1978; 41:1025–34.
A good overview of atrial pacing in the treatment of supraventricular tachycardias, including atrial flutter.

13. Vergara GS, Hildner FJ, Schoenfeld CB, Javier RP, Cohen LS, Samet P. Conversion of supraventricular tachycardias with rapid atrial stimulation. Circulation 1972; 46:788–93.
Rapid atrial stimulation can be used to revert atrial tachycardia, atrial flutter, or junctional tachycardia to either sinus rhythm or atrial fibrillation. It is safe in patients with digitalis intoxication, does not require anesthesia, and can be used repeatedly without cumulative effects.

14. Pittman DE, Makar JS, Kooros KS, Joyner CR. Rapid atrial stimulation: successful method of conversion of atrial flutter and atrial tachycardia. Am J Cardiol 1973; 32:700–06.
Many cases of atrial flutter can be converted to sinus rhythm with rapid atrial stimulation.

15. Waldo AL, Maclean WAH, Karp RB, Kouchoukos NT, James TN. Entrainment and interruption of atrial flutter with atrial pacing. Studies in man following open heart surgery. Circulation 1977; 56:737–45.
Atrial pacing at a constant rate for an average of 10 seconds is usually required to interrupt atrial flutter.

16. Wellens HJJ. Value and limitations of programmed electrical stimulation of the heart in the study and treatment of tachycardias. Circulation 1978; 57:845–53.
A thorough review of the use of programmed electrical stimulation in patients with various kinds of tachycardia.

17. Das G, Anand KM, Ankineedu K, Chinnavaso T, Talmers FN, Weissler AM. Atrial pacing for cardioversion of atrial flutter in digitalized patients. Am J Cardiol 1978; 41:308–12.
In a group of digitalized patients with atrial flutter, rapid atrial pacing reverted 98% to sinus rhythm or atrial fibrillation.

18. Orlando J, Cassidy J, Aronow WS. High reversion of atrial flutter to sinus rhythm after atrial pacing in patients with pulmonary disease. Chest 1977; 71:580–2.
In patients whose risk of direct current countershock is increased because of poor anesthetic tolerance and hypoxia, atrial pacing may be the treatment of choice for atrial flutter.

19. Resnekov L. Present status of electroversion in the management of cardiac dysrhythmias. Circulation 1973; 47:1356–63.
More than 90% of patients with atrial flutter are converted to sinus rhythm with less than 50 watt-seconds of direct current countershock.

20. Castellanos A, Lemberg L, Gosselin A, Fonseca EJ. Evaluation of countershock treatment of atrial flutter. Arch Int Med 1965; 115:426–33.
Direct current countershock successfully reverted 60 consecutive patients with atrial flutter to sinus rhythm. There were no failures of countershock therapy.

ATRIAL FIBRILLATION

Atrial fibrillation is characterized by irregular and chaotic atrial fibrillatory waves at a rate of 350 to 600 per minute. The ventricular response is irregular, usually at a rate of 120 to 160 per minute. Atrial fibrillation can occur in association with many different kinds of cardiac disease. It is a common and rather characteristic arrhythmia in patients with rheumatic mitral valve disease (stenosis or regurgitation); in these patients, its appearance is related directly to left atrial size and the duration of valvular disease. In general, aortic valve disease is not associated with atrial fibrillation until it is advanced enough to cause marked cardiomegaly. Atrial fibrillation occurs frequently in patients with primary myocardial disease, atherosclerotic coronary artery disease, pericarditis, long-standing systemic arterial hypertension, atrial septal defect, and thyrotoxicosis. It is a common occurrence during the 2 weeks after cardiac surgery (usually secondary to concomitant pericarditis). Its reported incidence in acute myocardial infarction is 7 to 16 percent when continuous electrocardiographic monitoring is used. Finally, it may rarely be the result of digitalis intoxication. At times, atrial fibrillation occurs in individuals with apparently normal hearts; these patients are referred to as "lone atrial fibrillators." Tobacco, alcohol, or other toxic substances may contribute to the appearance of atrial fibrillation in these individuals.

The patient with atrial fibrillation may complain of palpitations. If the ventricular response is rapid, cardiac output may fall, resulting in symptoms of cardiac congestion (dyspnea, orthopnea, and paroxysmal nocturnal dyspnea) or inadequate peripheral perfusion (angina pectoris or myocardial infarction, dizziness, or focal neurologic deficits). In patients with mitral valve disease or large and congested hearts, recurrent systemic arterial embolization may occur from the left atrium. On physical examination, the peripheral and precordial pulse is irregularly irregular. The ventricular rate varies, depending on the rapidity of AV junctional conduction. The presence of other physical findings depends on the patient's underlying cardiac disease.

On the ECG, discrete P wave activity is absent, and the baseline is irregular and somewhat chaotic. The QRS complexes occur irregularly and usually are morphologically normal. Regularization of the ventricular response is an electrocardiographic sign of digitalis intoxication. It is also reported to occur following verapamil administration, but this does not signify intoxication.

There is little doubt that atrial fibrillation with a rapid and poorly controlled ventricular response induces a decline in cardiac output in comparison to a much slower sinus rhythm. Even when the ventricular response is well controlled, however, the continued variability of the period of ventricular diastolic filling and the absence of atrial systole contribute to a diminished cardiac output. Several studies have demonstrated that in patients with atrial fibrillation a reversion to sinus rhythm is followed by a substantial increase in cardiac output.

In the patient with atrial fibrillation, the ventricular response can be controlled with the digitalis glycosides, propranolol, or verapamil. These agents usually slow the ventricular response but do not restore sinus rhythm. If mitral valve disease or a cardiomyopathy is present, the patient should be anticoagulated for at least 3 weeks prior to attempted cardioversion. Once this has been accomplished, pharmacologic conversion with quinidine or procainamide is attempted, and, if successful, the patient is continued on digitalis and quinidine (or procainamide). If pharmacologic cardioversion is unsuccessful, electrical conversion is attempted. Atrial fibrillation usually reverts to sinus rhythm with 100 to 200 watt-sec of DC countershock. Again, if electrical conversion is successful, the patient is continued on digitalis and quinidine (or procainamide). In some patients, especially those with mitral valve disease and an enlarged left atrium, reversion to sinus rhythm may not occur, even with adequate direct countershock. The success of conversion of atrial fibrillation to sinus rhythm is indirectly proportional, first, to left atrial size and, second, to the length of time the patient has been in atrial fibrillation. In addition, successful pharmacologic or electrical cardioversion requires that obvious precipitating factors be eliminated, such as severe mitral valve disease, thyrotoxicosis, hypoxemia, and poor left ventricular function.

Etiology and Associated Diseases

1. Aberg H. Atrial fibrillation. Acta Med Scand 1968; 184:425–31.
   A retrospective analysis of 463 patients with atrial fibrillation. The major underlying cardiac diseases were coronary artery disease (23%) and hypertension (34%); 6% were idiopathic.
2. DeSanctis RW, Block P, Hutter AM. Tachyarrhythmias in myocardial infarction. Circulation 1972; 45:681–702.
   In the setting of acute myocardial infarction, atrial fibrillation occurs in approximately 10% of patients.
3. Meltzer LE, Kitchell JB. The incidence of arrhythmias associated with acute myocardial infarction. Prog Cardiovasc Dis 1966; 9:50–63.
   In patients with acute myocardial infarction, atrial fibrillation occurs in 7–16%.
4. Probst P, Goldschlager N, Selzer A. Left atrial size and atrial fibrillation in mitral stenosis. Circulation 1973; 48:1282–7.
   Patient age appears to be a factor in the development of atrial fibrillation in the setting of mitral stenosis.
5. Selzer A, Katayama F. Mitral regurgitation: clinical patterns, pathophysiology, and natural history. Medicine 1972; 51:337–66.
   Of 61 patients whose mitral regurgitation was severe enough to require surgery, 46 (75%) had atrial fibrillation.
6. Glancy DL, O'Brien KP, Gold HK, Epstein SE. Atrial fibrillation in patients with idiopathic hypertrophic subaortic stenosis. Br Heart J 1970; 32:652–9.
   Atrial fibrillation was present in 10% of patients with IHSS. In each patient the onset of the arrhythmia was accompanied by severe clinical deterioration, emphasizing the importance of the "atrial kick" in these patients.
7. Weber DM, Phillips JH. A reevaluation of electrocardiographic changes accompanying acute pulmonary embolism. Am J Med Sci 1966; 251:381–98.
   Of 60 patients with documented pulmonary embolus, atrial fibrillation occurred in 10%; it comprised about one-quarter of all arrhythmias that occurred in this clinical setting.
8. Spodick DH. Arrhythmias during acute pericarditis. A prospective study of 100 consecutive cases. JAMA 1976; 235:39–41.
   In these 100 patients with pericarditis, 5 had accompanying atrial fibrillation.
9. Levine HD. Myocardial fibrosis in constrictive pericarditis: electrocardiographic and pathologic observations. Circulation 1973; 48:1268–81.
   Of 67 individuals with constrictive pericarditis, atrial fibrillation was present in 19.
10. Tikoff G, Schmidt AM, Hecht HH. Atrial fibrillation in atrial septal defect. Arch Intern Med 1968; 121:402–5.
    In a group of adult patients with ASD, atrial fibrillation was present in 19%.
11. Irons GV, Orgain ES. Digitalis-induced arrhythmias and their management. Prog Cardiovasc Dis 1966; 8:539–69.
    Occasionally, transient or permanent atrial fibrillation is encountered as a manifestation of digitalis toxicity.
12. Peter RH, Gracey JG, Beach TB. A clinical profile of idiopathic atrial fibrillation. Ann Intern Med 1968; 68:1288–95.
    Thirty military personnel, all under the age of 47, with lone atrial fibrillation are described.

13. Lamb LE, Pollard LW. Atrial fibrillation in flying personnel. Circulation 1964; 29:694–701.
    Sixty cases of lone atrial fibrillation in air force personnel are described. This article emphasizes the benign nature of this disorder.
14. Liberthson RR, Salisbury KW, Hutter AM Jr, DeSanctis RW. Atrial tachyarrhythmias in acute myocardial infarction. Am J Med 1976; 60:956–60.
    Of more than 900 patients with acute myocardial infarction, 11% had atrial fibrillation, atrial flutter, or paroxysmal supraventricular tachycardia. Occurrence was not related to the location or extent of infarction nor associated with an increased mortality.
15. Kramer RJ, Zeldis SM, Hamby RI. Atrial fibrillation—a marker for abnormal left ventricular function in coronary heart disease. Br Heart J 1982; 47:606–8.
    Of 1,176 patients with coronary artery disease, 10 (0.8%) had atrial fibrillation. Its presence was a marker of impaired left ventricular function.
16. Bauernfiend RA, Wyndham CRC, Swiryn SP, Palileo EV, Strasberg B, Lam W, Westveer D, Rosen KM. Paroxysmal atrial fibrillation in the Wolff-Parkinson-White syndrome. Am J Cardiol 1981; 47:562–9.
    Patients with preexcitation and documented spontaneous paroxysmal atrial fibrillation almost always have inducible reentrant tachycardia or heart disease, or both.
17. Wyndham CRC, Amat-y-Leon F, Wu D, Denes P, Dhingra R, Simpson R, Rosen KM. Effects of cycle length on atrial vulnerability. Circulation 1977; 55:260–7.
    A decrease in cycle length potentiates atrial vulnerability, leading to atrial flutter or fibrillation.
18. Killip T, Gault JH. Mode of onset of atrial fibrillation in man. Am Heart J 1965; 70:172–9.
    In most patients with atrial fibrillation, an atrial premature beat preceded the onset of fibrillation.

Hemodynamic Consequences

19. Rodman T, Pastor BH, Figueroa W. Effect on cardiac output of conversion from atrial fibrillation to normal sinus mechanism. Am J Med 1966; 41:249–58.
    Following conversion of atrial fibrillation to sinus rhythm, cardiac output increased substantially.
20. Morris JJ Jr, Entman M, North WC, Kong Y, McIntosh H. The changes in cardiac output with reversion of atrial fibrillation to sinus rhythm. Circulation 1965; 31:670–8.
    In 12 patients converted from atrial fibrillation to sinus rhythm, almost all showed a marked increase in cardiac output.

Therapy

21. Kastor JA. Digitalis intoxication in patients with atrial fibrillation. Circulation 1973; 47:888–96.
    In patients with atrial fibrillation, digitalis toxicity induces a regularization of the ventricular response.
22. Schamroth L. Immediate effects of intravenous verapamil on atrial fibrillation. Cardiovasc Res 1971; 5:419–24.
    Of 20 patients with atrial fibrillation, intravenous verapamil slowed the ventricular response in 19.
23. Schamroth L, Krikler DM, Garrett C. Immediate effects of intravenous verapamil in cardiac arrhythmias. Br Med J 1972; 1:660–2.
    In 115 individuals with atrial fibrillation, intravenous verapamil caused a reversion to sinus rhythm in 1 and a slowing of the ventricular response in 111.
24. Heng MK, Singh BN, Roche AHG, Norris RM, Mercer CJ. Effect of intravenous verapamil on cardiac arrhythmias and on the electrocardiogram. Am Heart J 1975; 90:487–98.
    When administered to patients with atrial fibrillation, intravenous verapamil both slows and regularizes the ventricular response. Such regularization is not a manifestation of verapamil intoxication.
25. Stern EH, Pitchon R, King BD, Guerrero J, Schneider RR, Wiener I. Clinical use of

oral verapamil in chronic and paroxysmal atrial fibrillation. Chest 1982; 81:308–11.

Oral verapamil, either alone or combined with digoxin, is effective in controlling the ventricular response in patients with atrial fibrillation.

26. Yahalom J, Klein HO, Kaplinsky E. Beta-adrenergic blockade as adjunctive oral therapy in patients with chronic atrial fibrillation. Chest 1977; 71:592–6.

     In patients with atrial fibrillation in whom digitalis does not completely control the ventricular response, propranolol can be added to the drug regimen for better rate control.

27. Weiner P, Bassan MM, Jarchovsky J, Iusim S, Plavnick L. Clinical course of acute atrial fibrillation treated with rapid digitalization. Am Heart J 1983; 105:223–7.

     Of 47 episodes of acute atrial fibrillation, 40 reverted to sinus rhythm within 96 hours following the institution of digoxin therapy.

28. Lang R, Klein HO, DiSegni E, Gefen J, Sareli P, Libhaber C, David D, Weiss E, Guerrero J, Kaplinsky E. Verapamil improves exercise capacity in chronic atrial fibrillation: double-blind crossover study. Am Heart J 1983; 105:820–5.

     In 20 digitalized patients with atrial fibrillation, oral verapamil substantially improved exercise capacity.

MULTIFOCAL ATRIAL TACHYCARDIA

Multifocal atrial tachycardia (also called chaotic atrial rhythm or chaotic atrial mechanism) is characterized by electrocardiographic evidence of at least three atrial foci; the absence of one dominant atrial pacemaker; variable P–P, P–R, and R–R intervals; and a ventricular rate greater than 100 per minute. It occurs almost exclusively in the setting of severe hypoxia, especially in patients with chronic lung disease. It can also appear in the patient with generalized sepsis or severe diabetes mellitus. As a result of these underlying conditions, patients with this tachyarrhythmia often have a severe derangement of arterial blood gases or electrolytes, and they are frequently being treated with theophylline or catecholamines. On physical examination, multifocal atrial tachycardia may be confused with atrial fibrillation, since the patient has a rapid and irregularly irregular ventricular response.

Multifocal atrial tachycardia is often preceded or followed by frequent premature atrial contractions, sinus tachycardia, atrial fibrillation, atrial flutter, paroxysmal supraventricular tachycardia, or paroxysmal supraventricular tachycardia with block. Some reports, in fact, have shown it to be preceded by or to have progressed to atrial fibrillation or flutter in over half the cases. The rhythm disturbance is usually transient, lasting no more than a few days, but recurrences are common.

The treatment of multifocal atrial tachycardia should center on the correction of the underlying hypoxia. Quinidine is sometimes successful in suppressing the ectopic atrial foci. Although this rhythm disturbance generally is not a manifestation of digitalis intoxication, it sometimes does occur in patients whose serum digoxin levels are at the upper limit of normal.

1. Shine KI, Kastor JA, Yurchak PM. Multifocal atrial tachycardia: clinical and electrocardiographic features in 32 patients. N Engl J Med 1968; 279:344–9.

   Of 32 patients with MAT, control of the arrhythmia paralleled improvement in ventilation and oxygenation, control of sepsis, correction of metabolic and electrolyte derangements, and reduction in chronotropic drugs used as bronchodilators.

2. Lipson MJ, Naimi S. Multifocal atrial tachycardia (chaotic atrial tachycardia). Circulation 1970; 42:397–407.

Of 31 patients with this tachyarrhythmia, atrial fibrillation or flutter evolved in 17 (55%).

3. Chung EK. Appraisal of multifocal atrial tachycardia. Br Heart J 1971; 33:500–4.
   This paper describes the specific electrocardiographic criteria for a diagnosis of MAT. The most common underlying causes are chronic lung disease and digitalis intoxication.
4. Phillips J, Spano J, Burch G. Chaotic atrial mechanism. Am Heart J 1969; 78:171–9.
   In most of the 31 patients described in this report, severe pulmonary disease and diabetes mellitus were present. Of these 31, 16 (52%) died during hospitalization, emphasizing the severity of their underlying disease.
5. Kones RJ, Phillips JH, Hersh J. Mechanism and management of chaotic atrial mechanism. Cardiology 1974; 59:92–101.
   Of 37 patients with this rhythm disturbance, 30 had chronic obstructive lung disease, 14 acute congestive heart failure, 5 acute pulmonary embolism, and 4 digitalis intoxication.
6. Berlinerblau R, Feder W. Chaotic atrial rhythm. J Electrocardiol 1972; 5:135–44.
   In this series of 31 patients with MAT, the most common underlying diseases were arteriosclerotic heart disease and bronchopulmonary disease. Digitalis intoxication was infrequent.

VENTRICULAR TACHYCARDIA, IDIOVENTRICULAR TACHYCARDIA, AND VENTRICULAR FIBRILLATION

Ventricular tachycardia is said to be present when three or more ventricular premature beats occur in rapid succession, usually at a rate of 140 to 200 per minute. The great majority of patients with ventricular tachycardia have underlying organic heart disease. First, it appears most commonly in patients with ischemic heart disease, especially in the minutes to hours following myocardial infarction. In fact, nonsustained ventricular tachycardia is reported to occur in as many as 40 percent of patients with myocardial infarction. Second, ventricular tachycardia occurs frequently in patients with congestive cardiomyopathy. It can also occur in conjunction with other cardiomyopathic processes, such as sarcoid involvement of the heart. Third, digitalis intoxication is a common cause of ventricular tachycardia. Other cardiac medications, such as quinidine and procainamide, also can induce it. Fourth, ventricular tachycardia can be caused by severe electrolyte abnormalities, such as hyperkalemia, hypokalemia, or hypercalcemia. Fifth, this tachyarrhythmia occasionally occurs in the patient with mitral valve prolapse or rheumatic or congenital cardiac disease. Finally, some patients' ventricular tachycardia has no identifiable etiology. The reported incidence of this idiopathic group varies from 5 to 12 percent.

Although an occasional patient tolerates ventricular tachycardia for hours or days, most become abruptly hypostensive during it, with resultant loss of consciousness. The occasional patient who maintains an adequate systemic arterial pressure during ventricular tachycardia may complain of palpitations or dyspnea. On physical examination, the systemic arterial pressure is usually low, and the peripheral pulse (if palpable) is rapid and regular. Since there is complete AV dissociation, the right atrium periodically contracts against a closed tricuspid valve, resulting in easily visible *a* waves in the jugular venous pulse (so-called cannon *a* waves) and an S_1 that varies in intensity from one beat to the next.

On the ECG, ventricular tachycardia is characterized by (1) abnormal ventricular complexes with a duration of at least 0.12 second, at times varying in morphology because of the episodic superimposition of P waves, (2) evidence of complete AV dissociation, and (3) a regular or only slightly irregular rhythm at a rate of 140 to 200 beats per minute. Although ventricular tachycardia is generally a very regular rhythm, some irregularity may be present at its initiation or termination, as well as after the administration of certain antiarrhythmic agents. The diagnosis of ventricular tachycardia is confirmed by the presence of fusion beats, that is, beats that are a combination of a ventricular ectopic beat and a normally conducted beat. In addition, in most episodes of ventricular tachycardia, the QRS axis shifts far to the left and is often between − 90 and − 180 degrees.

It is sometimes difficult to distinguish ventricular tachycardia from supraventricular tachycardia with aberrant conduction. On the routine 12-lead ECG, several clues may help to clarify which rhythm is present. First, the presence of AV dissociation is solid evidence of ventricular tachycardia. Second, certain features of QRS morphology may allow one to differentiate ventricular tachycardia from supraventricular tachycardia with aberrant conduction. Specifically, ventricular tachycardia is characterized by (1) an RR' configuration in lead V1, with the initial R wave taller than the ensuing R', (2) a QS or an rS complex in lead V6, (3) dominantly positive or dominantly negative QRS complexes in all six precordial leads, and (4) a bizarre frontal plane QRS axis. Conversely, supraventricular tachycardia with abberrancy is suggested by (1) a right bundle branch block pattern of conduction, (2) a triphasic rSR' complex in lead V1, or (3) a qR, qRs, or qRS complex in lead V6. If confusion persists despite a careful analysis of the 12-lead ECG, a His bundle recording should allow one to determine whether ventricular activation is preceded by atrial activity.

If ventricular tachycardia does not cause acute hemodynamic embarrassment, pharmacologic conversion to sinus rhythm may be attempted with intravenous lidocaine (50–100 mg by bolus injection), intravenous procainamide (25–50 mg/min to a total dose of 1.0–1.25 gm), or intravenous bretylium (5 mg/kg of body weight). If hemodynamic instability is present or if pharmacologic measures are unsuccessful, DC countershock should be administered. The direct current required to convert ventricular tachycardia to sinus rhythm is usually extremely small (i.e., 1 to 10 watt-sec). Once conversion to sinus rhythm has been accomplished, the patient should be maintained on an antiarrhythmic medication, such as quinidine or procainamide, to prevent recurrence of ventricular tachycardia.

Over the past 5 years, the induction of ventricular tachyarrhythmias (specifically ventricular tachycardia) by programmed electrical stimulation has become an important technique in evaluating antiarrhythmic drug therapy and in identifying those patients at risk of recurrent arrhythmias. Previous studies have demonstrated (1) that the induction of sustained ventricular tachycardia is specific for patients with this tachyarrhythmia and (2) that the induced arrhythmia is identical to the clinically observed arrhythmia in almost all patients. Furthermore, these studies have shown that programmed stimulation can be used effectively to assess the efficacy of antiarrhythmic agents, either alone or in combination, and that their success in suppressing ventricular tachycardia during programmed stimulation is an accurate indicator of their ability to do so during chronic oral therapy. (See Invasive Electrophysiologic Testing, p. 48, for a more detailed description of this technique.)

Some cases of recurrent ventricular tachycardia are not satisfactorily controlled with antiarrhythmic drug therapy, and these patients may therefore require surgical therapy. In most patients with sustained ventricular tachycardia, this tachyarrhythmia is related to fixed anatomic and electrophysiologic abnormalities resulting from previous myocardial infarction rather than ongoing myocardial ischemia. In the past few years, many of these patients have been treated successfully by localization of the area of origin of ventricular tachycardia (with intraoperative activation mapping) and direct resection or destruction of that site. Alternatively, an occasional patient with recurrent, sustained ventricular tachycardia can be treated effectively by overdrive ventricular pacing, that is, at a rate of 90 to 120 beats per minute.

Idioventricular tachycardia (also called slow ventricular tachycardia or accelerated idioventricular rhythm) occurs very commonly in patients with acute myocardial infarction (possibly as many as 50–60%). In addition, it has been observed in patients with digitalis intoxication, hypertensive heart disease, and cardiomyopathy, as well as rheumatic and congenital heart disease. The patient with this tachycardia usually has no symptoms referable to it. Most episodes are transient, lasting seconds to minutes. On physical examination, signs of complete AV dissociation may be observed (variability in the intensity of S_1, cannon *a* waves in the jugular venous pulse). The ECG reveals regular ventricular complexes at 90 to 110 per minute. There may be an occasional fusion beat, and there is evidence of independent atrial activity.

Idioventricular tachycardia is generally a benign rhythm, although in an occasional patient it serves as a prodrome of ventricular fibrillation. It usually does not cause hemodynamic compromise. As a result, it normally requires no therapy. If, for some reason, therapy is required, atropine is often effective in accelerating sinus activity and increasing the sinus rate so that the sinoatrial node becomes the dominant pacemaker. If atropine is unsuccessful, lidocaine may be efficacious.

Finally, *ventricular fibrillation* is recognized on the ECG as a coarse, undulating baseline without other electrical activity. Peripheral perfusion ceases immediately, and the patient loses consciousness. Recent reports have demonstrated that the intravenous bolus administration of bretylium tosylate (5 mg/ kg of body weight) may convert ventricular fibrillation to sinus rhythm. If this drug fails or is not available, DC countershock (with 400 watt-sec) is required to convert ventricular fibrillation to sinus rhythm.

Ventricular Tachycardia

1. Lown B, Temte JV, Arter WJ. Ventricular tachyarrhythmias: clinical aspects. Circulation 1973; 47:1364–81.
   A review of the pathogenesis, clinical features, electrocardiographic characteristics, and therapy of ventricular tachycardia and fibrillation.
2. Marriott HJL, Sandler IA. Criteria, old and new, for differentiating between ectopic ventricular beats and aberrant ventricular conduction in the presence of atrial fibrillation. Prog Cardiovasc Dis 1966; 9:18–28.
   A description of new criteria for differentiating ventricular beats from supraventricular beats with aberration.
3. DeSanctis RW, Block P, Hutter AM Jr. Tachyarrhythmias in myocardial infarction. Circulation 1972; 45:681–702.
   Ventricular tachycardia occurs in approximately 10% of patients with acute myocardial infarction.
4. Kistin AD. Problems in differentiation of ventricular arrhythmia from supraventricular arrhythmia with abnormal QRS. Prog Cardiovasc Dis 1966; 9:1–17.
   This paper describes other helpful clues to distinguishing ventricular tachycardia from supraventricular tachycardia with aberrancy.
5. Moss AJ, Schnitzler R, Green R, Decamilla J. Ventricular arrhythmias 3 weeks after acute myocardial infarction. Ann Intern Med 1971; 75:837–41.
   Of 100 patients who had electrocardiographic monitoring 3 weeks after infarction, 4 had one or more transient runs of ventricular tachycardia.

6. Samet P. Hemodynamic sequelae of cardiac arrhythmias. Circulation 1973; 47:399–407.
   Rapid ventricular tachycardia usually causes severe hypotension, a fall in cardiac output, and evidence of cerebral, coronary, and renal hypoperfusion.
7. Bigger JT, Dresdale RJ, Heissenbuttel RH, Weld FM, Wit AL. Ventricular arrhythmias in ischemic heart disease: mechanism, prevalence, significance, and management. Prog Cardiovasc Dis 1977; 19:255–300.
   A very thorough review of all aspects of ventricular ectopy, including 258 references.
8. Duvernoy WFC, Garcia R. Sarcoidosis of the heart presenting with ventricular tachycardia and atrioventricular block. Am J Cardiol 1971; 28:348–52.
   Direct involvement of the myocardium is a serious complication of sarcoidosis. This paper describes 2 such cases.
9. MacKenzie GJ, Pascual S. Paroxysmal ventricular tachycardia. Br Heart J 1964; 26:441–51.
   In this series of 83 patients with ventricular tachycardia, 60 (72%) had underlying ischemic heart disease. In 13 (22%) tachycardia was induced by digitalis.
10. Wei JY, Greene HL, Weisfeldt ML. Cough-facilitated conversion of ventricular tachycardia. Am J Cardiol 1980; 45:174–6.
    This paper describes a 64-year-old man who repeatedly converted drug-refractory ventricular tachycardia to sinus rhythm by abrupt and forceful coughing.
11. Vandepol CJ, Farshidi A, Spielman SR, Greenspan AM, Horowitz LN, Josephson ME. Incidence and clinical significance of induced ventricular tachycardia. Am J Cardiol 1980; 45:725–31.
    Ventricular tachycardia that resembles the clinical variety can be induced by programmed electrical stimulation in almost all patients with sustained clincial ventricular tachycardia, whereas it can be induced only rarely in patients with no previously documented ventricular tachycardia.
12. Wellens HJJ, Bar FW, Farre J, Ross DL, Wiener I, Vanagt EJ. Initiation and termination of ventricular tachycardia by supraventricular stimuli. Incidence and electrophysiologic determinants as observed during programmed stimulation of the heart. Am J Cardiol 1980; 46:576–82.
    Ventricular tachycardia was inducible by a single atrial premature stimulus in 7 of 43 patients with previous episodes of sustained ventricular tachycardia.
13. Strasberg B, Sclarovsky S, Erdberg A, Duffy CE, Lam W, Swiryn S, Agmon J, Rosen KM. Procainamide-induced polymorphous ventricular tachycardia. Am J Cardiol 1981; 47:1309–14.
    This paper presents 7 cases of procainamide-induced ventricular tachycardia.
14. Mason JW, Winkle RA. Accuracy of the ventricular tachycardia–induction study for predicting long-term efficacy and inefficacy of antiarrhythmic drugs. N Engl J Med 1980; 303:1073–7.
    In 51 patients with inducible ventricular tachycardia, the arrhythmia-induction technique accurately predicted the clinical effectiveness of drugs used in the long-term treatment of recurrent ventricular tachycardia.
15. Kastor JA, Horowitz LN, Harken AH, Josephson ME. Clinical electrophysiology of ventricular tachycardia. N Engl J Med 1981; 304:1004–20.
    A thorough review of the diagnosis and therapy of ventricular tachycardia. Includes 207 references.
16. Horowitz LN, Harken AH, Josephson ME, Kastor JA. Surgical treatment of ventricular arrhythmias in coronary artery disease. Ann Intern Med 1981; 95:88–97.
    An excellent review of surgical therapy in patients with recurrent, sustained ventricular tachycardia. Includes 107 references.

Idioventricular Tachycardia

17. Rothfeld EL, Zucker IR, Parsonnet V, Alinsonorin CA. Idioventricular rhythm in acute myocardial infarction. Circulation 1968; 37:203–9.
    This rhythm was noted in 36 of 100 consecutively monitored patients with acute myocardial infarction.
18. Lichstein E, Ribas-Meneclier C, Gupta PK, Chadda KD. Incidence and description of accelerated ventricular rhythm complicating acute myocardial infarction. Am J Med 1975; 58:192–8.

This rhythm is a common complication of both anterior and inferior infarction, occurring in about 13% of the patients in this series.

Ventricular Fibrillation

19. Surawicz B. Ventricular fibrillation. Am J Cardiol 1971; 28:268–87.
    A detailed review of factors that predispose to ventricular fibrillation. Includes 179 references.
20. Schaffer WA, Cobb LA. Recurrent ventricular fibrillation and modes of death in survivors of out-of-hospital ventricular fibrillation. N Engl J Med 1975; 293:259–62.
    Patients who are resuscitated from ventricular fibrillation are susceptible to early recurrence.

TORSADE DE POINTES

Torsade de pointes ("twisting about a point") is a polymorphous ventricular tachycardia in which the QRS axis undulates about the isoelectric line, changing its vector during runs of 5 to 20 beats. Such paroxysms may be brief, consisting of only a few complexes, or they may be prolonged, with resultant syncope. Rates greater than 150 beats per minute are frequently observed. Torsade de pointes may have one of several etiologies, including (1) bradycardia, often with atrioventricular or sinoatrial block, (2) hypokalemia, (3) hypomagnesemia, (4) antiarrhythmic drug excess (especially quinidine and procainamide), (5) acute myocardial infarction, and (6) myocarditis. In addition, patients with a prolonged Q–T interval and those receiving phenothiazines and tricyclic antidepressants in excess are at particular risk to develop this arrhythmia.

The treatment of torsade de pointes centers, first, on avoiding those pharmacologic agents that might further prolong the Q–T interval (especially quinidine and procainamide) and, second, on correcting any underlying abnormalities, such as hypokalemia and hypomagnesemia. Pharmacologic agents or maneuvers that shorten repolarization and increase heart rate may correct the arrhythmia, such as the administration of isoproterenol or the initiation of ventricular pacing at a rapid rate (100–120 beats/min). Occasionally, emergent cardioversion is necessary.

Torsade de Pointes

1. Krikler DM, Curry PVL. Torsade de pointes, an atypical ventricular tachycardia. Br Heart J 1976; 38:117–20.
   A thorough review of the clinical features of torsade de pointes.
2. Sclarovsky S, Strasberg B, Lewin RF, Agmon J. Polymorphous ventricular tachycardia: clinical features and treatment. Am J Cardiol 1979; 44:339–44.
   Thirty-four cases of polymorphous ventricular tachycardia (torsade de pointes) are described and the clinical features discussed. Patients with severe myocardial involvement receiving antiarrhythmic drugs for ventricular premature beats are at risk for this arrhythmia.
3. DiSegni E, Klein HO, David D, Libhaber C, Kaplinsky E. Overdrive pacing in quinidine syncope and other long QT-interval syndromes. Arch Intern Med 1980; 140:1036–40.
   Overdrive pacing suppressed recurrent ventricular tachycardia-fibrillation in 9 patients with a prolonged Q–T interval without appreciably shortening the corrected Q–T interval.
4. Jervell A, Lange-Nielsen F. Congenital deaf-mutism, functional heart disease with prolongation of the Q–T interval, and sudden death. Am Heart J 1957; 54:59–68.
   The early description of a combination of deaf-mutism and Q–T prolongation in 4 children in a family of 6.

5. Loeb HS, Pietras RJ, Gunnar RM, Tobin JR Jr. Paroxysmal ventricular fibrillation in two patients with hypomagnesemia. Treatment by transvenous pacing. Circulation 1968; 37:210–5.
   Marked Q–T prolongation and paroxysmal ventricular fibrillation occurred in 2 patients with profound hypomagnesemia (0.5 and 0.7 mEq/L).
6. Meltzer RS, Robert EW, McMorrow M, Martin RP. Atypical ventricular tachycardia as a manifestation of disopyramide toxicity. Am J Cardiol 1978; 42:1049–53.
   Torsade de pointes occurring in a patient with disopyramide toxicity is described.
7. Rossi L, Matturri L. Histopathological findings in two cases of torsade de pointes with conduction disturbances. Br Heart J 1976; 38:1312–8.
   Widespread damage to the conduction system was found in these 2 patients.
8. Smith WM, Gallagher JJ. "Les torsade de pointes": an unusual ventricular arrhythmia. Ann Int Med 1980; 93:578–84.
   A clinical review of torsade de pointes. Includes 98 references.
9. Horowitz LN, Greenspan AM, Spielman SR, Josephson ME. Torsades de pointes: electrophysiologic studies in patients without transient pharmacologic or metabolic abnormalities. Circulation 1981; 63:1120–8.
   Electrophysiologic studies were performed in 21 patients with torsade de pointes, suggesting that it is a rapid, reentrant ventricular tachycardia and a precursor of sudden death.
10. Keren A, Tzivoni D, Gavish D, Levi J, Gottlieb S, Benhorin J, Stern S. Etiology, warning signs, and therapy of torsade de pointes. A study of 10 patients. Circulation 1981; 64:1167–74.
    Isoproterenol or pacing is the therapy of choice for torsade. The conventional drugs used to treat typical ventricular tachycardia are not only ineffective but contraindicated.
11. Koenig W, Schinz AM. Spontaneous ventricular flutter and fibrillation during quinidine medication. Am Heart J 1983; 105:863–5.
    This report describes an episode of torsade precipitated by quinidine therapy.
12. Sclarovsky S, Lewin RF, Kracoff O, Strasberg B, Arditti A, Agmon J. Amiodarone-induced polymorphous ventricular tachycardia. Am Heart J 1983; 105:6–12.
    This article presents 5 cases of amiodarone-induced torsade de pointes.

SICK SINUS SYNDROME

The term *sick sinus syndrome* describes a group of clinical disorders that are due to an inability of the automatic cells in the sinus node to perform their pacemaking function or a failure of the sinus node impulse to activate the atria. The term *bradycardia-tachycardia* (or brady-tachy) *syndrome* is used to describe a subset of the sick sinus syndrome in which recurrent supraventricular tachyarrhythmias (including atrial fibrillation) occur in association with sinus bradycardia, other bradyarrhythmias, or sinus arrest. The most common cause of the sick sinus syndrome is an idiopathic degeneration of the conducting system frequently involving not only the sinus node but also the AV node and other portions of the conducting system; this is termed Lenegre's disease. Other causes include ischemic or rheumatic heart disease, myocarditis, connective tissue disorders, cardiac trauma, and infiltrative or congestive cardiomyopathies.

The patient with the sick sinus syndrome may present in several ways. The electrocardiographic manifestations may occur in some patients who are asymptomatic. These electrocardiographic abnormalities may be due to *impaired sinus node impulse generation* (including sinus arrest and bradycardia) or *sinoatrial block,* with or without accompanying tachyarrhythmias. The patient with the sick sinus syndrome may compain of a variety of symptoms, most of which are attributable to end-organ hypoperfusion during periods of either bradycardia or tachycardia. Thus, cerebral symptoms, including episodic light-headedness, dizziness, and syncope, are common. Less commonly, the patient may complain of transient episodes of pulmonary vascular congestion or angina pectoris, generalized fatigue, myalgias, periodic oliguria, or mild digestive disorders. Occasionally, systemic arterial embolization may occur, leading to a neurologic deficit, myocardial infarction, or visceral organ infarction.

The physical examination of the patient with the sick sinus syndrome may be totally normal. During periods of tachycardia or bradycardia, the peripheral pulses vary accordingly, and the systemic arterial pressure may decline transiently. *The diagnosis of symptomatic sick sinus syndrome rests on the demonstration of symptoms attributable to hypoperfusion during periods of arrhythmia.* Ancillary information can be obtained by assessing the heart rate response to atropine, isoproterenol, or vigorous physical exertion. In addition, detailed electrophysiologic testing can be used to determine sinus node recovery following rapid atrial pacing and to assess the integrity of the remainder of the conduction system.

In most patients, the sick sinus syndrome begins insidiously and progresses slowly over several years. Initially, the patient has periods of normal impulse initiation and conduction, interrupted only occasionally by periods of tachycardia or bradycardia. During this period, the randomly obtained 12-lead ECG may be completely normal. Gradually, the involved conducting tissue degenerates further, leading to more sustained periods of arrhythmia. The escape rhythms, at first only occasional rescuers, eventually become the predominant pacemaker mechanism. Atrial fibrillation can occur by default in patients with the sick sinus syndrome. Although it is impossible to distinguish atrial fibrillation that occurs in the presence of sinus node dysfunction from that which occurs in its absence, a strong clue to the presence of underlying sinus node dysfunction is the occurrence of *atrial fibrillation with a slow ventricular response* in the absence of drug therapy, a finding attributable to the strong association between sinus node and AV node dysfunction. In these patients, a temporary ventricular pacemaker should be inserted during attempted electrical cardioversion to prevent the appearance of severe sinus bradycardia or sinus arrest.

Only a small number of patients with the sick sinus syndrome have had detailed postmortem examination. In some, focal fibrosis is demonstrable in the cardiac conduction system, whereas in others, such fibrosis is more widespread. In most patients, histologic abnormalities are noted throughout the conduction system, from the sinoatrial node to the distal bundle branches.

The therapy of the sick sinus syndrome should be reserved for the patient with electrocardiographic documentation of bradyarrhythmia or tachyarrhythmia and symptoms during the periods of arrhythmia. The syndrome is most effectively treated with (1) a permanent pacemaker (to prevent symptomatic bradycardia) and (2) digitalis or propranolol (to prevent and control symptomatic tachycardia). Some patients may benefit from quinidine in combination with digitalis or propranolol to prevent or control recurrent tachyarrhythmias. In addition, because of the documented risk of systemic arterial embolization, serious thought should be given to long-term anticoagulation of the patient with the sick sinus syndrome, particularly if the patient has chronic atrial fibrillation or has frequent changes in cardiac rhythm.

1. Conde CA, Leppo J, Lipski J, Stimmel B, Litwak R, Donoso E, Dack S. Effectiveness of pacemaker treatment in the bradycardia-tachycardia syndrome. Am J Cardiol 1973; 32:209–14.

In 31 patients with sick sinus syndrome, insertion of a permanent pacemaker alleviated symptoms and allowed for the use of antiarrhythmic agents.

2. Bharati S, Nordenberg A, Bauernfiend RA, Varghese JP, Carvalho AG, Rosen KM, Lev M. The anatomic substrate for the sick sinus syndrome in adolescence. Am J Cardiol 1980; 46:163–72.
   Two young men—ages 16 and 17—with prolonged sinus nodal dysfunction are described. Post mortem, one demonstrated fibrosis and the other fatty infiltration of the cardiac conducting system.

3. Scott O, Macartney FJ, Deverall BP. Sick sinus syndrome in children. Arch Dis Child 1976; 51:100–5.
   Six patients, all between the ages of 10 and 15, with the sick sinus syndrome are described.

4. Yabek SM, Swensson RE, Jarmakani JM. Electrocardiographic recognition of sinus node dysfunction in children and young adults. Circulation 1977; 56:235–9.
   In this paper 24 children and young adults, all of whom had brady-tachy syndrome, are described. Although most of them had associated congenital or acquired heart disease (particularly following corrective cardiac surgery), some had no definable cardiac disease other than the conduction system abnormalities.

5. Jordan JL, Yamaguchi I, Mandel WJ. Studies on the mechanism of sinus node dysfunction in the sick sinus syndrome. Circulation 1978; 57:217–23.
   Pathophysiologically the sick sinus syndrome is not a homogeneous entity: some patients have intrinsic sinus node dysfunction, others have disturbed autonomic regulation.

6. Gomes JAC, Kang PS, Matheson M, Gough WB Jr, El-Sherif N. Coexistence of sick sinus rhythm and atrial flutter-fibrillation. Circulation 1981; 63:80–6.
   In this report, a 58-year-old man with atrial flutter-fibrillation is described. Sinus node function was assessed by overdrive stimulation of the area of sinus node activity, revealing an underlying sick sinus syndrome.

7. Kaplan BM, Langendorf R, Lev M, Pick A. Tachycardia-bradycardia syndrome (sick sinus syndrome). Pathology, mechanism, and treatment. Am J Cardiol 1973; 31:497–508.
   A pathologic study emphasizing that this syndrome often results from diffuse conduction system disease rather than from sinus node dysfunction alone.

8. Rubenstein JJ, Schulman CL, Yurchak PM, DeSanctis RW. Clinical spectrum of the sick sinus syndrome. Circulation 1972; 46:5–13.
   A series of 56 patients with sick sinus syndrome is described. Coronary artery disease was the most common definable etiology.

9. Ferrer MI. The sick sinus syndrome. Circulation 1973; 47:635–41.
   A review of the causes, physiologic and clinical manifestations, and therapy of this syndrome.

10. Ferrer MI. Sick sinus syndrome. J Cardiovasc Med 1981; 6:743–51.
    A thorough review of the clinical manifestations of this disease entity.

11. Moss AJ, Davis RJ. Brady-tachy syndrome. Prog Cardiovasc Dis 1974; 16:439–54.
    A general overview of this disease entity, including 88 references.

12. Radford DJ, Julian DG. Sick sinus syndrome: experience of a cardiac pacemaker clinic. Brit Med J 1974; 3:504–7.
    In 21 patients with sick sinus syndrome, a high incidence of cerebral embolization was observed, so that the routine use of anticoagulants in these patients merits serious consideration.

13. Wohl AJ, Laborde NJ, Atkins JM, Blomqvist CG, Mullins CB. Prognosis of patients permanently paced for sick sinus syndrome. Arch Intern Med 1976; 136:406–8.
    In 39 patients with sick sinus syndrome, the long-term prognosis was poor despite pacemaker treatment.

14. Aroesty JM, Cohen SI, Morkin E. Bradycardia-tachycardia syndrome: results in 28 patients treated by combined pharmacologic therapy and pacemaker implantation. Chest 1974; 66:257–63.
    In this series of 28 patients, permanent pacemaker implantation, when combined with drug therapy, was effective in the control of the brady-tachy syndrome.

15. Gillette PC, Shannon C, Garson A Jr, Porter CJ, Ott D, Cooley D, McNamara DG. Pacemaker treatment of sick sinus syndrome in children. JACC 1983; 1:1325–9.
    Permanent pacing for sick sinus syndrome in children is safe and effective.

PREEXCITATION SYNDROMES

In *preexcitation,* an impulse originating in the atria activates the ventricles earlier than would be anticipated if it traversed the normal route through the AV node to the bundle of His. Thus, the preexcitation syndromes are characterized by accelerated AV conduction. Such preexcitation can occur (1) through an accessory connection between the atria or AV node and the ventricles, (2) through a bypass tract connecting the atria to the His bundle or one portion of the AV node to another, or (3) through a so-called fasciculoventricular connection, which (as the name implies) originates in the bundle of His and inserts in the ventricular myocardium.

The *Wolff-Parkinson-White syndrome* is characterized anatomically by an accessory connection (or connections) between the atria or AV node and the ventricles. It occurs in about 1 percent of the population. Although most individuals with this syndrome have otherwise normal hearts, it may be associated with Ebstein's anomaly of the tricuspid valve, mitral valve prolapse, or idiopathic congestive cardiomyopathy. About 50 percent of those with the Wolff-Parkinson-White syndrome have periodic tachyarrhythmias, whereas the other 50 percent demonstrate evidence of preexcitation on a routine ECG but have no rhythm disturbances.

The patient with the Wolff-Parkinson-White syndrome usually comes to medical attention when a routine ECG is noted to be abnormal. Alternatively, the patient may seek medical advice because of recurrent episodes of palpitations and associated light-headedness. The physical examination is usually normal, unless the patient has the findings of an associated cardiac abnormality, such as mitral valve prolapse. The standard 12-lead ECG demonstrates (1) a shortened P–R interval (less than 0.12 sec), (2) a widened QRS complex (greater than 0.10 sec), and (3) a delta wave (i.e., a slurring of the initial 30–50 msec of the QRS complex), which is caused by the activation of ventricular myocardium through the accessory pathway. In some patients with this syndrome, the characteristic electrocardiographic features occur intermittently. When the Wolff-Parkinson-White syndrome is suspected, but the standard ECG is not diagnostic, maneuvers designed to alter the autonomic influences on AV conduction may elicit the typical electrocardiographic features. Thus, an augmentation of vagal tone or a withdrawal of sympathetic tone usually enhances conduction through an accessory pathway, providing ample electrocardiographic evidence of the Wolff-Parkinson-White syndrome.

On the standard 12-lead ECG, the patient with the Wolff-Parkinson-White syndrome can be classified as having a type A or type B pattern. Type A is characterized by an upright R wave in the anterior precordial leads (V1–3), simulating a right bundle branch block pattern. Those with type B have an upright R wave in the lateral precordial leads (V4–6), resembling the pattern of left bundle branch block.

Patients with the Wolff-Parkinson-White syndrome often have episodes of (1) paroxysmal supraventricular tachycardia and (2) atrial fibrillation. An episode of paroxysmal supraventricular tachycardia is initiated when a premature atrial impulse is blocked in one AV pathway (the normal or the accessory) and is propagated through the other. Most frequently, the premature impulse that initiates the tachycardia is blocked in the accessory pathway and is conducted through the AV node to the ventricles. Subsequently, it returns to the atrium through the accessory pathway, thus creating a reciprocating tachycardia in which antegrade conduction occurs through the normal pathway, and retrograde conduction takes place through the accessory pathway. Since antegrade conduction occurs through the normal pathway, the QRS complexes during supraventricular tachycardia appear normal. In an occasional individual, the supraventricular tachycardia is initiated and propagated in the opposite direction, so that antegrade conduction occurs through the accessory pathway, and retrograde conduction occurs through the normal pathway. During episodes of tachycardia in these patients, the QRS complexes are bizarre and widened.

The mechanism by which patients with the Wolff-Parkinson-White syndrome develop atrial fibrillation is not understood. If the accessory pathway has an especially short refractory period, an extremely rapid ventricular response may result, leading to ventricular fibrillation. The need to determine the refractory period of the accessory pathway and the ventricular response during induced atrial fibrillation is an important reason for these patients to undergo invasive electrophysiologic testing.

The acute therapy of the patient with the Wolff-Parkinson-White syndrome and either paroxysmal supraventricular tachycardia or atrial fibrillation is determined by the presence or absence of hemodynamic instability. If the tachyarrhythmia causes hypotension or venous congestion, DC countershock should be instituted without delay. On the other hand, if the patient is hemodynamically stable, propranolol, lidocaine, or procainamide may be administered. Digitalis and verapamil should *not* be given, since in some individuals they accelerate conduction through the accessory pathway. If the patient with the Wolff-Parkinson-White syndrome has frequent episodes of supraventricular tachycardia or atrial fibrillation, chronic maintenance antiarrhythmic therapy may be necessary. This can be accomplished with quinidine, procainamide, amiodarone, or propranolol. Alternatively, if invasive electrophysiologic testing has demonstrated that digoxin or verapamil does not accelerate conduction through the accessory pathway, these agents may be administered. If pharmacologic therapy is unsuccessful in preventing frequent tachyarrhythmias, a permanent pacemaker can be implanted to deliver rapid bursts of atrial stimulation during episodes. Finally, if neither pharmacologic nor pacemaker therapy is effective, the patient should be referred for surgical ablation or cryotherapy of the accessory pathway. In the operating room, specialized electrocardiographic mapping techniques are used to localize the accessory connection, after which it is ablated.

The *Lown-Ganong-Levine syndrome* is characterized anatomically by a bypass tract between the atria and the His bundle; alternatively, it can occur because of intranodal bypass connections from one portion of the AV node to another. Its exact frequency is unknown. Similar to the Wolff-Parkinson-White syndrome, this disorder usually occurs in individuals with otherwise normal hearts. The patient complains of occasional palpitations, and by electrocardiographic monitoring these individuals have episodes of paroxysmal supraventricular tachycardia and atrial fibrillation. The routine ECG of the patient with Lown-Ganong-Levine demonstrates a shortened P–R interval (less than 0.12 sec) and a normal QRS duration (0.08 sec). The patient with this syndrome should be treated—both acutely and chronically—in a similar manner to the individual with the Wolff-Parkinson-White syndrome.

Finally, a *nodoventricular* or *fasciculoventricular connection* is the rarest form of preexcitation. As the names imply, these syndromes are characterized anatomically by an accessory pathway that connects the distal AV node, the bundle of His, or the upper bundle branches to the ventricular myocardium. The resultant ECG demonstrates a normal P–R interval and a prolonged QRS complex with a typical delta wave. It is hypothesized that these anomalous pathways may be involved in ventricular tachycardia, but this is unproved. Thus, neither the incidence of tachyarrhythmias nor the overall prognosis is known in patients with nodoventricular or fasciculoventricular connections. As a result, optimal therapy for these patients is also unknown.

General

1. Gallagher JJ, Pritchett ELC, Sealy WC, Kasell J, Wallace AG. The preexcitation syndromes. Prog Cardiovasc Dis 1978; 20:285–327.
   An elegant and thorough review of the anatomy and electrophysiology of these syndromes. Includes 166 references.

Wolff-Parkinson-White Syndrome: Clinical and Electrophysiologic Characteristics

2. Bauernfiend RA, Wyndham CR, Swiryn SP, Palileo EV, Strasberg B, Lam W, Westveer D, Rosen KM. Paroxysmal atrial fibrillation in the Wolff-Parkinson-White syndrome. Am J Cardiol 1981; 47:562–9.
   Patients with preexcitation and spontaneous paroxysmal atrial fibrillation almost always have inducible AV reentrant tachycardia.
3. Newman BJ, Donoso E, Friedberg CK. Arrhythmias in the Wolff-Parkinson-White syndrome. Prog Cardiovasc Dis 1966; 9:147–65.
   A complete review of the incidence, diagnosis, and therapy of the tachyarrhythmias that accompany this syndrome. Includes 116 references.
4. Durrer D, Schoo L, Schuilenburg RM, Wellens HJJ. The role of premature beats in the initiation and termination of supraventricular tachycardia in the Wolff-Parkinson-White syndrome. Circulation 1967; 36:644–62.
   This electrophysiologic analysis in 4 patients establishes the mechanism by which episodes of reciprocating tachycardia are often initiated.
5. Denes P, Wu D, Amat-y-Leon F, Dhingra R, Wyndham C, Kehoe R, Ayres BF, Rosen KM. Paroxysmal supraventricular tachycardia induction in patients with Wolff-Parkinson-White syndrome. Ann Intern Med 1979; 90:153–7.
   Of patients with preexcitation, tachycardia induction was noted in 28 of 32 patients with previously documented supraventricular tachycardia or atrial fibrillation but in only 1 of 12 asymptomatic patients.
6. Strasberg B, Ashley WW, Wyndham CRC, Bauernfeind RA, Swiryn SP, Dhingra RC, Rosen KM. Treadmill exercise testing in the Wolff-Parkinson-White syndrome. Am J Cardiol 1980; 45:742–8.
   Because treadmill testing does not usually provoke arrhythmia in patients with preexcitation, the results of such testing cannot be used to ascertain the effectiveness (or lack thereof) of antiarrhythmic therapy.
7. German LD, Gallagher JJ, Broughton A, Guarnieri T, Trantham JL. Effects of exercise and isoproterenol during atrial fibrillation in patients with Wolff-Parkinson-White syndrome. Am J Cardiol 1983; 51:1203–6.
   Isoproterenol increased the rate of conduction over the accessory pathway during atrial fibrillation, thus allowing a good assessment of the risk of an excessively rapid ventricular response. Exercise was not an effective means of assessing this risk.

Wolff-Parkinson-White Syndrome: Drug Therapy

8. Wellens HJJ, Bar FW, Dassen WRM, Brugada P, Vanagt EJ, Farre J. Effect of drugs in the Wolff-Parkinson-White syndrome. Importance of initial length of effective refractory period of the accessory pathway. Am J Cardiol 1980; 46:665–9.
   When the effective refractory period of the accessory pathway is short and there is a documented episode of atrial fibrillation with a rapid ventricular response, the protection offered by drugs known to prolong the refractoriness must be individually assessed.
9. Sclarovsky S, Kracoff OH, Strasberg B, Lewin RF, Agmon J. Paroxysmal atrial flutter and fibrillation associated with preexcitation syndrome: treatment with ajmaline. Am J Cardiol 1981; 48:929–33.
   In 6 patients with the Wolff-Parkinson-White syndrome and paroxysmal atrial flutter or fibrillation, intravenous ajmaline was an effective agent for terminating these episodes.
10. Wellens HJJ, Durrer D. Effect of procaine amide, quinidine, and ajmaline on the Wolff-Parkinson-White syndrome. Circulation 1974; 50:114–20.

In 16 patients with this syndrome, procainamide proved to be the most effective drug for controlling the ventricular rate in patients with paroxysmal atrial fibrillation.

11. Mandel WJ, Laks MM, Obayashi K, Hayakawa H, Daley W. The Wolff-Parkinson-White syndrome: pharmacologic effects of procaine amide. Am Heart J 1975; 90:744–54.
    In 13 patients with the Wolff-Parkinson-White syndrome, intravenous procainamide eliminated the delta wave in 10 and modified it in the other 3. Thus, this drug should be beneficial in these patients.

12. Wellens HJJ, Lie KI, Bar FW, Wesdorp JC, Dohmen HJ, Duren DR, Durrer D. Effect of amiodarone in the Wolff-Parkinson-White syndrome. Am J Cardiol 1976; 38:189–94.
    In this study of 15 patients, the authors conclude that amiodarone is especially useful in patients with Wolff-Parkinson-White syndrome and atrial fibrillation.

13. Critelli G, Grassi G, Perticone F, Coltorti F, Monda V, Condorelli M. Transesophageal pacing for prognostic evaluation of preexcitation syndrome and assessment of protective therapy. Am J Cardiol 1983; 51:513–8.
    In 5 patients with the Wolff-Parkinson-White syndrome, decremental atrial pacing was performed with an esophageal lead to show that amiodarone provided good protection against life-threatening arrhythmias.

Wolff-Parkinson-White Syndrome: Pacemaker and Surgical Therapy

14. Krikler D, Curry P, Buffet J. Dual-demand pacing for reciprocating atrioventricular tachycardia. Br Med J 1976; 1:1114–6.
    The initial report of pacemaker therapy for 2 patients with reciprocating AV tachycardia.

15. Gillette PC, Garson A Jr, Kugler JD, Cooley DA, Zinner A, McNamara DG. Surgical treatment of supraventricular tachycardia in infants and children. Am J Cardiol 1980; 46:281–4.
    Ten patients with drug-resistant supraventricular tachycardia underwent surgical division of an accessory connection; in 8 the episodes of tachycardia were totally abolished by the operation.

16. Gallagher JJ, Gilbert M, Svenson RH, Sealy WC, Kasell J, Wallace AG. Wolff-Parkinson-White syndrome: the problem, evaluation, and surgical correction. Circulation 1975; 51:767–85.
    In selected patients, surgical correction of the Wolff-Parkinson-White syndrome can be accomplished, especially in those in whom free wall AV connections are present.

17. Sealy WC, Gallagher JJ, Wallace AG. The surgical treatment of Wolff-Parkinson-White syndrome: evolution of improved methods for identification and interruption of the Kent bundle. Ann Thorac Surg 1976; 22:443–57.
    Of 50 patients operated on for tachyarrhythmias, division of the Kent bundle was successful in 31.

18. Prystowsky EN, Pritchett ELC, Smith WM, Wallace AG, Sealy WC, Gallagher JJ. Electrophysiologic assessment of the atrioventricular conduction system after surgical correction of ventricular preexcitation. Circulation 1979; 59:789–96.
    In 19 patients who had undergone operative division of an accessory pathway, electrophysiologic testing showed no damage to the normal conduction system.

Lown-Ganong-Levine Syndrome

19. Benditt DG, Pritchett ELC, Smith WM, Wallace AG, Gallagher JJ. Characteristics of atrioventricular conduction and the spectrum of arrhythmias in Lown-Ganong-Levine syndrome. Circulation 1978; 57:454–65.
    Of 12 patients with this syndrome, 6 had a narrow-QRS tachycardia, 2 had atrial fibrillation, and 4 had ventricular tachycardia.

20. Mandel WJ, Danzig R, Hayakawa H. Lown-Ganong-Levine syndrome: a study of His bundle electrograms. Circulation 1971; 44:696–708.
    A detailed analysis of His bundle recordings in 3 patients with Lown-Ganong-Levine syndrome is presented in this paper.

21. Josephson ME, Kastor JA. Supraventricular tachycardia in Lown-Ganong-Levine syndrome: atrionodal versus intranodal reentry. Am J Cardiol 1977; 40:521–7.
    A detailed electrophysiologic analysis of 6 patients with this syndrome.

ATRIOVENTRICULAR BLOCK

Atrioventricular (AV) block generally is classified into three degrees. With *first degree AV block*, each atrial impulse is conducted to the ventricles, but there is a delay in AV conduction, so that the P–R interval on the standard ECG is prolonged (> 0.2 sec). First degree AV block may be caused by enhanced vagal stimulation, several pharmacologic agents (including digitalis, the beta-adrenergic blockers, and verapamil), or a number of disease entities, such as ischemic heart disease, infiltrative myocardial disease, acute myocardial infarction (especially inferior in location), myocarditis, adrenocortical insufficiency (i.e., Addison's disease), congenital heart disease (particularly atrial septal defect and Ebstein's anomaly), rheumatic fever, or streptococcal infections. A prolonged P–R interval occasionally is present in otherwise normal subjects and in well-trained athletes.

On physical examination, the patient with first degree AV block demonstrates a softened S_1, since the long P–R interval permits the AV valves to close prior to ventricular contraction. If the P–R interval is extremely long, atrial contraction may occur while the tricuspid and mitral valves are still closed, producing a prominent *a* wave in the jugular venous pulse. The mere presence of first degree AV block is not an indication for therapy. In the child receiving digitalis, first degree AV block may be a manifestation of digitalis excess, and its dosage should be reduced. In the adult on digitalis therapy, first degree AV block is not of itself an indication for the withdrawal or reduction in dosage of digitalis. Similarly, such first degree block in the presence of beta-blocker or verapamil therapy should not mandate an alteration in dosage or frequency of administration. In the setting of acute inferior myocardial infarction, first degree AV block requires no specific therapy, although it may serve as the harbinger of second or third degree AV block.

With *second degree AV block*, some atrial impulses are conducted to the ventricles, whereas others are not. Second degree AV block may be either Mobitz type I (Wenckebach) or Mobitz type II. *Mobitz I AV block* is characterized by progressive prolongation of the P–R interval, eventually culminating in a nonconducted P wave. In most patients, this block is located in the AV junction, although occasionally it is subjunctional in a bundle branch. It is believed to be due to AV junctional fatigue. Typically, the QRS morphology is normal, since there is no delay in intraventricular depolarization. However, if bundle branch block coexists with Mobitz I AV block, QRS prolongation is present. Mobitz I AV block can be caused by digitalis excess, acute myocardial ischemia or infarction (particularly inferior in location), acute rheumatic fever, myocardial disease, calcium deposition in the conduction system, or degenerative conduction system disease. Intense vagal stimulation also can produce Mobitz I AV block. Finally, it is occasionally present in very well-trained athletes.

Digitalis intoxication should be suspected as the cause of Mobitz I AV block if the patient is taking this agent at the time such block develops, in which case digitalis should be discontinued. As a general rule, neither temporary nor permanent pacing is necessary in the patient with Mobitz I AV block, provided the ventricular rate is adequate. However, if the ventricular response is sufficiently slow to induce angina, venous congestion, syncope, or frequent ventricular premature beats, temporary (and sometimes permanent) pacing is necessary. In the patient whose Mobitz I AV block occurs in the setting of an inferior myocardial infarction, complete heart block may develop, but it generally resolves within 5 to 6 days.

In contrast to Mobitz I AV block, *Mobitz II AV block* is intraventricular in location and is therefore associated with electrocardiographic QRS prolongation. The P–R interval in the conducted sinus beats is constant, and there are multiple P waves for each QRS complex. When only 2:1 AV block is present, it may be difficult to distinguish Mobitz type I from Mobitz type II block. If the P–R interval of the conducted beats is substantially prolonged (> 0.25 sec) and the QRS complexes are narrow, Mobitz I AV block is likely. In contrast, if the QRS complexes are widened, Mobitz II AV block is probably present. In addition, when the atrial rate is increased with exercise or atropine, the AV block in type I tends to decrease, whereas that in type II tends to increase. This distinction is important, since the etiology and treatment of Mobitz types I and II block are different. Specifically, Mobitz II AV block rarely occurs as a manifestation of digitalis intoxication, whereas Mobitz I AV block frequently does. Although Mobitz I AV block seldom requires pacemaker insertion (temporary or permanent), Mobitz II AV block should be treated with a pacemaker as soon as it is discovered. Initially, temporary ventricular pacing should be performed, after which a permanent pacemaker should be implanted.

With *third degree AV block* (complete heart block), atrial impulses are not conducted to the ventricles, and as a result, a totally independent ectopic ventricular pacemaker exists. In general, the ventricular rate is 30 to 40 beats per minute. On physical examination, the patient may have intermittent cannon *a* waves in the jugular venous pulse, as well as an S_1 that varies in intensity. A systolic ejection murmur often is present. Complete heart block can be caused by digitalis or potassium intoxication, acute myocardial infarction (usually inferior in location), acute myocarditis, tumors involving the heart, collagen diseases involving the heart (particularly rheumatoid arthritis), calcium deposition in the AV junction, or cardiac trauma. It also can occur as a complication of surgical closure of a ventricular septal defect. When it develops as a complication of an inferior myocardial infarction, it is usually temporary. In contrast, when it occurs as a complication of anterior infarction, it is usually permanent. Acquired complete heart block invariably requires pacemaker insertion. In contrast, congenital complete heart block is frequently associated with a near-normal escape heart rate and may not require pacemaker placement.

1. Kastor JA. Atrioventricular block. N Engl J Med 1975; 292:462–5, 572–4.
   A general discussion of both AV nodal block and fascicular block.
2. Langendorf R, Pick A. Atrioventricular block, type II (Mobitz): its nature and clinical significance. Circulation 1968; 38:819–21.
   Especially in the setting of acute MI, it is important—prognostically and therapeutically—to differentiate Mobitz I from Mobitz II AV block.
3. Langendorf R, Cohen H, Gozo EC Jr. Observations on second degree atrioventricular block, including new criteria for the differential diagnosis between type I and type II block. Am J Cardiol 1972; 29:111–9.
   Criteria are presented with which one can differentiate Mobitz I and II second degree block, even when there is consistent 2:1 block.
4. Norris RM: Heart block in posterior and anterior myocardial infarction. Br Heart J 1969; 31:352–6.
   Heart block in conjunction with an inferior (or posterior) infarction usually runs an uncomplicated course, resolving spontaneously in 1–3 days. In contrast, heart block with anterior infarction is usually permanent and, therefore, requires pacemaker insertion.
5. Kostuk WJ, Beanlands DS. Complete heart block associated with acute myocardial infarction. Am J Cardiol 1970; 26:380–4.
   In a series of 308 patients with acute MI, complete heart block occurred in 28 (9.1%). Those with anterior infarction had a very poor prognosis (mortality, 80%); those with inferior infarction had a mortality rate of 45%.
6. Damato AN, Lau SH, Helfant R, Stein E, Patton RD, Scherlag BJ, Berkowitz WD. A

study of heart block in man using His bundle recordings. Circulation 1969; 39:297–305.

The original description of the use of His bundle recordings to define the anatomic site of AV block.

7. Barold SS, Friedberg HD. Second degree atrioventricular block: matter of definition. Am J Cardiol 1974; 33:311–5.

   A review of the mechanisms by which one can differentiate Mobitz I and II second degree AV block.

8. Johnson RL, Averill KH, Lamb LE. Electrocardiographic findings in 67,375 asymptomatic subjects. VII. Atrioventricular block. Am J Cardiol 1960; 6:153–77.

   Of over 67,000 healthy male air force personnel, 350 had first degree AV block, 1 had Mobitz I second degree AV block, and 1 had third degree AV block.

9. Stock RJ, Macken DL: Observations on heart block during continuous electrocardiographic monitoring in myocardial infarction. Circulation 1968; 38:993–1005.

   Complete heart block occurred in 24 of 350 patients with myocardial infarction. With inferior infarction, such block occurred because of AV nodal malfunction. With anterior infarction, extensive conduction system necrosis was usually present.

10. Strasberg B, Amat-Y-Leon F, Dhingra RC, Palileo E, Swiryn S, Bauernfiend R, Wyndham C, Rosen KM. Natural history of chronic second-degree atrioventricular nodal block. Circulation 1981; 63:1043–9.

    This report describes 56 patients with chronic Mobitz I second degree AV block. This block had a relatively benign course in those without underlying heart disease; in contrast, in those with organic heart disease, prognosis was poor and was related to the severity of underlying cardiac disease.

11. Meytes I, Kaplinsky E, Yahini JH, Hanne-Paparo N, Neufeld HN. Wenckebach A-V block: a frequent feature following heavy physical training. Am Heart J 1975; 90:426–30.

    In a study of the literature, it was seen that Mobitz I second degree AV block was related to vigorous physical training in half of 32 patients who had no detectable organic disease. In this report of 126 Israeli athletes, 11 had first degree AV block, and 3 had Mobitz type I second degree block.

BUNDLE BRANCH AND FASCICULAR BLOCKS

In the normally depolarized heart, each electrical impulse from the atria is conducted through the AV node to the bundle of His. From this bundle the impulse is transmitted to the ventricles by the right and left bundle branches. The left bundle quickly divides into two divisions or *fascicles:* the anterior and the posterior. The former supplies Purkinje fibers to the anterior and lateral walls of the left ventricle, whereas the latter supplies the inferior and posterior walls. In essence, the interventricular conduction system is composed of three fascicles: the right bundle, the left anterior fascicle, and the left posterior fascicle. A conduction block in any of the three results in *unifascicular* block; a block in two of the three causes *bifascicular* block; and the blockage of all three leads to *trifascicular* block.

Right bundle branch block is caused by altered conduction of the right bundle with a resultant abnormal sequence of activation of the right ventricle. The left ventricle is depolarized in a normal fashion through the intact left bundle, but right ventricular activation is delayed, since it depends on impulses propagated from the left ventricle. The great majority of patients with right bundle branch block have organic heart disease, with coronary artery disease the most common cause. Alternatively, a complete right bundle branch block may be caused by acute myocarditis; degenerative conduction system disease; congenital heart disease, including atrial septal defect or any anomaly producing right ventricular outflow tract obstruction; or pulmonary hypertension. Finally, right bundle branch block can occur in patients without underlying cardiac disease.

The electrocardiographic criteria on which a diagnosis of right bundle branch block is made include (1) QRS prolongation to 0.12 seconds or greater, (2) an rSR' complex in the right precordial leads (V1 and V2), and (3) a slurred S wave in leads I, aVL, and V5 to V6. The prognosis of the patient with right bundle branch block is determined by the presence and severity of underlying cardiac disease. On the one extreme, those individuals without demonstrable organic heart disease have a benign course, and their survival is similar to that of the general population. On the other extreme, a right bundle branch block that appears in the setting of an acute myocardial infarction is associated with a 40 to 60-percent mortality. The patient with a right bundle branch block requires no specific therapy for this conduction abnormality.

Left anterior hemiblock is said to be present if the ECG demonstrates (1) a shift of the QRS axis leftward (to between -30 and $-90°$), (2) a normal or only minimally prolonged QRS duration, and (3) no evidence of an inferior myocardial infarction (i.e., residual R waves in leads II, III, and aVF). This conduction abnormality is most often caused by coronary artery disease, hypertensive heart disease, aortic valve disease, and cardiomyopathy, but it also occurs with some frequency (1.5–2.0%) in healthy persons. It can also be seen in those with acyanotic congenital heart disease, most commonly primum atrial septal defect, AV canal, common atrium, and ventricular septal defect. Similar to the patient with right bundle branch block, the prognosis of the individual with left anterior hemiblock depends on the presence and severity of organic heart disease. No specific therapy is needed for this conduction abnormality.

Left posterior hemiblock is characterized electrocardiographically by (1) a rightward shift of the QRS axis ($+90$–$+180°$), (2) a normal or only slightly prolonged QRS duration, and (3) Q waves in the inferior leads (II, III, and aVF). In contrast to left anterior hemiblock, left posterior hemiblock is considered rare, probably because the posterior fascicle of the left bundle is short and thick and receives blood from two coronary arteries. The most common underlying diseases include coronary artery disease, hypertension, cardiomyopathy, and aortic valve disease. The prognosis of left posterior hemiblock depends on the heart disease that underlies it, and like the other two kinds of unifascicular block, it requires no therapy.

If there is blockage of any two of the three fascicles, *bifascicular block* is said to be present. The most common type of bifascicular block is right bundle branch block and left anterior hemiblock. In a random population of hospitalized patients, it is present in about 1 percent. Electrocardiographically, it is characterized by (1) prolongation of the QRS complex (to greater than 0.12 sec), (2) an rSR' in leads V1 and V2, (3) a wide, slurred S wave in leads I, aVL, and V5 to V6, (4) a frontal QRS axis of -30 to -90 degrees, and (5) initial r waves in the inferior leads (i.e., no evidence of transmural inferior infarction). Similar to unifascicular block, this type of bifascicular block is most often caused by coronary artery disease, hypertensive heart disease, aortic valve disease, cardiomyopathy, congenital heart disease, and degenerative conduction system disease. Of these various etiologies, coronary heart disease is responsible for about half.

Over a several year period, a minority of patients with right bundle branch block and left anterior hemiblock progress to complete heart block. On the average, such progression occurs in 7 to 10 percent per year. The appearance of complete heart block in patients with this type of bifascicular block is distinctly more common in the setting of acute myocardial infarction, where the incidence of at least transient complete block is 25 to 40 percent. Based on these data, permanent pacemaker implantation is not recommended in the asymptomatic patient with chronic right bundle branch block and left anterior hemiblock. In the setting of acute myocardial infarction, the development of this type of bifascicular block requires placement of a temporary pacemaker. If, during the period of observation, complete heart block appears (even though transient), a permanent pacemaker should be implanted.

Right bundle branch block and left posterior hemiblock are an uncommon form of bifascicular block. The electrocardiographic characteristics include (1) a prolonged QRS duration (0.12 sec or greater), (2) rSR' complexes in V1 and V2, (3) wide, slurred S waves in I, aVL, and V5 to V6, and (4) a frontal QRS axis of +90 to +180 degrees. Coronary artery disease is the most common underlying disorder. Although there is some disagreement as to the frequency with which the patients with this type of bifascicular block develop complete heart block, it appears to occur with similar frequency as those with right bundle branch block and left anterior hemiblock, i.e., about 7 to 10 percent per year. The indications for temporary or permanent pacemaker implantation are similar to those of the more common type of bifascicular block.

Left bundle branch block is caused by a blockage of impulses to both fascicles of the left bundle, and, therefore, represents a type of bifascicular block. Although it occurs occasionally in individuals without underlying heart disease, it is most commonly caused by acute myocardial infarction (usually anterior), acute myocarditis, degenerative conduction system disease, cardiomyopathy, or aortic valve disease with extension of calcium into the specialized conduction tissue below the AV junction. Electrocardiographically, left bundle branch block is characterized by (1) a QRS duration greater than 0.12 second, (2) a broad monophasic R wave in leads I, V5, and V6, as well as the absence of Q waves in these leads, and (3) a displacement of the S–T segment and T wave in a direction opposite that of the major QRS deflection. The prognosis of the patient with left bundle branch block is dependent on the presence and severity of underlying cardiac disease. In the absence of demonstrable heart disease, left bundle branch block per se does not imply a poor prognosis. In contrast, the appearance of left bundle branch block in the setting of acute myocardial infarction signifies extensive left ventricular damage and, as a result, a poor outlook, i.e., a mortality of 40 to 70 percent. In the setting of acute infarction, the appearance of a left bundle branch block should be treated with placement of a temporary pacemaker.

If, in addition to bifascicular block, there is a prolonged P–R interval (>0.2 sec), *incomplete trifascicular block* is said to exist. This appears most often in individuals with coronary artery disease, cardiomyopathy, or degenerative conduction system disease. A minority of these patients progress to complete heart block, so that a permanent pacemaker implantation is not mandatory in the asymptomatic patient with incomplete trifascicular block.

Bilateral bundle branch block occurs most frequently in patients with acute myocardial infarction, degenerative conduction system disease, cardiomyopathy, calcific aortic stenosis, or myocarditis. Its appearance implies extensive conduction system abnormalities. If it occurs in a patient with acute myocardial infarction, its presence implies a large infarction and a substantial risk of complete heart block, i.e., 40 to 60 percent. In addition, these patients often have cardiogenic shock or severe congestive heart failure. The patient with bilateral bundle branch block in the setting of acute myocardial infarction should receive a temporary and then a permanent pacemaker. Despite pacing, many of these patients die of left ventricular dysfunction with resultant congestive heart failure.

Left Anterior Hemiblock

1. Hiss RG, Lamb LE, Allen MF. Electrocardiographic findings in 67,375 asymptomatic subjects. X. Normal values. Am J Cardiol 1960; 6:200–31.
   In this large survey, a QRS axis of −30° to −90° occurred in 1,280 (1.9%) patients.
2. Bahl OP, Walsh TJ, Massie E. Left axis deviation: an electrocardiographic study with post-mortem correlation. Br Heart J 1969; 31:451–6.
   Of 353 patients with left axis deviation, 300 (85%) had underlying coronary artery disease.
3. Waugh RA, Wagner GS, Haney TL, Rosati RA, Morris JJ Jr. Immediate and remote prognostic significance of fascicular block during acute myocardial infarction. Circulation 1973; 47:765–75.
   In the setting of acute myocardial infarction, the appearance of bifascicular block of any kind carries a guarded prognosis.
4. Rosenbaum MB, Elizari MV, Levi RJ, Nau GJ, Pisani N, Lazarri JO, Halpern MS. Five cases of intermittent left anterior hemiblock. Am J Cardiol 1969; 24:1–7.
   Of these 5 patients, 2 had clear evidence of coronary artery disease, 1 had probable coronary disease, 1 had a cardiomyopathy, and 1 had severe hypoxia as the only identifiable cause.
5. Ostrander LD. Left axis deviation—prevalence, associated conditions, and prognosis: an epidemiologic study. Ann Intern Med 1971; 75:23–28.
   Isolated left axis deviation (greater than −30°) is a common electrocardiographic finding that has no unfavorable prognostic implications.

Left Posterior Hemiblock

6. Bobba P, Salerno JA, Casari A. Transient left posterior hemiblock: report of four cases induced by exercise test. Circulation 1972; 46:931–8.
   Four patients, all with severe coronary artery disease, developed transient left posterior hemiblock during exercise-induced ischemia.
7. Rizzon P, Rossi L, Baissus C, Demoulin JC, DiBiase M. Left posterior hemiblock in acute myocardial infarction. Br Heart J 1975; 37:711–20.
   Of 15 patients with left posterior hemiblock (with or without right bundle branch block) in the setting of myocardial infarction, 13 (87%) died, usually as a result of severe left ventricular dysfunction.

Right Bundle Branch Block

8. Rotman M, Triebwasser JH. A clinical and follow-up study of right and left bundle branch block. Circulation 1975; 51:477–84.
   In a study of 237,000 air force personnel, 394 were found to have right bundle branch block. The majority with right bundle branch block had no underlying cardiac disease and, as a result, had an excellent prognosis.
9. Nimetz AA, Shubrooks SJ Jr, Hutter AM Jr, DeSanctis RW. The significance of bundle branch block during acute myocardial infarction. Am Heart J 1975; 90:439–44.
   Of 71 patients with bundle branch block in the setting of acute myocardial infarction, 40 (57%) had high-degree AV block, and 25 (35%) had severe left ventricular failure.
10. Schneider JF, Thomas HE Jr, Kreger BE, McNamara PM, Sorlie P, Kannel WB. Newly acquired right bundle branch block: the Framingham study. Ann Intern Med 1980; 92:37–44.
    Of 70 patients in this group who developed a new right bundle branch block, the incidence of coronary artery disease and congestive heart failure was 2.5–4 times greater than in a group of age-matched controls.
11. Fleg JL, Das DN, LaKatta EG. Right bundle branch block: long-term prognosis in apparently healthy men. JACC 1983; 1:887–92.
    Long-term cardiac morbidity and mortality of 24 healthy men with right bundle branch block were similar to morbidity and mortality in men without it.

Left Bundle Branch Block

12. Haft JI, Herman MV, Gorlin R. Left bundle branch block: etiologic, hemodynamic, and ventriculographic considerations. Circulation 1971; 43:279–87.
    Of 24 patients with left bundle branch block, 7 had severe coronary artery disease, 5 had cardiomyopathy, and 7 had valvular disease.

13. Smith S, Hayes WL. The prognosis of complete left bundle branch block. Am Heart J 1965; 70:157–9.

Of 146 patients with complete left bundle branch block, the average survival after recognition of the block was only 36 months.

14. Lev M, Unger PN, Rosen KM, Bharati S. The anatomic substrate of complete left bundle branch block. Circulation 1974; 50:479–86.

Of 8 patients with left bundle branch block examined at postmortem, all had ischemic damage of the left bundle.

Bifascicular Block

15. Watt TB Jr, Pruitt RD. Character, cause, and consequence of combined left axis deviation and right bundle branch block in human electrocardiograms. Am Heart J 1969; 77:460–5.

The mean age of 55 patients with right bundle branch block and left anterior hemiblock was 67. These 55 individuals comprised about 1% of all those whose electrocardiograms were available for analysis.

16. Surawicz B: Prognosis of patients with chronic bifascicular block. Circulation 1979; 60:40–2.

In patients with chronic bifascicular block, prognosis is better evaluated by a clinical assessment than by a measurement of the H–V interval.

17. Dhingra RC, Wyndham C, Bauernfiend R, Denes P, Wu D, Swiryn S, Rosen KM. Significance of chronic bifascicular block without apparent organic heart disease. Circulation 1979; 60:33–9.

Patients with chronic bifascicular block due to primary conduction system disease have a small chance of cardiovascular or sudden death.

18. Scanlon PJ, Pryor R, Blount SG Jr. Right bundle branch block associated with left superior or inferior intraventricular block—associated with acute myocardial infarction. Circulation 1970; 42:1135–42.

For the patient with bifascicular block in the setting of acute infarction, insertion of a temporary transvenous pacemaker is indicated.

19. Pine MB, Oren M, Ciafone R, Rosner B, Hirota Y, Rabinowitz B, Abelmann WH. Excess mortality and morbidity associated with right bundle branch and left anterior fascicular block. JACC 1983; 1:1207–12.

In 108 patients with this form of bifascicular block, cardiac deaths and progression to complete heart block were more frequent than in a group of matched controls.

Incomplete and Complete Trifascicular Block

20. Rosenbaum MB, Elizari MV, Lazzari JO, Nau GJ, Levi RJ, Halpern MS. Intraventricular trifascicular blocks: review of the literature and classification. Am Heart J 1969; 78:450–9.

A review of the various kinds of incomplete and complete trifascicular blocks, including excellent explanatory diagrams.

21. Levites R, Haft JI: Significance of first degree heart block (prolonged PR interval) in bifascicular block. Am J Cardiol 1974; 34:259–64.

In the patient with bifascicular block, a prolonged P–R interval does not necessarily mean that conduction through the remaining fascicle is abnormal, nor does a normal P–R interval exclude the possibility of conduction delay in the remaining fascicle.

PROLONGED Q–T INTERVAL

A prolonged Q–T interval can occur as a congenital or acquired abnormality. The heritable causes of a prolonged Q–T interval include (1) the Jervell and Lange-Nielsen syndrome (syncope, deafness, prolonged Q–T interval, and sudden death, inherited as an autosomal recessive trait) and (2) the Romano-Ward syndrome (these same clinical manifestations without deafness, inherited as an autosomal dominant trait). Prolongation of the Q–T interval can also occur

(1) with certain electrolyte abnormalities, including hypokalemia, hypomagnesemia, and hypocalcemia; (2) with the use of several antiarrhythmic and pharmacologic agents, including quinidine, procainamide, phenothiazines, tricyclic antidepressants, and amiodarone; (3) with intraventricular conduction defects; and (4) with myocardial ischemia. Finally, some patients have idiopathic Q–T interval prolongation.

The patient with a prolonged Q–T interval may be asymptomatic, in which case the electrocardiographic abnormality is an incidential finding. Alternatively, the patient may have life-threatening arrhythmias, syncope, or sudden death. Syncope in the patient with a prolonged Q–T interval is generally due to transient ventricular fibrillation.

There is some experimental evidence to suggest that an imbalance in stellate ganglion stimulation of the heart may produce or aggravate a prolonged Q–T interval. The ablation of the right stellate ganglion (with resultant dominance of the left cardiac sympathetic nerves) produces a prolonged Q–T interval, as well as an increase in the frequency of ischemia and exercise-induced ventricular arrhythmias. In addition, such an imbalance lowers the ventricular fibrillation threshold. Therefore, the patient with Q–T interval prolongation may have cardiac sympathetic innervation that is predominantly left-sided.

For the patient with a prolonged Q–T interval and recurrent ventricular arrhythmias, antiarrhythmic agents that further prolong the Q–T interval, such as quinidine, procainamide, and amiodarone, should be avoided. Beta-adrenergic blocking agents may be effective in reducing the frequency of syncope and sudden death. Alternatively, beneficial results are also reported with phenytoin and bretylium. Left cervicothoracic sympathetic ganglionectomy has been shown to prevent recurrent ventricular arrhythmias in patients with a prolonged Q–T interval, even though left stellectomy is often not associated with a reduction in the Q–T interval, thus suggesting that left stellectomy increases the ventricular fibrillation threshold as the mechanism for its protective effect against recurrent ventricular arrhythmias. Therefore, since potentially effective therapy is available, early identification and diagnosis of the hereditary and sporadic forms of a prolonged Q–T interval are important.

1. Moss AJ, Schwartz PJ. Sudden death and the idiopathic long QT syndrome. Am J Med 1979; 66:6–7.
   A detailed and thorough review of all aspects of this syndrome.
2. Moss AJ, McDonald J. Unilateral cervicothoracic sympathetic ganglionectomy for the treatment of long Q–T interval syndrome. N Engl J Med 1971; 285:903–4.
   A case report describing a new surgical approach for shortening the Q–T interval and for the prevention of potentially fatal ventricular arrhythmias in patients with this syndrome.
3. Schwartz PJ, Wolf S. QT interval prolongation as predictor of sudden death in patients with myocardial infarction. Circulation 1978; 57:1074–7.
   Fifty-five patients with recent myocardial infarction and 55 healthy controls were matched and an ECG obtained every 2 months for 7 years. The Q–T interval was prolonged in 1 control (2%), in 5 of 27 surviving patients with myocardial infarction (18%), and in 16 of 28 patients with myocardial infarction who died suddenly (57%). These investigators concluded that a constant prolongation of Q–T interval in patients with myocardial infarction may be a marker of a poor prognosis.
4. Schwartz PJ. Cardiac sympathetic innervation and the sudden infant death syndrome. Am J Med 1976; 60:167–72.
   This report describes a relationship between the sudden infant death syndrome and an abnormality in cardiac sympathetic innervation.
5. Schwartz PJ, Periti M, Malliani A. The long QT syndrome. Am Heart J 1975; 89:378–90.
   A thorough review of the syndrome, including 105 references.

6. Crampton R. Preeminence of the left stellate ganglion in the long QT syndrome. Circulation 1979; 59:769–78.
   In 7 patients with the Romano-Ward syndrome, left stellate ganglion block and right stellate ganglion stimulation shortened the Q–T interval and suppressed tachyarrhythmias.

7. Yanowitz F, Preston JB, Abildskov JA. Functional distribution of right and left stellate innervation to the ventricles: production of neurogenic electrocardiographic changes by unilateral alteration of sympathetic tone. Circ Res 1966; 18:416–28.
   The distribution of right and left stellate innervation to the ventricles is explored in this canine study. Right stellate ganglionectomy or left stellate stimulation produced a prolonged QT interval.

8. Jervell A, Lange-Nielsen F. Congenital deaf-mutism, functional heart disease with prolongation of the QT interval, and sudden death. Am Heart J 1957; 54:59–68.
   The initial description of deaf-mutism and syncope in a familial form.

9. Romano C. Congenital cardiac arrhythmia (letter.) Lancet 1965; 1:658–9.
   A letter calling attention to the original report of a long Q–T interval and syncope caused by a ventricular arrhythmia.

10. James TN, Froggatt P, Atkinson WJ, Lurie PR, McNamara DG, Miller WW, Schloss GT, Carroll JF, North RL. Observations on the pathophysiology of the long QT syndromes with special reference to the neuropathology of the heart. Circulation 1978; 57:1221–31.
    Detailed postmortem studies were performed in 8 patients with syncope and a long QT interval who died suddenly. The consistent histologic abnormality was focal neuritis and neural degeneration within the sinus node, AV node, His bundle, and ventricular myocardium.

11. Khan MM, Logan KR, McComb JM, Adgey AAJ. Management of recurrent ventricular tachyarrhythmias associated with QT prolongation. Am J Cardiol 1981; 47:1301–8.
    Eleven patients with acquired prolongation of the Q–T interval and recurrent ventricular arrhythmias were studied. Overdrive ventricular pacing or atrioventricular sequential pacing abolished the ventricular arrhythmias in every patient.

12. Mitsutake A, Takeshita A, Kuroiwa A, Nakamura M. Usefulness of the Valsalva maneuver in mangement of the long QT syndrome. Circulation 1981; 63:1029–35.
    In 8 patients with a prolonged Q–T interval, the Valsalva maneuver further prolonged the QT and induced short runs of ventricular tachycardia in some.

13. DeSilvey DL, Moss AJ. Primidone in the treatment of the long QT syndrome: QT shortening and ventricular arrhythmia suppression. Ann Intern Med 1980; 93:53–4.
    In 3 patients with Q–T interval prolongation, primidone (an antiepileptic agent) was effective in shortening the Q–T interval and suppressing ventricular arrhythmias.

CARDIOVERSION

Over the past 20 years, direct current (DC) shock has gained widespread acceptance as an effective and safe means of terminating various tachyarrhythmias and restoring sinus rhythm. Prior to the use of electrical cardioversion, tachyarrhythmias were controlled or terminated with various cardioactive medications, such as the digitalis glycosides, quinidine, and procainamide. Since these agents sometimes produce unwanted side effects or are unsuccessful in restoring sinus rhythm, synchronized DC shock has largely replaced them as the preferred treatment of certain rhythm disturbances, especially life-threatening atrial and ventricular tachyarrhythmias.

For the patient with *atrial fibrillation,* quinidine or procainamide may induce a reversion to sinus rhythm. However, even when these agents are administered to the point of toxicity, they accomplish reversion in only about half the patients, whereas DC shock is successful in about 90 percent. In patients with long-standing atrial fibrillation (i.e., in excess of 5 years) and in those whose left atria are substantially enlarged (usually secondary to mitral valve disease), attempts at conversion to sinus rhythm often fail, even with high-energy DC shock. The amount of electrical energy necessary to convert atrial fibrillation to sinus rhythm is variable, but averages about 150 watt-sec. In general, somewhat higher energies are required in those with the Wolff-Parkinson-White syndrome, congestive cardiomyopathy, severe coronary artery disease, or acute myocardial infarction. Although electrical cardioversion is more efficient than pharmacologic conversion, quinidine or procainamide are invaluable for maintenance therapy.

Electrical cardioversion is generally considered the treatment of choice for the patient with *atrial flutter*. The average energy requirement is only 25 watt-sec. Although DC shock usually converts atrial flutter to sinus rhythm, it occasionally converts it to atrial fibrillation. Direct current shock is almost always successful in converting *paroxysmal supraventricular tachycardia* to sinus rhythm. The energy required for such conversion is similar to that needed in the patient with atrial fibrillation (i.e., 100–200 watt-sec).

The electrical conversion of *ventricular tachycardia* to sinus rhythm is usually accomplished with very low energies, i.e., 1 to 10 watt-sec. Once conversion to sinus rhythm is accomplished, maintenance antiarrhythmic therapy with lidocaine, quinidine, or procainamide should be instituted in an attempt to stabilize the patient in sinus rhythm. *Ventricular fibrillation* requires immediate electrical cardioversion with high energies, i.e., 400 watt-sec. Once sinus rhythm is achieved, maintenance antiarrhythmic therapy should be started to prevent a recurrence.

Electrical cardioversion can be either an elective or an emergency procedure. As an elective procedure, it is used to treat an acute or chronic tachyarrhythmia that is not jeopardizing the patient's well-being. Those with atrial fibrillation or flutter are begun on quinidine 24 to 48 hours before attempted electrical conversion. A reversion to sinus rhythm occurs in a small number of patients (i.e., 10–15%) with quinidine alone; in the remainder, quinidine is helpful in maintaining sinus rhythm after electrical cardioversion. In addition, quinidine reduces the necessary number of shocks, decreases (by about 40%) the energy required to restore sinus rhythm, and diminishes the incidence of postcardioversion arrhythmias. The patient who is receiving maintenance digitalis is not given it on the day of elective cardioversion. If atrial fibrillation is present, full anticoagulation (with heparin or coumadin) is accomplished for 3 to 4 weeks prior to elective cardioversion to prevent systemic arterial embolism, which follows restoration of sinus rhythm in 1 to 2 percent of patients. Amnesia during elective electrical cardioversion is obtained with either diazepam or a short-acting barbiturate; both are given by intravenous injection.

If the tachyarrhythmia is life-threatening, DC shock should be performed without delay. The conscious patient should receive intravenous diazepam, but the unconscious patient need not receive any premedication; rather, the emphasis should be on rapid correction of the arrhythmia.

Although electrical cardioversion is generally a safe procedure, there are occasional complications. In the immediate postcardioversion period, ventricular arrhythmias (ventricular premature beats, ventricular tachycardia, or ventricular fibrillation) may occur, especially in patients with serum electrolyte abnormalities or digitalis intoxication. Often, these can be avoided by careful energy titration and by the precardioversion administration of lidocaine. Systemic arterial embolization occurs in 1 to 2 percent of patients in the minutes after conversion to sinus rhythm. In a rare patient, pulmonary congestion develops during the 12 to 24 hours after electrical cardioversion.

Several kinds of patients require especially meticulous management if electrical cardioversion is planned. First, in the patient with possible sick sinus syndrome, DC shock is dangerous, since the tachyarrhythmia may be replaced by extreme sinus bradycardia or even sinus arrest in the seconds to minutes following cardioversion. Therefore, electrical cardioversion in the patient with suspected or documented sick sinus syndrome should be performed with a temporary pacemaker in place. Second, electrical cardioversion in the patient already taking a beta-adrenergic blocker can result in severe bradycardia. Third, although the presence of a permanent pacemaker does not prevent electrical cardioversion, this procedure can damage temporary bipolar pacemakers; therefore, a temporary pacemaker should be momentarily disconnected during the conversion procedure. Fourth, patients in whom tachyarrhythmias develop immediately after valve replacement often do not maintain sinus rhythm even if it is restored electrically. Therefore, if the patient is tolerating the tachyarrhythmia without difficulty, electrical conversion should be postponed for 10 to 14 days after the operation. Finally, it should be emphasized that DC countershock should not be employed in the patient whose rhythm disturbance is due to digitalis intoxication, since attempted electrical cardioversion is likely to induce ventricular tachycardia or fibrillation.

Once DC shock has been used successfully to convert the patient from a tachyarrhythmia to sinus rhythm, long-term antiarrhythmic therapy is usually required to maintain the patient in sinus rhythm. For the individual in whom cardioversion was employed to terminate atrial flutter or fibrillation, digitalis and quinidine (or digitalis and procainamide) are administered to minimize the chance of a recurrence. For the patient who required DC shock for paroxysmal supraventricular tachycardia, long-term therapy with digitalis, a beta-adrenergic blocker, or verapamil may be indicated. Finally, the patient in whom DC shock was required to terminate ventricular tachycardia or fibrillation should be placed on maintenance quinidine, procainamide, disopyramide, or one of the newer antiarrhythmic agents presently under investigation.

1. Horn HR, Lown B. Cardioversion 1975: foremost therapy for tachyarrhythmias. Geriatrics 1975; 30:75–82.
   Extensive clinical experience indicates that electrical cardioversion is the most effective method available for terminating cardiac tachyarrhythmias. This paper reviews the energy levels needed to convert various tachyarrhythmias to sinus rhythm.
2. Resnekov L. Drug therapy before and after the electroversion of cardiac dysrhythmias. Prog Cardiovasc Dis 1974; 16:531–8.
   A thorough review of the use of anesthetics, digitalis, anticoagulants, and antiarrhythmics during the pericardioversion period.
3. Muenster JJ, Rosenberg MS, Carleton RA, Graettinger JS. Comparison between diazepam and sodium thiopental during DC countershock. JAMA 1967; 199:758–60.
   In this comparison, diazepam anesthesia was associated with less ventricular ectopy than was thiopental.
4. Lown B, Kleiger R, Williams J. Cardioversion and digitalis drugs: changed threshold to electric shock in digitalized animals. Circ Res 1965; 17:519–31.
   In the experimental animal, cardioversion is ineffective for arrhythmias induced by digitalis toxicity. In the presence of digitalis excess, electrical cardioversion may provoke serious rhythm disturbances.
5. Katz MJ, Zitnik RS. Direct current shock and lidocaine in the treatment of digitalis-induced ventricular tachycardia. Am J Cardiol 1966; 18:552–6.
   For digitalis-induced ventricular tachyarrhythmias, lidocaine is beneficial, whereas DC shock is detrimental.
6. Byrne-Quinn E, Wing AJ. Maintenance of sinus rhythm after DC reversion of atrial fibrillation. Br Heart J 1970; 32:370–6.
   After electrical cardioversion, long-term quinidine is more effective than placebo in maintaining the patient in sinus rhythm.

7. Lown B. Electrical reversion of cardiac arrhythmias (Thomas Lewis Lecture). Br Heart J 1967; 29:469–89.
   A complete review of the early experience—experimental and clinical—with electrical cardioversion.
8. DeSilva RA, Graboys TB, Podrid PJ, Lown B. Cardioversion and defibrillation. Am Heart J 1980; 100:881–95.
   A thorough discussion of the history, technique, use, and complications of electrical cardioversion. Includes 135 references.
9. Chun PKC, Davia JE, Donohue DJ. ST-segment elevation with elective DC cardioversion. Circulation 1981; 63:220–4.
   An occasional patient will develop transient S–T segment elevation immediately after electrical cardioversion. In this report, 3 patients are described who had such S–T segment elevation without enzymatic evidence of myocardial damage.
10. Kerber RE, Martins JB, Gascho JA, Marcus ML, Grayzel J. Effect of direct-current countershocks on regional myocardial contractility and perfusion: experimental studies. Circulation 1981; 63:323–32.
    In a dog model, high-energy transthoracic shocks exert no deleterious effect on myocardial perfusion or contraction.
11. Kerber RE, Jensen SR, Grayzel J, Kennedy J, Hoyt R. Elective cardioversion: influence of paddle-electrode location and size on success rates and energy requirements. N Engl J Med 1981; 305:658–62.
    In a prospective study of 173 patients with atrial fibrillation or flutter, neither paddle size nor location (anteroposterior vs. anterolateral) affected the success of electrical cardioversion.
12. Ditchey RV, Karliner JS. Safety of electrical cardioversion in patients without digitalis toxicity. Ann Intern Med 1981; 95:676–9.
    Patients receiving digoxin without clinical evidence of digitalis toxicity are a low risk for serious postcardioversion ventricular arrhythmias, even when serum digoxin levels are modestly elevated.
13. Babbs CF, Tacker WA, VanVleet JF, Bourland JD, Geddes LA. Therapeutic indices for transchest defibrillator shocks: effective, damaging, and lethal electrical doses. Am Heart J 1980; 99:734–8.
    Using experimental animals, this study attempted to distinguish between effective and damaging electrical doses.
14. Ditchey RV, LeWinter MM. Effects of direct-current electrical shocks on systolic and diastolic left ventricular function in dogs. Am Heart J 1983; 105:727–31.
    Three consecutive 50 joule DC shocks applied directly to the canine heart had only minor consequences on systolic and diastolic left ventricular performance.

TEMPORARY AND PERMANENT PACING

Cardiac pacing is indicated for the treatment of arrhythmias or their precursors that are unresponsive to medical management and that cause a reduction in cardiac output, with resultant cerebral, coronary, or renal insufficiency. The patient who requires pacemaker therapy may complain of dizziness or syncope, symptoms of pulmonary or peripheral venous congestion (dyspnea, orthopnea, and ankle edema), or angina pectoris. A *temporary* pacemaker is usually inserted transvenously through the subclavian, internal jugular, brachial, or femoral vein and is positioned in the right ventricular apex. In an emergency, a transthoracic approach may be utilized when immediate pacemaker therapy is needed. The indications for temporary pacemaker insertion include (1) symptomatic sinus bradycardia, usually due to drugs (propranolol, verapamil, reserpine, or aldomet) or occurring with a myocardial infarction (usually inferior in location); (2) second or third degree heart block, also most often caused by drugs (propranolol, verapamil, or digitalis) or myocardial infarction; (3) bifascicular or trifascicular block in association with infarction; and (4) sinus pauses or sinus arrest, usually associated with acute myocardial infarction or intrinsic conduction system disease (e.g., the sick sinus syndrome). In addition, temporary pacing may be used as "overdrive" therapy for malignant ventricular ectopic activity or as an effective means of converting paroxysmal supraventricular tachycardia or atrial flutter to sinus rhythm.

Temporary pacemaker therapy is potentially associated with many complications, but none of these occurs frequently. First, a transvenous electrode may be positioned incorrectly, so that it is left in the right atrium or coronary sinus. Second, right ventricular perforation may occur during pacemaker manipulation, occasionally resulting in hemopericardium with tamponade. In most instances, however, perforation of the right ventricular free wall with a pacemaker electrode is well tolerated. Third, if a transvenous temporary pacemaker electrode is left in place for many days, venous thrombosis and infection are likely. Fourth, several technical problems related to pacemaker function may arise, including breaks, loose connections, or poor contact within the pacemaker system. Finally, the pacing and sensing thresholds may be poor despite extensive efforts to position the temporary pacing electrode optimally.

A *permanent* pacemaker is inserted by the transvenous route in 90 percent of patients, whereas it is implanted directly on the epicardial surface in the remaining 10 percent. The transvenous method of implantation is usually preferred, since it does not require general anesthesia and is associated with a very low morbidity and mortality. Its major disadvantage is displacement of the endocardial electrode, but in experienced hands, this occurs in less than 5 percent of transvenous implantations. The epicardial method of implantation requires a thoracotomy and, therefore, carries a higher morbidity and mortality, especially in elderly patients. Its advantages center on the security of electrode placement and the very low threshold that is required to pace.

The indications for permanent pacemaker implantation include (1) intermittent or continuous complete AV block, either congenital or acquired; (2) chronic Mobitz II second degree AV block; (3) symptomatic (or potentially symptomatic) bifascicular or incomplete trifascicular block; and (4) symptomatic sick sinus syndrome. In addition, permanent pacemaker implantation may offer an effective therapy for patients with supraventricular or ventricular tachyarrhythmias that are resistant to antiarrhythmic drug therapy. With such a pacemaker, the patient with one of these tachyarrhythmias may initiate burst atrial or ventricular pacing during an episode of symptomatic tachycardia, causing a reversion to sinus rhythm. Recently developed devices even provide the capability of recognizing and converting ventricular fibrillation to sinus rhythm.

Once a permanent pacemaker is implanted, a regular evaluation of its function is necessary. Much of this periodic assessment can be performed by transtelephonic monitoring. The patient with a permanent pacemaker should be instructed to resume normal activities and should be informed that most electrical devices do not inhibit a pacemaker unless they are within inches of the pulse generator.

In general, the implantation and maintenance of a permanent pacemaker are associated with a low incidence of complications. First, an occasional patient becomes infected after a pacemaker is implanted. If infection occurs, it is best treated by removing the entire unit. Second, deep venous thrombosis occasionally occurs with transvenous pacemakers, but it is usually not associated with symptoms. Third, failure to pace may result from battery depletion or from breakage or displacement of the pacing electrode. If this occurs, its cause must be identified quickly and corrected. Finally, an occasional individual develops a so-called runaway pacemaker, a situation in which the pacemaker's intrinsic rate increases and cannot be controlled. If this occurs, the pulse generator must be replaced immediately.

Finally, there is intense interest at present about the advantages of so-called physiologic pacing in many patients who require a permanent pacemaker. Such an approach allows the patient to maintain the normal sequence of AV depolarization, with a resulting maintenance of cardiac output. Newer models may even allow the pacing rate to increase or decrease automatically in conjunction with respiratory rate or exercise.

Temporary Pacing: Indications

1. Escher DJW, Furman S. Emergency treatment of cardiac arrhythmias—emphasis on use of electrical pacing. JAMA 1970; 214:2028–34.
   A succinct review of the indications for emergency temporary pacing.
2. Beregovich J, Fenig S, Lasser J, Allen D. Management of acute myocardial infarction complicated by advanced atrioventricular block—role of artifical pacing. Am J Cardiol 1969; 23:54–65.
   Of 25 patients with acute myocardial infarction and advanced AV block treated with transvenous temporary pacing, 18 (72%) survived.
3. Gupta PK, Lichstein E, Chadda KD. Heart block complicating acute inferior wall myocardial infarction. Chest 1976; 69:599–604.
   Of 410 patients with inferior infarction, heart block (second or third degree) occurred in 60.
4. Chamberlain D, Leinbach R. Electrical pacing in heart block complicating acute myocardial infarction. Br Heart J 1970; 32:2–5.
   These authors express confidence that artifical pacing can improve prognosis in high-risk patients with myocardial infarction.
5. Hindman MC, Wagner GS, JaRo M, Atkins JM, Scheinman MM, DeSanctis RW, Hutter AM Jr, Yeatman L, Rubenfire M, Pujura C, Rubin M, Morris JJ. The clinical significance of bundle branch block complicating acute myocardial infarction. 2. Indications for temporary and permanent pacemaker insertion. Circulation 1978; 58:689–99.
   In the setting of acute myocardial infarction, patients at high risk of developing high degree AV block should receive prophylactic temporary pacing.

Temporary Pacing: Therapeutic Considerations

6. Orlando J, Cassidy J, Aronow WS. High reversion of atrial flutter to sinus rhythm after atrial pacing in patients with pulmonary disease. Chest 1977; 71:580–2.
   In 36 episodes of atrial flutter, 24 (67%) converted to sinus rhythm within 1 minute of atrial pacing.
7. Waldo AL, MacLean WAH, Karp RB, Kouchoukos NT, James TN. Continuous rapid atrial pacing to control recurrent or sustained supraventricular tachycardias following open heart surgery. Circulation 1976; 54:245–50.
   In postoperative patients, continuous rapid atrial pacing produced and sustained either atrial fibrillation or 2:1 AV block. This method was safe and effective.

Temporary Pacing: Technical Considerations

8. Weinstein J, Gnoj J, Mazzara JT, Ayres SM, Grace WJ. Temporary transvenous pacing via the percutaneous femoral vein approach. A prospective study of 100 cases. Am Heart J 1973; 85:695–705.
   The transfemoral approach provides a reliable, safe, and rapid technique for temporary pacemaker insertion.
9. Rosenberg AS, Grossman JI, Escher DJW, Furman S. Bedside transvenous cardiac pacing. Am Heart J 1969; 77:697–703.
   Of 111 patients who required temporary pacing, indications included high grade heart block in 37, bradycardia or heart block with acute infarction in 24, and cardiac arrest in 14.

Temporary Pacing: Complications

10. Lumia FJ, Rios JC. Temporary transvenous pacemaker therapy: an analysis of complications. Chest 1973; 64:604–8.
In this series of 142 patients with temporary pacing catheters, 29 (16%) had minor complications; however, no deaths were caused by pacemaker insertion or maintenance.

Permanent Pacing: Indications

11. Escher DJW, Furman S. Pacemaker therapy for chronic rhythm disorders. Prog Cardiovasc Dis 1972; 14:459–74.
A review of the indications for permanent pacing. Includes 101 references.

12. Wright KE Jr, McIntosh HD. Artifical pacemakers—indications and management. Circulation 1973; 47:1108–18.
This paper reviews the accepted indications for permanent pacemaker insertion.

13. Aroesty JM, Cohen SI, Morkin E. Bradycardia-tachycardia syndrome: results in 28 patients treated by combined pharmacologic therapy and pacemaker implantation. Chest 1974; 66:257–63.
The combination of drug therapy and permanent pacemaker insertion was an effective therapy in patients with the brady-tachy syndrome.

14. Hartel G, Talvensaari T. Treatment of sinoatrial syndrome with permanent cardiac pacing in 90 patients. Acta Med Scand 1975; 198:341–7.
In these 90 patients, permanent pacemaker implantation eliminated syncope in 48 of 49 and dizziness in 28 of 28.

Permanent Pacing: "Physiologic" Pacing

15. Sutton R, Perrins J, Citron P. Physiological cardiac pacing. PACE 1980; 3:207–19.
A thorough historical review of physiologic pacing is presented in this paper.

Permanent Pacing: Therapeutic Considerations

16. Hartzler GO, Holmes DR Jr, Osborn MJ. Patient-activated transvenous cardiac stimulation for the treatment of supraventricular and ventricular tachycardia. Am J Cardiol 1981; 47:903–9.
This article describes the use of a patient-activated burst pacemaker in 8 patients with refractory supraventricular tachycardia and in 9 with refractory ventricular tachycardia. This system was generally successful and well-tolerated by these 17 individuals.

17. Ruskin JN, Garan H, Poulin F, Harthorne JW. Permanent radiofrequency ventricular pacing for management of drug-resistant ventricular tachycardia. Am J Cardiol 1980; 46:317–21.
Three patients with frequent episodes of symptomatic, sustained ventricular tachycardia that often required physician intervention were treated with a permanent patient-activated radiofrequency ventricular pacemaker for self-termination of ventricular tachycardia.

18. Mirowski M, Reid PR, Mower MM, Watkins L, Gott VL, Schauble JF, Langer A, Heilman MS, Kolenik SA, Fischell RE, Weisfeldt ML. Termination of malignant ventricular arrhythmias with an implanted automatic defibrillator in human beings. N Engl J Med 1980; 303:322–4.
This article describes the experience in 3 patients who had an automatic defibrillator implanted to manage recurrent ventricular tachyarrhythmias refractory to medical therapy.

19. Reid PR, Mirowski M, Mower MM, Platia EV, Griffith LSC, Watkins L Jr, Bach SM Jr, Imran M, Thomas A. Clinical evaluation of the internal automatic cardioverter-defibrillator in survivors of sudden cardiac death. Am J Cardiol 1983; 51:1608–13.
This article describes the initial experience with this device in 12 patients.

Permanent Pacing: Complications

20. Choo MH, Holmes DR Jr, Gersh BJ, Maloney JD, Merideth J, Pluth JR, Trusty J. Permanent pacemaker infections: characterization and management. Am J Cardiol 1981; 48:559–64.
Over a 6 to 7 year time period, 46 patients were treated for infections of permanent

pacing systems. Optimal therapy for the large majority of patients requires the removal of the entire infected pacing system.

21. Peters RW, Scheinman MM, Raskin S, Thomas AN. Unusual complications of epicardial pacemakers. Recurrent pericarditis, cardiac tamponade and pericardial constriction. Am J Cardiol 1980; 45:1088–94.
    Recurrent pericarditis after insertion of an epicardial pacemaker requires careful medical follow-up because either life-threatening tamponade or chronic constrictive pericarditis may develop.

22. Nicolosi GL, Charmet PA, Zanuttini D. Large right atrial thrombosis: rare complication during permanent transvenous endocardial pacing. Br Heart J 1980; 43:199–201.
    In 2 elderly women, postmorten examination showed large right atrial thrombi around the transvenous pacing electrode.

23. Stoney WS, Addlestone RB, Alford WC Jr, Burrus GR, Frist RA, Thomas CS Jr. The incidence of venous thrombosis following long-term transvenous pacing. Ann Thorac Surg 1976; 22:166–70.
    In 32 patients whose transvenous pacemakers had been in place for at least 18 months, venography showed severe obstruction in 11.

INVASIVE ELECTROPHYSIOLOGIC TESTING

Although the standard ECG records the electrical activity of the heart from the body surface, the recent development of intracardiac electrophysiologic recording and stimulation techniques has led to an improved understanding of the mechanisms and management of both supraventricular and ventricular arrhythmias. With electrode catheters positioned in the ventricles, atria, and the region of the His bundle, several goals can be accomplished. First, sinus node function can be assessed by measuring the sinoatrial conduction time. The patient with the sick sinus syndrome often has a prolonged sinoatrial conduction time in conjunction with symptomatic and electrocardiographic evidence of conduction system disease.

Second, invasive electrophysiologic testing has provided a better understanding of the mechanisms underlying various supraventricular tachyarrhythmias, such as paroxysmal supraventricular tachycardia with block, atrial fibrillation, and atrial flutter. In addition, pacing-induced conversion of atrial flutter has been used in managing the patient in whom DC countershock is contraindicated, and recently developed endocardial and epicardial atrial mapping has made possible the successful surgical excision of a focal paroxysmal atrial tachycardia.

Third, invasive electrophysiologic testing has made possible a better understanding of normal and abnormal AV conduction. His bundle recordings have improved on the accuracy of the surface ECG in defining the site of block in patients with second degree AV block. They have also added to our knowledge of bifascicular block and its propensity (or lack thereof) to progress to complete heart block.

Fourth, intracardiac electrophysiologic recording techniques have greatly expanded our knowledge of the mechanisms responsible for the initiation and maintenance of supraventricular tachycardias. Using these techniques, AV nodal reentry has been identified as the electrophysiologic mechanism in most individuals with paroxysmal supraventricular tachycardia. In addition, these techniques have provided a full understanding of the preexcitation syndromes, allowing an examination of the electrophysiologic properties of the normal and accessory pathways of AV conduction. Armed with this in-depth understanding of electrophysiologic mechanisms in these patients, specially designed anti-tachycardiac pacemakers, as well as intraoperative mapping techniques to identify the location of the anomalous AV connection and to ablate it, have been developed.

Fifth, intracardiac electrophysiologic techniques have provided the means by which the pathophysiology of recurrent sustained ventricular tachycardia has been evaluated, and this detailed understanding of pathophysiology has made possible (1) a rational approach to antiarrhythmic drug therapy, (2) the development of antitachycardiac pacemakers, and (3) surgical endocardial ventriculotomy as a means of removing the anatomic site of recurrent tachycardia.

General

1. Denes P, Ezri MD. Clinical electrophysiology—a decade of progress. JACC 1983; 1:292–305.
   A succinct review of the indications for invasive electrophysiologic testing. Includes 125 references.

Assessment of Sinus Node and Atrial Function

2. Narula OS, Samet P, Javier RP. Significance of the sinus node recovery time. Circulation 1972; 45:140–58.
   The corrected sinus node recovery time provides a potentially useful clinical means of assessing the sinus node function, thereby helping in the diagnosis of sick sinus syndrome.

3. Watson RM, Josephson ME. Atrial flutter. I. Electrophysiologic substrates and modes of initiation and termination. Am J Cardiol 1980; 45:732–41.
   One or two atrial extrastimuli induced atrial flutter in 31 of 41 patients in whom atrial flutter could be induced by programmed electrical stimulation.

4. Waldo AL, MacLean WAH, Karp RB, Kouchoukos NT, James TN. Entrainment and interruption of atrial flutter with atrial pacing: studies in man following open heart surgery. Circulation 1977; 56:737–45.
   Atrial flutter was converted to sinus rhythm after atrial pacing in 30 patients following cardiac surgery.

5. Orlando J, Cassidy J, Aronow WS. High reversion of atrial flutter to sinus rhythm after atrial pacing in patients with pulmonary disease. Chest 1977; 71:580–2.
   Atrial pacing caused conversion to sinus rhythm in 14 of 17 patients with atrial flutter and pulmonary disease.

6. Wyndham CRC, Arnsdorf MF, Levitsky S, Smith TC, Dhingra RC, Denes P, Rosen KM. Successful surgical excision of focal paroxysmal atrial tachycardia. Observations in vivo and in vitro. Circulation 1980; 62:1365–72.
   This case illustrates the feasibility of direct surgical excision of an atrial focus producing tachycardia.

Assessment of Atrioventricular Conduction

7. Scheinman MM, Peters RW, Modin G, Brennan M, Mies C, O'Young J. Prognostic value of infranodal conduction time in patients with chronic bundle branch block. Circulation 1977; 56:240–4.
   Patients with chronic bundle branch block and a prolonged H–V interval often progress to second or third degree AV block. In addition, they have a high incidence of congestive heart failure and sudden death.

8. Strasberg B, Amat-y-Leon F, Dhingra RC, Palileo E, Swiryn S, Bauernfeind R, Wyndham C, Rosen KM. Natural history of chronic second-degree atrioventricular nodal block. Circulation 1981; 63:1043–9.
   Chronic second degree AV block proximal to the His bundle is, of itself, a benign lesion. In patients with it in the setting of organic heart disease, prognosis is related to the severity of underlying heart disease.

Evaluation of Supraventricular Tachycardia

9. Denes P, Wu D, Dhingra RC, Chuquimia R, Rosen KM. Demonstration of dual AV nodal pathways in patients with paroxysmal supraventricular tachycardia. Circulation 1973; 48:549–55.

This article presents electrophysiologic evidence of dual AV nodal pathways in 2 patients with normal P–R intervals and reentrant paroxysmal supraventricular tachycardia.

10. Wu D, Denes P, Amat-y-Leon F, Dhingra RC, Wyndham CRC, Bauernfiend R, Latif P, Rosen KM. Clinical, electrocardiographic, and electrophysiologic observations in patients with paroxysmal supraventricular tachycardia. Am J Cardiol 1978; 41:1045–51.

Of 79 patients without ventricular preexcitation but with documented paroxysmal supraventricular tachycardia, electrophysiologic study suggested AV nodal reentry in 50, reentrance using a concealed extranodal pathway in 9, sinus or atrial reentrance in 7, and ectopic automatic tachycardia in 3.

11. Gallagher JJ, Gilbert M, Svenson RH, Sealy WC, Kasell J, Wallace AG. Wolff-Parkinson-White syndrome: the problem, evaluation, and surgical correction. Circulation 1975; 51:767–85.

A thorough discussion of the electrophysiologic characteristics of this syndrome as well as a review of drug, pacemaker, and surgical therapy.

12. Wellens HJJ. Value and limitations of programmed electrical stimulation of the heart in the study and treatment of tachycardias. Circulation 1978; 57:845–53.

A discussion of the use of invasive electrophysiologic testing in patients with supraventricular and ventricular tachycardias. Includes 95 references.

13. Gallagher JJ, Kasell J, Sealy WC, Pritchett ELC, Wallace AG. Epicardial mapping in the Wolff-Parkinson-White syndrome. Circulation 1978; 57:854–66.

Epicardial mapping provides a method for defining antegrade and retrograde sites of preexcitation in the operating room, where the accessory atrioventricular pathway can be incised.

14. Klein GJ, Bashore TM, Sellers TD, Pritchett ELC, Smith WM, Gallagher JJ. Ventricular fibrillation in the Wolff-Parkinson-White syndrome. N Engl J Med 1979; 301:1080–5.

Based on the electrophysiologic findings in 31 patients with Wolff-Parkinson-White syndrome and a previous episode of ventricular fibrillation, this report proposes some guidelines for assessing the risk of ventricular fibrillation in this patient group.

Evaluation of Ventricular Tachycardia

15. Josephson ME, Horowitz LN. Electrophysiologic approach to therapy of recurrent sustained ventricular tachycardia. Am J Cardiol 1979; 43:631–42.

The efficacy of drug therapy for recurrent ventricular tachycardia can be assessed in sequential studies using programmed electrical stimulation; the efficacy of pacemaker therapy can be evaluated by examining the effects of stimulation on the tachycardia; and the site of tachycardia can be identified and approached surgically.

16. Vandepol CJ, Farshidi A, Spielman SR, Greenspan AM, Horowitz LN, Josephson ME. Incidence and clinical significance of induced ventricular tachycardia. Am J Cardiol 1980; 45:725–31.

Programmed electrical stimulation induced ventricular tachycardia in 52 (91%) of 57 patients with recurrent sustained ventricular tachycardia.

17. Horowitz LN, Harken AH, Kastor JA, Josephson ME. Ventricular resection guided by epicardial and endocardial mapping for treatment of recurrent ventricular tachycardia. N Engl J Med 1980; 302:589–93.

Surgical therapy of recurrent ventricular tachycardia can be improved through the identification of the endocardial origin of the arrhythmia followed by appropriately guided resection.

18. Ruskin JN, DiMarco JP, Garan H. Out-of-hospital cardiac arrest: electrophysiologic observations and selection of long-term antiarrhythmic therapy. N Engl J Med 1980; 303:607–13.

Ventricular arrhythmias can be initiated and reproduced by programmed ventricular stimulation in most patients who have been resuscitated after out-of-hospital cardiac arrest. Complete suppression of these arrhythmias with antiarrhythmic therapy is highly predictive of survival for at least 1 year.

19. Spielman SR, Farshidi A, Horowitz LN, Josephson ME. Ventricular fibrillation during programmed ventricular stimulation: incidence and clinical implications. Am J Cardiol 1978; 42:913–8.

Ventricular fibrillation occurred in only 10 of 300 patients undergoing programmed ventricular stimulation.

20. Mason JW, Winkle RA. Electrode-catheter arrhythmia induction in the selection and assessment of antiarrhythmic drug therapy for recurrent ventricular tachycardia. Circulation 1978; 58:971–85.
    In patients with recurrent ventricular tachycardia, drug efficacy trials using intracardiac pacing techniques provide an excellent means of selecting effective long-term antiarrhythmic therapy.

21. Horowitz LN, Josephson ME, Farshidi A, Spielman SR, Michelson EL, Greenspan AM. Recurrent sustained ventricular tachycardia. 3. Role of the electrophysiologic study in selection of antiarrhythmic regimens. Circulation 1978; 58:986–97.
    Serial electrophysiologic testing provides rapid identification of successful antiarrhythmic therapy and can predict in which patients conventional therapy will be ineffective, thereby identifying those individuals who require a more aggressive mode of therapy.

22. Josephson ME, Harken AH, Horowitz LN. Endocardial excision: a new surgical technique for the treatment of recurrent ventricular tachycardia. Circulation 1979; 60:1430–9.
    In 12 patients with medically refractory ventricular tachycardia secondary to ischemic heart disease, intraoperative mapping localized the tachycardia to the border of an aneurysm, and resection was accomplished. The 10 survivors remained free of sustained ventricular tachycardia for 9–20 months postoperatively.

MYOCARDIAL ISCHEMIA AND INFARCTION

CORONARY ARTERIAL SPASM

Coronary arterial spasm, superimposed on either obstructive arteriosclerotic coronary artery disease or radiographically normal coronary arteries, has been shown to be the cause of Prinzmetal's variant angina pectoris. More recently, some studies have incriminated spasm as a contributing factor in some patients with angina of effort, unstable angina, acute myocardial infarction, and even sudden death. Thus, coronary arterial spasm may play an important pathophysiologic role throughout the entire spectrum of ischemic heart disease.

In 1959, Prinzmetal et al. described a group of patients with so-called variant angina pectoris. These patients usually experienced chest discomfort at rest rather than during physical exertion or emotional excitement. The ECGs recorded during episodes of chest pain showed S–T segment elevation (rather than depression), which resolved completely as pain subsided. The episodes of chest discomfort were occasionally accompanied by various degrees of AV block as well as ventricular ectopic activity. Finally, the chest pain was quickly relieved by sublingual nitroglycerin. Although coronary arteriography was not performed in these patients, it was postulated that this clinical syndrome was due to spasm superimposed on a fixed atheromatous stenosis of the proximal portion of a major coronary artery.

Since this original description, numerous reports have confirmed the existence of variant angina pectoris as a distinct clinical entity and have clarified its underlying pathophysiology. Coronary arteriographic studies have demonstrated that many patients with this syndrome have severe proximal arteriosclerotic disease involving one or more major coronary arteries; however, other patients with the same clinical features have been shown to have angiographically normal coronary arteries. Thus, severe coronary arterial spasm, with resultant transmural myocardial ischemia and S–T segment elevation, can occur in the presence or absence of fixed atheromatous coronary artery disease.

If coronary arterial spasm is suspected clinically, several agents or maneuvers can be used in an attempt to provoke an episode. Ergonovine maleate, an ergot alkaloid and alpha-adrenergic agonist with a direct constrictive effect on vascular smooth muscle, can be administered to the patient with possible coronary arterial spasm under carefully controlled conditions, i.e., either in the coronary care unit or (more appropriately) in the cardiac catheterization laboratory at the time of selective coronary arteriography. When administered carefully, ergonovine can be given to patients with or without obstructive atherosclerotic coronary artery disease. It is given intravenously in small increments every 3 to 5 minutes, beginning with 0.02 to 0.05 mg and gradually increasing in size until a single dose of 0.1 to 0.2 mg is given. In the doses outlined, ergonovine is highly specific for provoking coronary arterial spasm in patients with variant angina, but its sensitivity in doing so may not be as good as was once believed. Many patients with coronary arterial spasm vary markedly in their sensitivity to ergonovine; the same patient that at times develops myocardial ischemia after very small amounts of ergonovine at other times does not develop chest pain or ECG alterations even after large doses.

Methacholine, a parasympathomimetic agent, has been used on occasion to induce coronary arterial spasm, as have exposure to cold (the so-called cold pressor test), the combination of vigorous hyperventilation and the intravenous administration of a buffer solution, and histamine administration. It is the subjective impression of most investigators in this country that ergonovine administration is the strongest available provocation, but no formal attempt has yet been made to compare these various methods.

Coronary arterial spasm is effectively relieved by nitroglycerin, administered either sublingually or intravenously. The therapeutic use of adrenergic stimulants and blockers is complicated and as yet unsettled. Prinzmetal observed that his patients obtained symptomatic relief with a beta-adrenergic agonist, nylidrin. This observation, in combination with scattered anecdotal reports that beta blockade may exacerbate variant angina, has led some investigators to discourage the use of beta-adrenergic blockers (such as propranolol) in the treatment of patients with possible coronary arterial spasm. At the same time, these data have encouraged the use of alpha-adrenergic antagonists, such as phentolamine. Finally, the calcium antagonists, such as verapamil, diltiazem, and nifedipine, have been found to be effective in preventing coronary arterial spasm. These agents inhibit the contraction of smooth muscle by decreasing the cellular uptake of calcium (a process that is fundamental to cellular contraction).

In the early reports of variant angina pectoris, there was a high incidence of myocardial infarction or death during the first 2 years after diagnosis. Recently, however, the growing use of the calcium antagonists has substantially altered the outlook of patients with this disease entity, with or without underlying obstructive coronary artery disease. Therefore, the prognosis of patients with variant angina receiving maximal medical therapy (calcium antagonists and nitrates) appears to be favorable, even in the presence of severe atherosclerosis.

Finally, coronary arterial spasm has been implicated as a possible contributing factor in patients with exertional angina, unstable angina, or acute myocardial infarction, and some authors have even suggested that such spasm may play a role in individuals with sudden death. Patients with underlying arteriosclerotic disease and angina of effort respond in an exaggerated fashion to alpha-adrenergic stimulation. In a series of carefully performed hemodynamic, scintigraphic, and coronary arteriographic studies in patients with various kinds of angina or myocardial infarction, Maseri et al. have implicated spasm as a contributor to these clinical syndromes. In short, there may be a broad spectrum of manifestations of coronary arterial spasm, including angina of effort (with S–T segment depression), variant angina pectoris (with S–T segment elevation), acute myocardial infarction, and sudden cardiac death.

Diagnosis, Clinical Characteristics, and Prognosis

1. Hillis LD, Braunwald E. Coronary artery spasm. N Engl J Med 1978; 299:695–702.
   A broad overview of the role of coronary artery spasm in the various ischemic heart disease syndromes.
2. Prinzmetal M, Kennamer R, Merliss R, Wada T, Bor N. Angina pectoris. I. A variant form of angina pectoris. Am J Med 1959; 27:375–88.
   The original description of variant angina.
3. Cheng TO, Bashour T, Kelser GA, Weiss L, Bacos J. Variant angina of Prinzmetal with normal coronary arteriograms: a variant of the variant. Circulation 1973; 47:476–85.
   This report describes 4 patients with angiographically normal coronary arteries and superimposed spasm.
4. Severi S, Davies G, Maseri A, Marzullo P, L'Abbate A. Long-term prognosis of "variant" angina with medical treatment. Am J Cardiol 1980; 46:226–32.
   The prognosis of patients with variant angina receiving appropriate medical therapy (calcium antagonists and nitrates) is reasonably good following the acute phase of the disease, even in the presence of severe coronary atherosclerosis.

Provocation of Coronary Arterial Spasm

5. Ginsburg R, Bristow MR, Kantrowitz N, Baim DS, Harrison DC. Histamine provocation of clinical coronary artery spasm: implications concerning pathogenesis of variant angina pectoris. Am Heart J 1981; 102:819–22.

   In a limited number of patients with variant angina, histamine successfully induced coronary arterial spasm.

6. Schroeder JS, Bolen JL, Quint RA, Clark DA, Hayden WG, Higgins CB, Wexler L. Provocation of coronary spasm with ergonovine maleate: new test with results in 57 patients undergoing coronary arteriography. Am J Cardiol 1977; 40:487–91.

   One of the earliest reports of ergonovine administration to induce spasm in the catheterization laboratory.

7. Heupler FA, Proudfit WL, Razavi M, Shirey EK, Greenstreet R, Sheldon WC. Ergonovine maleate provocative test for coronary arterial spasm. Am J Cardiol 1978; 41:631–40.

   This paper concludes that ergonovine administration is a safe, sensitive, and specific method for inducing coronary arterial spasm.

8. Endo M, Hirosawa K, Kaneko N, Hase K, Inoue Y, Konno S. Prinzmetal's variant angina: coronary arteriogram and left ventriculogram during angina attack induced by methacholine. N Engl J Med 1976; 294:252–5.

   In this report, 3 patients with variant angina had spasm induced by methacholine (0.13 mg/kg subcutaneously).

9. Raizner AE, Chahine RA, Ishimori T, Verani MS, Zacca N, Jamal N, Miller RR, Luchi RJ. Provocation of coronary artery spasm by the cold pressor test. Circulation 1980; 62:925–32.

   Although the cold pressor maneuver provoked episodes of spasm in 7 patients, the data from this report suggest that ergonovine is a more potent provoker than exposure to cold.

10. Yasue H, Nagao M, Omote S, Takizawa A, Miwa K, Tanaka S. Coronary arterial spasm and Prinzmetal's variant form of angina induced by hyperventilation and trisbuffer infusion. Circulation 1978; 58:56–62.

    In 8 of 9 patients with variant angina, vigorous hyperventilation (for 5 minutes) immediately after a 5-minute infusion of 100 mL of tris-buffer (pH 10) induced coronary arterial spasm.

11. Waters DD, Szlachcic J, Bonan R, Miller DD, Dauwe F, Theroux P. Comparative sensitivity of exercise, cold pressor, and ergonovine testing in provoking attacks of variant angina in patients with active disease. Circulation 1983; 67:310–5.

    The sensitivity of the ergonovine test appears to be high in patients with active variant angina, whereas the sensitivity of the cold pressor test is low.

Therapy

12. Winniford MD, Johnson SM, Mauritson DR, Rellas JS, Redish GA, Willerson JT, Hillis LD. Verapamil therapy for Prinzmetal's variant angina: comparison with placebo and nifedipine. Am J Cardiol 1982; 50:913–8.

    In 27 patients with documented vasospastic angina, verapamil was very effective. Nifedipine was also efficacious but was associated with more frequent adverse effects than verapamil.

13. Schroeder JS, Feldman RL, Giles TD, Friedman MJ, DeMaria AN, Kinney EL, Mallon SM, Pitt B, Meyer R, Basta LL, Curry RC Jr, Groves BM, MacAlpin RN. Multiclinic controlled trial of diltiazem for Prinzmetal's angina. Am J Med 1982; 72:227–32.

    In 48 patients with variant angina, diltiazem was better than placebo in the alleviation of angina and in reducing the need for nitroglycerin.

14. Hill JA, Feldman RL, Pepine CJ, Conti CR. Randomized double-blind comparison of nifedipine and isosorbide dinitrate in patients with coronary arterial spasm. Am J Cardiol 1982; 49:431–8.

    Both nifedipine and isosorbide dinitrate are effective in most patients with coronary arterial spasm.

15. Ginsburg R, Lamb IH, Schroeder JS, Hu M, Harrison DC. Randomized double-blind comparison of nifedipine and isosorbide dinitrate therapy in variant angina pectoris

due to coronary artery spasm. Am Heart J 1982; 103:44–8.
Both nifedipine and isosorbide are efficacious in patients with variant angina, but isosorbide is accompanied by more frequent and more troubling side effects.

16. Rutitzky B, Girotti AL, Rosenbaum MB. Efficacy of chronic amiodarone therapy in patients with variant angina pectoris and inhibition of ergonovine coronary constriction. Am Heart J 1982; 103:38–43.
In 3 patients with variant angina, amiodarone (an antiarrhythmic and vasodilator) was an effective antianginal agent.

17. Weber S, Donzêau-Gouge GP, Chauvaud S, Picard G, Guerin F, Carpentier A, Degeorges M. Assessment of plexectomy in the treatment of severe coronary spasm in patients with normal coronary arteries. Am J Cardiol 1983; 51:1072–5.
In 3 patients with variant angina and angiographically normal coronary arteries, plexectomy was not beneficial.

Spasm as a Cause of Other Ischemic Heart Disease Syndromes

18. Biagini A, Mazzei MG, Carpeggiani C, Testa R, Antonelli R, Michelassi C, L'Abbate A, Maseri A. Vasospastic ischemic mechanism of frequent asymptomatic transient ST–T changes during continuous electrocardiographic monitoring in selected unstable angina patients. Am Heart J 1982; 103:13–20.
This report documents coronary arterial spasm during chest pain in 6 of 11 patients hospitalized with unstable angina pectoris.

19. Johnson AD, Detwiler JH. Coronary spasm, variant angina, and recurrent myocardial infarctions. Circulation 1977; 55:947–50.
A 24-year-old man with 3 infarctions, 1 before and 2 after the demonstration of angiographically normal coronary arteries and ergonovine-induced spasm, is described.

20. Maseri A, L'Abbate A, Pesola A, Ballestra AM, Marzilli M, Maltinti G, Severi S, DeNes DM, Parodi O, Biagini A. Coronary vasospasm in angina pectoris. Lancet 1977; 1:713–7.
This paper suggests that many episodes of typical angina may be due to coronary arterial spasm.

21. Maseri A, Severi S, DeNes M, L'Abbate A, Chierchia S, Marzilli M, Ballestra AM, Parodi O, Biagini A, Distante A. "Variant" angina: one aspect of a continuous spectrum of vasospastic myocardial ischemia. Am J Cardiol 1978; 42:1019–35.
Vasospastic angina can occur in the presence of extremely variable degrees of coronary atherosclerosis and in any phase of ischemic heart disease.

EXERTIONAL ANGINA PECTORIS

In the normal myocardium, there is a balance between myocardial oxygen supply and demand at rest and during physical exertion or emotional excitement. In response to an increase in myocardial oxygen demand, adequate tissue oxygenation is maintained by an appropriate augmentation of oxygen supply. If oxygen supply is reduced or oxygen demands are increased in the setting of limited supply, myocardial ischemia results. Thus, although the patient with underlying atherosclerotic coronary artery disease may have adequate myocardial oxygenation *at rest,* he is unable to increase his oxygen supply during periods of enhanced demand. *Stable angina pectoris* (also called *exertional* angina pectoris or *angina of effort*) occurs when an increase in myocardial oxygen demand cannot be matched by an appropriate increase in oxygen supply because of atherosclerotic coronary artery disease.

The patient with exertional angina pectoris usually complains of a retrosternal "pressure" or "dull ache" during periods of enhanced myocardial oxygen demand, such as physical exertion or emotional excitement. Other adjectives that the patient may use to describe his chest discomfort include "viselike," "constricting," "crushing," "heavy," and "squeezing." In many patients, the retrosternal pain radiates to the jaw, neck, and left shoulder and arm. It is often accompanied by dyspnea and may be associated with diaphoresis and nausea. Although its duration varies considerably from one patient to another, it usually lasts from 3 to 10 minutes. On occasion, however, it may linger for as long as a half hour. It is typically relieved by sublingual nitroglycerin within 1 to 5 minutes.

At a time when the patient is not having angina, the physical examination is usually totally normal. During an episode of chest discomfort, the patient may become somewhat pale and diaphoretic, and his respiratory rate and effort may increase. The heart rate and systemic arterial pressure are usually greater than at rest. There may be some evidence of pulmonary vascular congestion (rales at both bases posteriorly). On auscultation of the heart, a loud S_4 is usually audible, and a transient S_3 may be present. In an occasional patient, a murmur of mitral regurgitation (due to ischemia-induced papillary muscle dysfunction) is audible at the cardiac apex. As the episode of angina resolves, the pulmonary rales, S_3, and systolic murmur may disappear quickly.

Several noninvasive techniques have been used to demonstrate transient episodes of myocardial ischemia in the patient with exertional angina pectoris. First, the resting ECG in these patients is often normal. During exercise-induced or spontaneous chest pain, however, the ECG usually shows S–T segment depression (reflective of subendocardial myocardial ischemia) and T wave alterations, both of which resolve within minutes after the pain has disappeared. Second, gated equilibrium blood pool scintigraphy or two-dimensional echocardiography performed in the resting state may demonstrate well-preserved global left ventricular function without segmental wall motion abnormalities. During exercise-induced angina, however, global left ventricular function is diminished, and segmental wall motion abnormalities develop. As with the electrocardiographic alterations, these segmental wall motion abnormalities may resolve within minutes after relief of pain. Third, myocardial perfusion can be assessed during exercise-induced angina by the intravenous injection of a radioactive tracer, such as thallium 201. This agent is distributed to the myocardium in direct proportion to coronary blood flow. At peak exercise, therefore, an area of ischemic myocardium is devoid of thallium 201 uptake, whereas the normally perfused myocardium has an adequate amount of the tracer. As the ischemia resolves, the thallium is redistributed, so that 2 to 6 hours later a repeat image shows a normal distribution of thallium.

With selective coronary arteriography, the patient with exertional angina pectoris is found to have substantial narrowing of at least one major epicardial coronary artery. Left ventricular function (assessed by left ventriculography) is often normal, since this evaluation is usually done in the resting state. With rapid atrial pacing at the time of cardiac catheterization, however, evidence of myocardial ischemia develops, with associated electrocardiographic alterations, increases in left ventricular filling pressure (caused by an ischemia-induced reduction in left ventricular compliance), and segmental wall motion abnormalities by contrast ventriculography.

The medical treatment of exertional angina pectoris centers on three classes of drugs. First, the patient should be given both short-acting and long-acting nitrate preparations. Sublingual nitroglycerin is recommended for the acute relief of anginal episodes, whereas long-acting nitrates (given topically or orally) are used as prophylactic medications. Although there is still uncertainty about their mechanism of action in patients with exertional angina, the nitrate preparations probably act both by reducing myocardial oxygen demands (by diminishing left ventricular wall tension) and by augmenting myocardial oxygen supply (by redistributing coronary blood flow from the epicardium to the endocardium). Second, the beta-adrenergic blocking agents, such as propranolol, have gained widespread popularity as maintenance therapy for the patient with exertional angina. This group of drugs probably does nothing to increase myocardial oxygen supply; instead, they reduce oxygen demands by diminishing heart rate, left ventricular contractility, and left ventricular wall tension. (See Beta-Adrenergic Blockers, p. 283, for more details.) Third, the calcium antagonists, such as verapamil, nifedipine, and diltiazem, are becoming increasingly popular as antianginal medications. These agents enhance myocardial oxygen supply and reduce demands, so that they favorably alter the oxygen supply-demand balance by acting on both sides of this ratio. (See Calcium Antagonists, p. 288, for more details.)

If the patient with exertional angina pectoris continues to have limiting angina despite maximal medical therapy, he should be referred for percutaneous transluminal coronary angioplasty (see p. 108) or coronary artery bypass grafting (see p. 105), provided, of course, that his coronary anatomy is suitable.

With the development of selective coronary arteriography and left ventriculography, it is now possible to relate the natural history of exertional angina to both the severity of coronary artery disease and the extent of left ventricular wall motion abnormalities. With medical therapy, those patients with well-preserved left ventricular performance and narrowing of only one major coronary artery have an annual mortality of 1 to 2 percent; those with good left ventricular function and narrowing of two major coronary arteries have a yearly mortality of 4 to 6 percent; whereas those with good left ventricular performance and narrowing of three major coronary arteries have an annual death rate of 8 to 10 percent. Substantial narrowing of the left main coronary artery is associated with a 1-year mortality of 25 to 30 percent and a 5-year mortality of 60 percent. Coronary artery bypass surgery clearly improves the prognosis in patients with exertional angina and left main coronary artery stenosis and may do so in patients with three-vessel coronary artery disease, but it has not proved to do so in patients with one- or two-vessel coronary artery narrowing.

Clinical Features and Prognosis

1. Herman MV. The clinical picture of ischemic heart disease. Prog Cardiovasc Dis 1971; 14:321–9.
   An overall review of exertional angina, unstable angina, and sudden death among patients with coronary artery disease.
2. Fowler NO. Angina pectoris: clinical diagnosis. Circulation 1972; 46:1079–97.
   A thorough discussion of the symptomatology and signs of exertional angina pectoris.
3. Sampson JJ, Cheitlin MD. Pathophysiology and differential diagnosis of cardiac pain. Prog Cardiovasc Dis 1971; 13:507–31.
   A detailed discussion of angina and those diseases that sometimes imitate it.
4. Proudfit WL, Shirey EK, Sheldon WC, Sones FM Jr. Certain clinical characteristics correlated with extent of obstructive lesions demonstrated by selective cine-coronary arteriography. Circulation 1968; 38:947–54.
   The duration of angina bears no relation to the severity of underlying coronary artery disease.
5. Cohen LS, Elliott WC, Klein MD, Gorlin R. Coronary heart disease: clinical, cinearteriographic, and metabolic correlations. Am J Cardiol 1966; 17:153–68.
   In 60 patients with exertional angina, the severity of pain had no value in predicting the degree of underlying disease.
6. Robinson BF. Relation of heart rate and systolic blood pressure to the onset of pain in angina pectoris. Circulation 1967; 35:1073–83.
   In 15 patients with exertional angina, chest pain could be reliably produced when the heart rate–systolic arterial pressure double product reached a certain level.
7. Proudfit WL, Hodgman JR. Physical signs during angina pectoris. Prog Cardiovasc Dis 1968; 10:283–6.

A description of various physical findings during angina.

8. Martin CE, Shaver JA, Leonard JJ. Physical signs, apexcardiography, phonocardiography, and systolic time intervals in angina pectoris. Circulation 1972; 46:1098–1114.
   A review of angina-induced changes in heart sounds, gallop sounds, and murmurs, as well as a discussion of angina's influence on systolic time intervals.

9. Bruschke AVG, Proudfit WL, Sones FM Jr. Progress study of 590 consecutive non-surgical cases of coronary disease followed 5–9 years. I. Arteriographic correlations. Circulation 1973; 47:1147–53.
   A detailed analysis of life expectancy in patients with 1-, 2-, and 3-vessel coronary artery disease who are treated medically.

10. Kannel WB, Feinleib M. Natural history of angina pectoris in the Framingham study: prognosis and survival. Am J Cardiol 1972; 29:154–63.
    Of 303 patients with angina followed long-term, the mortality averaged about 5% per year in men and 2–3% per year in women.

11. Borow KM, Alpert JS, Cohn PF. The natural history and treatment of coronary artery disease: a perspective. J Cardiovasc Med 1978; 3:87–102.
    A thorough review of the prognosis of patients with 1-, 2-, and 3-vessel coronary artery disease who are treated medically.

Diagnosis

12. Martinez-Rios MA, DaCosta BCB, Cecena-Seldner FA, Gensini GG. Normal electrocardiogram in the presence of severe coronary artery disease. Am J Cardiol 1970; 25:320–4.
    The authors report that excellent collateral flow was present in 19 of 21 patients with normal ECGs and severe disease of at least one major coronary artery.

13. Goldschlager N, Selzer A, Cohn K. Treadmill stress tests as indicators of presence and severity of coronary artery disease. Ann Intern Med 1976; 85:277–86.
    In a large study of treadmill exercise tests, the authors show that S–T segment changes that are marked and appear early are highly sensitive and specific in identifying those individuals with coronary artery disease.

14. Ellestad MH, Cooke BM Jr, Greenberg PS. Stress testing: clinical application and predictive capacity. Prog Cardiovasc Dis 1979; 21:431–60.
    An excellent general review of exercise tolerance testing, including a discussion of exercise testing with radioisotope imaging. Includes 144 references.

15. Dehmer GJ, Lewis SE, Hillis LD, Corbett J, Parkey RW, Willerson JT. Exercise-induced alterations in left ventricular volumes and the pressure-volume relationship: a sensitive indicator of left ventricular dysfunction in patients with coronary artery disease. Circulation 1981; 63:1008–18.
    In this study, gated blood pool imaging during exercise allowed a reliable identification of patients with 2- or 3-vessel coronary artery disease.

16. Berger HJ, Reduto LA, Johnstone DE, Borkowski H, Sands JM, Cohen LS, Langou RA, Gottschalk A, Zaret BL. Global and regional left ventricular response to bicycle exercise in coronary artery disease. Assessment by quantitative radionuclide angiocardiography. Am J Med 1979; 66:13–21.
    In normal patients, left ventricular ejection fraction increased during exercise. In most of those with coronary artery disease, it fell or was unchanged. Overall, global or regional evidence of exercise-induced left ventricular dysfunction was found in 48 of 60 patients with coronary artery disease.

17. Ritchie JL, Trobaugh GB, Hamilton GW, Gould KL, Narahara KA, Murray JA, Williams DL. Myocardial imaging with thallium-201 at rest and during exercise. Comparison with coronary arteriography and resting and stress electrocardiography. Circulation 1977; 56:66–71.
    In this study, thallium-201 imaging enhanced the diagnostic sensitivity of stress electrocardiography.

Therapy

18. Robinson BF. Mode of action of nitroglycerin in angina pectoris. Correlation between hemodynamic effects during exercise and prevention of pain. Br Heart J 1968; 30:295–302.

In 9 patients with angina pectoris, nitroglycerin reduced arterial pressure but did not change the rate-pressure product at which angina occurred.

19. Borer JS, Bacharach SL, Green MV, Kent KM, Johnston GS, Epstein SE. Effect of nitroglycerin on exercise-induced abnormalities of left ventricular regional function and ejection fraction in coronary artery disease. Assessment by radionuclide cineangiography in symptomatic and asymptomatic patients. Circulation 1978; 57:314–20.
    Exercise-induced abnormalities of left ventricular global and regional function can be mitigated by prophylactic nitroglycerin.

20. Warren SG, Brewer DL, Orgain ES. Long-term propranolol therapy for angina pectoris. Am J Cardiol 1976; 37:420–6.
    This paper describes the use of propranolol in 63 patients with severe angina for a follow-up period of 5–8 years.

21. Amsterdam EA, Gorlin R, Wolfson S. Evaluation of long-term use of propranolol in angina pectoris. JAMA 1969; 210:103–6.
    Of 95 patients with angina and underlying coronary artery disease, propranolol was effective in 83 (86%).

22. Johnson SM, Mauritson DR, Corbett JR, Woodward W, Willerson JT, Hillis LD. Double-blind, randomized, placebo-controlled comparison of propranolol and verapamil in the treatment of patients with stable angina pectoris. Am J Med 1981; 71:443–51.
    In 18 patients with exertional angina, propranolol and verapamil were each effective.

23. Strauss WE, McIntyre KM, Parisi AF, Shapiro W. Safety and efficacy of diltiazem hydrochloride for the treatment of stable angina pectoris: report of a cooperative clinical trial. Am J Cardiol 1982; 49:560–6.
    In patients with exertional angina, diltiazem was better than placebo.

24. Mueller HS, Chahine RA. Interim report of multicenter double-blind, placebo-controlled studies of nifedipine in chronic stable angina. Am J Med 1981; 71:645–57.
    In 66 patients, nifedipine was 50% more effective than placebo in reducing anginal frequency.

25. Mundth ED, Austen WG. Surgical measures for coronary heart disease. N Engl J Med 1975; 293:13–9, 75–80, 124–30.
    A detailed review of the indications and risks of coronary artery bypass grafting as a treatment for exertional angina.

UNSTABLE ANGINA PECTORIS

Unstable angina pectoris is a clinical syndrome intermediate between chronic, stable (exertional) angina and acute myocardial infarction. The patient with so-called unstable angina develops myocardial ischemia because of several possible mechanisms. On the one hand, these individuals may have transient subendocardial or transmural ischemia because of a reduction in coronary blood flow, due to coronary arterial spasm or enhanced platelet aggregability. On the other hand, they may develop ischemia because of an increase in myocardial oxygen requirements (induced by emotional excitement or physical activity) that cannot be met by an appropriate increase in coronary blood flow because of severe obstructive coronary artery disease. At present, the relative importance of these pathophysiologic mechanisms is unknown, but several recent studies have strongly suggested that a primary reduction in oxygen supply (again, due to either coronary arterial spasm or platelet aggregation at the site of a preexisting stenosis) occurs in most patients with this clinical syndrome.

The patient with unstable angina pectoris complains of retrosternal chest pain that is identical in character and consistency to that of the patient with stable, exertional angina. In contrast to the patient whose angina is stable, however, these individuals usually report that their anginal frequency, severity, and duration have recently worsened, and many of them have begun to have angina at rest. Furthermore, the patient may note that nitroglycerin is somewhat ineffective and slow in relieving his chest pain. On physical examination, the patient may have no visible or audible abnormalities at a time when he is pain-free. During an episode of angina, however, he may become anxious, diaphoretic, dyspneic, and tachycardic, and his cardiac examination may reveal an S_3 and a murmur of papillary muscle dysfunction.

If an ECG is obtained during an episode of chest pain, it often demonstrates S–T segment deviation (either elevation or depression) and T wave alterations. Continuous electrocardiographic (Holter) monitoring, if properly calibrated and meticulously performed, can also be used to show ST–T wave abnormalities, some of which occur during chest pain and some of which occur painlessly (and therefore reflect silent myocardial ischemia).

At cardiac catheterization, patients with unstable angina are found to have a spectrum of atherosclerotic coronary artery disease similar to those with stable, exertional angina. On the one extreme, some of these individuals have no obstructive coronary artery disease and are shown (by provocative maneuvers) to have coronary arterial spasm. On the other extreme, a small percentage have severe obstructive narrowing of all three major coronary arteries and even the left main coronary artery. Thus, the presence of clinical instability does not allow one to predict with any degree of certainty the severity or extent of underlying coronary artery disease.

The medical therapy of unstable angina pectoris includes a number of antianginal agents. First, the patient with this clinical syndrome should be hospitalized and placed on complete bed rest. Second, the short- and long-acting nitrate preparations (administered sublingually, orally, topically, or even intravenously) are the cornerstone of medical therapy. Topical nitrates are a particularly useful adjunct in some patients, since they are often tolerated better than the sublingual or oral forms. Third, the beta-adrenergic blocking agents have been used extensively in the management of unstable angina. On occasion, however they may exert a detrimental effect, especially in the patient whose unstable angina is vasospastic in etiology. Fourth, the calcium antagonists, administered either alone or in combination with a beta-adrenergic blocker, are efficacious in treating patients with this clinical entity. Lastly, if the patient with unstable angina continues to have chest pain despite maximal medical therapy, intra-aortic balloon counterpulsation can be instituted in an attempt to stabilize the patient.

Coronary artery bypass surgery is generally not recommended as an emergency procedure in patients with unstable angina pectoris. Although some authors advocate emergency surgery before the patient is stabilized on medical therapy, most prefer to stabilize the patient with intensive medical therapy, including intra-aortic balloon counterpulsation if necessary, before proceeding to selective coronary arteriography and surgery. Once coronary anatomy is defined, the patient's long-term therapy can be tailored accordingly: the patient with left main coronary artery disease should undergo bypass surgery, whereas the patient with less severe obstructive coronary artery disease (one-, two-, or three-vessel) should undergo surgery if a trial of intensive medical therapy fails.

Clinical Characteristics, Etiology, and Diagnosis

1. Bertolasi CA, Tronge JE, Carreno CA, Jalon J, Vega MR. Unstable angina--prospective and randomized study of its evolution, with and without surgery. Am J Cardiol 1974; 33:201–8.
   This paper demonstrates that surgical therapy is better than medical therapy in reducing mortality in patients with unstable angina.
2. Papapietro SE, Niess GS, Paine TD, Mantle JA, Rackley CE, Russell RO Jr, Rogers

WJ. Transient electrocardiographic changes in patients with unstable angina: relation to coronary arterial anatomy. Am J Cardiol 1980; 46:28–33.
In a substantial number of patients with unstable angina, S–T segment elevation develops. In addition, in patients with 3-vessel coronary artery disease, more ST-segment changes develop than in those with single or double vessel disease.

3. Johnson SM, Mauritson DR, Winniford MD, Willerson JT, Firth BG, Cary JR, Hillis LD. Continuous electrocardiographic monitoring in patients with unstable angina pectoris: identification of high-risk subgroup with severe coronary disease, variant angina, and/or impaired early prognosis. Am Heart J 1982; 103:4–12.
Two-channel Holter monitoring was used in a large number of unstable angina patients. It was able to identify a substantial percentage of those with especially severe coronary artery disease whose prognosis was guarded.

4. Scanlon PJ, Nemickas R, Moran JF, Talano JV, Amirparviz F, Pifarre R. Accelerated angina pectoris: clinical, hemodynamic, arteriographic, and therapeutic experience in 85 patients. Circulation 1973; 47:19–26.
Of 79 patients with unstable angina who underwent catheterization, 15 had no coronary artery disease.

5. Fischl SJ, Herman MV, Gorlin R. The intermediate coronary syndrome: clinical, angiographic, and therapeutic aspects. N Engl J Med 1973; 288:1193–8.
In 23 patients with unstable angina, coronary angiography revealed lesions similar to those seen during the chronic stage of coronary disease.

6. Mulcahy R, Daly L, Graham I, Hickey N, O'Donoghue S, Owens A, Ruane P, Tobin G. Unstable angina: natural history and determinants of prognosis. Am J Cardiol 1981; 48:525–8.
In a series of 101 patients with unstable angina, medical therapy was totally adequate (short-and long-term) in almost all.

7. Neill WA, Wharton TP Jr, Fluri-Lundeen J, Cohen IS. Acute coronary insufficiency—coronary occlusion after intermittent ischemic attacks. N Engl J Med 1980; 302:1157–62.
This paper provides inferential evidence that unstable angina is often caused by intermittent transient coronary artery occlusions (caused by spasm or platelet plugging).

8. Hirsh PD, Hillis LD, Campbell WB, Firth BG, Willerson JT. Release of prostaglandins and thromboxane into the coronary circulation in patients with ischemic heart disease. N Engl J Med 1981; 304:685–91.
Patients with unstable angina have serologic evidence of platelet hyperaggregability.

9. Pugh B, Platt MR, Mills LJ, Crumbo D, Poliner LR, Curry GC, Blomqvist GC, Parkey RW, Buja LM, Willerson JT. Unstable angina pectoris: a randomized study of patients treated medically and surgically. Am J Cardiol 1978; 41:1291–8.
Of 50 patients with unstable angina, 12 (25%) had either left main stenosis or no angiographically identifiable coronary artery disease.

10. Donsky MS, Curry GC, Parkey RW, Meyer SL, Bonte FJ, Platt MR, Willerson JT. Unstable angina pectoris: clinical, angiographic, and myocardial scintigraphic observations. Br Heart J 1976; 38:257–63.
One-third of patients with unstable angina pectoris have abnormal technetium-99m stannous pyrophosphate myocardial scintigrams, suggestive of small areas of myocardial necrosis.

Therapy

11. Firth BG, Hillis LD, Willerson JT. Unstable angina pectoris: medical versus surgical treatment. Herz 1980; 5:16–24.
A concise summary of medical and surgical therapy for this clinical syndrome.

12. Charles ED Jr, Kronenfeld JJ, Wayne JB, Kouchoukos NT, Oberman A, Rogers WJ, Mantle JA, Rackley CE, Russell RO Jr. Unstable angina pectoris: a comparison of the costs of medical and surgical treatment. Am J Cardiol 1979; 44:112–7.
Surgical therapy was more expensive than medical therapy, but those initially treated medically who later required surgery incurred the largest expense.

13. Parodi O, Maseri A, Simonetti I. Managment of unstable angina at rest by verapamil: a double-blind crossover study in coronary care unit. Br Heart J 1979; 41:167–74.
Verapamil was more effective than placebo in this clinical syndrome.

14. Mehta J, Pepine CJ, Day M, Guerrero JR, Conti CR. Short-term efficacy of oral ver-
    apamil in rest angina: a double-blind placebo controlled trial in CCU patients. Am J
    Med 1981; 71:977–82.
    *Again, verapamil was superior to placebo in a group of patients hospitalized with
    unstable angina.*
15. Gerstenblith G, Ouyang P, Achuff SC, Bulkley BH, Becker LC, Mellits ED, Baugh-
    man KL, Weiss JL, Flaherty JT, Kallman CH, Llewellyn M, Weisfeldt ML. Nifedi-
    pine in unstable angina: double-blind, randomized trial. N Engl J Med 1982;
    306:885–9.
    *A nifedipine-propranolol-nitrate combination was better than a placebo-propranolol-
    nitrate combination in patients with unstable angina.*
16. Gold HK, Leinbach RC, Sanders CA, Buckley MJ, Mundth ED, Austen WG. In-
    traaortic balloon pumping for control of recurrent myocardial ischemia. Circulation
    1973; 47:1197–1203.
    *In 11 patients with continued chest pain despite maximal therapy, intraaortic balloon
    pumping prevented ischemia in 9 and markedly reduced its frequency in the other 2.*
17. Selden R, Neill WA, Ritzmann LW, Okies JE, Anderson RP. Medical versus surgical
    therapy for acute coronary insufficiency: a randomized study. N Engl J Med 1975;
    293:1329–33.
    *This paper recommends that patients with unstable angina be stabilized with inten-
    sive medical therapy, since urgent bypass surgery does not offer a clear advantage in
    the prevention of early myocardial infarction or death.*
18. Kaplan K, Davison R, Parker M, Przybylek J, Teagarden JR, Lesch M. Intravenous
    nitroglycerin for the treatment of angina at rest unresponsive to standard nitrate
    therapy. Am J Cardiol 1983; 51:694–8.
    *In 35 patients with refractory angina at rest, intravenous nitroglycerin was markedly
    effective in reducing anginal frequency and analgesic use.*
19. Curfman GD, Heinsimer JA, Lozner EC, Fung HL. Intravenous nitroglycerin in the
    treatment of spontaneous angina pectoris: a prospective, randomized trial. Circula-
    tion 1983; 67:276–82.
    *Both intravenous and oral/topical nitroglycerin are effective in patients with severe
    angina, but the intravenous form offers a more consistent control of ischemic episodes.*
20. Rahimtoola SH, Nunley D, Grunkemeier G, Tepley J, Lambert L, Starr A. Ten-year
    survival after coronary bypass surgery for unstable angina. N Engl J Med 1983;
    308:676–81.
    *In 1,282 patients who underwent coronary artery bypass for unstable angina, the 5-
    and 10-year survival rates were 92% and 83%, respectively.*

ETIOLOGY, PATHOPHYSIOLOGY AND MORPHOLOGY
OF MYOCARDIAL INFARCTION

A myocardial infarction occurs when heart muscle dies as a result of inadequate oxygen availability for a prolonged period. Clinically, the patient usually
has chest pain that is similar to angina but is more severe and prolonged, often
lasting in excess of 30 mintues and requiring opiates for relief. It is often associated with diaphoresis, nausea, and dyspnea. In some patients, the pain is located in the back, the jaw or teeth, the epigastrium, or the left arm. On occasion, the patient with myocardial infarction has symptoms other than chest
pain. For example, syncope resulting from an arrhythmia may be the initial
clinical manifestation of infarction; alternatively, dyspnea, orthopnea, and
cough may result from severe left ventricular dysfunction. Rarely, a myocardial
infarction may be manifested by a systemic arterial embolus, with resultant
end-organ vascular insufficiency.

The pathophysiology of acute myocardial infarction is not completely understood. In most patients, the primary pathologic lesion is severe atherosclerotic narrowing of a coronary artery. Superimposed on this narrowing, blood flow may be further compromised by thrombosis, hemorrhage into an atherosclerotic plaque, coronary arterial spasm, or a complicated interaction among these events. Coronary thrombosis is considered the most likely cause because of the strong association between recent thrombus formation at the site of coronary arterial narrowing and infarction, but plaque hemorrhage or spasm may be important in initiating or perpetuating thrombus formation. In a minority of patients, it is difficult to implicate thrombosis as a pathophysiologic mechanism, since some infarctions occur without evidence of recent or remote thrombosis. In these individuals, coronary arterial spasm may play a pathogenetic role.

The first morphologic alterations that occur with infarction are present at 12 hours; they consist of early inflammatory changes and cellular infiltration. By 24 hours, the infarction is evident grossly as a pale or yellowish sharply demarcated area. On histologic examination, marked leukocytic infiltration is present. Necrosis is maximal at 3 to 4 days, with neovascularization and collagen accumulation appearing at 5 to 6 days. Fibrosis and scar formation begin during the third week and continue for 3 to 6 months.

1. Silver MD, Baroldi G, Mariani F. The relationship between acute occlusive coronary thrombi and myocardial infarction studied in 100 consecutive patients. Circulation 1980; 61:219–27.
   In this analysis, the authors conclude that an occlusive coronary thrombus has no primary role in the pathogenesis of myocardial infarction.
2. DeWood MA, Spores J, Notske R, Mouser LT, Burroughs R, Golden MS, Lang HT. Prevalence of total coronary occlusion during the early hours of transmural myocardial infarction. N Engl J Med 1980; 303:897–902.
   Total coronary occlusion is frequent during the early hours of transmural infarction, but it decreases in frequency over the initial 24 hours. This suggests that thrombus formation or coronary arterial spasm may be important in the evolution of infarction.
3. Oliva PB, Breckinridge JC. Arteriographic evidence of coronary arterial spasm in acute myocardial infarction. Circulation 1977; 56:366–74.
   In this group of 15 patients with acute myocardial infarction, 6 had evidence of coronary arterial spasm.
4. Buja LM, Willerson JT. Clinicopathologic correlates of acute ischemic heart disease syndromes. Am J Cardiol 1981; 47:343–56.
   Over 90% of transmural infarctions are associated with coronary thrombosis, whereas a much smaller percentage of subendocardial infarctions are associated with thrombosis.
5. Davies MJ, Woolf N, Robertson WB. Pathology of acute myocardial infarction with particular reference to occlusive coronary thrombi. Br Heart J 1976; 38:659–64.
   Of 469 patients with transmural infarctions who were examined post mortem, an occlusive coronary thrombus was present in 446 (95%).
6. Horie T, Sekiguchi M, Hirosawa K. Coronary thrombosis in pathogenesis of acute myocardial infarction. Histopathological study of coronary arteries in 108 necropsied cases using serial section. Br Heart J 1978; 40:153–61.
   Of these 108 patients with myocardial infarction, 86 (80%) had an intracoronary thrombus, and 78 (91%) of these were associated with a ruptured atheromatous plaque.
7. Ridolfi RL, Hutchins GM. The relationship between coronary artery lesions and myocardial infarcts: ulceration of atherosclerotic plaques precipitating coronary thrombosis. Am Heart J 1977; 93:468–86.
   In patients dying of myocardial infarction, thrombus was present in almost all, and over 90% had plaque ulceration, erosion, or rupture.
8. Chapman I. The cause-effect relationship between recent coronary artery occlusion and acute myocardial infarction. Am Heart J 1974; 87:267–71.
   In this author's opinion, coronary arterial occlusion by a thrombus leads to a myocardial infarction, not vice versa.

9. Davies MJ, Fulton WFM, Robertson WB. The relation of coronary thrombosis to ischemic myocardial necrosis. J Pathol 1979; 127:99–110.

   In most patients, myocardial infarction is caused by coronary thrombosis.

10. Hellstrom HR. Evidence in favor of the vasospastic cause of coronary artery thrombosis. Am Heart J 1979; 97:449–52.

    By causing intense vasoconstriction and stasis, coronary arterial spasm may initiate coronary artery thrombosis.

11. Oliva PB. Pathophysiology of acute myocardial infarction, 1981. Ann Intern Med 1981; 94:236–50.

    A dynamic interation among damaged arterial intima, platelet aggregates, and coronary arterial spasm is postulated to occur as a prelude to thrombosis in patients with acute transmural myocardial infarction.

12. Buja LM, Hillis LD, Petty CS, Willerson JT. The role of coronary arterial spasm in ischemic heart disease. Arch Pathol Lab Med 1981; 105:221–6.

    A review of the various pathogenetic mechanisms of angina and infarction. Includes 100 references.

13. Fishbein MC, Maclean D, Maroko PR. The histopathologic evolution of myocardial infarction. Chest 1978; 73:843–9.

    In a study of 1,155 patients dying of myocardial infarction, the pathologic alterations during the days to weeks after infarction are described.

DETECTION AND QUANTITATION OF MYOCARDIAL INFARCTION

Several methods are available for the recognition of myocardial necrosis, and some even allow a quantitation of tissue damage. With the standard 12-lead *electrocardiogram,* transmural myocardial ischemia and infarction are usually easily recognized. Within 1 minute of the onset of *transmural* ischemia, S–T segment elevation and T wave peaking occur in the involved leads, and R wave amplitude increases transiently. At the same time, S–T segment depression occurs in the electrocardiographic leads opposite the involved area of myocardium. If the ischemia is not relieved within 15 to 20 minutes, transmural infarction is initiated, reflected by Q wave appearance and a diminution in R wave voltage in the involved leads. Over a period of hours to days, Q wave development and R wave loss progress; at the same time, S–T segment elevation begins to resolve, and peaked T waves recede and eventually become inverted.

S–T segment elevation is not a specific electrocardiographic sign of transmural ischemia. It can be caused by pericarditis, normal early repolarization, a left ventricular aneurysm, or hyperkalemia. In addition, it can occur transiently following electrical cardioversion or in the setting of an intraventricular conduction defect.

The electrocardiographic alterations that occur with *subendocardial* ischemia and infarction are less specific than those of transmural infarction. S–T segment depression, as well as T wave flattening or inversion, may occur with ischemia or infarction. Unfortunately, these abnormalities can be induced by ventricular hypertrophy, digitalis, and various abnormalities in serum electrolytes, most notably hypokalemia and hyperkalemia.

The electrocardiographic recognition of infarction is limited in several ways. Evidence of extensive old infarction or the presence of an intraventricular conduction delay may impede or prevent the electrocardiographic recognition of new infarction. For example, a complete left bundle branch block makes the recognition of transmural or subendocardial infarction difficult. In the patient with right bundle branch block, a transmural infarction may be diagnosed by the appearance of Q waves, but a subendocardial infarction is difficult or impossible to recognize. Whether the infarction is transmural or subendocardial, there is substantial variability in how rapidly its electrocardiographic evolution occurs. On the one extreme, electrocardiographic alterations may not appear for several hours after the onset of infarction. On the other extreme, the entire sequence of electrocadiographic changes may occur within 3 to 4 hours of chest pain, making it difficult to determine the exact time of infarction or even to assess whether such infarction is new or old. Finally, although electrocardiographic techniques allow the recognition of most infarctions, they do not allow a precise quantitation of tissue damage.

When myocardial cells become irreversibly injured, the cell membranes become leaky, and certain intracellular *enzymes* appear in the blood. Their appearance in the blood allows one to recognize cellular damage, and their quantitation over a number of hours allows one to assess the amount of such damage. Creatine kinase (CK) and its "myocardial-specific" isoenzyme CK-MB have been used extensively both to detect and to measure myocardial necrosis. Following the onset of cellular injury, the CK and CK-MB concentrations begin to rise within 3 to 4 hours, peaking at 12 to 16 hours and returning to normal within 24 hours. Since CK is present in abundance in skeletal muscle and the brain, an injury to these organs, even one of minor proportion, may elevate the total CK. Hence, an increasing emphasis is now placed on the CK-MB isoenzyme, since its elevation is specific for myocardial injury.

In addition to creatine kinase, other enzymes have been used to detect myocardial infarction, including (1) serum glutamic-oxaloacetic transaminase (SGOT) and (2) lactic dehydrogenase (LDH). Similar to CK, SGOT is present in high concentration in the myocardium and is released from irreversibly damaged cells. Its peak serum concentration occurs 24 to 48 hours following infarction. Since the liver and skeletal muscle contain SGOT, heart failure with hepatic congestion or reduced oxygen delivery to skeletal muscle or the liver sometimes causes an elevation of SGOT. The LDH serum concentration begins to rise 36 to 48 hours after infarction, peaks at 4 to 7 days, and then gradually falls. LDH is also contained in the liver, skeletal muscle, kidney, and red blood cells, so that an abnormal serum concentration of LDH may result from irreversible damage to any of these tissues.

Recently, radioimmunoassays have become available for the detection of myoglobin and the light chain of myosin. In the experimental animal and man, these intracellular constituents are released into the circulation early after infarction (within 2 to 6 hr), peak in 4 to 6 hours, and return to normal within 12 to 24 hours. Since myoglobin is present in skeletal muscle, injury to this tissue can increase its serum concentration.

The enzymatic recognition of infarction is limited in certain ways. First, it has temporal limitations, such that if the patient's hospitalization is inordinately delayed, the serum CK and CK-MB concentrations may already have returned to normal. Second, except for CK-MB, the myocardial-specific isoenzyme of CK, the serum enzyme concentrations may rise after irreversible damage to other tissues, such as skeletal muscle or the liver, for example. Third, cardiac surgery of almost any kind causes an elevation of CK-MB, so that perioperative infarction may be difficult or impossible to detect enzymatically.

Myocardial *scintigraphy* can be used to detect and localize myocardial infarction. "Hot-spot" imaging agents, such as technetium 99m stannous pyrophosphate (^{99m}Tc-PYP), appear to be sensitive and capable of detecting an infarct as small as 3 gm. These scintigrams first become abnormal 10 to 12 hours after infarction, remain abnormal for 24 to 96 hours, and then fade and become normal at 6 to 7 days. Some patients, however, have "persistently positive" ^{99m}Tc-

PYP scintigrams, making it difficult to recognize new infarction. Those individuals whose scintigrams are positive for more than 3 months have an increased incidence of limiting angina, and at postmortem examination they have a histologic picture compatible with severe chronic ischemic heart disease.

"Cold-spot" myocardial scintigraphy using thallium 201 (^{201}Tl) can be used to recognize and localize myocardial infarction. This imaging is termed cold-spot because reductions in myocardial perfusion due to ischemia or necrosis cause a decrease in thallium uptake. Myocardial scintigraphy using ^{201}Tl is most useful in the detection of infarction when it is performed within 24 hours of symptoms. Thereafter, perfusion defects resulting from infarction may become smaller (probably as a result of an increase in collateral flow); if imaging is done 2 to 3 days after infarction, a perfusion deficit may no longer be present.

Finally, dynamic myocardial imaging with technetium 99m pertechnetate–labeled red blood cells or technetium-labeled albumin permits the noninvasive assessment of global and segmental left ventricular function. Such imaging allows one to assess the functional impact of an infarction on global and segmental performance.

Scintigraphic methods are useful to detect infarction, either transmural or subendocardial, but they are limited in their ability to quantitate the amount of damage. Although recent studies have demonstrated that anterior transmural infarctions can be measured accurately with ^{99m}Tc-PYP imaging, the quantitation of inferior transmural and subendocardial infarctions awaits the development of tomographic imaging techniques that allow three-dimensional visualization. Similarly, ^{201}Tl "cold-spot" imaging does not allow a precise quantitation of tissue injury.

Electrocardiographic Techniques

1. Hillis LD, Askenazi J, Braunwald E, Radvany P, Muller JE, Fishbein MC, Maroko PR. Use of changes in the epicardial QRS complex to assess interventions which modify the extent of myocardial necrosis following coronary artery occlusion. Circulation 1976; 54:591–8.

   The amount of Q wave development and loss of R wave in the 24 hours after infarction accurately reflect the magnitude of myocardial necrosis.

2. Prinzmetal M, Kennamer R, Maxwell M. Studies on the mechanism of ventricular activity. VIII. The genesis of the coronary QS wave in through-and-through infarction. Am J Med 1954; 17:610–3.

   The appearance of a QS wave is indicative of transmural necrosis.

3. Shaw CM^{c}K Jr, Goldman A, Kennamer R, Kimura N, Lindgren I, Maxwell MH, Prinzmetal M. Studies on the mechanism of ventricular activity. VII. The origin of the coronary QR wave. Am J Med 1954; 16:490–503.

   The appearance of a QR wave is reflective of a mixture of living and dead muscle within the more superficial layers of the myocardium. Pure subendocardial infarction does not alter the QRS complex.

4. Madias JE. The earliest electrocardiographic sign of acute transmural myocardial infarction. J Electrocardiol 1977; 10:193–6.

   An increase in R wave amplitude occurs soon after the onset of infarction but usually lasts only a few minutes.

5. Ribeiro LGT, Louie EK, Hillis LD, Davis MA, Maroko PR. Early augmentation of R wave voltage after coronary artery occlusion: a useful index of myocardial injury. J Electrocardiol 1979; 12:89–95.

   Following the induction of transmural ischemia, R wave voltage increases transiently; the magnitude of its rise is related to the severity of ischemia.

6. Muller JE, Maroko PR, Braunwald E. Evaluation of precordial electrocardiographic mapping as a means of assessing changes in myocardial ischemic injury. Circulation 1975; 52:16–27.

In the minutes to hours after transmural anterior or lateral infarction, precordial S–T segment alterations can be used to assess the severity of ischemic injury.

Enzymatic Techniques

7. Mathey D, Bleifeld W, Buss H, Hanrath P. Creatine kinase release in acute myocardial infarction: correlation with clinical, electrocardiographic, and pathological findings. Br Heart J 1975; 37:1161–8.
   In 40 patients with infarction, a CK release of short duration indicated infarction without extension; a CK release of longer duration indicated gradual infarct extension; and repeated CK release resulted from a sudden extension of infarction.
8. Goldberg DM, Winfield DA. Diagnostic accuracy of serum enzyme assays for myocardial infarction in a general hospital population. Br Heart J 1972; 34:597–604.
   Of the various cardiac enzymes, CK is the most reliable for the routine diagnosis of myocardial infarction.
9. Sobel BE, Bresnahan GF, Shell WE, Yoder RD. Estimation of infarct size in man and its relation to prognosis. Circulation 1972; 46:640–8.
   In this assessment of 33 patients with infarction, CK-quantitation of infarct size provided a useful diagnositc and prognostic index.
10. Wagner GS, Roe CR, Limbird LE, Rosati RA, Wallace AG. The importance of identification of the myocardial-specific isoenzyme of creatine phosphokinase (MB form) in the diagnosis of acute myocardial infarction. Circulation 1973; 47:263–9.
    In this group of 376 patients admitted to a coronary care unit, CK-MB was both a sensitive and specific marker of acute myocardial infarction.
11. Roberts R, Gowda KS, Ludbrook PA, Sobel BE. Specificity of elevated serum MB creatine phosphokinase activity in the diagnosis of acute myocardial infarction. Am J Cardiol 1975; 36:433–7.
    Elevated serum CK-MB is a highly specific and sensitive marker of myocardial injury. The myocardium is the only tissue containing sufficient CK-MB to account for substantial increases in CK-MB activity.
12. Shell WE, Kjekshus JK, Sobel BE. Quantitative assessment of the extent of myocardial infarction in the conscious dog by means of analysis of serial changes in serum creatine phosphokinase activity. J Clin Invest 1971; 50:2614–25.
    The original description of the technique by which one can calculate actual infarct size by serial measurements of serum CK.
13. Vasudevan G, Mercer DW, Varat MA. Lactic dehydrogenase isoenzyme determination in the diagnosis of acute myocardial infarction. Circulation 1978; 57:1055–7.
    The cardiac isoenzymes of LDH offer good specificity and sensitivity in the diagnosis of acute myocardial infarction.
14. Stone MJ, Willerson JT, Gomez-Sanchez CE, Waterman MR. Radioimmunoassay of myoglobin in human serum: results in patients with acute myocardial infarction. J Clin Invest 1975; 56:1334–9.
    This radioimmunoassay of serum myoglobin is a useful and sensitive test for the early detection of acute myocardial infarction.
15. Drexel H, Dworzak E, Kirchmair W, Milz MM, Puschendorf B, Dienstl F. Myoglobinemia in the early phase of acute myocardial infarction. Am Heart J 1983; 105:642–51.
    In 9 patients with myocardial infarction, myoglobin was detectable in the serum earlier than creatine kinase or its MB isoenzyme.

Scintigraphic Techniques

16. Wackers FJT, Sokole EB, Samson G, van der Schoot JB, Lie KI, Liem KL, Wellens HJJ. Value and limitations of thallium-201 scintigraphy in the acute phase of myocardial infarction. N Engl J Med 1976; 295:1–5.
    In this study of 200 patients with myocardial infarction, thallium-201 scintigraphy gave optimal diagnostic information when performed within 24 hours of the onset of symptoms.
17. Parkey RW, Bonte FJ, Meyer SL, Atkins JM, Curry GL, Stokely EM, Willerson JT. A new method for radionuclide imaging of acute myocardial infarction in humans. Circulation 1974; 50:540–6.
    The original clinical experience with technetium-99m stannous pyrophosphate imaging is reported in this article.

18. Wackers FJT, Becker AE, Samson G, Sokole EB, van der Schoot JB, Vet AJTM, Lie KI, Durrer D, Wellens H. Location and size of acute transmural myocardial infarction estimated from thallium-201 scintiscans. A clinicopathological study. Circulation 1977; 56:72–8.
    In this study of 23 patients who died of myocardial infarction, thallium-201 scintigraphy was an excellent means of localizing infarction (better than the electrocardiogram) and of estimating its size.

19. Willerson JT, Parkey RW, Bonte FJ, Meyer SL, Stokely EM. Acute subendocardial myocardial infarction in patients. Its detection by technetium 99-m stannous pyrophosphate myocardial scintigrams. Circulation 1975; 51:436–41.
    In this early study, pyrophosphate scanning was useful in identifying the presence of subendocardial infarction.

20. Poliner LR, Buja LM, Parkey RW, Bonte FJ, Willerson JT. Clinicopathologic findings in 52 patients studied by technetium-99m stannous pyrophosphate myocardial scintigraphy. Circulation 1979; 59:257–67.
    Pyrophosphate scintigraphy offers an excellent specificity and sensitivity in the diagnosis of acute infarction.

21. Buja LM, Poliner LR, Parkey RW, Pulido JI, Hutcheson D, Platt MR, Mills LJ, Bonte FJ, Willerson JT. Clinicopathologic study of persistently positive technetium-99m stannous pyrophosphate myocardial scintigrams and myocytolytic degeneration after myocardial infarction. Circulation 1977; 56:1016–23.
    Patients with persistently positive pyrophosphate scintigrams have a high incidence of postinfarction angina.

22. Silverman KJ, Becker LC, Bulkley BH, Burow RD, Mellits ED, Kallman CH, Weisfeldt ML. Value of early thallium-201 scintigraphy for predicting mortality in patients with acute myocardial infarction. Circulation 1980; 61:996–1003.
    In this study of 42 patients with infarction, thallium-201 scintigraphy provided an accurate method for separating the patients into high- and low-risk subgroups.

23. Sanford CF, Corbett J, Nicod P, Curry GL, Lewis SE, Dehmer GJ, Anderson A, Moses B, Willerson JT. Value of radionuclide ventriculography in the immediate characterization of patients with acute myocardial infarction. Am J Cardiol 1982; 49:637–44.
    In this study of 100 patients with acute infarction, radionuclide ventriculography was performed an average of 8 hours after the onset of chest pain. Its results added to the discriminant power of clinical and radiographic characterization of left ventricular function.

TACHYARRHYTHMIAS COMPLICATING MYOCARDIAL INFARCTION

Over the past decade, there has been a decline in the number of deaths that occur in hospitalized patients with acute myocardial infarction. In large part, this reduction in mortality can be attributed to better recognition and therapy of various infarct-related arrhythmias. *Ventricular premature beats* occur commonly during the first 72 hours after the onset of infarction, appearing in over 90 percent of individuals. They are generally not life-threatening and, therefore, require no therapy unless they (1) are frequent (>10/min), (2) are multifocal, (3) occur in close proximity to the preceding T wave, or (4) occur in pairs, triplets, or short runs. If any of these characteristics is present, immediate suppressive therapy is indicated to prevent ventricular tachycardia or fibrillation. An initial intravenous bolus of 50 to 100 mg of lidocaine should be followed by a sustained intravenous infusion of 1 to 4 mg per minute. If lidocaine is unsuccessful, intravenous procainamide (25–50 mg/min to a total loading dose of about 1gm, followed by a sustained infusion of 1–3 mg/min) should be administered.

Ventricular tachycardia at a rate greater than 100 beats per minute (so-called *paroxysmal* ventricular tachycardia) can occur in patients with acute myocardial infarction. If systemic arterial pressure is maintained during this tachyarrhythmia, intravenous lidocaine (in the same dose as that used for ventricular premature beats) may be administered in an attempt to convert it to sinus rhythm. If more immediate therapy is indicated, DC countershock should be used. "Slow" ventricular tachycardia (accelerated idioventricular rhythm) occurs transiently in 30 to 40 percent of patients with acute infarction. It is generally well tolerated hemodynamically and requires no therapy. In an occasional patient, it causes hemodynamic deterioration and, therefore, requires treatment with atropine (0.5–1.0 mg intravenously) or lidocaine.

Finally, *ventricular fibrillation* can occur in the setting of acute myocardial infarction and should be treated with DC countershock. Subsequent to successful cardioversion, the patient should be placed on an antiarrhythmic agent to prevent its recurrence.

In some patients with acute myocardial infarction, serious ventricular tachyarrhythmias—tachycardia or even fibrillation—occur without prior warning, that is, without the appearance of frequent or multiformed ventricular premature beats. Since previous studies have demonstrated that intravenous lidocaine reduces the frequency of ventricular fibrillation in patients with frequent or multiformed premature beats, some authors have suggested that a lidocaine infusion should be administered to all patients for 24 to 48 hours after infarction. However, the benefits of such prophylactic lidocaine administration must be weighed against the risk of lidocaine toxicity. Thus, if lidocaine prophylaxis is to be used, it must be employed with great care in patients with advanced age (>70 years), congestive heart failure, shock, or liver disease, since these individuals have a greatly increased risk of developing lidocaine intoxication. At present, the authors do not administer lidocaine prophylactically to all patients with acute myocardial infarction.

A variety of supraventricular rhythm disturbances can occur in patients with acute myocardial infarction. In most individuals, they are a consequence of (1) electrolyte abnormalities, including hypokalemia, (2) hypoxemia, often resulting from severe left ventricular failure, (3) atrial infarction or ischemia, (4) associated mitral valve disease, (5) concomitant pericarditis, or (6) extensive left ventricular damage. First, *atrial premature beats* ordinarily are benign and of no concern unless they are sufficiently frequent to lead to a sustained supraventricular tachyarrhythmia, such as atrial flutter or fibrillation. If therapy is required, propranolol or quinidine may be administered orally. Second, *paroxysmal supraventricular tachycardia* occurs occasionally in patients with acute infarction. It is best treated with intravenous verapamil, 5 to 10 mg by bolus injection. Third, *atrial flutter* occurs in 2 to 4 percent of patients with acute myocardial infarction, often in association with atrial infarction or infarction-related pericarditis. Intravenous verapamil can be used to slow the ventricular response within 5 to 15 minutes. If reversion to sinus rhythm is desired, DC countershock is generally necessary. Fourth, *atrial fibrillation* is reported to occur in 5 to 8 percent of individuals with infarction. As with atrial flutter, the ventricular response can be slowed quickly with intravenous verapamil. If reversion to sinus rhythm is desired, DC countershock must be used. Finally, *sinus tachycardia* in the setting of an acute myocardial infarction is often a subtle manifestation of extensive left ventricular dysfunction, but easily correctable causes, such as fever, anxiety, or volume depletion, should be identified and corrected expeditiously.

During the several hours after the onset of infarction, measures should be employed aggressively to minimize myocardial oxygen requirements, so that the oxygen supply-demand balance in ischemic myocardium is not influenced unfavorably. Since tachycardia increases myocardial oxygen demand, all supraventricular tachyarrhythmias should be treated without delay. Thus, in the patient with any of the above-named tachyarrhythmias, the ventricular response should be slowed quickly (with intravenous verapamil), or sinus rhythm should be restored (with DC countershock). The more traditional pharmacologic means of slowing the ventricular response (i.e., with digitalis) or inducing a reversion to sinus rhythm (i.e., with quinidine or procainamide) have little place in the treatment of these rhythm disturbances in the hours following acute myocardial infarction.

Ventricular Tachyarrhythmias

1. Roberts R, Husain A, Ambos HD, Oliver GC, Cox JR Jr, Sobel BE. Relation between infarct size and ventricular arrhythmia. Br Heart J 1975; 37:1169–75.
   In 31 patients, the severity of ventricular arrhythmias early after infarction was related to the extent of myocardial injury (estimated enzymatically).
2. Rothfeld EL, Zucker IR, Parsonnet V, Alinsonorin CA. Idioventricular rhythm in acute myocardial infarction. Circulation 1968; 37:203–9.
   In this report, "slow" ventricular tachycardia was noted in 36 of 100 consecutive patients with acute myocardial infarction.
3. Lichstein E, Ribas-Meneclier C, Gupta PK, Chadda KD. Incidence and description of accelerated ventricular rhythm complicating acute myocardial infarction. Am J Med 1975; 58:192–8.
   "Slow" ventricular tachycardia is a common occurrence in patients with both anterior and inferior infarctions.
4. Harrison DC. Should lidocaine be administered routinely to all patients after acute myocardial infarction? Circulation 1978; 58:581–4.
   This paper recommends lidocaine prophylaxis for all patients hospitalized with possible infarction.
5. Lie KI, Wellens HJ, vanCapelle FJ, Durrer D. Lidocaine in the prevention of primary ventricular fibrillation. A double-blind, randomized study of 212 consecutive patients. N Engl J Med 1974; 291:1324–6.
   Lidocaine (at 3 mg/min for 48 hours) was highly effective in preventing ventricular fibrillation, but 15% of the patients who received it manifested toxicity.
6. Valentine PA, Frew JL, Mashford ML, Sloman JG. Lidocaine in the prevention of sudden death in the pre-hospital phase of acute infarction. A double-blind study. N Engl J Med 1974; 291:1327–31.
   In this study, intramuscular lidocaine reduced mortality in patients with acute myocardial infarction.
7. Jones DT, Kostuk WJ, Gunton RW. Prophylactic quinidine for the prevention of arrhythmias after acute myocardial infarction. Am J Cardiol 1974; 33:655–60.
   Oral quinidine sulfate did not reduce infarction-associated ventricular fibrillation.
8. Ambos HD, Roberts R, Oliver GC, Cox JR Jr, Sobel BE. Infarct size: a determinant of persistence of severe ventricular dysrhythmia. Am J Cardiol 1976; 37:116.
   In patients with acute infarction, the complexity of ventricular ectopy is closely linked to the amount of damaged myocardium.

Supraventricular Tachyarrhythmias

9. Jewitt DE, Balcon R, Raftery EB, Oram S. Incidence and management of supraventricular arrhythmias after acute myocardial infarction. Lancet 1967; 2:734–8.
   Of 222 patients with infarction, 73 had sinus tachycardia, and 38 (52%) of these died. This emphasizes the fact that sinus tachycardia often is a reflection of underlying left ventricular dysfunction.
10. Lemberg L, Castellanos A Jr, Arcebal AG, Iyengar RNV. The treatment of arrhythmias following acute myocardial infarction. Med Clin North Am 1971; 55:273–93.
    Of the supraventricular tachyarrhythmias that occur in the setting of infarction, sinus tachycardia is most frequent, followed by atrial fibrillation.
11. DeSanctis RW, Block P, Hutter AM Jr. Tachyarrhythmias in myocardial infarction. Circulation 1972; 45:681–702.
    A thorough review of the incidence and therapy of the various tachyarrhythmias that may occur in patients with myocardial infarction.

12. Julian DG, Valentine PA, Miller GG. Disturbances of rate, rhythm, and conduction in acute myocardial infarction. A prospective study of 100 consecutive unselected patients with the aid of electrocardiographic monitoring. Am J Med 1964; 37:915–27.

   In this group of 100 patients, 43 had sinus tachycardia, 67 had ventricular premature beats, and 16 had atrial fibrillation.

13. Meltzer LE, Kitchell JB. The incidence of arrhythmias associated with acute myocardial infarction. Prog Cardiovasc Dis 1966; 9:50–63.

   Atrial flutter occurs uncommonly in patients with acute myocardial infarction. When it does occur, it is almost always in the setting of congestive heart failure.

14. Hagemeijer F. Verapamil in the management of supraventricular tachyarrhythmias occurring after a recent myocardial infarction. Circulation 1978; 57:751–5.

   In 8 patients with flutter and acute infarction, intravenous verapamil caused a reversion to sinus rhythm in 7.

15. Resnekov L. Present status of electroversion in the management of cardiac dysrhythmias. Circulation 1973; 47:1356–63.

   Over 90% of patients with flutter are converted to sinus rhythm with less than 50 watt-sec of direct current countershock.

ATRIOVENTRICULAR BLOCK COMPLICATING MYOCARDIAL INFARCTION

Atrioventricular (AV) block of some degree (first, second, or third) is reported to occur in 15 to 25 percent of patients hospitalized with acute myocardial infarction. *First degree block,* reflected by a prolongation of the P–R interval to greater than 0.2 second, occurs in 4 to 14 percent of patients with acute infarction. It usually occurs in the setting of acute inferior infarction and is the result of ischemic dysfunction of the AV node. Although the patient with first degree AV block requires no therapy, he should be carefully observed for the appearance of second or third degree block. In the setting of acute infarction, first degree block is almost always transient; within 24 to 48 hours, it generally resolves or progresses to a higher degree of AV block.

Second degree AV block occurs in 4 to 10 percent of patients hospitalized with acute myocardial infarction. It is most commonly of the Mobitz I (Wenckebach) type in the patient with an acute *inferior* infarction. It is characterized electrocardiographically by a progressive prolongation of the P–R interval and shortening of the R–R interval until a P wave is nonconducted. After the nonconducted beat, the next P wave is conducted normally, and its P–R interval is the shortest in the sequence. In the setting of inferior myocardial infarction, Wenckebach block is generally not permanent, resolving completely within 4 to 5 days. In an occasional patient, however, it may persist for as long as 2 weeks. The patient with Mobitz I AV block requires no specific therapy unless the ventricular rate is sufficiently slow to produce syncope, congestive heart failure, angina, or ventricular ectopy, in which case the patient should receive intravenous atropine, 1 mg as a bolus. This may be repeated once or twice, if necessary. If the patient's Mobitz I AV block is not abolished with atropine, a temporary pacemaker should be inserted. Permanent pacing is rarely necessary, since Wenckebach block eventually resolves in most patients.

In contrast to Mobitz I block, Mobitz II second degree AV block usually occurs in patients with acute *anterior* myocardial infarction. It occurs much less frequently than Mobitz I AV block. It is characterized electrocardiographically by multiple nonconducted P waves. Anatomically, it takes place below the AV junction and is a manifestation of extensive myocardial necrosis. As a result, it is often permanent. In the patient who develops Mobitz II AV block in the setting of an anterior infarction, a temporary pacemaker should be inserted, and the patient's hospital course should be monitored carefully for evidence of left ventricular dysfunction. If the AV block does not resolve within 1 week, a permanent pacemaker should be inserted.

Third degree AV block is reported to occur in 2 to 5 percent of patients hospitalized with acute myocardial infarction. There is complete independence of atrial and ventricular activity, so that the resultant cardiac pacemaker is usually an ectopic ventricular source with a rate of 30 to 40 beats per minute. In the great majority of patients, third degree AV block develops in the setting of acute *inferior* infarction, in which case it is usually transient and eventually reverts to sinus rhythm. It should be emphasized, however, that its resolution may require up to 2 weeks. In contrast to its transient existence in patients with inferior infarction, third degree AV block that appears in association with an acute *anterior* infarction is usually permanent and, therefore, requires pacemaker implantation.

In general, AV block of any degree that occurs in the setting of an acute *inferior* myocardial infarction is transient and is due to temporary ischemic dysfunction of the AV node. It does not necessarily reflect extensive myocardial necrosis. As a result, it is not associated with an increased mortality, provided, of course, that the acute episode is treated appropriately. In contrast, AV block that occurs in the setting of an *anterior* infarction is usually due to necrosis of conducting tissue below the AV node. It is most often permanent. In most patients, extensive myocardial necrosis is present, and as a result, the patient is frequently troubled by persistent left ventricular dysfunction or ventricular ectopy. Even when pacemaker therapy is employed appropriately, these individuals have a guarded prognosis because of the magnitude of infarction.

1. Norris RM. Heart block in posterior and anterior myocardial infarction. Br Heart J 1969; 31:352–6.
   Heart block in association with inferior infarction usually runs an uncomplicated course, resolving spontaneously in 1–3 days. In contrast, heart block with anterior infarction is usually permanent and, therefore, requires pacemaker insertion.
2. Beregovich J, Fenig S, Lasser J, Allen D. Management of acute myocardial infarction complicated by advanced atrioventricular block. Role of artificial pacing. Am J Cardiol 1969; 23:54–65.
   Temporary transvenous pacing is recommended for any patient who develops second or third degree AV block in the setting of an MI.
3. Kostuk WJ, Beanlands DS. Complete heart block associated with acute myocardial infarction. Am J Cardiol 1970; 26:380–4.
   In a series of 308 patients with acute MI, complete heart block occurred in 28 (9%). Those with anterior infarction had a poor prognosis (mortality, 80%); those with inferior infarction had a mortality of 45%.
4. Hatle L, Rokseth R. Conservative treatment of AV block in acute myocardial infarction. Results of 105 consecutive patients. Br Heart J 1971; 33:595–600.
   Of 1,665 patients with acute MI, second or third degree AV block occurred in 105. Many of these were treated with no therapy (44) or isoproterenol (47) and generally did well.
5. Biddle TL, Ehrich DA, Yu PN, Hodges M. Relation of heart block and left ventricular dysfunction in acute myocardial infarction. Am J Cardiol 1977; 39:961–6.
   Patients with anterior infarction who develop complete heart block have a greater degree of left ventricular dysfunction than those who do not develop complete heart block.
6. Friedberg CK, Cohen H, Donoso E. Advanced heart block as a complication of acute myocardial infarction. Role of pacemaker therapy. Prog Cardiovasc Dis 1968; 10:466–81.
   Second degree heart block occurs in about 10% of acute infarctions, whereas third degree is seen (at least transiently) in 8%.

7. Courter SR, Moffat J, Fowler NO. Advanced atrioventricular block in acute myocardial infarction. Circulation 1963; 27:1034–42.

   Of 15 patients with complete heart block and acute inferior infarction, 6 died during hospitalization.

8. Meltzer LE, Kitchell JB. The incidence of arrhythmias associated with acute myocardial infarction. Prog Cardiovasc Dis 1966; 9:50–63.

   Third degree AV block occurs in 2.5–8% of patients with acute myocardial infarction.

9. Stock RJ, Macken DL. Observations on heart block during continuous electrocardiographic monitoring in myocardial infarction. Circulation 1968; 38:993–1005.

   Complete heart block occurred in 24 of 350 patients with acute myocardial infarction who had continuous ECG monitoring.

10. Sutton R, Davies M. The conduction system in acute myocardial infarction complicated by heart block. Circulation 1968; 38:987–92.

   AV block in conjunction with inferior infarction is usually not due to structural damage to the conducting system; in contrast, AV block with anterior infarction is associated with major damage to both bundle branches.

BUNDLE BRANCH BLOCK COMPLICATING MYOCARDIAL INFARCTION

Bundle branch block occurs at some time during hospitalization in 12 to 15 percent of patients with acute myocardial infarction. Of the episodes of bundle branch block in this setting, approximately one-third are old (i.e., the bundle branch block was known to be present for several weeks or months before infarction), about one-third are clearly new, and the remaining third are indeterminate in age. Of the various kinds of bundle and fascicular block, left bundle branch block occurs most commonly with an infarction, followed closely in frequency by a combination of right bundle branch block and left anterior hemiblock. The other kinds of block—isolated right bundle branch block, alternating bundle branch block, and a combination of right bundle branch block and left posterior hemiblock—are uncommon in patients with acute myocardial infarction.

When bundle branch block complicates acute myocardial infarction, the site of infarction is usually anteroseptal, and the infarction is often large. As a result, the mortality of an acute myocardial infarction complicated by bundle or fascicular block is two to three times higher than that reported for patients without concomitant block. The increased mortality is the result of extensive myocardial damage with resultant congestive heart failure rather than the conduction disturbance per se. For this reason, it is uncertain if prophylactic temporary pacemaker insertion alters the overall outlook of this patient population.

The patient who presents with a known old bundle or fascicular block in the setting of a myocardial infarction should receive routine care, and a temporary pacemaker is not indicated. In contrast, if a patient is found to have a new left bundle branch block or bifascicular block (right bundle branch block plus left anterior hemiblock or right bundle branch block plus left posterior hemiblock) in association with infarction, a temporary pacemaker should be inserted. This is not necessary in the patient with only a right bundle branch block. If a patient presents with an infarction and bundle or bifascicular block of undetermined age, he or she should be managed as if the conduction abnormality is new (i.e., with insertion of a temporary pacemaker).

The hospital survivors of myocardial infarction complicated by bundle branch block have an increased mortality during the first year following infarction when compared to those who survive a myocardial infarction without bundle branch block. Furthermore, those individuals with left bundle branch block or alternating bundle branch block have a higher mortality during the first year of follow-up than those with isolated right bundle branch block or bifascicular block, perhaps because the extent and severity of their coronary artery disease are greater.

1. Hindman MC, Wagner GS, JaRo M, Atkins JM, Scheinman MM, DeSanctis RW, Hutter AM Jr, Yeatman L, Rubenfire M, Pujura C, Rubin M, Morris JJ. The clinical significance of bundle branch block complicating acute myocardial infarction. I. Clinical characteristics, hospital mortality, and one-year follow-up. Circulation 1978; 58:679–88.
   Of 432 patients with infarction and bundle branch block studied, 28% (121) died, compared to 12% of a control group without bundle branch block.
2. Godman MJ, Lassers BW, Julian DG. Complete bundle branch block complicating acute myocardial infarction. N Engl J Med 1970; 282:237–40.
   Bundle branch block complicated 68 of 806 cases of acute myocardial infarction and was associated with a 56% mortality.
3. Norris RM, Croxson MS. Bundle branch block in acute myocardial infarction. Am Heart J 1970; 79:728–33.
   Of 565 patients with infarction, 7% had right bundle branch block, with a mortality of 61%; 4% had left bundle branch block, with a mortality of 48%.
4. Roos JC, Dunning AJ. Right bundle branch block and left axis deviation in acute myocardial infarction. Br Heart J 1970; 32:847–51.
   Of 11 patients with bifascicular block and acute infarction, 7 died, most of cardiogenic shock.
5. Gould L, Venkataraman K, Mohammad N, Gomprecht RF. Prognosis of right bundle branch block in acute myocardial infarction. JAMA 1972; 219:502–3.
   Of 25 patients with infarction-associated bifascicular block, 18 died.
6. Scheidt S, Killip T. Bundle branch block complicating acute myocardial infarction. JAMA 1972; 222:919–24.
   In this series of patients with right or left bundle branch block and acute infarction, pacemaker therapy was generally unsuccessful in reducing mortality.
7. Gould L, Ramana CV, Gomprecht RF. Left bundle branch block. Prognosis in acute myocardial infarction. JAMA 1973; 225:625–7.
   This article concludes that left bundle branch block in acute myocardial infarction does not affect prognosis and is not an indication for temporary or permanent pacing.
8. Waugh RA, Wagner GS, Haney TL, Rosati RA, Morris JJ Jr. Immediate and remote prognostic significance of fascicular block during acute myocardial infarction. Circulation 1973; 47:765–75.
   Of 538 consecutive patients with infarction, 116 had fascicular block. This article analyzes their subsequent course and, based on this, recommends therapy.
9. Nimetz AA, Shubrooks SJ, Hutter AM Jr, DeSanctis RW. The significance of bundle branch block during acute myocardial infarction. Am Heart J 1975; 90:439–44.
   Of 71 patients with acute myocardial infarction and bundle branch block, there was a high incidence of AV block (42%) and severe pump failure (35%).
10. Atkins JM, Leshin SJ, Blomqvist G, Mullins CB. Ventricular conduction blocks and sudden death in acute myocardial infarction. Potential indications for pacing. N Engl J Med 1973; 288:281–4.
    This article suggests that temporary prophylactic pacing should be instituted in patients with right bundle branch block plus left anterior hemiblock and acute myocardial infarction; furthermore, a permanent pacemaker should be inserted if complete heart block develops, even though it is transient.
11. Gann D, Balachandran PK, Sherif NE, Samet P. Prognostic significance of chronic versus acute bundle branch block in acute myocardial infarction. Chest 1975; 67:298–303.
    Mortality was similar from myocardial infarction in patients with old and new bundle branch block.
12. Hindman MC, Wagner GS, JaRo M, Atkins JM, Scheinman MM, DeSanctis RW, Hutter AM Jr, Yeatman L, Rubenfire M, Pujura C, Rubin M, Morris JJ. The clini-

cal significance of bundle branch block complicating acute myocardial infarction.
2. Indications for temporary and permanent pacemaker insertion. Circulation
1978; 58:689–99.
*This article reviews the indications for temporary and permanent pacing in a large
group of 432 patients with bundle branch block and acute myocardial infarction.*
13. Hollander G, Nadiminti V, Lichstein E, Greengart A, Sanders M. Bundle branch
block in acute myocardial infarction. Am Heart J 1983; 105:738–43.
*Of 606 patients hospitalized with acute myocardial infarction, 47 (8%) had complete
bundle branch block.*

LEFT VENTRICULAR DYSFUNCTION RESULTING FROM MYOCARDIAL INFARCTION

About 50 percent of the deaths caused by acute myocardial infarction occur before hospitalization and are due to ventricular fibrillation, asystole, or sudden severe heart failure. In the patient who lives long enough to reach the hospital, death is most often the result of cardiac "power failure." Such cardiac failure develops when at least 40 percent of the functioning left ventricular muscle mass is irreversibly damaged, either as a consequence of new infarction or a combination of old and new infarctions. The extent of left ventricular dysfunction during the days following acute infarction provides an accurate prediction of the patient's short- and long-term prognosis.

The patient with an acute myocardial infarction and no evidence on physical examination or chest x-ray of left ventricular failure has an excellent prognosis, with only a 3- to 5-percent mortality (so-called Killip Class I). The individual with some evidence of pulmonary vascular congestion (basilar rales, S_3, and radiographic evidence of pulmonary venous congestion) is classified as Killip Class II and has a short-term mortality of 12 to 15 percent. In the patient with clear-cut pulmonary edema (by physical examination or chest x-ray), the expected mortality is 25 to 30 percent (Killip Class III). Finally, the patient with cardiogenic shock is said to be Killip Class IV and has a mortality in excess of 80 percent. In these individuals, infarction is associated with systemic arterial hypotension and diminished peripheral perfusion, as manifested by mental confusion, cold and clammy skin, peripheral cyanosis, and oliguria. Hemodynamically, the systemic arterial systolic pressure is below 90 mm Hg, the cardiac index less than $1.8L/min/m^2$, the systemic arteriolar resistance greatly increased ($>2,000$ dynes/sec/cm^{-5}), and the left ventricular filling pressure elevated (>20 mm Hg). The reduced systemic arterial pressure further diminishes coronary arterial perfusion pressure, increasing myocardial ischemia. The low cardiac output and systemic arterial pressure induce an intense sympathetic discharge that produces peripheral vasoconstriction, further decreasing tissue perfusion and causing a systemic lactic acidosis, which depresses myocardial function. In response to a reduced cardiac output, the heart rate increases, thus increasing myocardial oxygen demands and diminishing subendocardial blood flow. In short, the hemodynamic and metabolic consequences of cardiogenic shock cause worsening myocardial ischemic injury, which, in turn, leads to worsening left ventricular dysfunction. A "vicious cycle" of severe hemodynamic impairment and deteriorating myocardial oxygenation is established.

The therapy of the patient with an acute myocardial infarction and resultant left ventricular dysfunction depends on the extent of such dysfunction. The individual with symptoms and signs of Killip Class II congestive heart failure (mild orthopnea, basilar rales, and an S_3) should be placed on complete bed rest and given both a diet low in sodium and a diuretic (usually furosemide). Digitalis is often not necessary in such a patient. If symptoms and signs of Killip Class III congestive failure are present (orthopnea, paroxysmal nocturnal dyspnea, tachypnea, and possibly some dyspnea at rest; bibasilar rales and an S_3; and radiographic evidence of interstitial and alveolar pulmonary edema), the patient should receive a low-salt diet, digitalis, diuretics, and ventilatory support, such as that provided by intermittent positive pressure ventilation. If full-blown cardiogenic shock is present (evidence of pulmonary congestion as well as hypotension and poor organ perfusion), the patient should receive intravenous positive inotropic agents (usually dopamine or dobutamine). If a response is not immediately forthcoming, the intra-aortic balloon can be inserted for circulatory support, particularly in a young patient with a first infarction. Even when such aggressive measures are instituted, the mortality of patients with Killip Class IV congestive heart failure is 75 to 80 percent. Because of this continued high mortality, some of these patients are now treated with balloon counterpulsation and emergent coronary artery bypass grafting. The efficacy of this approach remains to be determined.

1. Dunkman WB, Leinbach RC, Buckley MJ, Mundth ED, Kantrowitz AR, Austen WG, Sanders CA. Clinical and hemodynamic results of intra-aortic balloon pumping and surgery for cardiogenic shock. Circulation 1972; 46:465–77.
   One of the initial descriptions of intra-aortic balloon counterpulsation in 40 patients with cardiogenic shock due to acute myocardial infarction.
2. Mundth ED, Yurchak PM, Buckley MJ, Leinbach RC, Kantrowitz A, Austen WG. Circulatory assistance and emergency direct coronary artery surgery for shock complicating acute myocardial infarction. N Engl J Med 1970; 283:1382–4.
   A case report of a 50-year-old man with cardiogenic shock who survived following balloon counterpulsation and emergency bypass grafting.
3. Crexells C, Chatterjee K, Forrester JS, Dikshit K, Swan HJC. Optimal level of filling pressure in the left side of the heart in acute myocardial infarction. N Engl J Med 1973; 289:1263–6.
   This paper established that the optimal pulmonary capillary wedge pressure for left ventricular performance and cardiac output is 14–18 mmHg.
4. Willerson JT, Curry GC, Watson JT, Leshin SJ, Ecker RR, Mullins CB, Platt MR, Sugg WL. Intraaortic balloon counterpulsation in patients in cardiogenic shock, medically refractory left ventricular failure, and/or recurrent ventricular tachycardia. Am J Med 1975; 58:183–91.
   Of 27 patients with these clinical manifestations of severe left ventricular dysfunction, intra-aortic balloon counterpulsation restored arterial pressure in 19. Of these, 9 were eventually weaned from balloon support, only 3 of whom left the hospital.
5. Page DL, Caulfield JB, Kastor JA, DeSanctis RW, Sanders CA. Myocardial changes associated with cardiogenic shock. N Engl J Med 1971; 285:133–7.
   Patients who manifest cardiogenic shock clinically have post-mortem evidence of extensive left ventricular damage (>40%).
6. Scheidt S, Wilner G, Mueller H, Summers D, Lesch M, Wolff G, Krakauer J, Rubenfire M, Fleming P, Noon G, Oldham N, Killip T, Kantrowitz A. Intraaortic balloon counterpulsation in cardiogenic shock. Report of a cooperative clinical trial. N Engl J Med 1973; 288:979–84.
   Of 87 patients with cardiogenic shock given balloon support, 35 survived long enough to have the balloon removed, and 15 lived long enough to be discharged from the hospital.
7. Bleifeld W, Hanrath P, Mathey D, Merx W. Acute myocardial infarction. V: left and right ventricular hemodynamics in cardiogenic shock. Br Heart J 1974; 36:822–34.
   A detailed assessment of intracardiac hemodynamics in 42 patients with cardiogenic shock due to myocardial infarction.
8. Bardet J, Masquet C, Kahn JC, Gourgon R, Bourdarias JP, Mathivat A, Bouvrain Y.

Clinical and hemodynamic results of intraaortic balloon counterpulsation and surgery for cardiogenic shock. Am Heart J 1977; 93:280–8.
Balloon counterpulsation was effective in reversing the hemodynamic alterations of cardiogenic shock but did little to improve the patients' long-term outlook.

9. Leinbach RC, Dinsmore RE, Mundth ED, Buckley MJ, Dunkman WB, Austen WG, Sanders CA. Selective coronary and left ventricular cineangiography during intraaortic balloon pumping for cardiogenic shock. Circulation 1972; 45:845–52.
Eleven patients underwent coronary and left ventricular angiography during balloon counterpulsation. The procedure was performed without problem.

10. Goldberg LI, Hsieh Y, Resnekov L. Newer catecholamines for treatment of heart failure and shock: an update on dopamine and a first look at dobutamine. Prog Cardiovasc Dis 1977; 19:327–40.
A thorough review of the pharmacodynamics of these 2 agents, including 97 references.

11. Holzer J, Karliner JS, O'Rourke RA, Pitt W, Ross J Jr. Effectiveness of dopamine in patients with cardiogenic shock. Am J Cardiol 1973; 32:79–84.
In 24 patients with cardiogenic shock, dopamine was an effective agent, particularly in patients with diminished urine output and hypotension after cardiopulmonary bypass.

12. DeWood MA, Notske RN, Hensley GR, Shields JP, O'Grady WP, Spores J, Goldman M, Ganji JH. Intraaortic balloon counterpulsation with and without reperfusion for myocardial infarction shock. Circulation 1980; 61:1105–12.
Counterpulsation and immediate surgery appear to be beneficial only if surgery is performed early, i.e., within 12–16 hours of onset of chest pain.

13. Killip T III, Kimball JT. Treatment of myocardial infarction in a coronary care unit. Am J Cardiol 1967; 20:457–64.
In the coronary care unit, mortality in patients with a recent infarction is directly linked to left ventricular function.

14. Richard C, Ricome JL, Rimailho A, Bottineau G, Auzepy P. Combined hemodynamic effects of dopamine and dobutamine in cardiogenic shock. Circulation 1983; 67:620–6.
In 8 patients with cardiogenic shock, a dopamine-dobutamine combination was hemodynamically beneficial.

15. Gunnar RM, Loeb HS. Shock in acute myocardial infarction: evolution of physiologic therapy. JACC 1983; 1:154–63.
A good review of the therapy of patients with severe left ventricular dysfunction in the setting of myocardial infarction.

ACUTE VENTRICULAR SEPTAL DEFECT AFTER MYOCARDIAL INFARCTION

Several complications of myocardial infarction may interfere with the mechanical function of the heart, including rupture of the ventricular septum (with resultant left-to-right shunting), rupture of a papillary muscle (causing acute mitral regurgitation), and the formation of a left ventricular aneurysm (resulting in a dyskinetic segment of ventricular myocardium). Any of these so-called mechanical complications can lead to severe left ventricular failure in the patient who has sustained a recent infarction. A ventricular septal defect (VSD) most often occurs in association with an anterior transmural myocardial infarction, although it can also occur in the patient with a transmural inferior infarction. It is usually located near the junction of the septum and the anterior or posterior left ventricular free wall. The patient is likely to have multivessel coronary artery disease, as a result of which there is limited collateral blood flow to the ventricular septum. As a result of the VSD, there is shunting of blood from the left to the right ventricle. The magnitude of the shunt is determined by the size of the defect, the pumping ability of the left ventricle, and the resistance to flow in the pulmonary vascular bed.

Clinically, the patient with an infarct-related VSD typically develops symptoms and radiographic evidence of left ventricular failure (dyspnea, orthopnea, as well as interstitial and alveolar edema) 1 to 7 days after acute transmural infarction. On physical examination, a holosystolic murmur is usually easily audible along the lower left sternal border, and it is often accompanied by a palpable thrill. If the left-to-right intracardiac shunt is large, the patient may also have a mid-diastolic rumble at the cardiac apex, the result of greatly increased antegrade blood flow across the mitral valve. Finally, an S_3 is usually audible. The ECG demonstrates an evolving transmural infarction (most commonly anteroseptal, less commonly inferior). The chest x-ray usually shows generalized cardiomegaly and evidence of pulmonary venous congestion. It may, in fact, demonstrate obvious pulmonary edema.

If a VSD is suspected on clinical grounds, right heart catheterization (with a Swan-Ganz catheter) should be performed to confirm its presence and to quantitate the intracardiac shunt. During passage of the catheter, serial blood samples are obtained from the right heart chambers and are analyzed for oxygen saturation. If a VSD is present, a distinct increase in oxygen saturation is demonstrable in the right ventricle. The pulmonary capillary wedge pressure may demonstrate prominent v waves due to marked antegrade left atrial filling. The presence of a left-to-right shunt also can be confirmed by dynamic myocardial scintigraphy using technetium ^{99m} pertechnetate–labeled albumin or red blood cells. With the patient in the left anterior oblique position, the isotope is injected through a Swan-Ganz catheter into the pulmonary artery, after which there is an early appearance of radioactivity in the right ventricle.

With medical management, a large infarct-related VSD (i.e., pulmonary-to-systemic flow ratio of 2:1 or greater) is associated with a high mortality (80–90%) during the first 2 weeks after infarction, but attempts to close the VSD surgically during this time period are also associated with a high mortality. Ideally, the patient should be stabilized hemodynamically with digitalis, diuretics, and various afterload reducing agents, such as sodium nitroprusside or hydralazine, thus reducing impedance to left ventricular ejection, increasing forward blood flow, and diminishing the magnitude of the left-to-right shunt. In addition, intra-aortic balloon counterpulsation has been used successfully to reduce systemic vascular resistance, left ventricular end-diastolic pressure, and as a result, the magnitude of the left-to-right shunt. If hemodynamic stability can be achieved with these techniques and corrective surgery delayed for 3 to 4 weeks, the operative risk is substantially reduced. If hemodynamic stabilization is impossible, immediate corrective surgery must be performed, even though its attendant risk is high.

1. Donahoo JS, Brawley RK, Taylor D, Gott VL. Factors influencing survival following post-infarction ventricular septal defects. Ann Thorac Surg 1975; 19:648–53.
   In the patient with an acute VSD in whom heart failure or shock develop, aggressive therapy—including intra-aortic balloon pumping and surgery—should be instituted.
2. Vlodaver Z, Edwards JE. Rupture of ventricular septum or papillary muscle complicating myocardial infarction. Circulation 1977; 55:815–22.
   Of 18 cases with ventricular septal rupture, 10 had anterior infarction, and 8 had inferior infarction; all were transmural.
3. Kaplan MA, Harris CN, Kay JH, Parker DP, Magidson O. Postinfarctional ventricular septal rupture. Clinical approach and surgical results. Chest 1976; 69:734–8.
   This paper argues for a very aggressive approach to the patient with a VSD in the setting of myocardial infarction.
4. Selzer A, Gerbode A, Kerth WJ. Clinical, hemodynamic, and surgical considerations

of rupture of the ventricular septum after myocardial infarction. Am Heart J 1969; 78:598–607.

Septal perforation occurring within days of myocardial infarction usually manifests itself as a dramatic event, often leading to cardiac failure, shock, or both.

5. Graham AF, Stinson EB, Dailey PO, Harrison DC. Ventricular septal defects after myocardial infarction. Early operative treatment. JAMA 1973; 225:708–11.
    Out of 12 patients with acute VSD and resultant shock, early surgical therapy was accomplished successfully in 6.

6. Buckley MJ, Mundth ED, Daggett WM, DeSanctis RW, Sanders CA, Austen WG. Surgical therapy for early complications of myocardial infarction. Surgery 1971; 70:814–20.
    The authors report a reasonably good survival for patients with VSD operated acutely.

7. Montoya A, McKeever L, Scanlon P, Sullivan HJ, Gunnar RM, Pifarre R. Early repair of ventricular septal rupture after infarction. Am J Cardiol 1980; 45:345–8.
    Of 27 patients with an infarction-related VSD, 7 were treated without surgery, and all died. In contrast, of the 20 operated on, 11 survived. Operative survival was lowest in those operated within 48 hours of infarction and highest in those operated at least 4 weeks postinfarction.

8. Meister SG, Helfant RH. Rapid bedside differentiation of ruptured interventricular septum from acute mitral insufficiency. N Engl J Med 1972; 287:1024–5.
    Use of a Swan-Ganz catheter can quickly differentiate these 2 entities.

9. Farcot JC, Boisante L, Rigaud M, Bardet J, Bourdarias JP. Two dimensional echocardiographic visualization of ventricular septal rupture after acute anterior myocardial infarction. Am J Cardiol 1980; 45:370–7.
    In 3 consecutive patients with an infarction-related VSD, wide angle 2-dimensional echocardiography readily visualized the defect, permitting estimation of its location and size.

10. Radford MJ, Johnson RA, Daggett WM, Fallon JT, Buckley MJ, Gold HK, Leinbach RC. Ventricular septal rupture: a review of clinical and physiologic features and an analysis of survival. Circulation 1981; 64:545–53.
    Of 41 patients with VSD in the setting of infarction, all 13 unoperated patients died. Of the 28 operated, 21 (76%) survived.

11. Gold HK, Leinbach RC, Sanders CA, Buckley MJ, Mundth ED, Austen WG. Intraaortic balloon pumping for ventricular septal defect or mitral regurgitation complicating acute myocardial infarction. Circulation 1973; 47:1191–6.
    In 5 patients with acute VSD and resultant cardiogenic shock, intra-aortic balloon counterpulsation caused clinical and hemodynamic improvement in all cases.

12. Tecklenberg PL, Fitzgerald J, Allaire BI, Alderman EL, Harrison DC. Afterload reduction in the management of postinfarction ventricular septal defect. Am J Cardiol 1976; 38:956–8.
    In 2 patients with acute VSD, nitroprusside improved cardiac output without reducing arterial pressure. In 1 of the 2, the magnitude of the intracardiac shunt was diminished.

13. Fox AC, Glassman E, Isom OW. Surgically remediable complications of myocardial infarction. Prog Cardiovasc Dis 1979; 21:461–84.
    A succinct review of infarction-related VSD, free wall rupture, and papillary muscle abnormalities. Includes 148 references.

14. Chandraratna PAN, Balachandran PK, Shah PM, Hodges M. Echocardiographic observations on ventricular septal rupture complicating acute myocardial infarction. Circulation 1975; 51:506–10.
    By M-mode echo, 3 patients with infarction-related VSDs showed right ventricular dilatation and mitral valve motion suggestive of increased blood flow.

15. Campion BC, Harrison CE Jr, Giuliani ER, Schattenberg TT, Ellis FH Jr. Ventricular septal defect after myocardial infarction. Ann Intern Med 1969; 70:251–61.
    In this relatively early report, the authors urge that surgical closure of the VSD should be delayed at least 2 months after infarction to allow proper healing in the region of the VSD.

16. Bishop HL, Gibson RS, Stamm RB, Beller GA, Martin RP. Role of two-dimensional echocardiography in the evaluation of patients with ventricular septal rupture postmyocardial infarction. Am Heart J 1981; 102:965–71.

Two-dimensional echocardiography allows detection and localization of a postmyocardial infarction VSD. In addition, one can assess left ventricular function, making it possible to determine the patient's prognosis.

17. Grose R, Spindola-Franco H. Right ventricular dysfunction in acute ventricular septal defect. Am Heart J 1981; 101:67–74.

    In 8 patients with acute VSD, right ventricular function was severely depressed, contributing to death in 5.

18. Drobac M, Gilbert B, Howard R, Baigrie R, Rakowski H. Ventricular septal defect after myocardial infarction: diagnosis by two-dimensional contrast echocardiography. Circulation 1983; 67:335–41.

    In 13 patients with VSD after myocardial infarction, the defect was directly visualized in 6 by two-dimensional echo, whereas an analysis of microbubble movement allowed a diagnosis in all 13.

MITRAL REGURGITATION AFTER MYOCARDIAL INFARCTION

An acute myocardial infarction can involve the left ventricular papillary muscles in a number of ways. First, the entire papillary muscle can rupture as a consequence of acute myocardial infarction, quickly leading to massive mitral regurgitation. Second, the head of a papillary muscle can rupture. This is usually not associated with fulminant hemodynamic or clinical deterioration, thus allowing time for evaluation and possible surgical correction. Finally, either infarction without rupture or ischemic dysfunction of a papillary muscle can produce acute mitral regurgitation, but this, too, is usually less severe than that caused by a rupture of a papillary muscle. The mitral regurgitation that results from papillary muscle dysfunction may be transient (due to myocardial ischemia) or permanent (related to structural damage of the papillary muscle or ventricular myocardium into which it is inserted).

The patient with rupture of an entire papillary muscle usually develops symptoms and radiographic evidence of severe left ventricular failure (dyspnea, orthopnea, and pulmonary edema) 1 to 7 days after myocardial infarction. In most individuals, the onset of symptoms is abrupt. On physical examination, the systemic arterial pressure is often low, the pulse rapid, and the extremities cold and clammy, all evidence of reduced peripheral perfusion. The lungs demonstrate inspiratory rales. On cardiac examination, an S_3 is usually present. A holosystolic murmur, loudest at the apex and radiating to the axilla, the left sternal border, and the base, is audible in almost all patients, although an occasional patient with a ruptured papillary muscle, overwhelming mitral regurgitation, and severe left ventricular failure has no audible murmur. Rarely, a systolic thrill is palpable at the cardiac apex, but this is more common with an acute VSD.

The patient with papillary muscle dysfunction often has symptoms of only mild left ventricular failure, and the chest x-ray demonstrates only interstitial pulmonary edema. On physical examination, the peripheral pulse and blood pressure are usually normal. On cardiac auscultation, the systolic murmur of mitral regurgitation begins after S_1; it may be either holosystolic or ejection in quality, in which case it peaks in mid- to late systole.

Papillary muscle dysfunction or rupture usually occurs in association with inferior ischemia or infarction, so that the posteromedial papillary muscle is involved. Less frequently, the anterolateral papillary muscle develops dysfunction or rupture because of anterior ischemia or infarction. Therefore, the ECG usually demonstrates the ST–T wave abnormalities of inferior ischemia or subendocardial infarction or the QRS changes of an evolving transmural inferior infarction. It is important to note that papillary muscle dysfunction or even rupture can occur with only subendocardial (as opposed to transmural) infarction.

To confirm the diagnosis of papillary muscle rupture, right heart catheterization (with a flow-directed, balloon-tipped catheter) is performed and demonstrates, first, the absence of an oxygen "step-up" in the right ventricle (thus excluding the presence of an acute VSD) and, second, large regurgitant waves in the phasic pulmonary capillary wedge tracing. Since some patients with acute VSDs have prominent v waves in the pulmonary capillary wedge tracing (due to augmented antegrade filling of the left atrium), oximetric blood sampling in the right atrium, right ventricle, and pulmonary artery is necessary to distinguish an acute VSD from acute mitral regurgitation.

The medical management of the patient with severe left ventricular failure or cardiogenic shock due to papillary muscle rupture is similar to that described for the patient with a VSD: digitalis, diuretics, and, if hemodynamically tolerated, afterload reducing agents. In addition, intra-aortic balloon counterpulsation is used to stabilize the patient hemodynamically. In most individuals, papillary muscle rupture requires emergent mitral valve replacement. The rupture of a small head of a papillary muscle usually causes less severe heart failure, thus allowing medical therapy to be more efficacious. Finally, since papillary muscle dysfunction most often causes only mild to moderate mitral regurgitation, medical management (with digitalis and diuretics) ordinarily is successful. However, an occasional patient with papillary muscle dysfunction and resultant mitral regurgitation may require mitral valve replacement.

Papillary Muscle Dysfunction
1. Cheng TO. Some new observations on the syndrome of papillary muscle dysfunction. Am J Med 1969; 47:924–45.
   A thorough review of the clinical characteristics of this disease.
2. Burch GE, DePasquale NP, Phillips JH. The syndrome of papillary muscle dysfunction. Am Heart J 1968; 75:399–415.
   This paper emphasizes that the murmur of papillary muscle dysfunction may vary considerably depending on the nature of the dysfunction and the time course of papillary muscle and left ventricular activation.
3. Phillips JH, Burch GE, DePasquale NP. The syndrome of papillary muscle dysfunction: its clinical recognition. Ann Intern Med 1963; 59:508–20.
   In patients with this entity, the characteristic auscultatory finding is a systolic murmur, loudest at the apex, with delayed onset after S_1, and a tendency to an "ejection" or "diamond-shaped" configuration.

Papillary Muscle Rupture
4. Gold HK, Leinbach RC, Sanders CA, Buckley MJ, Mundth ED, Austen WG. Intraaortic balloon pumping for ventricular septal defect or mitral regurgitation complicating acute myocardial infarction. Circulation 1973; 47:1191–6.
   Of 6 patients with papillary muscle rupture and cardiogenic shock, intra-aortic balloon counterpulsation induced substantial clinical and hemodynamic improvement.
5. Vlodaver Z, Edwards JE. Rupture of ventricular septum or papillary muscle complicating myocardial infarction. Circulation 1977; 55:815–22.
   Of 20 patients with rupture of a papillary muscle, 11 had subendocardial infarction. Of the 20 infarctions, 14 were inferior in location.
6. Austen WG, Sokol DM, DeSanctis RW, Sanders CA. Surgical treatment of papillary-muscle rupture complicating myocardial infarction. N Engl J Med 1968; 278:1137–41.
   Of 5 patients requiring mitral valve replacement because of a ruptured papillary muscle, 4 were long-term survivors.

7. Nishimura RA, Schaff HV, Shub C, Gersh BJ, Edwards WD, Tajik AJ. Papillary muscle rupture complicating acute myocardial infarction: analysis of 17 patients. Am J Cardiol 1983; 51:373–7.
The authors recommend early surgical repair for the patient with this complication of myocardial infarction.

LEFT VENTRICULAR ANEURYSM

Although the formation of a scar after myocardial infarction is an expected event, the development of a large area of dyskinesis (i.e., a segment of myocardium that moves paradoxically during systole) is relatively uncommon. When a dyskinetic segment develops, it can lead to congestive heart failure, systemic embolization (due to mural thrombus formation), or recurrent ventricular tachyarrhythmias. On physical examination, the patient with an anterior left ventricular aneurysm often has a double left ventricular apical impulse. If the anterior aneurysm is especially large, the patient may have a diffuse and sustained apical impulse extending upward and medially over several interspaces or an ectopic impulse well removed from the point of maximal impulse. Alternatively, a left ventricular aneurysm resulting from an inferior infarction may not produce an abnormal precordial pulsation.

A left ventricular aneurysm is suggested electrocadiographically by persistent S–T segment elevation weeks or months following myocardial infarction. However, many patients with aneurysms do not demonstrate such S–T segment elevation. Similarly, although some individuals with aneurysms have radiographic alterations, such as an unusual bulge in the cardiac silhouette or the presence of intracardiac calcification, the majority of patients with left ventricular aneurysms do not demonstrate these findings. Radionuclide ventriculography can be used to assess the presence and location of a left ventricular aneurysm, and contrast ventriculography (performed during cardiac catheterization) demonstrates a discrete area of dyskinesis with a wide "neck."

A *true* aneurysm of the left ventricle should be distinguished from a *false* aneurysm. Although left ventricular rupture following myocardial infarction usually precipitates a massive hemopericardium and resultant pericardial tamponade, adherent pericardial tissue may confine the hemopericardium to a small area in an occasional patient, leading to a distended, thin-walled sack called a false aneurysm or pseudoaneurysm. Radiographically, it is impossible to distinguish a true from a false aneurysm. Two-dimensional echocardiography or gated equilibrium blood pool imaging may allow one to visualize the aneurysmal outpouching and assess the size of the orifice connecting it to the true left ventricular cavity. A false aneurysm characteristically has a narrow connecting orifice, whereas a true aneurysm has a wide orifice. Left ventricular contrast angiography also can be used to visualize the aneurysm and its neck.

Surgical resection of a true left ventricular aneurysm should be performed in the patient with medically refractory left ventricular failure, recurrent systemic embolization despite adequate anticoagulation, or medically refractory ventricular arrhythmias in whom invasive electrophysiologic testing suggests that the aneurysm is the arrhythmogenic focus. If a false aneurysm is present, surgical resection should be performed even in the absence of symptoms or complications, since such aneurysms are likely to rupture. In contrast, a true left ventricular aneurysm does not rupture and therefore does not constitute an indication for surgical resection.

Clinical and Pathological Manifestations of True Left Ventricular Aneurysms

1. Dubnow MH, Burchell HB, Titus JL. Postinfarction ventricular aneurysm. A clinicomorphologic and electrocardiographic study of 80 cases. Am Heart J 1965; 70:753–60.
   Of 2,293 autopsied patients with previous myocardial infarction, left ventricular aneurysms occurred in 80 (3.5%).
2. Gorlin R, Klein MD, Sullivan JN. Prospective correlative study of ventricular aneurysm: mechanistic concept and clinical recognition. Am J Med 1967; 42:512–31.
   A thorough discussion of the clinical and angiographic features of 24 patients with left ventricular aneurysm.
3. Abrams DL, Edelist A, Luria MH, Miller AJ. Ventricular aneurysm: A reappraisal based on a study of 65 consecutive autopsied cases. Circulation 1963; 27:164–9.
   The survival rate of patients with ventricular aneurysm is not different from that of all patients with myocardial infarction.
4. Baur HR, Daniel JA, Nelson RR. Detection of left ventricular aneurysm on two dimensional echocardiography. Am J Cardiol 1982; 50:191–6.
   Two-dimensional echo is an accurate method that allows differentiation of left ventricular aneurysm from diffuse left ventricular dilatation. In addition, this technique provides information regarding the resectability of the aneurysm.
5. Visser CA, Kan G, David GK, Lie KI, Durrer D. Echocardiographic-cineangiographic correlation in detecting left ventricular aneurysm: a prospective study of 422 patients. Am J Cardiol 1982; 50:337–41.
   Two-dimensional echocardiography can detect or exclude a left ventricular aneurysm with a high degree of sensitivity and specificity.
6. Cohen M, Wiener I, Pichard A, Holt J, Smith H Jr, Gorlin R. Determinants of ventricular tachycardia in patients with coronary artery disease and ventricular aneurysm: clinical, hemodynamic and angiographic factors. Am J Cardiol 1983; 51:61–4.
   Septal involvement by left ventricular aneurysm appears to be a major determinant of ventricular tachycardia in patients with coronary artery disease and left ventricular aneurysms.

Left Ventricular Pseudoaneurysms

7. Martin RH, Almond CH, Saab S, Watson LE. True and false aneurysms of the left ventricle following myocardial infarction. Am J Med 1977; 62:418–24.
   Since false aneurysms are likely to rupture, they should be resected, regardless of their size.
8. Vlodaver Z, Coe JI, Edwards JE. True and false left ventricular aneurysms: propensity for the latter to rupture. Circulation 1975; 51:567–72.
   Although rupture of true left ventricular aneurysms occurs rarely, spontaneous rupture of false aneurysms is common.
9. Hurst CO, Fine G, Keyes JW. Pseudoaneurysm of the heart: report of a case and review of literature. Circulation 1963; 28:427–36.
   The patient reported herein survived almost 6 years after a left ventricular false aneurysm was clinically recognized.
10. Gueron M, Wanderman KL, Hirsch M, Borman J. Pseudoaneurysm of the left ventricle after myocardial infarction: a curable form of myocardial rupture. J Thorac Cardiovasc Surg 1975; 69:736–42.
    Left ventricular false aneurysm is amenable to surgical correction if it is recognized.
11. Botvinick EH, Shames D, Hutchinson JC, Roe BB, Fitzpatrick M. Noninvasive diagnosis of a false left ventricular aneurysm with radioisotope gated cardiac blood pool imaging: differentiation from true aneurysm. Am J Cardiol 1976; 37:1089–93.
    The initial report of a false aneurysm visualized and diagnosed by gated blood pool imaging.
12. Catherwood E, Mintz GS, Kotler MN, Parry WR, Segal BL. Two-dimensional echocardiographic recognition of left ventricular pseudoaneurysm. Circulation 1980; 62:294–303.

In 5 patients with false aneurysms and 22 with true aneurysms, two-dimensional echocardiography was a useful method for identifying the presence of the false aneurysms and distinguishing them from true aneurysms.

13. Chesler E, Korns ME, Semba T, Edwards JE. False aneurysms of the left ventricle following myocardial infarction. Am J Cardiol 1969; 23:76–82.
    A false aneurysm has a wall consisting of fibrous tissue and is sharply demarcated from the left ventricular cavity. The rarity of false aneurysm is related to the usual occurrence of fatal hemopericardium following rupture of the left ventricular wall.

14. Ersek RA, Chesler E, Korns ME, Edwards JE. Spontaneous rupture of a false left ventricular aneurysm following myocardial infarction. Am Heart J 1969; 77:677–80.
    An elderly man is described who died of a ruptured left ventricular false aneurysm.

15. Roelandt J, vandenBrand M, Vletter WB, Nauta J, Hugenholtz PG. Echocardiographic diagnosis of pseudoaneurysm of the left ventricle. Circulation 1975; 52:466–72.
    The original description of the M-mode echocardiographic diagnosis of a left ventricular false aneurysm.

16. Gould L, Yang DCS, Martinucci L. Radionuclide diagnosis of left ventricular pseudoaneurysm. Am Heart J 1982; 104:1377–8.
    The authors visualized a pseudoaneurysm in a 79-year-old man using gated blood pool scintigraphy.

Therapy of True Left Ventricular Aneurysms

17. Loop FD, Effler DB, Navia JA, Sheldon WC, Groves LK. Aneurysms of the left ventricle: survival and results of a ten-year surgical experience. Ann Surgery 1973; 178:399–405.
    Of 400 consecutive patients undergoing aneurysmectomy, symptoms of congestive heart failure were markedly improved. In addition, angina and ventricular tachyarrhythmias were helped in most patients.

18. Favaloro RG, Effler DB, Groves LK, Westcott RN, Suarez E, Lozado J. Ventricular aneurysm—clinical experience. Ann Thorac Surg 1968; 6:227–45.
    Of 130 patients undergoing aneurysmectomy, 17 died.

19. Cohen M, Packer M, Gorlin R. Indications for left ventricular aneurysmectomy. Circulation 1983; 67:717–22.
    A succinct review of the specific reasons for aneurysmectomy.

Prognosis of True Left Ventricular Aneurysm

20. Faxon DP, Ryan TJ, Davis KB, McCabe CH, Myers W, Lesperance J, Shaw R, Tong TGL. Prognostic significance of angiographically documented left ventricular aneurysm from the coronary artery surgery study (CASS). Am J Cardiol 1982; 50:157–64.
    In patients with left ventricular aneurysms, mortality is related to age, overall left ventricular function, and clinical severity of heart failure. The presence of an aneurysm does not independently alter survival.

RUPTURE OF THE HEART AFTER MYOCARDIAL INFARCTION

Rupture of the left ventricular free wall, with resultant pericardial tamponade, can occur as a complication of acute myocardial infarction. Like rupture of the interventricular septum or a papillary muscle, it ordinarily occurs 1 to 7 days following infarction. It is most likely to occur in the patient with a first infarction and in the individual with postinfarction hypertension. Rupture of the left ventricular free wall usually leads to the sudden loss of blood pressure despite continued electrical activity on the ECG (so-called electromechanical dissociation). In most instances, surgical therapy cannot be mobilized rapidly enough to save the patient. In an occasional patient, however, the leakage of blood into the pericardial space is sufficiently slow to allow time for pericardiocentesis and attempted surgical repair.

Ventricular rupture usually precipitates massive hemopericardium and sudden death from cardiac tamponade. In rare instances, however, adherent pericardial tissue confines the hemopericardium to a small adjacent area. Subsequent organization of the contained hematoma results in a distended, thin-walled sac called a *false aneurysm* or *pseudoaneurysm,* which is connected to the left ventricular cavity by a narrow neck. As a result of a false aneurysm, the patient may have symptoms of pulmonary congestion (dyspnea and orthopnea). Alternatively, the false aneurysm can cause ventricular tachyarrhythmias or systemic embolization. In addition, a pseudoaneurysm has a tendency toward delayed rupture, even if it is small.

By chest x-ray, it is usually impossible to distinguish a true from a false aneurysm. Two-dimensional echocardiography or gated equilibrium blood pool imaging may allow for the direct visualization of the aneurysmal outpouching as well as the characteristic narrow orifice connecting it to the true left ventricular cavity. Left ventriculography at the time of cardiac catheterization also can be used to visualize the aneurysmal cavity and its narrow connection with the left ventricle. It is important to determine if a false aneurysm is present, since spontaneous rupture is common, and once identified, it should be resected.

Catastrophic Left Ventricular Rupture

1. Griffith GC, Hedge B, Oblath RW. Factors in myocardial rupture: an analysis of 204 cases at Los Angeles County Hospital between 1924 and 1959. Am J Cardiol 1961; 8:792–8.
   In this series, rupture was more common in women and in Caucasians.
2. London RE, London SB. Rupture of the heart: a critical analysis of 47 consecutive autopsy cases. Circulation 1965; 31:202–8.
   In 1,001 consecutive autopsies of patients with recent myocardial infarction, the incidence of left ventricular rupture was 4.7%.
3. Lewis AJ, Burchell HB, Titus JL. Clinical and pathologic features of postinfarction cardiac rupture. Am J Cardiol 1969; 23:43–53.
   In this series, rupture occurred in 8.6% of fatal myocardial infarctions. Hypertension had been present in 70% of the patients.
4. Hagemeijer F, Verbaan CJ, Sonke PCF, DeRooij CH. Echocardiography and rupture of the heart. Br Heart J 1980; 43:45–6.
   In 4 patients with left ventricular free wall rupture, the diagnosis was made at the bedside with a portable cross-sectional echocardiograph.

Left Ventricular Pseudoaneurysm

5. Martin RH, Almond CH, Saab S, Watson LE. True and false aneurysms of the left ventricle following myocardial infarction. Am J Med 1977; 62:418–24.
   Since false aneurysms are likely to rupture, they should be resected, regardless of their size.
6. Vlodaver Z, Coe JI, Edwards JE. True and false left ventricular aneurysms: propensity for the latter to rupture. Circulation 1975; 51:567–72.
   Although rupture of true left ventricular aneurysms occurs rarely, spontaneous rupture of false aneurysms is common.
7. Hurst CO, Fine G, Keyes JW. Pseudoaneurysm of the heart: report of a case and review of literature. Circulation 1963; 28:427–36.
   A patient with a left ventricular false aneurysm survived almost 6 years after the condition was clinically recognized.
8. Gueron M, Wanderman KL, Hirsch M, Borman J. Pseudoaneurysm of the left ventricle after myocardial infarction: a curable form of myocardial rupture. J Thorac Cardiovasc Surg 1975; 69:736–42.
   Left ventricular false aneurysm is amenable to surgical correction if it is recognized.
9. Botvinick EH, Shames D, Hutchinson JC, Roe BB, Fitzpatrick M. Noninvasive diagnosis of a false left ventricular aneurysm with radioisotope gated cardiac blood

pool imaging. Am J Cardiol 1976; 37:1089–93.

The initial report of a false aneurysm visualized and diagnosed by gated blood pool imaging.

10. Catherwood E, Mintz GS, Kotler MN, Parry WR, Segal BL. Two-dimensional echocardiographic recognition of left ventricular pseudoaneurysm. Circulation 1980; 62:294–303.

In 5 patients with false aneurysms and 22 with true aneurysms, two-dimensional echocardiography was a useful method for identifying the presence of false aneurysms and distinguishing them from true aneurysms.

11. Chesler E, Korns ME, Semba T, Edwards JE. False aneurysms of the left ventricle following myocardial infarction. Am J Cardiol 1969; 23:76–82.

A false aneurysm has a wall consisting of fibrous tissue and is sharply demarcated from the left ventricular cavity. The rarity of false aneurysm is related to the usual occurrence of fatal hemopericardium following rupture of the left ventricular wall.

12. Ersek RA, Chesler E, Korns ME, Edwards JE. Spontaneous rupture of a false left ventricular aneurysm following myocardial infarction. Am Heart J 1969; 77:677–80.

An elderly man who died of a ruptured left ventricular false aneurysm is described.

13. Roelandt J, vandenBrand M, Vletter WB, Nauta J, Hugenholtz PG. Echocardiographic diagnosis of pseudoaneurysm of the left ventricle. Circulation 1975; 52:466–72.

The original description of the M-mode echocardiographic diagnosis of a left ventricular false aneurysm.

14. Gould L, Yang DCS, Martinucci L. Radionuclide diagnosis of left ventricular pseudoaneurysm. Am Heart J 1982; 104:1377–8.

In a 79-year-old man, these authors visualized a pseudoaneurysm by gated blood pool scintigraphy.

RECURRENT CHEST PAIN AFTER MYOCARDIAL INFARCTION

The development of chest pain in the 2 weeks following myocardial infarction can be caused by (1) extension of myocardial infarction, (2) angina pectoris, (3) postinfarction pericarditis, (4) acute pulmonary embolism, or (5) pneumonia. Myocardial infarct extension occurs in 20 to 25 percent of patients hospitalized with acute infarction. Clinically, it is characterized by a recurrence of chest pain in association with further electrocardiographic alterations and a reelevation of myocardial enzymes during the 1 to 2 weeks after the initial event. It occurs with similar frequency in patients with transmural and subendocardial infarctions, as well as those whose infarctions are located anteriorly and inferiorly. Myocardial infarct extension should be treated with strict bed rest, supplemental oxygen, and morphine sulfate for pain relief. In addition, long-acting nitrate preparations and beta-adrenergic blockers should be given if they are not contraindicated.

Recurrent angina pectoris may occur during the 2 weeks after myocardial infarction; it is particularly likely to appear as the patient begins to increase his physical activity. It is caused by ischemia in the peri-infarction area or in an area remote from the recent infarction. In either event, it should be treated with long-acting nitrates, beta-adrenergic blockade, and calcium blockade, depending on the specific needs of the patient. If, despite medical therapy, angina persists, the patient should undergo coronary arteriography and subsequent saphenous vein grafting, provided that coronary anatomy is suitable.

The patient in whom recurrent chest pain represents pericarditis usually has a large transmural infarction. Often he complains of chest pain that is exacerbated by the supine position and partially or completely relieved by sitting. In many patients, a pericardial friction rub may not be audible, but the presence of pericarditis is suspected because of pleuritic pain with classic positional characteristics. The therapy of infarction-related pericarditis should include salicylates or another nonsteroidal anti-inflammatory agent, such as indomethacin. Anticoagulants should be avoided because of the risk of a hemorrhagic pericardial effusion or pericardial tamponade.

An acute pulmonary embolism should be suspected in the acutely ill patient, especially one with cardiomegaly and congestive heart failure. This diagnosis should be suspected if the patient develops pleuritic chest pain with dyspnea, anxiety, and tachycardia, and a fall in arterial oxygen tension below 80 mm Hg supports the clinical diagnosis. A lung scan following the intravenous injection of radioactively labeled albumin demonstrates a segmental perfusion defect.

Myocardial Infarct Extension

1. Rothkopf M, Boerner J, Stone MJ, Smitherman TC, Buja LM, Parkey RW, Willerson JT. Detection of myocardial infarct extension by CK-B radioimmunoassay. Circulation 1979; 59:268–74.

   Using the radioimmunoassay for CK-B, these authors detected infarct extension in 23% of patients. It was found in 32% of those with anterior transmural infarction, 14% with inferior transmural infarction, and 20% with subendocardial infarction.

2. Reid PR, Taylor DR, Kelley DT, Weisfeldt ML, Humphries JO, Ross RS, Pitt B. Myocardial infarct extension detected by precordial ST-segment mapping. N Engl J Med 1974; 290:123–8.

   Of 19 patients with acute myocardial infarction, infarct extension was demonstrated in 16 (86%) by precordial S–T segment mapping.

3. Mathey D, Bleifeld W, Buss H, Hanrath P. Creatine kinase release in acute myocardial infarction: correlation with clinical, electrocardiographic, and pathologic findings. Br Heart J 1975; 37:1161–8.

   In this series, infarct extension occurred in 62% of patients.

Recurrent Angina After Myocardial Infarction

4. Gold HK, Leinbach RC, Sanders CA, Buckley MJ, Mundth ED, Austen WG. Intraaortic balloon pumping for control of recurrent myocardial ischemia. Circulation 1973; 47:1197–1203.

   In 11 patients with recurrent pain after infarction, balloon counterpulsation abolished it in 9 and markedly reduced its frequency in the other 2.

Infarct-related Pericarditis

5. Liem KL, Lie KI, Durrer D, Wellens HJJ. Pericarditis in acute myocardial infarction. Lancet 1975; 2:1004–6.

   Of 300 patients with infarction, pericarditis occurred in 44 (14.7%).

6. Lichstein E, Liu HM, Gupta P. Pericarditis complicating acute myocardial infarction: incidence of complications and significance of electrocardiogram on admission. Am Heart J 1974; 87:246–52.

   In patients with infarct-related pericarditis, the incidence of ventricular arrhythmias, congestive heart failure, and death are slightly greater than in those without pericarditis.

7. Thadani U, Chopra MP, Aber CP, Portal RW. Pericarditis after acute myocardial infarction. Br Med J 1971; 2:135–7.

   Of 779 patients with myocardial infarction, 52 (6.8%) developed a pericardial friction rub. Mortality was not influenced by the presence of pericarditis.

POSTMYOCARDIAL INFARCTION (DRESSLER'S) SYNDROME

The postmyocardial infarction syndrome occurs in a small percentage (2–3%) of patients after myocardial infarction. It usually becomes manifest 2 to 4 weeks following infarction, at a time when most patients are convalescing at home. Clinically, it is heralded by the appearance of fever (as high as 40°C) and both pericardial and pleural pain, which varies from a mild generalized discomfort to a severe and crushing pain. The discomfort may be well localized (usually in the retrosternal area) or diffuse. On physical examination, the patient is febrile. A pericardial friction rub is usually audible, but it may wax and wane from minute to minute, so that its absence on one examination does not exclude pericardial involvement. In addition, breath sounds are often diminished at one or both lung bases, and there may even be an audible pleural rub.

The chest x-ray typically shows an enlarged cardiac silhouette (due to a pericardial effusion) and pleural effusions. A minority of patients also have an interstitial pulmonary infiltrate due to pneumonitis. The ECG is indicative of pericarditis with a pericardial effusion: diffuse S–T segment elevation, diminished R wave voltage, and, in an occasional patient, electrical alternans. Echocardiography (M-mode or two-dimensional) confirms the presence of a pericardial effusion.

The etiology of Dressler's syndrome is unknown, but it is believed to represent an autoimmune process, since antiheart antibodies have been demonstrated in the sera of some patients. Histologically, the pericardium and pleura show a nonspecific inflammatory reaction. There are no laboratory tests diagnostic of this syndrome. Instead, the diagnosis depends on the appearance of a pleuropericarditis several weeks after a myocardial infarction.

The patient with the postmyocardial infarction syndrome should be treated first with a nonsteroidal anti-inflammatory agent, such as aspirin or ibuprofen. Since indomethacin exerts a deleterious effect on coronary blood flow and ischemic injury in patients with coronary artery disease, it is uncertain if this agent should be administered to patients with Dressler's. If the syndrome is not adequately controlled with these agents, glucocorticosteroids should be administered. Heparin and coumadin should be avoided, since they can convert a serous pericardial effusion into a large and bloody one, leading to tamponade.

Either treated or untreated, Dressler's syndrome is self-limited. Chronic pericardial effusions and recurrent episodes occur only rarely.

1. Dressler W. A complication of myocardial infarction resembling idiopathic recurrent benign pericarditis. Circulation 1955; 12:697.
   The original report of this syndrome, in which 10 patients are briefly described.
2. Dressler W. A postmyocardial infarction syndrome: preliminary report of a complication resembling idiopathic, recurrent benign pericarditis. JAMA 1956; 160:1379–83.
   An early description of the postmyocardial infarction syndrome.
3. Tew FT, Mantle JA, Russell RO Jr, Rackley CE. Cardiac tamponade with nonhemorrhagic pericardial fluid complicating Dressler's syndrome. Chest 1977; 72:93–5.
   A 39-year-old man with tamponade due to Dressler's syndrome is reported, and the rarity of this development is discussed.
4. Van der Geld H. Anti-heart antibodies in the post-pericardiotomy and the post-myocardial infarction syndrome. Lancet 1964; 2:617–21.
   Anti-heart antibodies were detected in 8 of 14 patients with the postmyocardial infarction syndrome.
5. Dressler W. The post-myocardial infarction syndrome: a report on 44 cases. Arch Intern Med 1959; 103:28–42.
   Most commonly, Dressler's syndrome must be distinguished clinically from a myocardial infarct extension or a pulmonary embolus.
6. Levin EJ, Bryk D. Dressler's syndrome (post-myocardial infarction syndrome). Radiology 1966; 87:731–6.
   The radiographic features of Dressler's syndrome are described.
7. Das SK, Cassidy JT, Petty RE. The significance of heart-reactive antibodies in heart disease. Chest 1974; 66:179–81.
   The rarity of Dressler's syndrome, the time interval between infarction and onset of

symptoms, the antibody response and its relation to clinical symptomatology, and the dramatic response of these patients to therapy with corticosteroids all suggest that this syndrome has an autoimmune basis.

8. Versey JMB, Gabriel R. Soluble-complex formation after myocardial infarction. Lancet 1974; 2:493–4.

Of 45 patients with acute myocardial infarction, 4 had evidence of an activated complement cascade; 3 subsequently developed Dressler's syndrome. This suggests that the postmyocardial infarction syndrome may be mediated by soluble complexes.

RIGHT VENTRICULAR INFARCTION

Since acute myocardial infarction predominantly involves the left ventricle, the hemodynamic derangements produced by infarction almost invariably present as *left* ventricular dysfunction. Recently, however, it has become clear that *right* ventricular infarction, with resultant dysfunction, occurs in a minority of patients, and in some of these the hemodynamic alterations produced by such infarction are catastrophic. Large postmortem studies have demonstrated that right ventricular infarction occurs in 15 to 25 percent of patients dying of acute myocardial infarction, and its clinical incidence in patients surviving infarction appears to be about the same. In light of these data, it is surprising that this clinical entity has not received more attention.

Pathologically, isolated right ventricular infarction is rare, and the vast majority of cases occur in association with inferior left ventricular infarction. Since the right coronary artery supplies both the right ventricular free wall and the inferior left ventricular wall in 85 to 90 percent of patients, it is not surprising that total occlusion of this artery is responsible for right ventricular infarction in most patients. Although early postmortem studies suggested that right ventricular infarction occurred with increased frequency in patients with right coronary artery occlusion and preexisting right ventricular hypertrophy, more recent studies have failed to support this observation.

Clinically, the patient with right ventricular infarction complains of retrosternal chest discomfort, which is often accompanied by nausea, vomiting, and diaphoresis. In contradistinction to the patient with extensive left ventricular infarction, dyspnea is an uncommon symptom. On physical examination, the patient usually manifests prominent peripheral venous congestion (jugular venous distention and hepatojugular reflux), a reduced cardiac output (with resultant hypotension and peripheral vasoconstriction), and no evidence of pulmonary vascular congestion. If right ventricular dysfunction is severe, the patient may have pulsus alternans or even a murmur of tricuspid regurgitation. In short, the physical findings in the patient with right ventricular infarction are similar to those of pericardial tamponade or constrictive pericarditis in that there is peripheral venous congestion in the absence of pulmonary edema. In fact, some patients with right ventricular infarction are initially misdiagnosed as having pericardial disease.

Electrocardiographically, right ventricular infarction is almost always associated with transmural inferior left ventricular infarction. Thus, the patient typically presents with S–T segment elevation, as well as evolving Q and R wave alterations in the inferior leads (II, III, and aVF). Although these electrocardiographic findings are diagnostic of inferior left ventricular infarction, they are not specific for right ventricular involvement. However, recent studies have demonstrated that S–T segment elevation in one or more *right* precordial leads is a highly specific and sensitive criterion for identifying acute right ventricular infarction.

Right ventricular infarction can be diagnosed accurately with several different scintigraphic techniques. First, technetium 99m stannous pyrophosphate has been used to identify patients with recent infarction of the right ventricular free wall. Second, thallium 201 scintigraphy during the 24 hours after the onset of infarction has been used to demonstrate that perfusion of the right ventricular free wall is diminished. Finally, gated equilibrium blood pool scintigraphy has been employed in these patients to allow an assessment of right ventricular size and function. Similarly, both M-mode and two-dimensional echocardiography have been used successfully to diagnose right ventricular infarction; by echocardiography, right ventricular chamber size and wall motion can be assessed.

The hemodynamic sequelae of right ventricular infarction with resultant dysfunction can be assessed accurately with a flow-directed, balloon-tipped catheter. These patients usually have (1) elevated right-sided filling pressures, (2) normal or only minimally elevated left-sided filling pressures, and (3) a reduced cardiac output. As noted previously, some of these patients are initially thought to have pericardial tamponade. Both gated equilibrium blood pool scintigraphy and echocardiography are extremely helpful in distinguishing right ventricular dysfunction from tamponade.

The therapy of the patient with right ventricular infarction and resultant dysfunction should center on the following procedures. First, intravascular volume should be expanded substantially in an attempt to increase left-sided filling pressures and, as a result, to improve left-sided output. This is usually accomplished only by raising right-sided filling pressures to very high levels. This is the cornerstone of therapy in these patients. Various pressor agents, such as dopamine, isoproterenol, and dobutamine, are usually not effective unless intravascular volume has been greatly expanded. Second, an occasional patient may respond beneficially to an unloading agent, such as nitroprusside, but it must be administered cautiously to the patient whose systemic arterial pressure is borderline or low. Third, intra-aortic balloon counterpulsation has been employed in some patients with right ventricular infarction and dysfunction, but its salutary effect is not proved.

With improved recognition of right ventricular infarction has come improved therapy, and with this has come a good prognosis, so that several recent studies have demonstrated that these patients have a good long-term outlook. In fact, if initial right ventricular dysfunction is treated appropriately (with vigorous volume expansion), the patient's long-term prognosis is usually dependent only on the extent of left ventricular dysfunction.

Pathologic and Clinical Features

1. Isner JM, Roberts WC. Right ventricular infarction complicating left ventricular infarction secondary to coronary heart disease: frequency, location, associated findings, and significance from analysis of 236 necropsy patients with acute or healed myocardial infarction. Am J Cardiol 1978; 42:885–94.
   At postmortem examination, 33 (14%) of 236 patients with transmural infarction had right ventricular involvement. All had inferior left ventricular infarction.
2. Cohn JN, Guiha NH, Broder MI, Limas CJ. Right ventricular infarction. Clinical and hemodynamic features. Am J Cardiol 1974; 33:209–14.
   One of the early characterizations of hemodynamics in 6 patients with right ventricular infarction. Right atrial pressure in these 6 individuals averaged 20 mm Hg.
3. Lorell B, Leinbach RC, Pohost GM, Gold HK, Dinsmore RE, Hutter AM Jr, Pastore JO, DeSanctis RW. Right ventricular infarction: clinical diagnosis and differentiation from cardiac tamponade and pericardial constriction. Am J Cardiol 1979; 43:465–71.

Of 12 patients with right ventricular infarction and dysfunction, 4 were originally misdiagnosed as having pericardial tamponade.

4. Ratliff NB, Hackel DB. Combined right and left ventricular infarction: pathogenesis and clinicopathologic correlations. Am J Cardiol 1980; 45:217–21.
   Of 102 consecutive cases of fatal infarction examined at necropsy, 35 (34%) had right ventricular involvement.
5. Rotman M, Ratliff NB, Hawley J. Right ventricular infarction: a hemodynamic diagnosis. Br Heart J 1974; 36:941–4.
   The case report of a 61-year-old man who died of a massive right ventricular infarction.
6. Coma-Canella I, Lopez-Sendon J, Gamallo C. Low output syndrome in right ventricular infarction. Am Heart J 1979; 98:613–20.
   In 10 patients with right ventricular infarction, right atrial pressure averaged 16 mm Hg, and the wave contour was often suggestive of constrictive pericarditis.
7. Raabe DS, Chester AC. Right ventricular infarction. Chest 1978; 73:96–9.
   A 49-year-old woman with a massive right ventricular infarction was treated with fluid therapy and nitroprusside and did well.
8. Jensen DP, Goolsby JP Jr, Oliva PB. Hemodynamic pattern resembling pericardial constriction after acute inferior myocardial infarction with right ventricular infarction. Am J Cardiol 1978; 42:858–61.
   Two patients with right ventricular infarction and a hemodynamic picture resembling constrictive pericarditis are described.
9. Cintron GB, Hernandez E, Linares E, Aranda JM. Bedside recognition, incidence, and clinical course of right ventricular infarction. Am J Cardiol 1981; 47:224–7.
   Of 44 consecutive patients with inferior left ventricular infarction, 16 had clinical evidence of right ventricular dysfunction. The long-term prognosis of these patients was good (all 16 survived at least 3 months postinfarction).
10. Rackley CE, Russell RO Jr, Mantle JA, Rogers WJ, Papapietro SE, Schwartz KM. Right ventricular infarction and function. Am Heart J 1981; 101:215–8.
    A concise review of the recognition and diagnosis of this entity.

Diagnosis

11. Croft CH, Nicod P, Corbett JR, Lewis SE, Huxley R, Mukharji J, Willerson JT, Rude RE. Detection of acute right ventricular infarction by right precordial electrocardiography. Am J Cardiol 1982; 50:421–7.
    S–T segment elevation in one or more right precordial leads is both highly sensitive and specific in identifying acute right ventricular infarction.
12. Wackers FJT, Lie KI, Sokole EB, Res J, Van der Schoot JB, Durrer D. Prevalence of right ventricular involvement in inferior wall infarction assessed with myocardial imaging with thallium-201 and technetium-99m pyrophosphate. Am J Cardiol 1978; 42:358–62.
    Scintigraphic studies with thallium-201 and technetium-99m showed right ventricular involvement in 24 (38%) of 78 consecutive patients with acute inferior left ventricular infarction.
13. Rigo P, Murray M, Taylor DR, Weisfeldt ML, Kelly DT, Strauss HW, Pitt B. Right ventricular dysfunction detected by gated scintiphotography in patients with acute inferior myocardial infarction. Circulation 1975; 52:268–74.
    Using gated equilibrium blood pool scintigraphy, these authors examined end-diastolic right and left ventricular areas. Many of the patients with recent inferior left ventricular infarction had right ventricular dilatation, suggesting a high incidence of right ventricular involvement.
14. Tobinick E, Schelbert HR, Henning H, LeWinter M, Taylor A, Ashburn WL, Karliner JS. Right ventricular ejection fraction in patients with acute anterior and inferior myocardial infarction assessed by radionuclide angiography. Circulation 1978; 57:1078–84.
    Of 19 patients with inferior left ventricular infarction, 7 had scintigraphic evidence of right ventricular dysfunction.
15. Elkayam U, Halprin SL, Frishman W, Strom J, Cohen MN. Echocardiographic findings in cardiogenic shock due to right ventricular myocardial infarction. Cathet Cardiovasc Diagn 1975; 5:289–94.

In a 62-year-old woman with right ventricular infarction, M-mode echocardiography revealed right ventricular dilatation and abnormal septal motion.

16. Sharpe DN, Botvinick EH, Shames DM, Schiller NB, Massie BM, Chatterjee K, Parmley WW. The noninvasive diagnosis of right ventricular infarction. Circulation 1978; 57:483–90.
    In 6 patients with inferior left ventricular infarction and right ventricular radio-nuclide uptake, echocardiographic right ventricular end-diastolic dimension was increased.

17. Chou T, VanDer Bel-Khan J, Allen J, Brockmeier L, Fowler NO. Electrocardiographic diagnosis of right ventricular infarction. Am J Med 1981; 70:1175–80.
    When acute inferior left ventricular infarction is accompanied by S–T segment elevation in the right precordial leads, the coexistence of right ventricular infarction should be suspected.

18. Lopez-Sendon J, Coma-Canella I, Gamallo C. Sensitivity and specificity of hemodynamic criteria in the diagnosis of acute right ventricular infarction. Circulation 1981; 64:515–25.
    This paper assesses the sensitivity and specificity of intracardiac pressures and waveforms in the diagnosis of right ventricular dysfunction.

19. Candell-Riera J, Figueras J, Valle V, Alvarez A, Gutierrez L, Cortadellas J, Cinca J, Salas A, Rius J. Right ventricular infarction: relationships between ST segment elevation in V_{4R} and hemodynamic, scintigraphic, and echocardiographic findings in patients with acute inferior myocardial infarction. Am Heart J 1981; 101:281–7.
    S–T segment elevation in a right precordial lead is an excellent diagnostic criterion for right ventricular infarction.

20. Klein HO, Tardjman T, Ninio R, Sareli P, Oren V, Lang R, Gefen J, Pauzner C, Segni ED, David D, Kaplinksy E. The early recognition of right ventricular infarction: diagnostic accuracy of the electrocardiographic V_{4R} lead. Circulation 1983; 67:558–65.
    In 58 patients with right ventricular infarction, changes in lead V_{4R} were sensitive (83%) and reasonably specific (77%).

21. Trappler B, Abkiewicz SR, Millar RNS, Obel IWP. Hemodynamics and treatment of right ventricular infarction. S Afr Med J 1976; 50:1135–7.
    Optimal therapy of this condition entails vigorous volume administration, either alone or in conjunction with inotropic agents.

22. Erhardt LR. Right ventricular involvement in acute myocardial infarction. Eur J Cardiol 1976; 4:411–8.
    Treatment of these patients must be done with close hemodynamic monitoring.

23. Haffajee CI, Ockene IS, Dalen JE. Cardiogenic shock due to right ventricular infarction. Chest 1978; 74:601–2.
    The report of a 69-year-old woman with this disease entity who was treated successfully with volume infusion and intra-aortic balloon counterpulsation.

24. Lloyd EA, Gersh BJ, Kennelly BM. Hemodynamic spectrum of "dominant" right ventricular infarction in 19 patients. Am J Cardiol 1981; 48:1016–22.
    In 19 patients with right ventricular infarction and resultant dysfunction, right atrial pressure averaged 15 mm Hg, and 13 patients were hypotensive. A combination of fluid administration and nitroprusside was effective in this group; only 1 patient died.

TREATMENT OF MYOCARDIAL INFARCTION

The patient with acute myocardial infarction should be hospitalized immediately, preferably in a facility where continuous electrocardiographic monitoring can be performed. Subsequently, care should center on (1) restriction of physical activity, (2) sedation and relief of pain, and (3) prevention or proper therapy of complications. Strict bed rest should be enforced for at least 2 to 3 days after hospitalization. Thereafter, the patient is allowed to ambulate progressively over the next 4 to 10 days. The patient with an uncomplicated infarction can be discharged after 7 to 14 days in the hospital, provided that his home environment will allow a continued gradual progression of physical activity.

Opiates (specifically morphine or meperidine) should be employed to relieve chest pain and to sedate the patient with an acute myocardial infarction. These agents are usually given intravenously to ensure complete and immediate onset of action and to avoid an elevation of serum enzymes (creatine kinase, glutamic-oxaloacetic transaminase) caused by intramuscular injections. These analgesics should be administered cautiously, since they may induce hypotension, respiratory depression, or bradycardia. The authors routinely administer 2 to 5 mg of morphine every 5 minutes until chest pain is relieved, observing the systemic arterial pressure at frequent intervals.

If chest pain continues despite large doses of opiates, intravenous nitroglycerin should be initiated, provided the patient's arterial pressure is not low. If pain persists, the intra-aortic balloon should be inserted for counterpulsation. If continued chest pain is present in spite of these aggressive measures, emergent coronary arteriography and, if feasible, coronary artery bypass surgery should be performed.

In the patient without a relative or absolute contraindication, low-dose heparin (i.e., 5,000 units subcutaneously every 12 hr) often is administered in the setting of acute myocardial infarction to minimize the chance of a thromboembolic event. Among the contraindications to the use of heparin are uncontrolled hypertension, a history of gastrointestinal bleeding, a known bleeding diathesis, and the presence of a pericardial friction rub. Administration of heparin is discontinued when the patient becomes mobile.

Previous studies have shown that intravenous lidocaine reduces the frequency of ventricular fibrillation in patients with frequent or multiformed premature beats, and therefore, some authors have suggested that a lidocaine infusion should be administered to all patients for 24 to 48 hours after infarction. However, the benefits of such prophylactic lidocaine administration must be weighed against the risk of lidocaine toxicity. Thus, if lidocaine prophylaxis is to be used, it must be employed with great care in patients with advanced age (>70 years), congestive heart failure, shock, or liver disease, since individuals with these entities are at a greatly increased risk of developing lidocaine intoxication. At present, the authors do not administer lidocaine prophylactically to all patients with acute myocardial infarction.

Finally, the various complications of myocardial infarction should be identified and treated promptly. Supraventricular tachyarrhythmias should be treated with verapamil, digitalis, propranolol, or DC countershock; ventricular tachyarrhythmias should be treated with lidocaine, procainamide, or countershock; and bradyarrhythmias should be treated with atropine or, if necessary, temporary transvenous pacing. Left ventricular dysfunction with resultant venous congestion should be treated with a diuretic, digitalis, and, if needed, inotropic support with an agent such as dobutamine. If cardiogenic shock develops, the intra-aortic balloon should be inserted, after which emergent coronary arteriography and bypass surgery should be considered.

Restriction of Activity After Myocardial Infarction

1. McNeer JF, Wagner GS, Ginsburg PB, Wallace AG, McCants CB, Conley MJ, Rosati RA. Hospital discharge one week after acute myocardial infarction. N Engl J Med 1978; 298:229–32.
   Patients with uncomplicated infarctions can be discharged from the hospital at 1 week without problems.
2. Hutter AM Jr, Sidel VW, Shine KI, DeSanctis RW. Early hospital discharge after myocardial infarction. N Engl J Med 1973; 288:1141–4.

There is no additional benefit to the patient with an uncomplicated myocardial infarction from a 3-week as compared to a 2-week hospital stay.

3. Chaturvedi NC, Walsh MJ, Evans A, Munro P, Boyle DM, Barber JM. Selection of patients for early discharge after acute myocardial infarction. Br Heart J 1974; 36:533–5.
   Those individuals without complications can be safely discharged 7 days after infarction.

4. Tucker HH, Carson PHM, Bass NM, Sharratt GP, Stock JPP. Results of early mobilization and discharge after myocardial infarction. Br Med J 1973; 1:10–13.
   Of 342 patients with myocardial infarction, the average hospital stay was 8.4 days.

5. Block A, Maeder JP, Haissly JC, Felix J, Blackburn H. Early mobilization after myocardial infarction: a controlled study. Am J Cardiol 1974; 34:152–7.
   A carefully performed study demonstrating that early mobilization is not detrimental in patients with uncomplicated infarction.

6. McNeer JF, Wallace AG, Wagner GS, Starmer CF, Rosati RA. The course of acute myocardial infarction: feasibility of early discharge of the uncomplicated patient. Circulation 1975; 51:410–3.
   One of the initial articles demonstrating that it is feasible and ethically justified to discharge those with uncomplicated infarction after 7 days.

Prophylactic Antiarrhythmic Therapy

7. Harrison DC. Should lidocaine be administered routinely to all patients after acute myocardial infarction? Circulation 1978; 58:581–4.
   This paper recommends lidocaine prophylaxis for all patients hospitalized with possible infarction.

8. Lie KI, Wellens HJ, vanCapelle FJ, Durrer D. Lidocaine in the prevention of primary ventricular fibrillation: a double-blind, randomized study of 212 consecutive patients. N Engl J Med 1974; 291:1324–6.
   Lidocaine, administered for 48 hours, was effective in preventing ventricular fibrillation; however, the drug had a toxic effect on 15% of those receiving it.

9. Valentine PA, Frew JL, Mashford ML, Sloman JG. Lidocaine in the prevention of sudden death in the pre-hospital phase of acute infarction: a double-blind study. N Engl J Med 1974; 291:1327–31.
   Intramuscular lidocaine reduced mortality in patients with myocardial infarction.

10. Jones DT, Kostuk WJ, Gunton RW. Prophylactic quinidine for the prevention of arrhythmias after acute myocardial infarction. Am J Cardiol 1974; 33:655–60.
    Oral quinidine sulfate did not reduce infarction-associated ventricular fibrillation.

Prophylactic Anticoagulation

11. Wray R, Maurer B, Shillingford J. Prophylactic anticoagulant therapy in the prevention of calf-vein thrombosis after myocardial infarction. N Engl J Med 1973; 288:815–7.
    Although anticoagulation reduces the frequency of calf-vein thrombosis, the authors recommend that such therapy be reserved for patients with venous thromboses or patients who are confined to bed for more than a week.

12. Chalmers TC, Matta RJ, Smith H Jr, Kunzler AM. Evidence favoring the use of anticoagulants in the hospital phase of acute myocardial infarction. N Engl J Med 1977; 297:1091–6.
    This review of the literature concludes that all patients who present no specific contraindication should receive anticoagulants during hospitalization for infarction.

Therapy for Complications of Myocardial Infarction

13. Epstein SE, Goldstein RE, Redwood DR, Kent KM, Smith ER. The early phase of acute myocardial infarction: pharmacologic aspects of therapy. Ann Intern Med 1973; 78:918–36.
    A review of the preferred approach to the various arrhythmic complications of infarction.

14. Willerson JT, Curry GC, Watson JT, Leshin SJ, Ecker RR, Mullins CB, Platt MR, Sugg WL. Intraaortic balloon counterpulsation in patients in cardiogenic shock, medically refractory left ventricular failure, and/or recurrent ventricular tachycardia. Am J Med 1975; 58:183–91.

Intra-aortic balloon counterpulsation is a useful adjunct to currently existing medical measures in patients with cardiogenic shock or medically refractory left ventricular failure; however, most patients have such extensive underlying disease that they cannot be weaned from balloon support.

PROTECTION OF ISCHEMIC MYOCARDIUM

Over the past 10 to 15 years, studies in experimental animals have shown that only some of the myocardial tissue perfused by a recently occluded coronary artery becomes irreversibly damaged within 20 to 30 minutes of the occlusion, whereas a substantial portion of myocardium (the so-called border zone) is only reversibly injured for a number of hours after occlusion. The eventual extent of infarction depends on the balance between oxygen supply and demand within the border zone. Thus, any intervention that favorably influences the border zone's supply-demand ratio may reduce the extent of ischemic injury; in contrast, any intervention that unfavorably alters this ratio may worsen such injury. In the experimental animal, a number of metabolic, pharmacologic, and hemodynamic interventions have been shown to reduce ischemic injury in its reversible phase, thus diminishing the extent of subsequent infarction. Furthermore, preliminary investigations in patients with acute myocardial infarction have demonstrated that some of these interventions are effective in reducing morbidity and mortality. The following will consider those agents or maneuvers whose use in patients appears especially promising.

In the experimental animal with coronary artery occlusion, *supplemental oxygen* inhalation has proved beneficial in reducing ischemic injury. In patients with acute myocardial infarction, high-flow supplemental oxygen has been demonstrated to reduce the magnitude and extent of precordial S–T segment elevation (an electrocardiographic marker of ischemia) but to exert no effect (beneficial or detrimental) on the overall clinical course. Since pulmonary oxygen toxicity usually results only from prolonged inhalation of an oxygen concentration in excess of 50%, the supplemental oxygen usually given to patients with acute infarction is neither concentrated nor prolonged enough to result in toxicity.

Numerous experimental and clinical studies have suggested that an infusion of *glucose, insulin, and postassium* in the setting of myocardial ischemia exerts a beneficial effect, presumably through both an enhancement of anaerobic glycolysis by the ischemic cells and a reduction in the concentration of circulating free fatty acids. In the dog and baboon with coronary artery occlusion, the infusion of a glucose-insulin-potassium solution reduces the magnitude of eventual myocardial necrosis. In patients with acute myocardial infarction, such an infusion has been shown (1) to be safe and well tolerated, (2) to increase the myocardial utilization of glucose and to diminish the utilization of free fatty acids, (3) to induce no change in left ventricular filling pressure or cardiac index, (4) to decrease the frequency and complexity of ventricular ectopic activity, and (5) to diminish mortality in those individuals whose left ventricular function is initially impaired.

In both experimental animals and man, *glucocorticosteroids* have been shown to diminish the magnitude of myocardial ischemic injury but, at the same time, to inhibit proper healing of ischemic damage, leading to an increased frequency of left ventricular aneurysm formation or rupture. The *nonsteroidal anti-inflammatory agents* ibuprofen and flurbiprofen have been shown to reduce infarct size in experimental animals, but their effects on infarct healing are unknown, as is their influence on ischemic injury in man. Interestingly, aspirin exerts no effect on ischemic injury, and indomethacin actually worsens it, even though all these agents act by inhibiting cyclo-oxygenase, the enzyme involved in prostaglandin synthesis.

Many studies have shown that the intravenous administration of the enzyme *hyaluronidase* diminishes the magnitude of myocardial ischemic injury. Preliminary studies have shown that it reduces electrocardiographic evidence of myocardial necrosis when it is administered to patients within 8 hours of symptoms, and a smaller study has demonstrated a trend toward less creatine kinase release in patients given hyaluronidase. Hyaluronidase may exert its beneficial effect on the ischemic myocardium by improving the transport of nutrients (i.e., oxygen and glucose) to the ischemic tissue, enhancing the washout of toxic metabolic substances that accumulate during ischemia (e.g., lactate and free fatty acids), and increasing collateral blood flow to the ischemic area.

Numerous experimental studies have demonstrated that the *beta-adrenergic blocking agents* diminish myocardial ischemic injury. In patients with acute myocardial infarction, propranolol has been shown to reduce precordial electrocardiographic and enzymatic evidence of injury, and similar results have been reported for several other beta-adrenergic blocking agents, including atenolol, alprenolol, and metoprolol. In addition, the chronic administration of the beta-adrenergic blocking agents during the weeks to months following infarction has been shown to lower mortality, but it is not clear whether the mechanism of this beneficial long-term effect is a limitation of acute ischemic injury, a prevention of subsequent infarction, or an antiarrhythmic effect.

In patients with acute myocardial infarction, several studies have shown that *nitroglycerin* diminishes the extent of myocardial ischemic injury, whether administered alone or concomitantly with an alpha-adrenergic agonist (e.g., phenylephrine) to reverse the nitroglycerin-induced fall in systemic arterial pressure. In addition, nitroglycerin has been shown to improve myocardial perfusion (as measured by thallium 201 scintigraphy) and to reduce the frequency of subsequent infarct extension as well as late ventricular arrhythmias.

Intra-aortic balloon counterpulsation exerts a salutary influence on the myocardial oxygen suppy-demand balance by augmenting supply and reducing demand. In patients with acute infarction but without associated shock, counterpulsation markedly diminishes precordial electrocardiographic evidence of ischemic injury, especially in those individuals whose infarction is caused by only a subtotal coronary occlusion. Since such balloon counterpulsation carries a substantial risk of complications, it should probably be reserved for patients with continuing myocardial ischemia or pump failure. (See Intra-aortic Balloon Counterpulsation, p. 323, for more details.)

Several studies in dogs have demonstrated that early *coronary artery reperfusion* (within 3 hr of coronary artery occlusion) reduces the magnitude of ischemic injury. Although the reported clinical experience with urgent surgical revascularization for evolving myocardial infarction is limited, the results have been surprisingly good. More recently, acute thrombolysis (with intracoronary or intravenous streptokinase) has been shown to reduce the magnitude of precordial S–T segment elevation, to relieve chest pain, and possibly even to improve left ventricular performance. (See Thrombolytic Therapy of Myocardial Infarction, p. 102.)

General
1. Hillis LD, Braunwald E. Myocardial ischemia. N Engl J Med 1977; 296:971–8, 1034–41, 1093–6.

An exhaustive review of those agents that have been shown to worsen or improve myocardial ischemic injury.

2. Rude RE, Muller JE, Braunwald E. Efforts to limit the size of myocardial infarcts. Ann Intern Med 1981; 95:736–61.
   An especially good discussion of those interventions that have been shown to be beneficial in patients with acute myocardial infarction.

Supplemental Oxygen

3. Maroko PR, Radvany P, Braunwald E, Hale SL. Reduction of infarct size by oxygen inhalation following acute coronary occlusion. Circulation 1975; 52:360–8.
   In the dog with coronary artery occlusion, 40% inspired oxygen decreases acute ischemic injury and reduces the eventual development of necrosis.

4. Madias JE, Madias NE, Hood WB Jr. Precordial ST segment mapping. 2. Effects of oxygen inhalation on ischemic injury in patients with acute myocardial infarction. Circulation 1976; 53:411–7.
   In 17 patients with acute anterior infarction, supplemental oxygen reduced the magnitude of precordial S-T segment elevation by an average of 16%.

Glucose-Insulin-Postassium

5. Maroko PR, Libby P, Sobel BE, Bloor CM, Sybers HD, Shell WE, Covell JW, Braunwald E. Effect of glucose-insulin-potassium infusion on myocardial infarction following experimental coronary artery occlusion. Circulation 1972; 45:1160–75.
   In the dog with coronary artery occlusion, a solution of glucose-insulin-potassium begun 30 minutes after occlusion diminished the amount of myocardial necrosis 24 hours later.

6. Rogers WJ, Segall PH, McDaniel HG, Mantle JA, Russell RO Jr, Rackley CE. Prospective randomized trial of glucose-insulin-potassium in acute myocardial infarction: effects on myocardial hemodynamics, substrates, and rhythm. Am J Cardiol 1979; 43:801–9.
   In patients with acute myocardial infarction, a glucose-insulin-potassium infusion does not adversely alter hemodynamics, reduces circulating free fatty acids, and diminishes the frequency of ventricular arrhythmias.

Anti-inflammatory Agents

7. Libby P, Maroko PR, Bloor CM, Sobel BE, Braunwald E. Reduction of experimental myocardial infarct size by corticosteroid administration. J Clin Invest 1973; 52:599–607.
   In the dog with acute coronary artery occlusion, hydrocortisone reduced the extent of ischemic injury, as assessed electrocardiographically and enzymatically.

8. Roberts R, deMello V, Sobel BE. Deleterious effects of methylprednisolone in patients with myocardial infarction. Circulation 1976; 53 (Suppl I):204–6.
   In 22 patients with myocardial infarction given methylprednisolone, infarct size was extended and ventricular dysrhythmias worsened.

9. Bulkley BH, Roberts WC. Steroid therapy during acute myocardial infarction: a cause of delayed healing and of ventricular aneurysm. Am J Med 1974; 56:244–50.
   An interesting case report demonstrating that corticosteroids markedly impede the healing process after myocardial infarction.

10. Jugdutt BI, Hutchins GM, Bulkley BH, Becker LC. Salvage of ischemic myocardium by ibuprofen during infarction in the conscious dog. Am J Cardiol 1980; 46:74–82.
    In the conscious dog with coronary artery occlusion, ibuprofen diminished ischemic injury without altering collateral blood flow or myocardial oxygen demands, suggesting that ibuprofen's cellular and metabolic effects are of importance.

Hyaluronidase

11. Hillis LD, Fishbein MC, Braunwald E, Maroko PR. The influence of the time interval between coronary artery occlusion and the administration of hyaluronidase on salvage of ischemic myocardium in dogs. Circ Res 1977; 41:26–31.
    In the dog with coronary artery occlusion, hyaluronidase given as late as 6 hours after occlusion reduced the magnitude of ischemic injury.

12. Maroko PR, Hillis LD, Muller JE, Tavazzi L, Heyndrickx GR, Ray M, Chiariello M, Distante A, Askenazi J, Salerno J, Carpentier J, Reshetnaya NI, Radvany P, Libby P, Raabe DS, Chazov EI, Bobba P, Braunwald E. Favorable effects of hyaluronidase on electrocardiographic evidence of necrosis in patients with acute myocardial infarction. N Engl J Med 1977; 296:898–903.
In 46 patients with acute anterior transmural infarction given hyaluronidase, electrocardiographic evidence of necrosis was diminished.

Beta-Adrenergic Blocking Agents
13. Gold HK, Leinbach RC, Maroko PR. Propranolol-induced reduction of signs of ischemic injury during acute myocardial infarction. Am J Cardiol 1976; 38:689–95.
In 12 patients given intravenous propranolol within 8 hours of the onset of chest pain, electrocardiographic evidence of transmural ischemia was decreased.
14. Norwegian Multicenter Study Group. Timolol-induced reduction in mortality and reinfarction in patients surviving acute myocardial infarction. N Engl J Med 1981; 304:801–7.
In a study involving almost 2000 patients who had recently suffered an infarction, timolol reduced mortality by 45% and reinfarction by 28%.

Nitroglycerin
15. Borer JS, Redwood DR, Levitt B, Cagin N, Bianchi C, Vallin H, Epstein SE. Reduction in myocardial ischemia with nitroglycerin or nitroglycerin plus phenylephrine administered during acute myocardial infarction. N Engl J Med 1975; 293:1008–12.
In 12 patients with acute infarction, nitroglycerin, alone or with phenylephrine, reduced myocardial ischemic injury. The response to phenylephrine was dependent on the presence or absence of left ventricular failure before treatment.

Intra-aortic Balloon Counterpulsation
16. Maroko PR, Bernstein EF, Libby P, DeLaria GA, Covell JW, Ross J Jr, Braunwald E. Effects of intraaortic balloon counterpulsation on the severity of myocardial ischemic injury following acute coronary occlusion. Circulation 1972; 45:1150–9.
In the dog with coronary occlusion, balloon counterpulsation, even when begun 3 hours after occlusion, reduced electrocardiographic evidence of ischemia.
17. Leinbach RC, Gold HK, Harper RW, Buckley MJ, Austen WG. Early intraaortic balloon pumping for anterior myocardial infarction without shock. Circulation 1978; 58:204–10.
In 11 patients with anterior infarction but without shock, balloon counterpulsation was used. In those individuals in whom there was residual antegrade blood flow in the involved artery, counterpulsation markedly reduced the amount of S-T segment elevation.

Coronary Artery Reperfusion
18. Phillips SJ, Kongtahwarn C, Zeff RH, Benson M, Iannone L, Brown T, Gordon DF. Emergency coronary artery revascularization: a possible therapy for acute myocardial infarction. Circulation 1979; 60:241–6.
Coronary artery bypass was performed on 75 patients with acute infarction. One patient (1%) died during surgery; and two (3%) died later.
19. Mathey DG, Kuck KH, Tilsner V, Krebber HJ, Bleifeld W. Nonsurgical coronary artery recanalization in acute transmural myocardial infarction. Circulation 1981; 63:489–97.
One of the early reports of intracoronary streptokinase for patients with acute evolving myocardial infarction. Of the 41 patients included in this report, streptokinase was successful in causing clot lysis in 30 (73%).
20. Markis JE, Malagold M, Parker JA, Silverman KJ, Barry WH, Als AV, Paulin S, Grossman W, Braunwald E. Myocardial salvage after intracoronary thrombolysis with streptokinase in acute myocardial infarction: assessment by intracoronary thallium-201. N Engl J Med 1981; 305:777–82.
In 9 patients with acute infarction, thrombolysis led to improved regional perfusion in 7.

THROMBOLYTIC THERAPY OF MYOCARDIAL INFARCTION

In patients with acute myocardial infarction who reach the hospital, extensive myocardial necrosis—with resultant heart failure, myocardial rupture, and associated ventricular tachyarrhythmias—remains the principal cause of morbidity and mortality. Although numerous pharmacologic interventions designed to limit the amount of necrosis have provided promising results in experimental animals, their ability to reduce morbidity and mortality in patients has not been convincingly demonstrated. At the same time, however, these animal studies have shown that early (i.e., within 3–4 hr of the onset of infarction) restoration of coronary blood flow can substantially reduce the amount of necrosis, and preliminary studies in patients with acute myocardial infarction have suggested that a clinically meaningful limitation of myocardial necrosis can be achieved with early restoration of blood flow to the jeopardized myocardium. The reestablishment of blood flow in the patient with an acute myocardial infarction can be achieved either surgically (i.e., with emergency coronary artery bypass grafting) or nonsurgically (i.e., with pharmacologic lysis of the occluding coronary arterial thrombus using a fibrinolytic agent, such as streptokinase). Autopsy studies have demonstrated that 85 to 95 percent of patients dying of transmural myocardial infarction have a fresh thrombotic occlusion of a large epicardial coronary artery, and angiographic studies within several hours of transmural infarction have shown a similar incidence of total occlusion. In short, it seems clear that coronary artery occlusion by a fresh thrombus is the cause of most transmural infarctions. Therefore, if the thrombus could, in some way, be dissolved within 3 to 6 hours of its formation, the amount of myocardial necrosis might be markedly limited.

In the patient with an acute transmural myocardial infarction, streptokinase can be administered intravenously or directly into the thrombosed coronary artery. Intravenous streptokinase carries the distinct advantage that it can be administered quickly and without the associated morbidity or cost of emergent cardiac catheterization. Over the past 20 years, numerous studies have been performed to assess the efficacy of intravenous streptokinase in patients with myocardial infarction, but none has demonstrated a beneficial effect. However, in most of these trials, streptokinase was administered in relatively small doses (e.g., an initial loading dose of 250,000 units, followed by an infusion of 100,000 units/hr for 12–24 hr), it was sometimes given as long as 48–72 hours after the onset of infarction, and its effects on variables other than mortality (e.g., left ventricular function, functional class) were not evaluated. More recently, intravenous streptokinase has been given only to patients whose transmural infarction began within 6 hours of arrival at the hospital. In juxtaposition to the aforementioned studies, it has been administered in a dose of 500,000 to 1,500,000 units over a 20- to 60-minute period of time. In the more recent studies, the success rate of restoring blood flow to the jeopardized myocardium following intravenous streptokinase is 50 to 65 percent, and in these patients, clot lysis usually occurs within 1 hour following intravenous streptokinase.

The intracoronary administration of streptokinase has several advantages over the intravenous route. First, it allows a higher concentration of the fibrinolytic material to be delivered to the thrombus; at the same time, however, a smaller total amount of streptokinase may be necessary to achieve clot lysis. Therefore, systemic fibrinolysis may be avoided, and with it the hemorrhagic complications may be reduced in number and magnitude. Second, it allows the physician the opportunity to promote the dissolution of a thrombus by mechanically fragmenting it with a soft guide wire or selective infusion catheter. Finally, it allows a direct visual assessment of whether recanalization of the occluded coronary artery actually occurs. Its disadvantages are (1) the morbidity of arterial catheterization in a patient receiving fibrinolytic therapy and (2) the requirement that a cardiac catheterization laboratory, with all its equipment and personnel, be immediately available at the time the patient arrives at the hospital. In recent studies, intracoronary streptokinase has been administered as a 15,000- to 20,000-unit bolus followed by 2,000 to 3,000 units per minute. Successful recanalization has been noted in 80 to 85 percent of patients following an average infusion time of 30 minutes.

Streptokinase administration by the intravenous or intracoronary route may be associated with several adverse effects. When it is administered in large doses (such as those given intravenously), it frequently induces an allergic reaction. To combat this occurrence, most centers in which intravenous streptokinase is employed administer hydrocortisone and diphenhydramine several minutes before the infusion is begun. Hemorrhagic complications occur in 5 to 15 percent of patients receiving streptokinase, although they seldom cause major morbidity or mortality.

Once dissolution of the intracoronary thrombus has been achieved with streptokinase, a coronary stenosis of variable severity remains whose endothelial surface is ulcerated and denuded. To prevent rethrombosis as the fibrinolytic potency of streptokinase disappears, the patient should receive (1) heparin for 10 to 14 days, followed by oral anticoagulation for 3 to 4 months, or (2) aspirin and dipyridamole for 3 to 4 months to prevent the reaccumulation of platelets on the denuded endothelium. The long-term prevention of rethrombosis is a crucial part of thrombolytic therapy. After 3 to 4 months have elapsed, the nidus for thrombus formation (in most patients, an ulcerated atherosclerotic plaque whose endothelial surface was exposed) has healed completely, and the patient is no longer at risk of rethrombosis at that site.

Although thrombolysis can be achieved in 50 to 85 percent of patients who receive intravenous or intracoronary streptokinase within 3 to 6 hours of transmural infarction, its beneficial effects on morbidity and mortality are unproved. Preliminary controlled studies demonstrate that intracoronary streptokinase exerts a beneficial effect on left ventricular function, but its influence on functional class and death will require properly designed, randomized, and large studies.

Intravenous Streptokinase

1. Schroder R. Systemic versus intracoronary streptokinase infusion in the treatment of acute myocardial infarction. JACC 1983; 1:1254–61.
   A succinct review of the advantages and limitations of intravenous and intracoronary streptokinase.
2. European Cooperative Study Group for Streptokinase Treatment in Acute Myocardial Infarction. Streptokinase in acute myocardial infarction. N Engl J Med 1979; 301:797–802.
   Intravenous streptokinase reduced mortality from myocardial infarction when given to a group of medium-risk patients.
3. Schroder R, Biamino G, Leitner ER, Linderer T, Bruggemann T, Heitz J, Vohringer HF, Wegscheider K. Intravenous short-term infusion of streptokinase in acute myocardial infarction. Circulation 1983; 67:536–48.
   In this study of 93 patients, high-dose (500,000 to 1,500,000 units over a 30–60 minute period) intravenous streptokinase was an effective method of restoring coronary blood flow.
4. Spann JF, Sherry S, Carabello BA, Mann RH, McCann WD, Gault JH, Gentzler RD, Rosenberg KM, Maurer AH, Denenberg BS, Warner HF, Rubin RN, Malmud LS,

Comerota A. High-dose, brief intravenous streptokinase early in acute myocardial infarction. Am Heart J 1982; 104:939–45.

Of 13 patients given intravenous streptokinase (850,000 units), coronary reperfusion was achieved in 6 within 1 hour of beginning the infusion.

5. Stampfer MJ, Goldhaber SZ, Yusuf S, Peto R, Hennekens CH. Effect of intravenous streptokinase on acute myocardial infarction: pooled results from randomized trials. N Engl J Med 1982; 307:1180–2.

This article suggests that intravenous streptokinase after acute myocardial infarction reduces mortality over the subsequent few weeks by about 20%.

Intracoronary Streptokinase

6. Anderson JL, Marshall HW, Bray BE, Lutz JR, Frederick PR, Yanowitz FG, Datz FL, Klausner SC, Hagan AD. A randomized trial of intracoronary streptokinase in the treatment of acute myocardial infarction. N Engl J Med 1983; 308:1312–8.

In comparison to standard therapy, intracoronary streptokinase improved Killip class and left ventricular ejection fraction.

7. Khaja F, Walton JA Jr, Brymer JF, Lo E, Osterberger L, O'Neill WW, Colfer HT, Weiss R, Lee T, Kurian T, Goldberg AD, Pitt B, Goldstein S. Intracoronary fibrinolytic therapy in acute myocardial infarction: report of a prospective randomized trial. N Engl J Med 1983; 308:1305–11.

In comparison to placebo, intracoronary streptokinase exerted no effect on left ventricular function.

8. Ganz W, Geft I, Maddahi J, Berman D, Charuzi Y, Shah PK, Swan HJC. Nonsurgical reperfusion in evolving myocardial infarction. JACC 1983; 1:1247–53.

Intracoronary thrombolysis appears to be an effective and relatively safe method for reopening the coronary artery in patients with acute myocardial infarction, but the clinical impact of successful reperfusion depends on how soon after occlusion this is achieved.

9. Rentrop P, Blanke H, Karsch KR, Kaiser H, Kostering H, Leitz K. Selective intracoronary thrombolysis in acute myocardial infarction and unstable angina pectoris. Circulation 1981; 63:307–17.

In 29 patients with infarction, intracoronary streptokinase successfully achieved recanalization in 22 (76%).

10. Mathey DG, Kuck KH, Tilsner V, Krebber HJ, Bleifeld W. Nonsurgical coronary artery recanalization in acute transmural myocardial infarction. Circulation 1981; 63:489–97.

Of 41 consecutive patients with acute transmural infarction, intracoronary streptokinase successfully recanalized the occluded artery within 1 hour in 30 (73%).

11. Reduto LA, Smalling RW, Freund GC, Gould KL. Intracoronary infusion of streptokinase in patients with acute myocardial infarction: effects of reperfusion on left ventricular performance. Am J Cardiol 1981; 48:403–9.

In this uncontrolled study, reperfusion with intracoronary streptokinase led to an improvement in left ventricular ejection fraction (0.44 on admission to 0.55 at hospital discharge).

12. Markis JE, Malagold M, Parker JA, Silverman KJ, Barry WH, Als AV, Paulin S, Grossman W, Braunwald E. Myocardial salvage after intracoronary thrombolysis with streptokinase in acute myocardial infarction: assessment by intracoronary thallium-201. N Engl J Med 1981; 305:777–82.

In 9 patients successfully reperfused with intracoronary streptokinase, improved regional perfusion (by thallium-201 imaging) was observed in 7.

13. Goldberg S, Greenspon AJ, Urban PL, Muza B, Berger B, Walinsky P, Maroko PR. Reperfusion arrhythmia: a marker of restoration of antegrade flow during intracoronary thrombolysis for acute myocardial infarction. Am Heart J 1983; 105:26–32.

Accelerated idioventricular rhythm is a common transient occurrence when thrombolysis occurs.

14. Cowley MJ, Hastillo A, Vetrovec GW, Fisher LM, Garrett R, Hess ML. Fibrinolytic effects of intracoronary streptokinase administration in patients with acute myocardial infarction and coronary insufficiency. Circulation 1983; 67:1031–8.

In 25 patients given intracoronary streptokinase, systemic fibrinolysis occurred in 22.

15. de Feyter PJ, van Eenige MJ, van der Wall EE, Bezemer PD, van Engelen CLJ,

Funke-Kupper AJ, Kerkkamp HJJ, Visser FC, Roos JP. Effects of spontaneous and streptokinase-induced recanalization on left ventricular function after myocardial infarction. Circulation 1983; 67:1039–44.

In this uncontrolled study, intracoronary streptokinase exerted a beneficial effect on left ventricular function.

16. Schwarz F, Schuler G, Katus H, Hofmann M, Manthey J, Tillmanns H, Mehmel HC, Kubler W. Intracoronary thrombolysis in acute myocardial infarction: duration of ischemia as a major determinant of late results after recanalization. Am J Cardiol 1982; 50:933–7.

Intracoronary streptokinase administered less than 4 hours after the onset of pain was beneficial in comparison to its administration more than 4 hours after the onset of infarction.

17. Smalling RW, Fuentes F, Freund GC, Reduto LA, Wanta-Matthews M, Gaeta JM, Walker W, Sterling R, Gould KL. Beneficial effects of intracoronary thrombolysis up to eighteen hours after onset of pain in evolving myocardial infarction. Am Heart J 1982; 104:912–20.

These investigators report that intracoronary streptokinase can be of benefit even when given up to 18 hours after the onset of chest pain.

18. Rentrop KP, Blanke H, Karsch KR. Effects of nonsurgical coronary reperfusion on the left ventricle in human subjects compared with conventional treatment: study of 18 patients with acute myocardial infarction treated with intracoronary infusion of streptokinase. Am J Cardiol 1982; 49:1–8.

This uncontrolled series suggests that intracoronary streptokinase preserved jeopardized myocardium in patients with myocardial infarction.

19. Schwarz F, Faure A, Katus H, Olshausen KV, Hofmann M, Schuler G, Manthey J, Kubler W. Intracoronary thrombolysis in acute myocardial infarction: an attempt to quantitate its effect by comparison of enzymatic estimate of myocardial necrosis with left ventricular ejection fraction. Am J Cardiol 1983; 51:1573–8.

Myocardial infarct size was significantly reduced in patients in whom coronary artery reperfusion occurred within 4 hours of pain.

CORONARY ARTERY SURGERY

Coronary artery bypass grafting is one of the most common surgical procedures performed in the United States. In patients with obstructive coronary artery disease, such bypass surgery is performed (1) to relieve limiting angina in those individuals who continue to have chest pain despite maximal medical therapy and (2) to improve longevity in those with especially severe coronary artery narrowing. Undoubtedly the most striking beneficial effect of coronary bypass grafting is a reduction in anginal frequency and severity, which occurs in about 85 percent of operative survivors. Of these, most have complete relief of angina, and the remainder report that their angina occurs less frequently and is more difficult to induce. Coronary bypass surgery clearly improves longevity (when compared to medical therapy) in patients with substantial narrowing of the left main coronary artery, and it may do so in those with more than 70-percent narrowing of all three major epicardial coronary arteries. In contrast, bypass grafting does not improve longevity in patients with narrowing of only one or two coronary arteries. Although bypass surgery is occasionally performed for other reasons, such as prevention of myocardial infarction, abolition of ventricular ectopic activity, improvement of left ventricular performance, or an improved chance for the patient to return to gainful employment, few controlled studies have demonstrated that it is effective in accomplishing these goals.

Coronary artery bypass grafting is most frequently performed using saphenous veins harvested from the patient's legs. These saphenous vein grafts are anastomosed to the ascending aorta and the distal portion of a diseased coronary artery. Occasionally the internal mammary artery is used, especially for grafting the left anterior descending coronary artery. Its advantages center (1) on the fact that a proximal anastomosis is not required, (2) on its high patency rate during the months to years after surgery, and (3) on the fact that intimal proliferation and subsequent narrowing does not occur postoperatively. Its disadvantages are (1) its limited length (making it difficult to use a mammary graft for a distal circumflex marginal artery or the posterior descending artery) and (2) the amount of time required to dissect it free from the anterior pleural surface. In this respect, even though the surgeon is required to perform only a distal anastomosis, the time required for arterial dissection is usually greater than that needed to perform a proximal anastomosis with a segment of autologous saphenous vein.

Perioperatively, myocardial infarction occurs in about 10 percent of patients undergoing coronary artery bypass grafting, and it is the most common cause of perioperative death. It is especially likely to occur when the procedure is complicated by hypotension or when operative time is prolonged. In most institutions, the operative mortality is 1 to 3 percent, although it is somewhat higher in patients with depressed left ventricular function or recent myocardial infarction.

Postoperatively, a small percentage (i.e., about 10%) of saphenous vein grafts become occluded within 2 weeks of bypass surgery, and an additional 10 to 20 percent do so within 1 year, so that the graft patency rate 1 year after surgery averages about 75 percent. These occlusions are almost always caused by acute thrombosis of the graft. The tendency to graft thrombosis appears to be dependent on the size of the coronary artery to which the graft is connected and the amount of myocardium supplied by that artery (i.e., the amount of so-called distal run-off). Recent studies have demonstrated that the pharmacologic inhibition of platelet function (with aspirin and dipyridamole) reduces the incidence of saphenous graft thrombosis during the weeks to months following bypass surgery. After 1 year postoperatively, graft occlusion is uncommon. When it occurs, it is usually due to intimal fibrosis of the graft and not to thrombosis. Coronary bypass grafting appears to induce an acceleration of arteriosclerotic disease in the proximal portions of grafted arteries, often leading to complete occlusion within months. The recurrence of angina several years after bypass grafting is usually due to progression of "native" disease and not to late graft occlusion.

1. McIntosh HD, Garcia JA. The first decade of aorto-coronary bypass grafting, 1967–77: a review. Circulation 1978; 57:405–31.
   A complete and critical review of the indications for bypass grafting. Includes 220 references.
2. Kloster FE, Kremkau EL, Ritzmann LW, Rahimtoola SH, Rosch J, Kanarek PH. Coronary bypass for stable angina: a prospective randomized study. N Engl J Med 1979; 300:149–57.
   Bypass surgery is better than medical therapy in improving functional class and minimizing the occurrence of unstable angina, but it exerts no effect on longevity.
3. Loop FD, Lytle BW, Cosgrove DM, Sheldon WC, Irarrazaval M, Taylor PC, Groves LK, Pichard AD. Atherosclerosis of the left main coronary artery: 5 year results of surgical treatment. Am J Cardiol 1979; 44:195–201.
   Of 300 consecutive patients with left main coronary artery narrowing subjected to bypass grafting, operative mortality was 4%. Of the remainder, 88% had patent grafts; 75% had no angina; and 94% were employed or fully active.
4. Knapp WS, Douglas JS Jr, Craver JM, Jones EL, King SB III, Bone DK, Bradford JM, Hatcher CR Jr. Efficacy of coronary artery bypass grafting in elderly patients with coronary artery disease. Am J Cardiol 1981; 47:923–30.

In a series of 121 patients over age 70 undergoing bypass grafting, the results were generally good, although the complication rate was somewhat higher than that for younger patients.

5. Josa M, Lie JT, Bianco RL, Kaye MP. Reduction of thrombosis in canine coronary bypass vein grafts with dipyridamole and aspirin. Am J Cardiol 1981; 47:1248–54.
   In dogs with saphenous vein grafting, a regimen of dipyridamole and aspirin effectively reduced early graft thrombosis.

6. Chesebro JH, Clements IP, Fuster V, Elveback LR, Smith HC, Bardsley WT, Frye RL, Holmes DR Jr, Vliestra RE, Pluth JR, Wallace RB, Puga FJ, Orszulak TA, Piehler JM, Schaff HV, Danielson GK. A platelet-inhibitor-drug trial in coronary-artery bypass operations: benefit of perioperative dipyridamole and aspirin therapy on early postoperative vein-graft patency. N Engl J Med 1982; 307:73–8.
   In 407 patients undergoing coronary bypass grafting, dipyridamole and aspirin were better than placebo in preventing graft occlusion early after operation.

7. Chaitman BR, Fisher LD, Bourassa MG, Davis K, Rogers WJ, Maynard C, Tyras DH, Berger RL, Judkins MP, Ringqvist I, Mock MB, Killip T. Effect of coronary bypass surgery on survival patterns in subsets of patients with left main coronary artery disease: report of the collaborative study in coronary artery surgery (CASS). Am J Cardiol 1981; 48:765–77.
   Of 1,492 patients with left main disease, the 3-year survival was 91% for those treated surgically and 69% for those treated medically.

8. Lytle BW, Loop FD, Thurer RL, Groves LK, Taylor PC, Cosgrove DM. Isolated left anterior descending coronary atherosclerosis: long-term comparison of internal mammary artery and venous autografts. Circulation 1980; 61:869–74.
   At recatheterization 20–24 months after surgery, 91% of mammary grafts were patent, whereas 79% of saphenous vein grafts were patent.

9. Norris RM, Agnew TM, Brandt PWT, Graham KJ, Hill DG, Kerr AR, Lowe JB, Roche AHG, Whitlock RML, Barratt-Boyes BG. Coronary surgery after recurrent myocardial infarction: progress of a trial comparing surgical with nonsurgical management for asymptomatic patients with advanced coronary disease. Circulation 1981; 63:785–92.
   In the absence of disabling angina or left main coronary artery stenosis, coronary bypass grafting need not be advised for survivors of recurrent infarction, even if they have severe coronary artery disease.

10. Kennedy JW, Kaiser GC, Fisher LD, Fritz JK, Myers W, Mudd JG, Ryan TJ. Clinical and angiographic predictors of operative mortality from the collaborative study in coronary artery surgery (CASS). Circulation 1981; 63:793–802.
    In this large multicenter study, operative mortality for elective bypass surgery was 1.7%. Advanced age, female sex, symptoms of heart failure, left main coronary artery stenosis, impaired left ventricular function, and nonelective surgery were each associated with a higher operative mortality.

11. Peduzzi P, Hultgren HN. Effect of medical vs. surgical treatment on symptoms in stable angina pectoris: the Veterans Administration cooperative study of surgery for coronary arterial occlusive disease. Circulation 1979; 60:888–900.
    In this large randomized study, bypass surgery was better than medical therapy at relieving angina.

12. Hammermeister KE, DeRouen TA, English MT, Dodge HT. Effect of surgical versus medical therapy on return to work in patients with coronary artery disease. Am J Cardiol 1979; 44:105–11.
    In this large study of about 1400 patients, surgical therapy was not more effective than medical therapy in maintaining full-time employment. Work status 3 months before surgery or catheterization was the best predictor of continued employment 15 months later.

13. Seides SF, Borer JS, Kent KM, Rosing DR, McIntosh CL, Epstein SE. Long-term anatomic fate of coronary artery bypass grafts and functional status of patients five years after operation. N Engl J Med 1978; 298:1213–7.
    Most saphenous vein grafts that are patent several months after operation remain so for at least 4½ years. Although most patients improve symptomatically postoperatively, symptomatic deterioration is common in the succeeding years and is usually due to progression of disease in ungrafted vessels.

14. Campeau L, Lesperance J, Hermann J, Corbara F, Grondin CM, Bourassa MG. Loss of the improvement of angina between 1 and 7 years after aortocoronary bypass surgery: correlations with changes in vein grafts and in coronary arteries. Circulation 1979; 60(Suppl I):1–5.
   In 75 patients undergoing bypass surgery, 61 (81%) were improved symptomatically 1 year after operation. Over the next 5 years, however, loss of improvement occurred in 22 (36%) of the 61. In most of these patients, this deterioration of results was related to a progression of atherosclerosis, particularly in ungrafted coronary arteries.

15. Murphy ML, Hultgren HN, Detre K, Thomsen J, Takaro T. Treatment of chronic stable angina: a preliminary report of survival data of the randomized Veterans Administration cooperative study. N Engl J Med 1977; 297:621–7.
   In patients with 1-, 2-, and 3-vessel coronary artery disease randomized to medical or surgical therapy, there was no difference in survival 36 months later.

16. Pantely GA, Goodnight SH Jr, Rahimtoola SH, Harlan BJ, DeMots H, Calvin L, Rosch J. Failure of antiplatelet and anticoagulant therapy to improve patency of grafts after coronary artery bypass: a controlled, randomized study. N Engl J Med 1979; 301:962–6.
   Neither an aspirin-dipyridamole combination nor coumadin improved graft patency when they were initiated 3 days postoperatively.

17. Favaloro RG. Direct myocardial revascularization: a ten year journey. Myths and realities. Am J Cardiol 1979; 43:109–29.
   A thorough review of the indications and results of bypass surgery.

18. Hurst JW, King SB III, Logue RB, Hatcher CR Jr, Jones EL, Craver JM, Douglas JS Jr, Franch RH, Dorney ER, Cobbs BW Jr, Robinson PH, Clements SD Jr, Kaplan JA, Bradford JM. Value of coronary bypass surgery. Controversies in cardiology: Part I. Am J Cardiol 1978; 42:308–29.
   The authors recommend bypass surgery in patients with 2- and 3-vessel disease to improve longevity, but those recommendations are not based on data from randomized studies.

19. Jones EL, Craver JM, Guyton RA, Bone DK, Hatcher CR Jr, Riechwald N. Importance of complete revascularization in performance of the coronary bypass operation. Am J Cardiol 1983; 51:7–12.
   Long-term relief of angina and survival are both dependent on complete revascularization.

20. Hamilton WM, Hammermeister KE, DeRouen TA, Zia MS, Dodge HT. Effect of coronary artery bypass grafting on subsequent hospitalization. Am J Cardiol 1983; 51:353–60.
   In comparison to those treated medically, the patients who underwent coronary bypass grafting had a 26% reduction in cardiovascular hospitalizations.

21. Gersh BJ, Kronmal RA, Frye RL, Schaff HV, Ryan TJ, Gosselin AJ, Kaiser GC, Killip T III, and participants in the coronary artery surgery study. Coronary arteriography and coronary artery bypass surgery: morbidity and mortality in patients ages 65 years or older. A report from the coronary artery surgery study. Circulation 1983; 67:483–91.
   In patients over age 65 undergoing coronary bypass surgery, operative mortality was higher (5.2%) than those under age 65 (1.9%).

22. Loop FD, Golding LR, MacMillan JP, Cosgrove DM, Lytle BW, Sheldon WC. Coronary artery surgery in women compared with men: analyses of risks and long-term results. JACC 1983; 1:383–90.
   In comparison to men, women undergoing coronary bypass grafting had a lower graft patency rate and a lower percentage of freedom from angina. However, overall survival was similar for women and men.

PERCUTANEOUS TRANSLUMINAL ANGIOPLASTY

About 20 years ago, the technique of transluminal angioplasty for the treatment of atherosclerotic obstruction of the femoral artery was introduced, and throughout the late 1960s and 1970s it was employed in a limited number of medical centers in this country. In the late 1970s, the equipment for angioplasty was modified and refined to allow dilatation of the renal artery and the coronary artery. Over the past 5 years, percutaneous transluminal angioplasty of the coronary arteries has been performed successfully in many patients with one-, two-, and even three-vessel coronary artery disease.

The ideal candidate for transluminal coronary angioplasty is a patient with a relatively brief history of angina, i.e., several weeks in duration. The recent onset of symptoms increases the likelihood that the patient's atherosclerotic coronary arterial narrowings are not calcified and are therefore compressible with an intraluminal balloon catheter. At the time of coronary arteriography, the patient ideally should have a single, isolated stenosis of one coronary artery that is less than 1.0 to 1.5 cm in length. Finally, the patient should meet all requirements as a reasonable candidate for coronary artery bypass surgery, since surgical revascularization may be necessary if angioplasty is unsuccessful or if it creates an emergent problem (e.g., dissection of a coronary artery). As experience with coronary angioplasty is gathered, some physicians have begun to perform multiple dilatations in the same patient. For the most part, however, the technique still appears best suited for patients with isolated and relatively proximal single-vessel coronary artery disease.

Percutaneous transluminal coronary angioplasty involves the inflation of a distensible balloon within a significant coronary stenosis, with subsequent compression or disruption of the atheromatous lesion. After baseline coronary arteriography, a large-bore guiding catheter is advanced to the appropriate coronary ostium, through which a smaller sized balloon dilatation catheter is advanced over a soft guide wire. Once the guide wire has been advanced beyond the stenosis that is to be dilated, the balloon dilation catheter is gently advanced over it. Once within the stenosis, the balloon is fully inflated for 5 to 15 seconds with 5 to 6 atm of pressure, after which it is deflated. The brief inflation of the balloon may be repeated several times within a period of several minutes. The balloon initially is seen to expand at both ends, with a central indentation due to the profile of the coronary stenosis. This central indentation typically resolves as the stenosis is successfully dilated.

In experienced hands, percutaneous transluminal coronary angioplasty appears to be an effective therapeutic modality in patients with limiting angina who would otherwise require coronary artery bypass grafting for symptomatic relief. Its overall success rate is dependent on patient selection, but in most series it averages about 70 percent. Although complications are reported to occur in 15 to 20 percent of patients undergoing angioplasty, most are correctable by emergent coronary bypass surgery, so that the overall mortality for the procedure is 0.9 percent in patients in whom one vessel is dilated and 1.9 percent in those in whom two or more vessels are dilated. During the first 4 to 6 months after successful angioplasty, about 30 percent of the stenoses recur, but these are usually amenable to repeat angioplasty. At present, its longer term effects are unknown, since most patients who have undergone this procedure have done so within the past 2 to 3 years.

1. Gruntzig AR, Senning A, Siegenthaler WE. Nonoperative dilatation of coronary artery stenosis: percutaneous transluminal coronary angioplasty. N Engl J Med 1979; 301:61–8.
   Of 50 patients having this procedure, 32 had a good result, emergency coronary bypass was necessary in 5, and 3 had angioplasty-induced infarction.
2. Cowley MJ, Vetrovec GW, Wolfgang TC. Efficacy of percutaneous transluminal coronary angioplasty: technique, patient selection, salutary results, limitations, and complications. Am Heart J 1981; 101:272–80.
   This article describes the authors' early angioplasty experience in 25 patients.

3. Kent KM, Bentivoglio LG, Block PC, Cowley MJ, Dorros G, Gosselin AJ, Gruntzig A, Myler RK, Simpson J, Stertzer SH, Williams DO, Fisher L, Gillespie MJ, Detre K, Kelsey S, Mullin SM, Mock MB. Percutaneous transluminal coronary angioplasty: report from the registry of the National Heart, Lung, and Blood Institute. Am J Cardiol 1982; 49:2011–20.

   Of 631 patients in whom angioplasty was performed, it was successful in 373 (59%) of the stenosed arteries. Emergency bypass surgery was required in 40 (6%); myocardial infarction occurred in 29 (4%).

4. Hirzel HO, Nuesch K, Gruentzig AR, Luetolf UM. Short- and long-term changes in myocardial perfusion after percutaneous transluminal coronary angioplasty assessed by thallium-201 exercise scintigraphy. Circulation 1981; 63:1001–7.

   In 49 patients in whom angioplasty was performed, thallium-201 exercise scintigraphy demonstrated improved flow to the myocardium distal to the dilated stenosis.

5. Kent KM, Bonow RO, Rosing DR, Ewels CJ, Lipson LC, McIntosh CL, Bacharach S, Green M, Epstein SE. Improved myocardial function during exercise after successful percutaneous transluminal coronary angioplasty. N Engl J Med 1982; 306:441–6.

   Of 59 consecutive patients subjected to angioplasty, a successful result was achieved in 38 (64%).

6. Sigwart U, Grbic M, Essinger A, Bischof-Delaloye A, Sadeghi H, Rivier JL. Improvement of left ventricular function after percutaneous transluminal coronary angioplasty. Am J Cardiol 1982; 49:651–7.

   In 7 patients with severe stenoses of the left anterior descending artery, successful coronary angioplasty greatly improved left ventricular ejection fraction during exercise.

7. Simpson JB, Baim DS, Robert EW, Harrison DC. A new catheter system for coronary angioplasty. Am J Cardiol 1982; 49:1216–22.

   A detailed description of the technical aspects of coronary angioplasty.

8. David PR, Waters DD, Scholl JM, Crepeau J, Szlachcic J, Lesperance J, Hudon G, Bourassa MG. Percutaneous transluminal coronary angioplasty in patients with variant angina. Circulation 1982; 66:695–702.

   Although coronary angioplasty is technically feasible in patients with variant angina and organic coronary arterial stenoses, symptoms due to coronary spasm usually persist or recur.

9. Meier B, Gruentzig AR, Hollman J, Ischinger T, Bradford JM. Does length or eccentricity of coronary stenoses influence the outcome of transluminal dilatation? Circulation 1983; 67:497–9.

   In 526 patients undergoing a first coronary angioplasty, stenoses that were long and eccentric had the highest incidence of complications, and stenoses that were short and concentric had the lowest.

10. Dorros G, Cowley MJ, Simpson J, Bentivoglio LG, Block PC, Bourassa M, Detre K, Gosselin AJ, Gruentzig AR, Kelsey SF, Kent KM, Mock MB, Mullin SM, Myler RK, Passamani ER, Stertzer SH, Williams DO. Percutaneous transluminal coronary angioplasty: report of complications from the National Heart, Lung, and Blood Institute PTCA registry. Circulation 1983; 67:723–30.

    Of the first 1,500 coronary angioplasties performed in this country, 945 (63%) were successful. Complications occurred in 315 (21%); the most frequent were prolonged angina, myocardial infarction, and coronary occlusion. The overall mortality was 13 (0.85%).

11. Goldberg S, Urban PL, Greenspon A, Lebenthal M, Walinsky P, Maroko P. Combination therapy for evolving myocardial infarction: intracoronary thrombolysis and percutaneous transluminal angioplasty. Am J Med 1982; 72:994–7.

    The case report of a 50-year-old woman in whom both intracoronary streptokinase infusion and angioplasty were performed emergently.

12. Meltzer RS, vanden Brand M, Serruys PW, Fioretti P, Hugenholtz PG. Sequential intracoronary streptokinase and transluminal angioplasty in unstable angina with evolving myocardial infarction. Am Heart J 1982; 104:1109–11.

    This case report demonstrates that intracoronary streptokinase and coronary angioplasty can be used sequentially to provide reperfusion in the setting of impending myocardial infarction.

REHABILITATION AFTER MYOCARDIAL INFARCTION

Following a myocardial infarction, the patient should be encouraged (1) to accept and understand his underlying disease process, (2) to minimize (as much as possible) the various risk factors of atherosclerotic disease, and (3) to return eventually (if possible) to independence and productivity. An acceptance and understanding of coronary artery disease should begin as soon as the patient has left the intensive care unit for an intermediate facility, that is, on day 3 or 4 of hospitalization. At the same time, the patient should be encouraged to discontinue smoking and to lose weight, if needed. During the initial 3 to 7 days of hospitalization, the patient may require a good deal of emotional support and encouragement, since an illness of catastrophic potential (such as a myocardial infarction) can lead to severe anxiety and depression.

After several days in the hospital, the patient should begin a gradual increase in physical activity, so that by the seventh to tenth day after infarction he is walking in the corridor without problems. About 10 to 14 days after infarction, just before hospital discharge, the patient should undergo submaximal exercise tolerance testing. If it is markedly abnormal in any respect (e.g., the appearance of angina, severe dyspnea, arrhythmias, hypotension, or marked S–T segment shifts), the patient should be referred for catheterization before discharge. In contrast, if the patient has no problem with the submaximal exercise test, he should be discharged, after which a graduated exercise program should be continued. The patient should avoid isometric activities, such as lifting. He should be given fresh nitroglycerin tablets and should be familiar with their use. The patient may return to part-time work 4 to 6 weeks after infarction and to full-time employment at 2 to 3 months.

Three to four months after myocardial infarction, the patient should undergo maximal exercise tolerance testing. If it is normal, the patient should be encouraged to take part in a medically supervised, formal rehabilitation program in which he gradually increases the level of exertion. Although such exercise programs improve the patient's sense of well-being, they have not been proved to alter the incidence of reinfarction or death during the 2 years after infarction, nor have they been shown to modify myocardial perfusion or function. Thus, the principal indication for exercise rehabilitation is the feeling of self-confidence and optimism gained by the patient.

1. Wenger NK, Hellerstein HK, Blackburn H, Castranova SJ. Uncomplicated myocardial infarction: current physician practice in patient management. JAMA 1973; 224:511–4.
   In a large group of postinfarction patients, 87% returned to work 2–4 months after uncomplicated myocardial infarction.
2. Hellerstein HK, Friedman EH. Sexual activity and the postcoronary patient. Arch Int Med 1970; 125:987–99.
   Over 80 % of patients who have sustained a myocardial infarction can fulfill the physiologic demands of most jobs and of sexual activity without symptoms of ischemic heart disease.
3. Bilodeau CB, Hackett TP. Issues raised in a group setting by patients recovering from myocardial infarction. Am J Psych 1971; 128:73–8.
   Group psychotherapy was very helpful in this group of 5 male patients after a myocardial infarction.
4. Lee AP, Ice R, Blessey R, Sanmarco ME. Long-term effects of physical training on coronary patients with impaired ventricular function. Circulation 1979; 60:1519–26.
   In 18 patients with coronary heart disease and a left ventricular ejection fraction below 0.40, exercise training was beneficial, as reflected by an improvement in functional aerobic capacity and both resting and submaximal heart rates.

5. Jensen D, Atwood JE, Froelicher V, McKirnan MD, Battler A, Ashburn W, Ross J Jr. Improvement in ventricular function during exercise studied with radionuclide ventriculography after cardiac rehabilitation. Am J Cardiol 1980; 46:770–7.

In a group of 19 consecutive patients with coronary artery disease, exercise training for 6 months induced an improvement in left ventricular function.

6. Shaw LW. Effects of a prescribed supervised exercise program on mortality and cardiovascular morbidity in patients after a myocardial infarction: the national exercise and heart disease project. Am J Cardiol 1981; 48:39–46.

The results of this study suggest that a program of prescribed supervised physical activity for patients after myocardial infarction may be beneficial in reducing subsequent cardiac mortality, but the evidence is not convincing.

7. Magder S, Linnarsson D, Gullstrand L. The effect of swimming on patients with ischemic heart disease. Circulation 1981; 63:979–86.

In 8 patients with ischemic heart disease, swimming, even at a comfortable speed, required near-maximal effort. Poor swimmers with ischemic heart disease should avoid swimming as an exercise unless properly supervised.

8. Naughton J, Bruhn J, Lategola MT, Whitsett T. Rehabilitation following myocardial infarction. Am J Med 1969; 46:725–34.

A succinct review of the advantages and design of a cardiac rehabilitation program.

9. Kellermann JJ. Rehabilitation of patients with coronary heart disease. Prog Cardiovasc Dis 1975; 17:303–28.

A thorough review of cardiac rehabilitation. Includes 97 references.

10. Redwood DR, Rosing DR, Epstein SE. Circulatory and symptomatic effects of physical training in patients with coronary artery disease and angina pectoris. N Engl J Med 1972; 286:959–65.

In 7 patients with ischemic heart disease, an organized exercise program improved exercise performance by reducing the responses of heart rate and arterial pressure to exercise.

11. Mead WF, Pyfer HR, Trombold JC, Frederick RC. Successful resuscitation of two near simultaneous cases of cardiac arrest with a review of fifteen cases occurring during supervised exercise. Circulation 1976; 53:187–9.

Individuals with known coronary artery disease should participate in exercise training under proper supervision, since ventricular fibrillation occurs in a small number.

12. Letac B, Cribier A, Desplanches JF. A study of left ventricular function in coronary patients before and after physical training. Circulation 1977; 56:375–8.

In 15 subjects recovering from myocardial infarction, training exerted no effect on myocardial function.

13. Haskell WL. Cardiovascular complications during exercise training of cardiac patients. Circulation 1978; 57:920–4.

During more than 1.6 million hours of exercise by patients enrolled in a group of cardiac rehabilitation programs, there were 50 cardiac arrests, 8 of which were fatal.

14. Kavanagh T, Shephard RJ, Tuck JA. Depression after myocardial infarction. Can Med Assoc J 1975; 113:23–7.

Of 101 patients studied by psychologic testing 16–18 months after a myocardial infarction, 34 were clearly depressed. These individuals tended to be older and to have a greater tendency to hypertension and angina.

15. Kavanagh T, Shephard RJ. Sexual activity after myocardial infarction. Can Med Assoc J 1977; 116:1250–3.

Of 161 patients surveyed 3 years after myocardial infarction, about half continued the same amount of sexual activity as before infarction. In the other half, sexual activity was reduced.

16. McLane M, Krop H, Mehta J. Psychosexual adjustment and counseling after myocardial infarction. Ann Intern Med 1980; 92:514–9.

This article emphasizes that resumption of sexual activity is important to the rehabilitation of patients and their partners.

17. Shephard RJ. Recurrence of myocardial infarction in an exercising population. Br Heart J 1979; 42:133–8.

A small percentage of patients sustain reinfarction during an exercise rehabilitation program, but there is no way to identify these individuals prospectively.

18. Nagle R, Gangola R, Picton-Robinson I. Factors influencing return to work after myocardial infarction. Lancet 1971; 2:454–6.

    Of those patients who do not return to work after sustaining an infarction, about half are limited by cardiac symptoms, whereas the other half are limited by anxiety and depression.

19. Oldridge NB, Donner AP, Buck CW, Jones NL, Andrew GM, Parker JO, Cunningham DA, Kavanagh T, Rechnitzer PA, Sutton JR. Predictors of dropout from cardiac exercise rehabilitation: Ontario exercise-heart collaborative study. Am J Cardiol 1983; 51:70–4.

    In this study of 733 men during rehabilitation after myocardial infarction, smoking and a blue collar occupation were predictors of dropout.

20. Vermeulen A, Lie KI, Durrer D. Effects of cardiac rehabilitation after myocardial infarction: changes in coronary risk factors and long-term prognosis. Am Heart J 1983; 105:798–801.

    In this analysis of 98 men with myocardial infarction, rehabilitation was beneficial and was associated with a lowering of serum cholesterol.

21. Murray GC, Beller GA. Cardiac rehabilitation following coronary artery bypass surgery. Am Heart J 1983; 105:1009–18.

    A succinct review of the advantages of an exercise program for patients who have recently had coronary artery bypass surgery. Includes 95 references.

MYOCARDIAL AND PERICARDIAL DISEASES

HYPERTROPHIC CARDIOMYOPATHY

Hypertrophic cardiomyopathy is characterized by an increased left ventricular wall thickness of unknown etiology. It can be *nonobstructive* or *obstructive,* depending on whether there is obstruction to left ventricular outflow, with a resultant pressure gradient between the left ventricular cavity and the aorta. *Nonobstructive hypertrophic cardiomyopathy* is characterized by concentric left ventricular hypertrophy of unknown cause. Systolic left ventricular performance is usually normal, but diastolic function is distinctly abnormal, since the hypertrophied left ventricle is stiff and noncompliant. As a result, left-sided filling pressures are elevated. Often, therefore, the patient with nonobstructive hypertrophic cardiomyopathy complains of dyspnea on exertion, since an exercise-induced augmentation of cardiac output causes an increase in left ventricular diastolic and left atrial pressures. Less commonly, these individuals may complain of chest pain suggestive of angina pectoris.

The noninvasive evaluation of the patient with nonobstructive hypertrophic cardiomyopathy reveals a normal sized but diffusely thickened left ventricle with normal systolic wall motion. The ECG reveals evidence of left ventricular hypertrophy. At cardiac catheterization, left ventricular filling pressures are elevated, and systolic left ventricular function is normal. The coronary arteries are often widely patent.

The patient with nonobstructive hypertrophic cardiomyopathy should be treated with a pharmacologic agent that promotes myocardial relaxation. The drug of choice is verapamil, 120 mg 3 or 4 times daily. If, for some reason, the patient cannot tolerate this agent, diltiazem, another calcium antagonist, should be administered in a dosage of 90 mg 3 or 4 times daily. Alternatively, the calcium antagonist nifedipine can be given in a dosage of 20 mg 3 or 4 times daily. These calcium blockers promote left ventricular relaxation during diastole, thus reducing left ventricular filling pressures, promoting left ventricular filling, and improving cardiac output.

Obstructive hypertrophic cardiomyopathy is much more commonly encountered than the nonobstructive variety. In the past, it has been termed idiopathic hypertrophic subaortic stenosis (IHSS), asymmetric septal hypertrophy (ASH), familial hypertrophic subaortic stenosis, and muscular subaortic stenosis. In most patients, this disorder is inherited as an autosomal dominant trait with a high degree of penetrance, although an occasional patient with it does not have a familial association. Pathophysiologically, obstructive hypertrophic cardiomyopathy is characterized by (1) a greatly thickened interventricular septum, which, on microscopic examination, demonstrates a characteristic disarray of myocardial fibers, (2) a variable and dynamic obstruction to left ventricular outflow in association with some degree of systolic anterior motion of the anterior mitral valve leaflet, (3) some degree of mitral regurgitation, and (4) a restriction to left ventricular filling, presumably the result of increased wall stiffness because of myocardial hypertrophy.

Although symptomatic obstructive hypertrophic cardiomyopathy is most frequently a disease of young adults, one-third of all patients coming to cardiac catheterization with this entity are older than 60 years. Most commonly, the patient with this disorder complains of symptoms of pulmonary vascular congestion: dyspnea, orthopnea, and paroxysmal nocturnal dyspnea, which result from the elevated left ventricular diastolic pressure. Alternatively, the patient may note angina pectoris, which may be due to concomitant atherosclerotic coronary artery disease or to an inadequate coronary vascular reserve even without intrinsic stenoses. An occasional individual with this disorder complains of syncope or near-syncope, due to an inability to increase cardiac output during exertion because of left ventricular outflow tract obstruction. Finally, some patients with obstructive hypertropic cardiomyopathy manifest their disease by dying suddenly.

On physical examination, the patient with obstructive hypertrophic cardiomyopathy has a rapid carotid upstroke. The carotid pulse may be bisferiens in configuration or may simply be characterized by a rapid upstroke, a prolonged ejection time, and an identifiable second dicrotic notch in its descent. The peripheral pulse is almost always regular, since most of these patients are in normal sinus rhythm. On cardiac examination, the apical impulse is often displaced laterally and is abnormally forceful and enlarged. An especially prominent a wave may be palpable at the cardiac apex, resulting in a double apical impulse. On occasion, a triple apical impulse may be palpable, with the third component representing a late systolic bulge that occurs when the dynamic left ventricular obstruction is marked. A systolic thrill may be palpable at the apex or along the left lower sternal border.

On auscultation, the S_1 is usually normal. The S_2 is often normal, but in patients with severe obstruction it may be paradoxically split. A prominent S_4 is present. Systolic ejection clicks are absent. A systolic ejection murmur is audible along the left sternal border; it usually radiates to the base of the heart but is not well appreciated in the carotids. The murmur increases in intensity with any physiologic or pharmacologic maneuver that reduces left ventricular cavitary size or increases contractility: the Valsalva maneuver, amyl nitrite, nitroglycerin, hypovolemia, digitalis, or catecholamines. Conversely, the murmur is diminished in intensity with any maneuver that increases left ventricular volume or decreases contractility, such as squatting, volume loading, isometric exertion (handgrip), or the administration of a beta-adrenergic blocking agent. Apart from the murmur of left ventricular outflow obstruction, many patients with obstructive hypertrophic cardiomyopathy have an apical holosystolic murmur of mitral regurgitation.

The ECG usually demonstrates left ventricular hypertrophy. About 10 to 15 percent of these patients have a "pseudoinfarct" pattern of poor R wave progression across the precordium. Although an occasional patient has atrial fibrillation, most are in sinus rhythm. Atrial fibrillation is often poorly tolerated hemodynamically, since these patients are especially dependent on atrial contraction to fill a stiff and noncompliant ventricle. For this reason, the patient with obstructive hypertrophic cardiomyopathy in whom atrial fibrillation develops may require emergent cardioversion. Echocardiographically, the patient demonstrates left ventricular hypertrophy, which preferentially involves the interventricular septum, so that the ratio of septal thickness to posterior left ventricular wall thickness is at least 1 : 1.3. The left ventricular outflow tract is narrowed, and there is systolic anterior motion of the anterior leaflet of the mitral valve. Radionuclide blood pool imaging may demonstrate left ventricular cavitary obliteration during systole as well as disproportionate upper septal thickening. Thallium 201 scintigraphy may show asymmetric septal thickening.

At cardiac catheterization, the patient with obstructive hypertrophic cardiomyopathy has diminished left ventricular compliance and a pressure gradient within the body of the left ventricle that may be labile. Some patients with this disorder have no gradient in the baseline state, but one is provoked during an infusion of isoproterenol. About 15 percent of patients also have hemodynamic evidence of right ventricular outflow tract obstruction. On angiography, the left ventricular wall appears thickened, and there is a variable amount of mitral regurgitation. Left ventricular systolic function is usually vigorous, resulting in virtual obliteration of the cavity at end-systole.

The medical treatment of the patient with obstructive hypertrophic cardiomyopathy involves the administration of propranolol (a beta-adrenergic blocker) or verapamil (a calcium antagonist). Both agents reduce the magnitude of left ventricular outflow obstruction and diminish symptoms. Digitalis, diuretics, and nitrates are contraindicated. In addition to propranolol or verapamil, antiarrhythmic therapy is probably indicated if ambulatory electrocardiographic monitoring demonstrates complex ventricular ectopy, since patients with such ectopy are at high risk of sudden death. If medical therapy is unsuccessful in alleviating symptoms, the patient should be referred for surgical treatment. The most popular operation for this disorder is a septal myectomy, whereby a portion of the hypertrophied septum is excised. Although mitral valve replacement has been advocated by some as the procedure of choice, septectomy alone usually cures the mitral regurgitation and relieves the outflow obstruction. The operative mortality is 5 to 10 percent.

Etiology

1. Clark CE, Henry WL, Epstein SE. Familial prevalence and genetic transmission of idiopathic hypertrophic subaortic stenosis. N Engl J Med 1973; 289:709–14.
   Most cases of this disorder are due to a genetic defect that is transmitted as an autosomal dominant trait with a high degree of penetrance.

Pathology

2. Ferrans VJ, Morrow AG, Roberts WC. Myocardial ultrastructure in idiopathic hypertrophic subaortic stenosis. A study of operatively excised left ventricular outflow tract muscle in 14 patients. Circulation 1972; 45:769–92.
   In 14 patients with this disease, the septal muscle cells were severely disorganized, with cells running in different directions instead of in parallel.
3. Bulkley BH, Weisfeldt ML, Hutchins GM. Asymmetric septal hypertrophy and myocardial fiber disarray: features of normal, developing, and malformed hearts. Circulation 1977; 56:292–8.
   In addition to obstructive hypertrophic cardiomyopathy, marked muscle fiber disarray may occur in certain congenital disorders characterized by abnormal systolic contraction, such as aortic atresia with intact ventricular septum.
4. Pomerance A, Davies MJ. Pathological features of hypertrophic obstructive cardiomyopathy (HOCM) in the elderly. Br Heart J 1975; 37:305–12.
   Of 15 elderly patients with this disorder whose hearts were examined at postmortem, two-thirds demonstrated substantial hypertrophy of the left ventricular free wall, thus making the diagnosis of asymmetric septal hypertrophy difficult during life.
5. Maron BJ, Sato N, Roberts WC, Edwards JE, Chandra RS. Quantitative analysis of cardiac muscle cell disorganization in the ventricular septum. Comparison of fetuses and infants with and without congenital heart disease and patients with hypertrophic cardiomyopathy. Circulation 1979; 60:685–96.
   Extensive ventricular septal disorganization is a highly sensitive and specific finding for hypertrophic cardiomyopathy. However, small areas of disorganization may occur in infants with other heart diseases, including aortic and pulmonary valve atresia.
6. Maron BJ, Epstein SE. Hypertrophic cardiomyopathy—recent observations regarding the specificity of three hallmarks of the disease: asymmetric septal hypertrophy, septal disorganization, and systolic anterior motion of the anterior mitral leaflet. Am J Cardiol 1980; 45:141–54.
   Although cell disorganization in the ventricular septum may occur with other cardiac malformations, extensive disorganization is present in about 90% of patients with hypertrophic cardiomyopathy and in only about 5% of patients with other cardiac diseases.
7. Isner JM, Maron BJ, Roberts WC. Comparison of amount of myocardial cell disorganization in operatively excised septectomy specimens with amount observed at

necropsy in 18 patients with hypertrophic cardiomyopathy. Am J. Cardiol 1980; 46:42–7.
Histologic examination of operatively excised septectomy specimens is of limited value in confirming the diagnosis of hypertrophic cardiomyopathy.

Clinical Characteristics and Natural History

8. Whiting RB, Powell WJ Jr, Dinsmore RE, Sanders CA. Idiopathic hypertrophic subaortic stenosis in the elderly. N Engl J Med 1971; 285:196–200.
Of 44 patients found to have this disorder, 14 (32%) were over age 60.

9. Frank S, Braunwald E. Idiopathic hypertrophic subaortic stenosis: clinical analysis of 126 patients with emphasis on the natural history. Circulation 1968; 37:759–88.
Of 126 patients with this disorder followed for up to 12 years, 10 died, 6 suddenly.

10. Adelman AG, Wigle ED, Ranganathan N, Webb GD, Kidd BSL, Bigelow WG, Silver MD. The clinical course in muscular subaortic stenosis: a retrospective and prospective study of 60 hemodynamically proved cases. Ann Intern Med 1972; 77:515–25.
Once symptoms begin, this disorder tends to be progressive.

11. McKenna WJ, Chetty S, Oakley CM, Goodwin JF. Arrhythmia in hypertrophic cardiomyopathy: exercise and 48-hour ambulatory electrocardiographic assessment with and without beta adrenergic blocking therapy. Am J Cardiol 1980; 45:1–5.
Asymptomatic ventricular ectopy is common in these patients and is usually not suppressed by beta blockers. This ectopy may contribute to sudden death in these patients.

12. Canedo MI, Frank MJ, Abdulla AM. Rhythm disturbances in hypertrophic cardiomyopathy: prevalence, relation to symptoms, and management. Am J Cardiol 1980; 45:848–55.
Of 33 patients with this disorder, arrhythmias were found in 29 (88%) and were potentially life-threatening in 13 (39%).

13. McKenna W, Deanfield J, Faruqui A, England D, Oakley C, Goodwin J. Prognosis in hypertrophic cardiomyopathy: role of age and clinical, electrocardiographic, and hemodynamic features. Am J Cardiol 1981; 47:532–8.
In a large group of patients with hypertrophic myopathy, the combination of young age, syncope at the time of diagnosis, severe dyspnea at follow-up, and a family history of sudden death best predicted sudden death.

14. Maron BJ, Savage DD, Wolfson JK, Epstein SE. Prognostic significance of 24-hour ambulatory electrocardiographic monitoring in patients with hypertrophic cardiomyopathy: a prospective study. Am J Cardiol 1981, 48:252–7.
The finding of ventricular tachycardia on a 24-hour Holter monitor identifies a subgroup of patients at high risk of sudden death.

Diagnosis

15. Angoff GH, Wistran D, Sloss LJ, Markis JE, Come PC, Zoll PM, Cohn PF. Value of a noninvasively induced ventricular extrasystole during echocardiographic and phonocardiographic assessment of patients with idiopathic hypertrophic subaortic stenosis. Am J Cardiol 1978; 42:919–24.
In patients with obstructive hypertrophic cardiomyopathy, the noninvasive induction of a ventricular extrasystole is a useful and easily performed procedure for diagnosis and evaluation of the pressure gradient.

16. Savage DD, Seides SF, Clark CE, Henry WL, Maron BJ, Robinson FC, Epstein SE. Electrocardiographic findings in patients with obstructive and nonobstructive hypertrophic cardiomyopathy. Circulation 1978; 58:402–8.
Of 134 patients with hypertrophic cardiomyopathy, repolarization abnormalities and left ventricular hypertrophy were the most common abnormalities, occurring in 109 (81%) and 83 (62%), respectively.

17. Henry WL, Clark CE, Glancy DL, Epstein SE. Echocardiographic measurement of the left ventricular outflow gradient in idiopathic hypertrophic subaortic stenosis. N Engl J Med 1973; 288:989–93.
Echocardiography demonstrates that the pressure gradient in this disorder is caused by narrowing of the left ventricular outflow tract; furthermore, echocardiography can be used to quantitate the gradient.

18. Rossen RM, Goodman DJ, Ingham RE, Popp RL. Echocardiographic criteria in the

diagnosis of idiopathic hypertrophic subaortic stenosis. Circulation 1974; 50:747–51. *In 4 individuals with this disorder, systolic anterior motion of the mitral valve was present in the absence of a pressure gradient across the left ventricular outflow tract.*

19. Martin RP, Rakowski H, French J, Popp RL. Idiopathic hypertrophic subaortic stenosis viewed by wide-angle, phased-array echocardiography. Circulation 1979; 59:1206–17.
    A detailed description of the two-dimensional echocardiographic features of this disorder.

20. Doi YL, McKenna WJ, Gehrke J, Oakley CM, Goodwin JF. M mode echocardiography in hypertrophic cardiomyopathy: diagnostic criteria and prediction of obstruction. Am J Cardiol 1980; 45:6–14.
    In this series of 70 patients with obstructive hypertrophic cardiomyopathy, a combination of ventricular septal thickness of at least 13 mm and systolic anterior motion of the mitral valve best differentiated obstructive from non-obstructive hypertrophic myopathy.

21. Spirito P, Maron BJ. Significance of left ventricular outflow tract cross-sectional area in hypertrophic cardiomyopathy: a two-dimensional echocardiographic assessment. Circulation 1983; 67:1100–8.
    The cross-sectional outflow tract area (measured by 2-D echo) is closely related to the presence or absence of subaortic obstruction in patients with hypertrophic cardiomyopathy.

Therapy

22. Fiddler GI, Tajik AJ, Weidman WH, McGoon DC, Ritter DG, Giuliani ER. Idiopathic hypertrophic subaortic stenosis in the young. Am J Cardiol 1978; 42:793–9.
    Of 36 patients with an average age of 11.3 years, surgery was performed in 16, 12 of whom were long-term survivors. All 7 treated with propranolol did well. Of the 13 receiving no therapy, 7 died, 6 suddenly.

23. Stenson RE, Flamm MD Jr, Harrison DC, Hancock EW. Hypertrophic subaortic stenosis. Clinical and hemodynamic effects of long-term propranolol therapy. Am J Cardiol 1973; 31:763–73.
    In 13 patients with obstructive hypertrophic cardiomyopathy, long-term propranolol therapy had a favorable effect on symptoms but did not appear to alter the course of the disease.

24. Frank MJ, Abdulla AM, Canedo MI, Saylors RE. Long-term medical management of hypertrophic obstructive cardiomyopathy. Am J Cardiol 1978; 42:993–1001.
    Complete beta-blockade is the treatment of choice for individuals with this disorder. Most patients do not require surgery.

25. Rosing DR, Kent KM, Borer JS, Seides SF, Maron BJ, Epstein SE. Verapamil therapy: a new approach to the pharmacologic treatment of hypertrophic cardiomyopathy. I. Hemodynamic effects. Circulation 1979; 60:1201–7.
    Verapamil significantly reduces left ventricular outflow obstruction in patients with this disorder.

26. Rosing DR, Kent KM, Maron BJ, Epstein SE. Verapamil therapy: a new approach to the pharmacologic treatment of hypertrophic cardiomyopathy. II. Effects on exercise capacity and symptomatic status. Circulation 1979; 60:1208–13.
    In many patients with hypertrophic cardiomyopathy, verapamil improves exercise capacity and symptomatic status.

27. Maron BJ, Merrill WH, Freier PA, Kent KM, Epstein SE, Morrow AG. Long-term clinical course and symptomatic status of patients after operation for hypertrophic subaortic stenosis. Circulation 1978; 57:1205–13.
    Of 124 patients operated on for this disorder, 10 (8%) died perioperatively, 14 (11%) had persistent or recurrent functional limitation, and 11 (9%) died up to 13 years later of hypertrophic cardiomyopathy.

28. Morrow AG, Reitz BA, Epstein SE, Henry WL, Conkle DM, Itscoitz SB, Redwood DR. Operative treatment in hypertrophic subaortic stenosis: techniques, and the results of pre and postoperative assessments in 83 patients. Circulation 1975; 52:88–102.
    Of those patients with this disorder who survived ventriculomyotomy, symptomatic and hemodynamic improvement were uniformly present.

29. Morrow AG, Koch JP, Maron BJ, Kent KM, Epstein SE. Left ventricular myotomy

and myectomy in patients with obstructive hypertrophic cardiomyopathy and previous cardiac arrest. Am J Cardiol 1980; 46:313–6.

This article suggests that myectomy may prevent sudden death in patients with this disorder.

30. Koch JP, Maron BJ, Epstein SE, Morrow AG. Results of operation for obstructive hypertrophic cardiomyopathy in the elderly: septal myotomy and myectomy in 20 patients 65 years of age or older. Am J Cardiol 1980; 46:963–6.

Advanced age in itself is not a contraindication to operative intervention in patients with this disorder.

31. Canedo MI, Frank MJ. Therapy of hypertrophic cardiomyopathy: medical or surgical? Clinical and pathophysiologic considerations. Am J Cardiol 1981; 48:383–8.

An excellent review of the therapies available for patients with this disease.

32. Bonow RO, Frederick TM, Bacharach SL, Green MV, Goose PW, Maron BJ, Rosing DR. Atrial systole and left ventricular filling in hypertrophic cardiomyopathy: effect of verapamil. Am J Cardiol 1983; 51:1386–91.

Many patients with hypertrophic cardiomyopathy are at risk of hemodynamic decompensation if atrial fibrillation occurs. This risk may be reduced during verapamil therapy.

33. Beahrs MM, Tajik AJ, Seward JB, Giuliani ER, McGoon DC. Hypertrophic obstructive cardiomyopathy: ten- to 21-year follow-up after partial septal myectomy. Am J Cardiol 1983; 51:1160–6.

Of 36 consecutive survivors of septal myectomy, 28 (77%) were alive after 10 years.

CONGESTIVE CARDIOMYOPATHY

Congestive cardiomyopathy is characterized by biventricular dilatation and impaired systolic performance, with resultant heart failure. It is caused by severe, generalized myocardial damage, which in turn may be induced by a variety of toxic substances or inflammatory processes. The chronic and excessive consumption of ethanol is probably the major cause of congestive cardiomyopathy in the United States. Ethanol may cause myocardial damage in several ways: (1) it has a direct toxic effect on the myocardium; (2) those individuals who consume large amounts of ethanol often have associated nutritional deficiencies that can affect myocardial integrity, such as thiamine deficiency; and (3) some alcoholic beverages contain additives that are toxic to the myocardium, such as the small amounts of cobalt that, at one time, were added to beer.

Viral myocarditis may lead to a congestive cardiomyopathy. The patient initially develops an acute viral syndrome due most often to a Coxsackie B virus—fever, myalgias, and cough. Over the course of 1 to 2 weeks, these acute symptoms resolve, but they are replaced by symptoms of pulmonary and peripheral venous congestion. In essence, the acute Coxsackie B viral myocarditis has progressed to a more chronic congestive cardiomyopathy. Although this hypothesis is an attractive one, it remains largely unsupported, since there have been few patients actually observed to develop a congestive cardiomyopathy after a documented episode of viral myocarditis.

Peripartum cardiomyopathy is a congestive myopathy that appears sometime between the last month of pregnancy and the first 3 to 4 months after delivery. Its etiology is unknown, but it is most common in older women (>30 years), in women who have had several previous pregnancies, and in women with a past history of associated toxemia. There is a tendency for recurrence of the syndrome in subsequent pregnancies, especially in women with persistent cardiomegaly.

Congestive cardiomyopathy may occasionally be caused by a variety of endocrinologic or immunologic abnormalities. Thus, it may appear in association with acromegaly, Cushing's disease, pheochromocytoma, and diabetes mellitus. It may result from exposure to various toxins, including doxorubicin, lead, chloroquine, certain hydrocarbons, mercury, lithium, and the toxins contained in the venom of certain snakes. Finally, in many patients, congestive cardiomyopathy has no discernible or identifiable etiologic agent and is therefore termed idiopathic.

The patient with a congestive cardiomyopathy usually complains of dyspnea on exertion, orthopnea, paroxysmal nocturnal dyspnea, and ankle edema. Fatigue and generalized weakness are frequently severe. Less commonly, he complains of palpitations or chest pain similar in character to angina pectoris. On occasion, the patient may come to medical attention after a syncopal episode or an asymmetric neurologic event caused by a systemic arterial embolization of a left ventricular thrombus. On physical examination, the patient often has a resting tachycardia and a narrow arterial pulse pressure. A pulsus alternans may be prominent and is indicative of severe left ventricular dysfunction. Jugular venous distention is usually present, and there may be prominent V waves in the jugular venous contour (reflective of tricuspid regurgitation). Moist rales over both lung fields are often present, and there may be evidence of unilateral or bilateral pleural effusions. There is generalized cardiomegaly, with the point of maximal intensity palpable in the axilla. Both right and left ventricular third heart sounds are frequently audible. Murmurs of mitral and tricuspid regurgitation, due to anular dilatation caused by ventricular enlargement, are usually present. If the tricuspid regurgitation is marked, the patient may have a tender, enlarged, and pulsatile liver.

The ECG often demonstrates sinus tachycardia and nonspecific ST–T wave abnormalities. Atrial and ventricular ectopic activity is frequent, and intraventricular conduction abnormalities are often present. About 10 to 15 percent of patients with a congestive cardiomyopathy have Q waves in the anterior or inferior leads suggestive of an old myocardial infarction; in fact, no infarction has occurred, and these Q waves are said to represent a pseudoinfarction pattern. The chest x-ray demonstrates moderate to severe generalized cardiomegaly. Pulmonary vascular congestion is usually prominent, and unilateral or even bilateral pleural effusions may be present. By echocardiography and gated equilibrium blood pool scintigraphy, both ventricles appear dilated and poorly contractile, so that the ejection fraction is substantially depressed.

At cardiac catheterization, elevated filling pressures are present bilaterally, the cardiac output is usually diminished, and left and right ventricular systolic dysfunction is marked (as reflected by a depressed ejection fraction). There is usually cineangiographic evidence of mitral regurgitation. The coronary arteries are widely patent. There may be a suggestion on the left ventriculogram of a thrombus within the ventricular cavity.

In general, the prognosis of the patient with a congestive cardiomyopathy is poor, despite maximal medical therapy. Over a 1- to 5-year period after the diagnosis is established, these patients will likely have (1) gradually worsening biventricular congestive heart failure, (2) recurrent pulmonary or systemic arterial embolization, or (3) worsening ventricular ectopic activity, often culminating in sudden death. The patient should therefore be treated with (1) digitalis, diuretics, salt restriction, and afterload reduction (in an attempt to control the symptoms of congestive heart failure); (2) long-term anticoagulation with coumadin (in an attempt to prevent recurrent embolization), provided there is no contraindication to such therapy; and (3) antiarrhythmic agents in those with frequent or complex ventricular ectopy (in an attempt to prevent sudden death). Recent studies have demonstrated that the new positive inotropic agent amrinone is beneficial in these patients, and others have shown the salutary effect of captopril, a specific inhibitor of the enzyme that converts angiotensin to its active form. Finally, if the patient continues to pursue a deteriorating course despite maximal medical therapy, cardiac transplantation may be attempted.

Etiology

1. Brown AK, Doukas N, Riding WD, Jones EW. Cardiomyopathy and pregnancy. Br Heart J 1967; 29:387–93.
   These authors hypothesize that peripartum cardiomyopathy is, in fact, idiopathic cardiomyopathy made worse by the intravascular volume expansion induced by pregnancy.
2. Goodwin JF, Oakley CM. The cardiomyopathies. Br Heart J 1972; 34:545–52.
   A concise review of both congestive and hypertrophic cardiomyopathy, including a good discussion of etiologic factors.
3. Morin YL, Foley AR, Martineau G, Roussel J. Quebec beer-drinkers' cardiomyopathy: forty-eight cases. Can Med Assoc J 1967; 97:881–3.
   Cardiomyopathy affected 48 habitual beer drinkers who consumed large amounts of a particular beer containing certain additives.
4. Burch GE, DePasquale NP. Alcoholic cardiomyopathy. Am J Cardiol 1969; 23:723–31.
   Many patients with alcoholic cardiomyopathy escape detection until irreversible cardiac damage has developed.
5. Grist NR, Bell EJ. Coxsackie viruses and the heart. Am Heart J 1969; 77:295–300.
   Because of improved hygiene, it is to be expected that many persons will reach older and even adult years without having been infected by Coxsackie B virus, thus making it likely that periodic outbreaks of this infection will occur in adults.
6. Abelmann WH. Virus and the heart. Circulation 1971; 44:950–6.
   Of the many viruses that may cause an acute myocarditis, only influenza, Coxsackie, and poliomyelitis have been isolated from heart tissue with any regularity.
7. Spodick DH, Pigott VM, Chirife R. Preclinical cardiac malfunction in chronic alcoholism: comparison with matched normal controls and with alcoholic cardiomyopathy. N Engl J Med 1972; 287:677–80.
   In 26 patients with chronic alcoholism but no clinical evidence of heart disease, left ventricular function (determined noninvasively) was depressed.

Clinical Manifestations

8. Shirey EK, Proudfit WL, Hawk WA. Primary myocardial disease: correlation with clinical findings, angiographic, and biopsy diagnosis. Follow-up of 139 patients. Am Heart J 1980; 99:198–206.
   Of 113 patients with congestive cardiomyopathy, the 5-year mortality in those with congestive heart failure was 52%.
9. Artenstein MS, Cadigan FC Jr, Buescher EL. Clinical and epidemiological features of Coxsackie group B virus infections. Ann Intern Med 1965; 63:597–603.
   Of 180 patients with serologic evidence of Coxsackie virus group B infection, aseptic meningitis was the most common clinical manifestation. In addition, pleurodynia, cardiac involvement, orchitis, and nonspecific febrile illnesses were also common.
10. Smith WG. Coxsackie heart disease in adults. Am Heart J 1967, 73:439–40.
    Unlike neonates, adults with viral myocarditis usually recover completely.
11. Baker G, Zeller NH, Weitzner S, Leach JK. Pheochromocytoma without hypertension presenting as cardiomyopathy. Am Heart J 1972; 83:688–93.
    Occasionally the predominant manifestation of a pheochromocytoma is congestive heart failure associated with primary myocardial disease in the absence of hypertension.
12. Rose HD. Recurrent illness following acute Coxsackie B 4 myocarditis. Am J Med 1973; 54:544–8.

The case report of a 59-year-old man who died of fulminant, recurrent Coxsackie B4 myocarditis.

13. Leier CV, Schaal SF, Leighton RF, Whayne TF Jr. Heart block in alcoholic cardiomyopathy. Arch Intern Med 1974; 134:766–8.
    This article describes a patient with alcoholic congestive cardiomyopathy and complete heart block.

14. Woods JD, Nimmo MJ, Mackay-Scollay EM. Acute transmural myocardial infarction associated with active Coxsackie virus B infection. Am Heart J 1975; 89:283–7.
    Of 233 patients with infarction, 20 had serologic evidence of active Coxsackie B infection. Although the infection could have been coincidental, it is possible that the virus may have played some part in the illness.

15. Demakis JG, Rahimtoola SH, Sutton GC, Meadows WR, Szanto PB, Tobin JR, Gunnar RM. Natural course of peripartum cardiomyopathy. Circulation 1971; 44:1053–61.
    Of 27 women with this entity, half had normal-sized hearts 6 months after delivery, whereas half still had cardiomegaly. In those with normal heart size, the long-term prognosis was excellent. In those with persistent cardiomegaly, the prognosis was poor.

16. Oakley C. Diagnosis and natural history of congested (dilated) cardiomyopathies. Postgrad Med J 1978; 54:440–7.
    The natural history of congestive cardiomyopathy appears to be highly variable and depends on the etiology.

17. Benjamin IJ, Schuster EH, Bulkley BH. Cardiac hypertrophy in idiopathic dilated congestive cardiomyopathy: a clinicopathologic study. Circulation 1981; 64:442–7.
    Patients with congestive cardiomyopathy in whom compensatory ventricular hypertrophy occurs appear to have a more favorable prognosis than those in whom it does not occur.

18. Fuster V, Gersh BJ, Giuliani ER, Tajik AJ, Brandenburg RO, Frye RL. The natural history of idiopathic dilated cardiomyopathy. Am J Cardiol 1981; 47:525–31.
    Of 104 patients with this disease entity, 80 (77%) had an accelerated course of death, and 53 (two-thirds) of the deaths occurred within the first 2 years.

19. Demakis JG, Proskey A, Rahimtoola SH, Jamil M, Sutton GC, Rosen KM, Gunnar RM, Tobin JR Jr. The natural course of alcoholic cardiomyopathy. Ann Intern Med 1974; 80:293–7.
    Patients with ethanolic cardiomyopathy who abstain from ethanol have a reasonably good prognosis; those that continue to drink do poorly.

Therapy

20. Goodwin JF. Treatment of the cardiomyopathies. Am J Cardiol 1973; 32:341–51.
    In congestive cardiomyopathy, treatment is directed toward improvement of contractile function with removal of possible toxic agents (such as alcohol), use of digitalis and diuretics, and prolonged rest.

21. Schwartz L, Sample KA, Wigle ED. Severe alcoholic cardiomyopathy reversed with abstention from alcohol. Am J Cardiol 1975; 36:963–6.
    In a 49-year-old man with a severe congestive cardiomyopathy, the cardiomyopathy was completely reversed by 1 year of abstinence.

22. Abelmann WH. Treatment of congestive cardiomyopathy. Postgrad Med J 1978; 54:477–84.
    The therapy of congestive cardiomyopathy is centered on digitalis, diuretics, salt restriction, and afterload reducing agents.

Prognosis

23. Franciosa JA, Wilen M. Ziesche S, Cohn JN. Survival in men with severe chronic left ventricular failure due to either coronary heart disease or idiopathic dilated cardiomyopathy. Am J Cardiol 1983; 51:831–6.
    In men with congestive cardiomyopathy, the 1- and 2-year mortality rates were 23% and 48%, respectively.

RESTRICTIVE CARDIOMYOPATHY

Of the three major kinds of cardiomyopathy—congestive, restrictive, and hypertrophic—the restrictive is the least common in the United States. In the patient with this disease entity, the right and left ventricular myocardia are excessively rigid, so that diastolic filling of both ventricles is distinctly abnormal. In contradistinction to abnormal diastolic function, the systolic function of both ventricles may be preserved.

A variety of disease processes may cause an infiltration of the ventricular myocardium with an abnormal substance, leading to stiffened and noncompliant right and left ventricles. First, amyloidosis is a disorder of unknown cause characterized by the deposition of an eosinophilic fibrous protein in various tissues of the body, including the heart. Most often, extensive cardiac amyloidosis is found in elderly men. Second, hemochromatosis is characterized by an excessive deposition of iron in a variety of tissues, one of which is the heart. Third, an occasional patient develops a restrictive cardiomyopathy because of glycogen deposition in the myocardium. Fourth, sarcoidosis may extensively infiltrate the myocardium, leading to a restrictive picture. With this disease process, conduction system involvement is especially common, so that AV block, intraventricular conduction delays, and complex ventricular ectopy are frequent. Fifth, in other parts of the world, endomyocardial fibroelastosis is a frequent cause of restrictive cardiomyopathy, especially in infants. Sixth, extensive metastatic infiltration of the ventricular myocardium may result in a restrictive cardiomyopathy. Finally, in some individuals, restrictive cardiomyopathy occurs without an identifiable cause and is therefore termed idiopathic.

The clinical and hemodynamic features of restrictive cardiomyopathy closely resemble those of chronic constrictive pericarditis. The right- and left-sided filling pressures are markedly elevated, and the cardiac output is usually substantially reduced. Because of the abnormally elevated right atrial and ventricular filling pressures, cardiac filling is diminished. As a result, the clinical manifestations of restrictive cardiomyopathy are usually predominantly right-sided. Pulmonary congestion is unusual, since the impediment to right ventricular filling prevents an excessive amount of the intravascular volume from reaching the pulmonary vasculature. Thus, the patient with a restrictive cardiomyopathy most frequently complains of fatigue, especially with exertion, and peripheral edema. In addition, he may note dyspnea on exertion (due to a diminished cardiac output, not to pulmonary vascular congestion) and abdominal discomfort (due to hepatic congestion). Chest pain occurs uncommonly. On physical examination, jugular venous distention is usually evident, as are hepatomegaly and peripheral edema. The apical impulse is usually easily palpable (in contrast to chronic constrictive pericarditis) and is not greatly displaced laterally. The S_1 and S_2 are usually normal, and an S_3 and S_4 may be audible. Since marked cardiomegaly is uncommon, murmurs of mitral or tricuspid regurgitation are not usually heard.

The ECG often demonstrates diffuse low voltage in all leads, especially when the restrictive process is due to extensive infiltration of the right and left ventricles. The routine chest x-ray usually shows a normal sized or only minimally enlarged heart. Pulmonary venous congestion is not marked, but pleural effusions may be present. Echocardiography is helpful in excluding the presence of (1) a pericardial effusion and (2) a thickened and sclerotic pericardium, both of which would suggest that the patient's disease is pericardial and not myocardial. At cardiac catheterization, the right and left ventricular pressure tracings demonstrate a characteristic "square root sign"—a deep and rapid early decline at the onset of diastole followed by a rise to a plateau. The right and left atrial pressures show a prominent Y descent and a very prominent a wave. In contrast to chronic constrictive pericarditis, the left-sided filling pressures are usually higher (3–7 mm Hg) than those on the right side. The cardiac output is depressed. On left ventriculography, the end-diastolic volume is usually normal or low, and the end-systolic volume may be normal, so that the ejection fraction may be well preserved. Some patients with restrictive cardiomyopathy, however, especially those in whom the underlying disease process is amyloidosis, have left ventricular systolic dysfunction due to extensive infiltration of the ventricular myocardium.

The therapy of the patient with a restrictive cardiomyopathy is extremely difficult. Digitalis may exert no beneficial effect, since left ventricular systolic function may be reasonably normal. In fact, patients with cardiac amyloidosis are extremely sensitive to digitalis, and they may develop toxicity at low serum concentrations. Salt restriction and diuretics may reduce cardiac filling, further lowering cardiac output and even leading to life-threatening hypotension. In short, the usual measures that are used to treat congestive heart failure are not only ineffective but also potentially deleterious. The patient with a restrictive cardiomyopathy due to hemochromatosis may improve following repeated venesections, and the patient with extensive tumor infiltration of the myocardium may improve after appropriate radiotherapy or chemotherapy. In any event, the prognosis of most individuals with restrictive cardiomyopathy—regardless of its cause—is extremely poor, with most patients dying within 1 to 2 years of diagnosis.

1. Meaney E, Shabetai R, Bhargava V, Shearer M, Weidner C, Mangiardi LM, Smalling R, Peterson K. Cardiac amyloidosis, constrictive pericarditis, and restrictive cardiomyopathy. Am J Cardiol 1976; 38:547–56.
   Cardiac amyloidosis sometimes simulates constrictive pericarditis, but in other patients it resembles a congestive cardiomyopathy.
2. Kyle RA, Bayrd ED. Amyloidosis: review of 236 cases. Medicine 1975; 54:271–99.
   A complete review of this disease entity, including 220 references.
3. Buja LM, Khoi NB, Roberts WC. Clinically significant cardiac amyloidosis. Am J Cardiol 1970; 26:394–405.
   Clinical and necropsy findings are presented for 15 patients with cardiac amyloidosis.
4. Ridolfi RL, Bulkley BH, Hutchins GM. The conduction system in cardiac amyloidosis: clinical and pathologic features in 23 patients. Am J Med 1977; 62:677–86.
   Although conduction and rhythm disturbances are frequent in patients with cardiac amyloidosis, direct amyloid infiltration of the specialized conduction tissue of the heart is unusual; it occurred in only 3 of 23 individuals examined at postmortem.
5. Schroeder JS, Billingham ME, Rider AK. Cardiac amyloidosis: diagnosis by transvenous endomyocardial biopsy. Am J Med 1975; 59:269–73.
   In many patients, it is difficult to distinguish constrictive pericarditis from restrictive cardiomyopathy. An endomyocardial biopsy may be of great help in these individuals.
6. Child JS, Krivokapich J, Abbasi AS. Increased right ventricular wall thickness on echocardiography in amyloid infiltrative cardiomyopathy. Am J Cardiol 1979; 44:1391–5.
   In 6 patients with clinically significant amyloid infiltrative cardiomyopathy, echocardiographic right ventricular anterior wall thickness was increased.
7. Bharati S, Lev M, Denes P, Modlinger J, Wyndham C, Bauernfeind R, Greenblatt M, Rosen KM. Infiltrative cardiomyopathy with conduction disease and ventricular arrhythmia: electrophysiologic and pathologic correlations. Am J Cardiol 1980; 45:163–73.
   The findings of two cases—one of cardiac sarcoidosis and the other of cardiac amyloidosis—during electrophysiologic study bore a good relationship with those at postmortem examination.
8. Tyberg TI, Goodyer AVN, Hurst VW III, Alexander J, Langou RA. Left ventricular

filling in differentiating restrictive amyloid cardiomyopathy and constrictive pericarditis. Am J Cardiol 1981; 47:791–6.

*Using a sophisticated analysis of left ventricular filling during the first half of dias-
tole, these disease entities can sometimes be distinguished from one another.*

9. Benotti JR, Grossman W, Cohn PF. Clinical profile of restrictive cardiomyopathy.
Circulation 1980; 61:1206–12.

*A detailed description of the hemodynamic findings in 9 patients with restrictive car-
diomyopathy.*

10. Siqueira-Filho AG, Cunha CLP, Tajik AJ, Seward JB, Schattenberg TT, Giuliani
ER. M-mode and two-dimensional echocardiographic features in cardiac amyloidosis. Circulation 1981; 63:188–96.

*The M-mode echocardiogram can suggest amyloid heart disease when it shows thick-
ened ventricular walls in the presence of a small or normal-sized left ventricle and a
dilated left atrium. Furthermore, two-dimensional echocardiography can define the
exact extent of cardiac involvement.*

11. Rubinow A, Skinner M, Cohen AS. Digoxin sensitivity in amyloid cardiomyopathy.
Circulation 1981; 63:1285–8.

*In an in vitro study, isolated amyloid fibrils bind digoxin; this may explain why pa-
tients with amyloid heart disease are sensitive to this medication.*

12. Cassidy JT. Cardiac amyloidosis: two cases with digitalis sensitivity. Ann Intern
Med 1961; 55:989–94.

*Two patients with amyloid infiltration of the heart both had marked sensitivity to dig-
italis.*

13. Cutler DJ, Isner JM, Bracey AW, Hufnagel CA, Conrad PW, Roberts WC, Kerwin
DM, Weintraub AM. Hemochromatosis heart disease: an unemphasized cause of potentially reversible restrictive cardiomyopathy. Am J Med 1980; 69:923–8.

*Hemochromatosis is the only cause of restrictive cardiomyopathy that is potentially
reversible by medical therapy.*

14. Short EM, Winkle RA, Billingham ME. Myocardial involvement in idiopathic hemochromatosis: morphologic and clinical improvement following venesection. Am J
Med 1981; 70:1275–9.

*The case report of a 31-year-old man with a restrictive cardiomyopathy due to hemo-
chromatosis shows repeated venesection successfully depleted his myocardium of iron.*

15. Silverman KJ, Hutchins GM, Bulkley BH. Cardiac sarcoid: a clinicopathologic study
of 84 unselected patients with systemic sarcoidosis. Circulation 1978; 58:1204–11.

*Although myocardial involvement occurs in about 25% of patients with sarcoid, it is
usually clinically silent. Only an occasional patient has extensive cardiac involvement.*

16. Lorell B, Alderman EL, Mason JW. Cardiac sarcoidosis: diagnosis with endomyocardial biopsy and treatment with corticosteroids. Am J Cardiol 1978; 42:143–6.

*A 27-year-old woman with biopsy-proved cardiac sarcoidosis responded nicely to ste-
roid therapy.*

17. Saffitz JE, Sazama K, Roberts WC. Amyloidosis limited to small arteries causing
angina pectoris and sudden death. Am J Cardiol 1983; 51:1234–5.

*Of 54 patients with cardiac amyloidosis, 53 had amyloid deposits of both the myocar-
dial interstitium and blood vessels; in the remaining patient amyloid deposits were
limited to the blood vessels.*

18. Falk RH, Lee VW, Rubinow A, Hood WB Jr, Cohen AS. Sensitivity of technetium-
99m-pyrophosphate scintigraphy in diagnosing cardiac amyloidosis. Am J Cardiol
1983; 51:826–30.

*Technetium-99m-pyrophosphate scanning is a sensitive and specific test for the diag-
nosis of cardiac amyloidosis in patients with congestive heart failure of obscure origin.*

ANTHRACYCLINE-INDUCED CARDIOMYOPATHY

The anthracycline drugs doxorubicin (Adriamycin) and daunorubicin (dauno-
mycin) are two of the most effective chemotherapeutic agents available for the

treatment of acute leukemia, lymphoma, breast cancer, Hodgkin's disease, ovarian cancer, several forms of lung cancer, and a variety of sarcomas. Their administration is associated with the appearance of a congestive cardiomyopathy, the incidence of which is directly proportional to the cumulative dose administered. Thus, for doxorubicin, clinically evident cardiotoxicity occurs in 2 percent of patients receiving less than 400 mg/m^2 and in over 20 percent of those receiving more than 700 mg/m^2. When the total dose exceeds 550 mg/m^2, there is a marked increase in the incidence of congestive heart failure, so that the present recommendations for doxorubicin administration call for limiting the total dose to 550 mg/m^2. Although the appearance of cardiotoxicity is directly related to total dose, there is substantial individual variability. Furthermore, morphologic evidence of cardiotoxicity usually precedes the appearance of congestive heart failure, so that pathologic alterations may be visualized in some patients who have received only 350 to 400 mg/m^2. Finally, concomitant or previous radiation therapy potentiates the development of doxorubicin-associated cardiotoxicity, as does concurrent cyclophosphamide therapy.

The patient with anthracycline-induced cardiotoxicity usually complains of the same symptoms that are noted by individuals with congestive cardiomyopathy of other causes: dyspnea, orthopnea, paroxysmal nocturnal dyspnea, peripheral edema, and easy fatigability. On physical examination, there is often evidence of pulmonary and peripheral venous congestion (bilateral inspiratory rales and peripheral edema), cardiac enlargement (lateral displacement of the apical impulse), and poor left ventricular function (resting tachycardia and a prominent S$_3$). If left ventricular function is severely compromised, a pulsus alternans may be evident. On chest x-ray, the heart is enlarged, and there is pulmonary vascular congestion. Unilateral or bilateral pleural effusions may be present. Echocardiography and radionuclide ventriculography demonstrate an enlarged and poorly contractile left ventricle. If cardiotoxicity is suspected, endomyocardial biopsy can be performed to allow a direct histologic assessment of cardiac damage. Although the results of a biopsy appear superior to some noninvasive techniques of assessing toxicity, the results of radionuclide ventriculography appear to correlate closely with those of endomyocardial biopsy.

Anthracycline-induced cardiotoxicity appears to persist indefinitely after its development. The cardiac glycosides digoxin and acetylstrophanthidin have been reported to lessen the cardiotoxicity of doxorubicin, as have verapamil, a slow channel calcium antagonist, and vitamin E. Coenzyme Q10 has also been reported to reduce toxicity caused by these agents. At present, it seems wise to monitor left ventricular performance (preferably with radionuclide ventriculography) in all patients receiving the anthracycline compounds (1) at baseline (i.e., before the initiation of chemotherapy) and (2) at regular intervals after a total dose of 350 mg/m^2 has been administered. If left ventricular function clearly begins to deteriorate, endomyocardial biopsy can be performed to confirm the diagnosis of anthracycline-induced cardiomyopathy, after which the offending agent should be discontinued.

1. Young RC, Ozols RF, Myers CE. The anthracycline antineoplastic drugs. N Engl J Med 1981; 305:139–53.
   A comprehensive review of the cardiac toxicity of these agents. Including 166 references.
2. Bristow MR, Mason JW, Billingham ME, Daniels JR. Doxorubicin cardiomyopathy: evaluation by phonocardiography, endomyocardial biopsy, and cardiac catheterization. Ann Intern Med 1978; 88:168–75.
   Previous mediastinal irradiation and an age ≥ 70 years appeared to be risk factors for doxorubicin-associated heart failure.
3. Gottdiener JS, Mathisen DJ, Borer JS, Bonow RO, Myers CE, Barr LH, Schwartz DE, Bacharach SL, Green MV, Rosenberg SA. Doxorubicin cardiotoxicity: assess-

ment of late left ventricular dysfunction by radionuclide cineangiography. Ann Intern Med 1981; 94:430–5.

Left ventricular dysfunction was evident in over half the asymptomatic patients long after "acceptable" cumulative doses of doxorubicin were given.

4. Isner JM, Ferrans VJ, Cohen SR, Witkind BG, Virmani R, Gottdiener JS, Beck JR, Roberts WC. Clinical and morphologic cardiac findings after anthracycline chemotherapy: analysis of 64 patients studied at necropsy. Am J Cardiol 1983; 51:1167–74.

This article emphasizes the fact that clinical evidence of anthracycline toxicity may be present without histologic signs of toxicity, and vice versa.

5. von Hoff DD, Layard MW, Basa P, Davis HL Jr, von Hoff AL, Rozencweig M, Muggia FM. Risk factors for doxorubicin-induced congestive heart failure. Ann Intern Med 1979; 91:710–7.

Of 4,018 patients given this agent, 88 (2.2%) developed congestive heart failure. It was especially likely to appear in (1) elderly patients and (2) those receiving large doses.

6. von Hoff DD, Rozencweig M, Layard M, Slavik M, Muggia FM. Daunomycin-induced cardiotoxicity in children and adults: a review of 110 cases. Am J Med 1977; 62:200–8.

With this drug, children seemed more susceptible to drug-induced cardiomyopathy than adults.

7. Bristow MR, Thompson PD, Martin RP, Mason JW, Billingham ME, Harrison DC. Early anthracycline cardiotoxicity. Am J Med 1978; 65:823–32.

Eight patients are described in whom small doses of these agents induced a pericarditis (4 patients) or cardiomyopathy.

8. Rinehart JJ, Lewis RP, Balcerzak SP. Adriamycin cardiotoxicity in man. Ann Intern Med 1974; 81:475–8.

This early study demonstrated that the noninvasive assessment of cardiac function is valuable in detecting early cardiotoxicity.

9. Alexander J, Dainiak N, Berger HJ, Goldman L, Johnstone D, Reduto L, Duffy T, Schwartz P, Gottschalk A, Zaret BL. Serial assessment of doxorubicin cardiotoxicity with quantitative radionuclide angiocardiography. N Engl J Med 1979; 300:278–83.

The assessment of radionuclide left ventricular ejection fraction during doxorubicin therapy may make it possible to avoid congestive heart failure.

10. Billingham ME, Mason JW, Bristow MR, Daniels JR. Anthracycline cardiomyopathy monitored by morphologic changes. Cancer Treat Rep 1978; 62:865–72.

In 60 patients receiving chemotherapy with an anthracycline compound, endomyocardial biopsy was a safe and reliable method for monitoring cardiac damage.

11. Cortes EP, Gupta M, Chow C, Amin VC, Folker K. Adriamycin cardiotoxicity: early detection by systolic time interval and possible prevention by coenzyme Q10. Cancer Treat Rep 1978; 62:887–91.

In this preliminary evaluation, coenzyme Q10 exerted a beneficial effect in patients receiving adriamycin, as reflected by measurement of the systolic time intervals.

12. Merrill J, Greco FA, Zimbler H, Brereton HD, Lamberg JD, Pomeroy TC. Adriamycin and radiation; synergistic cardiotoxicity. Ann Intern Med 1975; 82:122–3.

The initial report of two cases in which anthracycline-induced cardiotoxicity occurred at low total doses when anthracycline was administered in combination with mediastinal irradiation.

ACUTE PERICARDITIS

Acute inflammation of the pericardium, with or without a resultant pericardial effusion, can occur with a variety of disease processes. Most commonly, pericarditis is idiopathic, that is, it has no discernible etiology. Alternatively, it can occur (1) following an acute transmural myocardial infarction, (2) as an infectious process (which may be viral, bacterial, fungal, or tuberculous), (3) in conjunction with a dissecting aortic aneurysm (in which the dissection leaks or ruptures into the pericardial space), (4) following blunt or sharp trauma to the chest, (5) as a result of direct pericardial invasion by an adjacent tumor (most commonly from the breast or lung), (6) following large doses of irradiation to the chest (usually given to patients with lymphoma or solid tumors of the breast or lung), and (7) in association with uremia. Finally, acute pericarditis with effusion can result (1) from certain pharmacologic agents (most commonly hydralazine and procainamide), (2) from connective tissue disorders (most frequently rheumatoid arthritis, systemic lupus erythematosus, and scleroderma), and (3) as a part of Dressler's syndrome.

The patient with acute pericarditis complains of retrosternal chest pain, which may vary in severity. It is classically worsened by deep inspiration and by the patient's lying supine, whereas it is improved when the patient sits upright. In addition, the patient may complain of dyspnea, cough, hoarseness, or dysphagia, symptoms that are usually caused by pericardial compression of the bronchi, recurrent laryngeal nerve, and esophagus. Fever, chills, and weakness may be present.

On physical examination, the cardiac impulse is sometimes shifted leftward, but it may be difficult to palpate. An S_1 and S_2 are usually muffled and distant. A scraping, scratchy, and grating pericardial friction rub is usually audible over the entire precordium, but it may appear and disappear from one minute to the next. The chest x-ray usually shows an enlarged heart with a globular configuration. Fluoroscopically, the pulsations of the cardiac margin may be diminished or even absent. On the ECG, diffuse S–T segment elevation is usually present, and T wave flattening may be prominent. If a pericardial effusion is present, the QRS voltage may be diminished in all leads, and the echocardiogram (M-mode or two-dimensional) shows an echo-free space between the ventricular epicardium and the pericardium.

The course and prognosis of the patient with acute pericarditis depend on its underlying disease process. If the cause is remediable, the pericardial inflammation and accumulation of fluid usually resolve within days to weeks. The therapy of pericarditis and effusion is also aimed at the control or elimination of the underlying disease. Pericardiocentesis is indicated (1) as a *diagnostic* procedure in the patient who is suspected of having bacterial pericarditis and (2) as a *therapeutic* procedure in the patient with hemodynamic evidence of tamponade. At our institution, we prefer that a pericardial window (rather than a simple pericardiocentesis) be performed in the patient with pericarditis and effusion if a diagnosis is desired, since this procedure allows one to collect pericardial fluid and to examine a piece of pericardial tissue.

1. Ball GV, Schrohenloher R, Hester R. Gamma globulin complexes in rheumatoid pericardial fluid. Am J Med 1975; 58:123–8.
   In a 52-year-old man with rheumatoid arthritis, pericardiocentesis yielded fluid containing gamma globulin complexes similar to those found in rheumatoid synovial fluid.
2. Comty CM, Cohen SL, Shapiro FL. Pericarditis in chronic uremia and its sequels. Ann Intern Med 1971; 75:173–83.
   Uremic pericarditis was noted in 25 of 152 patients on chronic dialysis. Inadequate dialysis, infection, and hyperparathyroidism appeared to be contributing factors.
3. Kerber RE, Sherman B. Echocardiographic evaluation of pericardial effusion in myxedema: incidence and biochemical and clinical correlations. Circulation 1975; 52:823–7.
   In 33 hypothyroid patients, echocardiography revealed evidence of pericardial effusion in 10 (30%).
4. Klacsmann PG, Bulkley BH, Hutchins GM. The changed spectrum of purulent pericarditis: an 86 year autopsy experience in 200 patients. Am J Med 1977; 63:666–73.

In the modern era, purulent pericarditis occurs in older patients, is most likely due to Staphylococcus aureus *or gram negative bacilli, and often spreads to the pericardium from intrathoracic foci of infection.*

5. Krikorian JG, Hancock EW. Pericardiocentesis. Am J Med 1978; 65:808–14.
   A review of the benefits and risks of pericardiocentesis in 123 patients over a 6-year period.
6. Rubin RH, Moellering RC Jr. Clinical, microbiologic and therapeutic aspects of purulent pericarditis. Am J Med 1975; 59:68–78.
   Of 26 patients with purulent pericarditis, immunosuppressive therapy, extensive thermal burns, lymphoproliferative diseases, and other systemic disease processes affecting host resistance were present in half.
7. Silverberg S, Oreopoulos DG, Wise DJ, Uden DE, Meindok H, Jones M, Rapoport A, deVeber GA. Pericarditis in patients undergoing long-term hemodialysis and peritoneal dialysis: incidence, complications, and management. Am J Med 1977; 63:874–80.
   Of 218 patients on chronic dialysis followed over an 8-year period, 43 (20%) had episodes of uremic pericarditis.
8. Tajik AJ. Echocardiography in pericardial effusion. Am J Med 1977; 63:29–40.
   A thorough review of the advantages and limitations of M-mode echocardiography in the diagnosis of pericardial effusion.
9. Horowitz MS, Schultz CS, Stinson EB, Harrison DC, Popp RL. Sensitivity and specificity of echocardiographic diagnosis of pericardial effusion. Circulation 1974; 50:239–47.
   M-mode echocardiography was able to identify pericardial effusions as small as 15–25 ml.
10. Eng RHK, Sen P, Browne K, Louria DB. Candida pericarditis. Am J Med 1981; 70:867–9.
    A case report of a 39-year-old man who developed Candida tropicalis *pericarditis and was treated successfully with amphotericin B but later died of other causes.*
11. Martin RP, Bowden R, Filly K, Popp RL. Intrapericardial abnormalities in patients with pericardial effusion: findings by two-dimensional echocardiography. Circulation 1980; 61:568–72.
    By two-dimensional echocardiography, one can often identify loculation of pericardial fluid and a thickened pericardium.
12. Morse JR, Oretsky MI, Hudson JA. Pericarditis as a complication of meningococcal meningitis. Ann Intern Med 1971; 74:212–7.
    Of 32 patients with meningococcal meningitis, 6 developed acute pericarditis, an incidence of 19%.
13. Spodick DH. Differential diagnosis of acute pericarditis. Prog Cardiovasc Dis 1971; 14:192–209.
    A comprehensive review of the causes and differential diagnosis of acute pericarditis.
14. Spodick DH. Differential characteristics of the electrocardiogram in early repolarization and acute pericarditis. N Engl J Med 1976; 295:523–6.
    Some helpful clues for the ECG diagnosis of acute pericarditis.
15. Tomoda H, Hoshiai M, Furuya H, Oeda Y, Matsumoto S, Tanabe T, Tamachi H, Sasamoto H, Koide S, Kuribayashi S, Matsuyama S. Evaluation of pericardial effusion with computed tomography. Am Heart J 1980; 99:701–6.
    In 11 patients with pericardial effusions, computed tomography identified the effusion in all; the amount of fluid ranged from 25–585 ml.

PERICARDIAL TAMPONADE

Pericardial tamponade is caused by an accumulation of fluid within the pericardial space. Such a collection of fluid—a so-called pericardial effusion—can occur in association with several disease processes, including (1) infectious pericarditis (viral, bacterial, or tuberculous), (2) an acute transmural myocardial infarction, (3) blunt or sharp trauma to the chest, (4) invasion of the pericardium by an adjacent tumor (most commonly from the lung or breast), (5) a number of connective tissue diseases, and (6) uremia. The accumulation of pericardial fluid increases pericardial pressure, which, in turn, increases intracardiac filling pressures, eventually diminishing venous return to the right atrium. Stroke volume declines, and heart rate increases in an attempt to sustain cardiac output. Eventually, however, even a brisk sinus tachycardia cannot maintain a normal output, and systemic arterial pressure falls.

The amount of pericardial fluid needed to induce tamponade depends on the time course over which it accumulates. Thus, the rapid accumulation of as little as 100 to 200 ml can cause tamponade, since the pericardium has not had sufficient time to distend. In contrast, a pericardial effusion of 1 to 2 L can accumulate slowly without causing tamponade.

The patient with pericardial tamponade usually complains of symptoms attributable to a reduced cardiac output: dyspnea, fatigue, dizziness, and even syncope. He may note retrosternal chest pain. Orthopnea and paroxysmal nocturnal dyspnea are uncommon symptoms, since pulmonary vascular congestion does not occur. Finally, the patient with an especially large pericardial effusion may complain of cough, dysphagia, hoarseness, or hiccoughs, all attributable to impingement of the enlarged pericardial sac on adjacent intrathoracic structures (e.g., the bronchi, esophagus, or vagus or recurrent laryngeal nerves). On physical examination, the patient with pericardial tamponade is often anxious, restless, and pale. He usually prefers to sit upright and even to lean slightly forward. The peripheral pulse is rapid and may be thready. The systemic arterial pressure is normal or diminished, and during inspiration it falls substantially (i.e., >20 mm Hg)—a so-called paradoxical pulse. This marked fall in systemic blood pressure during inspiration is not specific for pericardial tamponade; it can occur in patients with severe congestive heart failure, chronic obstructive pulmonary disease, hypovolemia, acute pulmonary embolism, or shock. The jugular venous pressure is elevated, and, therefore, the neck veins are distended. They may distend further during inspiration. The cardiac examination usually reveals quiet heart sounds; a pericardial friction rub may be audible.

The chest x-ray often reveals an enlarged heart with a globular configuration. The lung fields are clear. The ECG may show generalized low QRS voltage in the six limb leads, and nonspecific ST–T wave abnormalities are often present. Total electrical alternans is a pathogomonic electrocardiographic sign of pericardial tamponade. The echocardiogram demonstrates an echo-free space between the ventricular epicardium and the pericardium. Gated blood pool scintigraphy reveals a generous distance between the intracardiac blood pool and the lungs.

Although the chest x-ray and echocardiogram demonstrate that a pericardial *effusion* is present, a diagnosis of *tamponade* is made in the cardiac catheterization laboratory, where right heart catheterization reveals elevated and equal filling pressures in all chambers: right atrium, right ventricle, and pulmonary capillary wedge (which equals left atrium). If a left-sided catheterization is performed, the left ventricular filling pressure is also equal to those on the right side. A pericardiocentesis reveals a high intrapericardial pressure equal to the filling pressures on both sides of the heart. As the pericardial fluid is removed, the pericardial pressure and intracardiac filling pressures decline and eventually reach normal.

Since pericardial tamponade of any cause is a life-threatening entity, it must be treated quickly and effectively. This is accomplished by a pericardiocentesis or a so-called pericardial window (created through a small subxiphoid incision). Until such pericardial drainage can be performed, the patient should receive a generous intravenous infusion of normal saline in an attempt to raise intracardiac filling pressures and, therefore, to augment cardiac output. Pressor amines are of limited value in the patient with tamponade. Once the tamponade is relieved, the course and prognosis depend on the cause of the pericardial effusion, which must be identified and treated appropriately.

1. Baldwin JJ, Edwards JE. Uremic pericarditis as a cause of cardiac tamponade. Circulation 1976; 53:896–901.

   Tamponade is more common in dialyzed than in nondialyzed patients with chronic renal failure.

2. Ofori-Krakye SK, Tyberg TI, Geha AS, Hammond GL, Cohen LS, Langou RA. Late cardiac tamponade after open heart surgery: incidence, role of anticoagulants in its pathogenesis and its relationship to the postpericardiotomy syndrome. Circulation 1981; 63:1323–8.

   Of 1,290 consecutive patients undergoing heart surgery, postoperative tamponade occurred in 10 (0.8%). Of the 10, 9 responded to pericardiocentesis alone, and the remaining patient required pericardial stripping.

3. Martins JB, Manuel WJ, Marcus ML, Kerber RE. Comparative effects of catecholamines in cardiac tamponade: experimental and clinical studies. Am J Cardiol 1980; 46:59–66.

   In animals and human patients with tamponade, intravenous catecholamines were of limited benefit, even as interim therapy.

4. Guberman BA, Fowler NO, Engel PJ, Gueron M, Allen JM. Cardiac tamponade in medical patients. Circulation 1981; 64:633–40.

   Of 56 medical patients with tamponade, the most common causes were metastatic tumor in 18, idiopathic pericarditis in 8, and uremia in 5.

5. Reddy PS, Curtiss EI, O'Toole JD, Shaver JA. Cardiac tamponade: hemodynamic observations in man. Circulation 1978; 58:265–72.

   In patients with tamponade, the venous pressure required to maintain a given cardiac volume is determined by pericardial compliance.

6. Wei JY, Taylor GJ, Achuff SC. Recurrent cardiac tamponade and large pericardial effusions: management with an indwelling pericardial catheter. Am J Cardiol 1978; 42:281–2.

   A technique is described which allows for continuous pericardial drainage in patients with effusions that reaccumulate rapidly.

7. Stein L, Shubin H, Weil MH. Recognition and management of pericardial tamponade. JAMA 1973; 225:503–6.

   A review of the clinical characteristics, recognition, and therapy of tamponade.

8. Spodick DH. Acute cardiac tamponade: pathologic physiology, diagnosis, and management. Prog Cardiovasc Dis 1967; 10:64–96.

   A complete review of pericardial tamponade, including 70 references.

9. Metcalfe J, Woodbury JW, Richards V, Burwell CS. Studies in experimental pericardial tamponade: effects on intravascular pressures and cardiac output. Circulation 1952; 5:518–23.

   As tamponade develops, intracardiac filling pressures rise, and cardiac output falls.

10. D'Cruz IA, Cohen HC, Prabhu R, Glick G. Diagnosis of cardiac tamponade by echocardiography: changes in mitral valve motion and ventricular dimensions, with special reference to paradoxical pulse. Circulation 1975; 52:460–5.

    In patients with tamponade, inspiration induces certain characteristic changes in mitral valve motion and in right and left ventricular dimensions.

11. Sotolongo RP, Horton JD. Total electrical alternans in pericardial tamponade. Am Heart J 1981; 101:853–5.

    Total electrical alternans is seen only in patients with pericardial tamponade.

CONSTRICTIVE PERICARDITIS

Constrictive pericarditis can result from one of several disease processes. First, an acute viral pericarditis can eventually cause scarring and contraction of the pericardium, but this is distinctly uncommon. Second, tuberculous pericarditis can lead to constriction. In the preantibiotic era, this was by far the most common cause of pericardial constriction, and it continues to occur frequently in relatively underdeveloped areas of the world. Third, pericardial involvement with certain connective tissue disorders (e.g., rheumatoid arthritis, systemic lupus erythematosus, and scleroderma) can eventually lead to constriction. Fourth, an occasional patient with uremic pericarditis may develop constriction. Fifth, constriction of the pericardium can result from irradiation of the heart or from involvement by a malignant tumor (most commonly of the lung or breast). Sixth, constrictive pericarditis has been reported to occur during the months to years following cardiac surgery. Finally, many patients' pericardial constriction has no discernible etiology and is therefore termed idiopathic.

The patient with constrictive pericarditis often complains of the insidious appearance of abdominal swelling (due to ascites) and peripheral edema. He may note fatigue or dyspnea, both resulting from a diminished cardiac output. Symptoms of pulmonary venous congestion, such as orthopnea and paroxysmal nocturnal dyspnea, are uncommon. Dizziness or, on occasion, true syncope may occur. The patient may have a vague, nonspecific retrosternal chest pain. On physical examination, the peripheral pulse is usually normal. The systemic arterial pressure may be normal or may demonstrate a narrowed pulse pressure (<30 mm Hg), and the systolic pressure may decline markedly during inspiration (so-called paradoxical pulse). The jugular veins are distended, with especially prominent X and Y descents, and the jugular venous pressure usually *increases* during inspiration (Kussmaul's sign). The liver is usually palpable, and there is peripheral edema. On cardiac examination, the S_1 and S_2 are quiet, and a loud protodiastolic sound—the so-called pericardial knock—may be heard 0.10 to 0.18 second after the S_2.

The chest x-ray of the patient with constrictive pericarditis usually shows a heart of normal size, but an enlarged cardiac silhouette—due to pericardial thickening and effusion—may be present in some patients. Pericardial calcification is present in some and usually indicates a tuberculous etiology. Cardiac pulsations (visible fluoroscopically) are greatly diminished or absent. The lung fields are usually clear. Electrocardiographically, the QRS voltage is diminished in almost all patients with pericardial constriction, and nonspecific ST–T wave abnormalities are frequent. Although most patients are in sinus rhythm, many have atrial ectopy, and an occasional patient develops atrial fibrillation. By M-mode echocardiography, the pericardium may appear thickened and calcified.

At cardiac catheterization, left- and right-sided diastolic pressures are elevated and similar to one another. The right atrial pressure demonstrates prominent X and Y descents. It usually has no respiratory variation. The right and left ventricular pressure curves are characterized by a rapid, early diastolic dip followed by a high diastolic plateau, leading to an elevated end-diastolic pressure (the so-called square root sign). This sign may be abolished or less evident in the presence of tachycardia. The pulmonary arterial systolic pressure is usually only mildly elevated (i.e., 35–40 mm Hg). The cardiac index is often decreased, and the left ventricular end-diastolic volume is small.

Although it is sometimes difficult (or even impossible) to distinguish constrictive pericarditis from restrictive cardiomyopathy, several clues may be helpful in making this differentiation. In the patient with pericardial constriction, the respiratory variation in right atrial pressure is usually absent, whereas it may be present in the individual with restrictive cardiomyopathy. The pulmonary arterial systolic pressure is almost always below 50 mm Hg in the patient with constriction, but it is often above 50 mm Hg in the setting of restriction. Similarly, the pulmonary capillary wedge pressure is frequently below 18 mm Hg with constrictive pericarditis, while it is usually above 18 mm Hg with restrictive cardiomyopathy. Finally, the patient with pericardial constriction usually has an equilibration of all intracardiac filling pressures, whereas the patient with restrictive cardiomyopathy often has higher pressures in the left ventricle and atrium than in the right. Despite these guidelines, it is sometimes impossible to distinguish constrictive pericarditis from restrictive cardiomyopathy, and pericardial stripping is indicated as a diagnostic and therapeutic procedure.

The patient with constrictive pericarditis should undergo pericardiectomy, and the cause of the constriction should be identified and treated appropriately. If the patient is known to have constrictive pericarditis of tuberculous etiology, he should receive antituberculous chemotherapy for 2 to 3 weeks before surgery. Postoperatively, this chemotherapy is continued for 1 year. In addition, corticosteroids may be beneficial in the patient with tuberculous pericarditis, since they diminish the amount of inflammation.

Etiology

1. Marsa R, Mehta S, Willis W, Bailey L. Constrictive pericarditis after myocardial revascularization: report of 3 cases. Am J Cardiol 1979; 44:177–83.
   Although postoperative constrictive pericarditis is rare, it should be considered when unexplained right-sided heart failure develops after cardiac surgery.
2. Cohen MV, Greenberg MA. Constrictive pericarditis: early and late complication of cardiac surgery. Am J Cardiol 1979; 43:657–61.
   Constrictive pericarditis should be considered in postoperative patients who do not recuperate satisfactorily after surgery or whose condition deteriorates after initial recovery.
3. Kutcher MA, King SB III, Alimurung BN, Craver JM, Logue RB. Constrictive pericarditis as a complication of cardiac surgery: recognition of an entity. Am J Cardiol 1982; 50:742–8.
   Among 5,207 adult patients who had cardiac surgery, constrictive pericarditis was recognized postoperatively in 11 (0.2%).
4. Rooney JJ, Crocco JA, Lyons HA. Tuberculous pericarditis. Ann Intern Med 1970; 72:73–8.
   Since cardiovascular complications of the inflammatory exudate in the pericardium are the major causes of death with tuberculous pericarditis, corticosteroids should be given to suppress inflammation and to enhance reabsorption of the effusion.
5. Thadani U, Iveson JMI, Wright V. Cardiac tamponade, constrictive pericarditis, and pericardial resection in rheumatoid arthritis. Medicine 1975; 54:261–70.
   Four patients with rheumatoid constrictive pericarditis and 2 patients with rheumatoid cardiac tamponade are presented, and 60 previously reported cases are reviewed.
6. Yurchak PM, Levine SA, Gorlin R. Constrictive pericarditis complicating disseminated lupus erythematosus. Circulation 1965; 31:113–8.
   A 58-year-old man is described with constriction due to SLE.
7. Stanley RJ, Subramanian R, Lie JT. Cholesterol pericarditis terminating as constrictive calcific pericarditis: follow-up study of patient with 40 year history of disease. Am J Cardiol 1980; 46:511–4.
   The case report of a patient with recurrent pericardial effusions since 1939 who died of calcific constrictive pericarditis 40 years later.
8. Applefeld MM, Slawson RG, Hall-Craigs M, Green DC, Singleton RT, Wiernik PH. Delayed pericardial disease after radiotherapy. Am J Cardiol 1981; 47:210–3.
   Delayed chronic constrictive pericarditis developed in 7 patients 51–268 months after radiotherapy.

9. Orlando RC, Moyer P, Burnett TB. Methysergide therapy and constrictive pericarditis. Ann Intern Med 1978; 88:213–4.

   A case report of a 77-year-old woman who developed constrictive pericarditis during methysergide therapy.

Clinical Characteristics

10. Tyberg TI, Goodyer AVN, Langou RA. Genesis of pericardial knock in constrictive pericarditis. Am J Cardiol 1980; 46:570–5.

    Sudden cessation of left ventricular filling generates the pericardial knock of constrictive pericarditis.

11. Shabetai R, Fowler NO, Guntheroth WG. The hemodynamics of cardiac tamponade and constrictive pericarditis. Am J Cardiol 1970; 26:480–9.

    A detailed comparison of the hemodynamic characteristics of tamponade and constriction.

12. Lewis BS, Gotsman MS. Left ventricular function in systole and diastole in constrictive pericarditis. Am Heart J 1973; 86:23–41.

    A detailed analysis of left ventricular function in 30 patients with constriction. Diastolic left ventricular performance was markedly abnormal.

13. Wood P. Chronic constrictive pericarditis. Am J Cardiol 1961; 7:48–61.

    A concise review of the etiology, clinical features, hemodynamics, and therapy of constrictive pericarditis.

14. Hancock EW. On the elastic and rigid forms of constrictive pericarditis. Am Heart J 1980; 100:917–23.

    A concise review of the clinical characteristics of pericardial constriction.

Diagnosis

15. Schnittger I, Bowden RE, Abrams J, Popp RL. Echocardiography: pericardial thickening and constrictive pericarditis. Am J Cardiol 1978; 42:388–95.

    There is no specific echocardiographic pattern of pericardial thickening pathognomonic of constriction.

16. Nicholson WJ, Cobbs BW Jr, Franch RH, Crawley IS. Early diastolic sound of constrictive pericarditis. Am J Cardiol 1980; 45:378–82.

    Squatting may be a valuable maneuver to elicit or intensify the early diastolic sound of constrictive pericarditis.

17. Tyberg TI, Goodyer AVN, Hurst VW III, Alexander J, Langou RA. Left ventricular filling in differentiating restrictive amyloid cardiomyopathy and constrictive pericarditis. Am J Cardiol 1981; 47:791–6.

    This study shows a different profile of diastolic left ventricular filling volume and ventricular filling rate curves during the first half of diastole in patients with restrictive cardiomyopathy and those with constrictive pericarditis.

18. Voelkel AG, Pietro DA, Folland ED, Fisher ML, Parisi AF. Echocardiographic features of constrictive pericarditis. Circulation 1978; 58:871–5.

    Of 12 patients with pericardial constriction, flattening of the left ventricular posterior endocardium was present in 11.

19. Bush CA, Stang JM, Wooley CF, Kilman JW. Occult constrictive pericardial disease: diagnosis by rapid volume expansion and correction by pericardiectomy. Circulation 1977; 56:924–30.

    In 19 patients, occult constriction was identified by rapid volume expansion during cardiac catheterization.

20. Candell-Riera J, del Castillo HG, Permanyer-Miralda G, Soler-Soler J. Echocardiographic features of the interventricular septum in chronic constrictive pericarditis. Circulataion 1978; 57:1154–8.

    In 7 of 8 patients with constrictive pericarditis, an early septal diastolic motion (consisting of a sudden anterior displacement followed by a brisk posterior rebound) was recorded on echo.

Therapy

21. Glenn F, Diethelm AG. Surgical treatment of constrictive pericarditis. Ann Surg 1962; 155:883–93.

Pericardiectomy was performed in 33 patients with pericardial constriction; the re-sults were "excellent" or "good" in 28 (85%).

22. Copeland JG, Stinson EB, Griepp RB, Shumway NE. Surgical treatment of chronic constrictive pericarditis using cardiopulmonary bypass. J Thorac Cardiovasc Surg 1975; 69:236–8.

    Eleven patients are described in whom pericardiectomy for constrictive pericarditis was performed on cardiopulmonary bypass, and its advantages are discussed.

23. Effler DB. Chronic constrictive pericarditis treated with pericardiectomy. Am J Cardiol 1961; 7:62–8.

    A review of the early surgical experience with 26 patients with constrictive pericarditis.

RADIATION-INDUCED PERICARDIAL AND MYOCARDIAL DISEASES

Large doses of mediastinal irradiation are often administered to patients with Hodgkin's disease and non-Hodgkin's lymphoma; these individuals are usually treated with 4000 to 5000 rads delivered to the hila of both lungs and mediastinal lymph nodes. The exposure of the heart to this amount of irradiation can cause several pathologic conditions. First, acute or chronic *pericarditis* is the most common cardiac complication of radiation therapy. A transient pericardial effusion may appear in as many as 30 percent of patients undergoing mediastinal irradiation, whereas acute pericarditis—manifested clinically by fever, pleuritic chest pain, a pericardial friction rub, and typical electrocardiographic alterations—occurs in 10 to 15 percent of patients receiving over 4000 rads to the mediastinum. The time period from completion of radiotherapy to the appearance of acute pericarditis varies from 0 to 85 months, with the peak incidence occurring at 5 to 9 months. Chronic constrictive pericarditis can become clinically manifest as long as 20 to 25 years after mediastinal irradiation. The overall incidence of pericarditis is dependent on (1) the total dose of radiotherapy and (2) the extent of mediastinal tumor involvement. Thus, pericarditis occurs frequently in patients in whom the entire radiation dose is delivered through an anterior port, whereas it is relatively infrequent when an anterior and posterior port are employed and proper shielding is ensured.

The patient with chronic constrictive pericarditis usually complains of gradually worsening dyspnea, and some may note peripheral edema. On physical examination, jugular venous distention is usually evident, and the heart sounds are distant. A pericardial knock may be audible. The ECG usually demonstrates diffusely diminished QRS voltage.

The patient with symptomatic acute pericarditis due to irradiation should be treated with a nonsteroidal anti-inflammatory agent, such as aspirin, indomethacin, or ibuprofen. If these are inadequate, corticosteroids may be required to control chest discomfort. The individual with radiation-induced chronic constrictive pericarditis may require a pericardiectomy for the alleviation of symptoms.

Second, large amounts of irradiation can cause *endocardial* or *myocardial fibrosis* as well as dysfunction of the cardiac conducting system. The patient with extensive endomyocardial fibrosis usually manifests the symptoms and signs of a restrictive cardiomyopathy: fatigue and dyspnea (both due to a diminished cardiac output) as well as evidence on physical examination of peripheral venous congestion. An occasional patient has been reported to have radiation-induced complete heart block.

Third, large doses of irradiation cause a marked acceleration of the atherosclerotic process, with resultant *coronary artery disease*. Such accelerated atherogenesis is especially likely to occur in a patient who is consuming a diet high in cholesterol and saturated fats. Therefore, mediastinal irradiation can be followed by the typical symptoms of ischemic heart disease—angina pectoris and myocardial infarction. Such radiation-induced atherosclerotic coronary artery disease usually becomes clinically manifest 6 to 12 years following radiotherapy. If the atherosclerotic narrowings are severe, coronary artery bypass grafting may be necessary for the relief of angina.

Pericardial Disease
1. Applefeld MM, Cole JF, Pollock SH, Sutton FJ, Slawson RG, Singleton RT, Wiernik PH. The late appearance of chronic pericardial disease in patients treated by radiotherapy for Hodgkin's disease. Ann Intern Med 1981; 94:338–41.
   This report describes 9 patients in whom radiation-induced chronic pericardial disease was recognized 53–124 months after radiotherapy.
2. Applefeld MM, Slawson RG, Hall-Craigs M, Green DC, Singleton RT, Wiernik PH. Delayed pericardial disease after radiotherapy. Am J Cardiol 1981; 47:210–3.
   Delayed chronic constrictive pericarditis developed in 7 patients 51–268 months following radiotherapy.
3. Brosias FC III, Waller BF, Roberts WC. Radiation heart disease. Analysis of 16 young (aged 15–33 years) necropsy patients who received over 3500 rads to the heart. Am J Med 1981; 70:519–30.
   Of the 16 patients, 15 had thickened pericardia, 5 of whom had evidence of tamponade.
4. Haas JM. Symptomatic constrictive pericarditis developing 45 years after radiation therapy to the mediastinum: a review of radiation pericarditis. Am Heart J 1969; 77:89–95.
   This report describes a 54-year-old woman who developed symptomatic constrictive pericarditis 45 years after radiotherapy to the mediastinum.
5. Keelan MH, Rudders RA. Successful treatment of radiation pericarditis with corticosteroids. Arch Intern Med 1974; 134:145–7.
   A 47-year-old woman is described in whom postirradiation pericarditis developed; both symptoms and pleuropericardial effusions resolved following prednisone therapy.
6. Morton DL, Glancy DL, Joseph WL, Adkins PC. Management of patients with radiation-induced pericarditis with effusion: a note on the development of aortic regurgitation in two of them. Chest 1973; 64:291–7.
   Experience with pericardiectomy was favorable in a series of patients with radiation-induced pericardial disease.
7. Schneider JS, Edwards JE. Irradiation-induced pericarditis. Chest 1979; 75:560–4.
   The necropsy findings in 3 patients with radiation-induced pericarditis are described.
8. Gottdiener JS, Katin MJ, Borer JS, Bacharach SL, Green MV. Late cardiac effects of therapeutic mediastinal irradiation: assessment by echocardiography and radionuclide angiography. N Engl J Med 1983; 308:569–72.
   Within 2 years of irradiation in these 25 patients, 7 had demonstrable pericardial effusions.
9. Applefeld MM, Wiernik PH. Cardiac disease after radiation therapy for Hodgkin's disease: analysis of 48 patients. Am J Cardiol 1983; 51:1679–81.
   Of 48 patients who received radiotherapy to the chest, 46 had cardiac abnormalities; of these, 24 had constrictive or occult constrictive pericarditis.

Myocardial and Conduction System Disease
10. Burns RJ, Bar-Shlomo BZ, Druck MN, Herman JG, Gilbert BW, Perrault DJ, McLaughlin PR. Detection of radiation cardiomyopathy by gated radionuclide angiography. Am J Med 1983; 74:297–302.
    With rest and exercise radionuclide angiography, the incidence of radiation-induced myocardial damage is shown to be higher than previously believed.

11. Botti RE, Driscol TE, Pearson OH, Smith JC. Radiation myocardial fibrosis simulating constrictive pericarditis. Cancer 1968; 22:1254–61.
    A 59-year-old woman who received thoracic irradiation for carcinoma of the breast is described. Subsequently, she developed myocardial fibrosis that clinically mimicked constrictive pericarditis.
12. Cohn KE, Stewart JR, Fajardo LF, Hancock EW. Heart disease following radiation. Medicine 1967; 46:281–98.
    This report provides a detailed analysis of 21 patients who developed heart or pericardial disease following radiotherapy of the chest.
13. Cohen SI, Bharati S, Glass J, Lev M. Radiotherapy as a cause of complete atrioventricular block in Hodgkin's disease: an electrophysiological-pathological correlation. Arch Intern Med 1981; 141:676–9.
    A 20-year-old man treated with radiotherapy for Hodgkin's disease developed complete heart block 11 years later.

Coronary Artery Disease

14. McReynolds RA, Gold GL, Roberts WC. Coronary heart disease after mediastinal irradiation for Hodgkin's disease. Am J Med 1976; 60:39–45.
    Therapeutic levels of irradiation can produce or hasten coronary atherosclerosis.
15. Tracy GP, Brown DE, Johnson LW, Gottlieb AJ. Radiation-induced coronary artery disease. JAMA 1974; 228:1660–2.
    This article describes a 35-year-old woman who developed severe angina 19 months after radiotherapy to the mediastinum. Coronary angiography revealed extensive coronary artery disease.
16. Iqbal SM, Hanson EL, Gensini GG. Bypass graft for coronary arterial stenosis following radiation therapy. Chest 1977; 71:664–6.
    A 48-year-old man developed symptoms of progressive angina 12 years after chest irradiation. Catheterization revealed an isolated severe stenosis of the left anterior descending coronary artery, for which he underwent bypass grafting.

CHRONIC PERICARDIAL EFFUSION

In some patients, a pericardial effusion accumulates and remains for several weeks or months without causing the hemodynamic alterations of tamponade. Such a chronic pericardial effusion can be caused by (1) a chronic, indolent infectious process, which can be viral, tuberculous, or fungal, (2) uremia, (3) neoplastic invasion of the pericardium, most commonly the result of direct extension of a carcinoma of the lung or breast, (4) involvement of the pericardium by one of several connective tissue diseases, most frequently systemic lupus erythematosus and rheumatoid arthritis, (5) blunt or sharp trauma to the pericardium, (6) biventricular congestive heart failure, and (7) hypothyroidism. In addition, a chronic pericardial effusion can appear (1) following large doses of irradiation to the chest (most often for mediastinal malignancy), (2) following cardiac surgery, and (3) during long-term therapy with hydralazine or procainamide.

The patient with a chronic pericardial effusion but without tamponade is generally asymptomatic from a cardiac standpoint. He or she may complain of symptoms referable to the underlying disease process (e.g., tuberculosis, rheumatoid arthritis, hypothyroidism). If the pericardial effusion is large, the patient may note a vague fullness in the anterior chest, and he may have cough, hoarseness, or dysphagia if the effusion is large enough to impinge on the phrenic nerve, the recurrent laryngeal nerve, or the esophagus, respectively. On physical examination, the apical impulse is difficult or impossible to palpate, and the heart sounds are muffled. A pericardial friction rub may be audible. There is no evidence of venous engorgement (distended neck veins, hepatomegaly, and peripheral edema) or a diminished cardiac output (tachycardia and a peripheral pulse of low amplitude).

The ECG usually demonstrates diminished voltage of all QRS complexes, and there may be partial electrical alternans. The T waves are often flattened diffusely. The chest x-ray shows cardiomegaly without pulmonary vascular congestion. By echocardiography, the pericardial effusion can be visualized posteriorly and (if it is sizable) anteriorly.

The prognosis of the patient with a chronic pericardial effusion depends on the disease process causing it. Thus, the individual in whom the pericardial effusion is caused by neoplastic invasion has a guarded outlook. In contrast, the patient in whom the effusion is due to a treatable infection has an excellent prognosis provided, of course, that appropriate antimicrobial agents are administered. In general, these authors do not recommend pericardiocentesis and catheter drainage of a chronic pericardial effusion. Such drainage is not indicated for *therapeutic* reasons, since tamponade is not present. At the same time, if pericardial fluid is needed for *diagnostic* reasons (to establish the cause of the effusion), a subxiphoid pericardial window is preferable to a pericardiocentesis. With this procedure, a piece of the pericardium can be obtained for pathologic examination, and complete drainage of the effusion can be accomplished. Such tissue examination is especially important in the patient in whom a chronic infectious process is considered a possibility, since the pericardial fluid alone will allow the identification of the organism in only a minority of patients.

1. Tajik AJ. Echocardiography in pericardial effusion. Am J Med 1977; 63:29–40.
   An excellent review of the echocardiographic technique and pitfalls of visualizing pericardial effusions.
2. Martin RP, Bowden R, Filly K, Popp RL. Intrapericardial abnormalities in patients with pericardial effusion: findings by two-dimensional echocardiography. Circulation 1980; 61:568–72.
   M-mode echocardiography is unquestionably a useful technique for detecting pericardial effusions, but wide-angle, two-dimensional echocardiography allows better recognition of the distribution of fluid and other structures within the pericardial sac.
3. Santos GH, Frater RWM. The subxiphoid approach in the treatment of pericardial effusion. Ann Thorac Surg 1977; 23:467–70.
   A subxiphoid pericardial "window" is a safe, easily performed procedure that allows one to obtain pericardial tissue as well as fluid.
4. Berger M, Bobak L, Jelveh M, Goldberg E. Pericardial effusion diagnosed by echocardiography: clinical and electrocardiographic findings in 171 patients. Chest 1978; 74:174–9.
   In this large group of patients, congestive heart failure was the most common cause of pericardial effusion, occurring in 37 patients. Other frequently noted conditions were neoplasms, acute idiopathic pericarditis, renal failure, and acute myocardial infarction.
5. Lemire F, Tajik AJ, Giuliani ER, Gau GT, Schattenberg TT. Further echocardiographic observations in pericardial effusion. Mayo Clin Proc 1976; 51:13–8.
   If a pericardial effusion is large, it may be visualized echocardiographically behind the left atrium.
6. Alfrey AC, Goss JE, Ogden DA, Vogel JHK, Holmes JH. Uremic hemopericardium. Am J. Med 1968; 45:391–400.
   The clinical features, cardiovascular effects, and changes induced by dialysis were studied in 12 patients with uremic pericardial effusion.
7. Kleiman JH, Motta J, London E, Pennell JP, Popp RL. Pericardial effusions in patients with end-stage renal disease. Br Heart J 1978; 40:190–3.
   Of 35 stable, asymptomatic patients on chronic hemodialysis, 4 (11%) had echocardiographic evidence of pericardial effusion.

8. Biran S, Brufman G, Klein E, Hochman A. The management of pericardial effusion in cancer patients. Chest 1977; 71:182–6.
   This article emphasizes that an aggressive approach to malignant pericardial effusions is indicated, since clinical improvement often results from such an approach.

9. Flannery EP, Gregoratos G, Corder MP. Pericardial effusions in patients with malignant diseases. Arch Intern Med 1975; 135:976–7.
   Short-term catheter drainage is a safe and effective alternative to a surgical pericardial window in patients with malignant pericardial effusions.

10. Smith FE, Lane M, Hudgins PT. Conservative management of malignant pericardial effusion. Cancer 1974; 33:47–57.
    In patients with malignant pericardial effusions, conservative management (with the local instillation of chemotherapeutic agents or focal radiotherapy) is often successful in causing the effusion to disappear.

11. Berger HW, Seckler SG. Pleural and pericardial effusions in rheumatoid disease. Ann Intern Med 1966; 64:1291–7.
    Two patients with pleural effusions due to rheumatoid arthritis are described; one also had a pericardial effusion.

12. Marks PA, Roof BS. Pericardial effusion associated with myxedema. Ann Intern Med 1953; 39:230–40.
    Two patients are described with myxedema and very large pericardial effusions.

13. Tomoda H, Hoshiai M, Furuya H, Oeda Y, Matsumoto S, Tanabe T, Tamachi H, Sasamoto H, Koide S, Kuribayashi S, Matsuyama S. Evaluation of pericardial effusion with computed tomography. Am Heart J 1980; 99:701–6.
    In 11 patients, computed tomography allowed the identification and quantitative estimation of pericardial effusion.

SYSTEMIC ARTERIAL HYPERTENSION

For the adult patient, a systolic arterial pressure above 150 mm Hg and a diastolic pressure above 90 mm Hg are considered abnormal, and therefore, the patient with one or both is said to have arterial hypertension. According to these criteria, approximately 15 to 20 percent of adults in the United States have arterial hypertension. An abnormally high systolic arterial pressure (with a normal diastolic pressure) is termed *systolic hypertension*. It is usually a manifestation of either peripheral arteriosclerosis (with a reduced elasticity of the arteries) or a hyperdynamic cardiovascular state (e.g., hyperthyroidism, fever, anemia, or any disorder in which substantial arteriovenous shunting occurs). In contrast, *diastolic hypertension* is a disease entity in itself and therefore requires careful evaluation of its etiology and close attention to therapy.

Diastolic hypertension can result from one of several remediable disorders, in which case it is called *secondary* hypertension. About 10 percent of all hypertensive patients have secondary hypertension. Alternatively, the other 90 percent of hypertensive individuals do not have a definable cause of their abnormally elevated arterial pressure; these individuals are said to have *primary* or *essential* hypertension. A number of disease entities can cause secondary hypertension. First, renal parenchymal disease of any cause, including chronic glomerulonephritis and chronic pyelonephritis, can lead to systemic hypertension. Second, diminished renal perfusion due to unilateral or bilateral arteriosclerotic renal arterial stenoses can lead to a marked elevation of systemic arterial pressure. Both of these disease entities are believed to induce hypertension by activating the renin-angiotensin system. Third, primary aldosteronism (due to an adrenal adenoma that secretes aldosterone) causes mild to moderate systemic arterial hypertension in conjunction with hypokalemia;

the excessive amount of aldosterone causes both sodium retention (with resultant hypertension) and potassium diuresis. Fourth, the patient with Cushing's syndrome develops hypertension because of the sodium-retaining effect of large amounts of glucocorticosteroids. Fifth, the individual with a pheochromocytoma often has an elevated systemic arterial pressure, particularly if the tumor secretes an excessive amount of norepinephrine. Finally, the patient with coarctation of the aorta often presents with severe hypertension in the upper extremities and head, whereas the arterial pressure distal to the aortic narrowing (i.e., in the abdominal viscera and legs) is low.

Whether the hypertension is primary or secondary, most patients have no symptoms referable to the blood pressure elevation per se. Rather, they are discovered to have hypertension on a routine physical examination. When symptoms are present, they are usually related to (1) the elevated pressure itself (headache, dizziness, palpitations, and easy fatigability), (2) the resultant hypertensive vascular disease (epistaxis, hematuria, changes in visual acuity, angina pectoris, or symptoms of cardiac failure), or (3) the underlying disease in patients with secondary hypertension (e.g., weakness due to the hypokalemia of primary aldosteronism; headache, palpitations, diaphoresis, and postural dizziness due to pheochromocytoma). On physical examination, the systemic arterial pressure is elevated and—except for the patient with coarctation of the aorta—is similar in all four extremities. The ocular fundi may reveal vascular changes of long-standing hypertension. The heart may be of normal size, or it may be enlarged. An S_4 is usually audible. The ECG may show evidence of left ventricular hypertrophy, and the chest x-ray may demonstrate mild or even moderate cardiomegaly.

There is an abundance of statistical evidence to demonstrate that untreated hypertension shortens life expectancy. Before the development of effective antihypertensive therapy, the average life expectancy of the hypertensive patient from the time of onset of the hypertension was approximately 20 years: an uncomplicated phase, lasting about 15 years, and a final phase, lasting 5 years, during which vascular complications became manifest and eventually caused death. The vascular complications of hypertension consist of arteriosclerotic changes in large arteries as well as thickening of the walls of the small arteries and arterioles. These occur most frequently in the brain (leading to cerebrovascular insufficiency), heart (leading to angina pectoris, acute myocardial infarction, and congestive heart failure), and kidneys (leading to progressive azotemia). Effective antihypertensive therapy has been shown to alter this prognosis substantially.

The therapy of secondary hypertension usually involves surgical correction of the causative abnormality—for example, excision of an adrenal adenoma or pheochromocytoma, correction of an aortic coarctation, or relief of a renal arterial stenosis. The therapy of primary (essential) hypertension is centered on (1) restriction of the dietary intake of sodium and (2) one or more antihypertensive agents (these are discussed in detail under Antihypertensive Agents, p. 318).

An occasional patient with primary or secondary hypertension may enter an accelerated phase characterized by severe systemic arterial hypertension and papilledema, a condition known as *malignant hypertension*. In addition to papilledema, many of individuals with this condition have concomitant headache, vomiting, visual disturbances (including transient blindness), paralyses, convulsions, stupor, or even coma. The patient may have active congestive heart failure or rapidly deteriorating renal function.

The pathogenesis of malignant hypertension is unknown. The vascular lesion characteristic of this condition is fibrinoid necrosis of the walls of small arteries and arterioles, but the inciting factors are not understood. Many patients with this condition have evidence of a microangiopathic hemolytic anemia, but this appears to be the result—not the cause—of malignant hypertension.

Malignant hypertension is a medical emergency and, therefore, requires immediate therapy. Several agents can be used to lower diastolic arterial pressure quickly to around 90 mm Hg. Diazoxide, sodium nitroprusside, and trimethaphan have each been used with good success in the acute therapy of the patient with malignant hypertension. Once arterial pressure is acutely controlled with one of these parenteral agents, a powerful oral antihypertensive, such as hydralazine or minoxidil in combination with a beta-adrenergic blocker, can be administered for longer-term blood pressure control.

Secondary Hypertension

1. Vertes V, Cangiano JL, Berman LB, Gould A. Hypertension in end-stage renal disease. N Engl J Med 1969; 280:978–81.

   In most patients with end-stage renal disease, blood pressure can be well-controlled if the patient is maintained at dry weight.

2. Fraley EE, Feldman BH. Renal hypertension. N Engl J Med 1972; 287:550–2.

   It is important to recognize renal hypertension early, since experimental data suggest its potential curability may be related to its duration.

3. Shapiro AP, McDonald RH Jr, Scheib E. Renal arterial stenosis and hypertension: II. Current criteria for surgery. Am J Cardiol 1976; 37:1065–8.

   Medical therapy is the initial treatment of choice in patients over 50 to 55 years of age with atherosclerotic renal artery narrowing. The outcome of surgery is often satisfactory in younger individuals.

4. Youngberg SP, Sheps SG, Strong CG. Management of the patient with renovascular hypertension. Am Heart J 1977; 94:785–94.

   The treatment of choice for the patient with severe hypertension and a renovascular stenosis is surgical.

5. George JM, Wright L, Bell NH, Bartter FC. The syndrome of primary aldosteronism. Am J Med 1970; 48:343–56.

   A thorough review of the metabolic balance studies in 19 patients operated on for this disorder.

6. Conn JW. Primary aldosteronism. J Lab Clin Med 1955; 45:661–4.

   In the original patient described with this disorder, all the chemical abnormalities became normal within 10 days following removal of the adrenal tumor.

7. Krakoff L, Nicolis G, Amsel B. Pathogenesis of hypertension in Cushing's syndrome. Am J Med 1975; 58:216–20.

   Patients with Cushing's syndrome have hypertension because (1) vascular responsiveness to pressor agents is enhanced by large amounts of glucocorticosteroids, and (2) elevated plasma renin concentrations lead to increased amounts of angiotensin.

8. Cheitlin MD. Coarctation of the aorta. Med Clin North Am 1977; 61:655–73.

   A thorough review of this disease entity. Includes 79 references.

9. Lindesmith GG, Stanton RE, Stiles QR, Meyer BW, Jones JC. Coarctation of the thoracic aorta. Ann Thorac Surg 1971; 11:482–97.

   This review gives details of the operative technique employed to repair a coarctation of the aorta. Includes 87 references.

10. Duston HP, Tarazi RC, Bravo EL. Differential diagnosis of etiologic types of hypertension. Prog Cardiovasc Dis 1971; 14:210–24.

    A succinct review of the differential diagnosis of the various causes of secondary hypertension.

Clinical Manifestations and Prognosis

11. Freis ED. The clinical spectrum of essential hypertension. Arch Intern Med 1974; 133:982–7.

    The patient with mild hypertension should be treated only if other factors—such as age, sex, race, target organ damage, family history, or the presence of concomitant hyperglycemia or hypercholesterolemia—render him or her at especially high risk.

12. Kannel WB, Castelli WP, McNamara PM, McKee PA, Feinleib M. Role of blood pressure in the development of congestive heart failure: the Framingham study. N Engl J Med 1972; 287:781–7.

   In 142 patients who developed heart failure, the dominant etiologic factor in those aged 30 to 62 was hypertension. Of these individuals, 50% died over a 5-year period.

13. Roberts WC. The hypertensive diseases: evidence that systemic hypertension is a greater risk factor to the development of other cardiovascular diseases than previously suspected. Am J Med 1975; 59:523–32.
   Hypertension by itself is the sole underlying factor in most cases of nontraumatic cerebral arterial or aortic rupture. In association with hyperlipidemia, it clearly accelerates atherosclerosis and its devastating consequences.

14. Cohn JN, Limas CJ, Guiha NH. Hypertension and the heart. Arch Intern Med 1974; 133:969–79.
   A complete review of the effects of essential hypertension on ventricular performance and the development of coronary artery disease.

15. Veterans Administration Cooperative Study Group on Antihypertensive Agents. Effects of treatment on morbidity in hypertension: II. Results in patients with diastolic blood pressure averaging 90 through 114 mmHg. JAMA 1970; 213:1143–52.
   In 380 male hypertensive patients whose diastolic blood pressures were in this range, antihypertensive therapy lowered the risk of a morbid event from 55% to 18%.

16. Kannel WB, Dawber TR, McGee DL. Perspectives on systolic hypertension: the Framingham study. Circulation 1980; 61:1179–82.
   Isolated systolic hypertension may not be a benign phenomenon; it appears to be related to all the complications of diastolic hypertension, including atherosclerotic sequelae.

Malignant Hypertension

17. Koch-Weser J. Hypertensive emergencies. N Engl J Med 1974; 290:211–4.
   Hypertensive emergencies require immediate and intensive treatment. The complications are largely reversible, but the degree of reversibility is a function of how soon effective treatment is instituted.

18. Gifford RW Jr, Westbrook E. Hypertensive encephalopathy: mechanisms, clinical features, and treatment. Prog Cardiovasc Dis 1974; 17:115–24.
   This article reviews the pathogenesis, clinical features, and therapy of this disorder.

19. Keith TA III. Hypertension crisis: recognition and management. JAMA 1977; 237:1570–7.
   Several drugs are useful in acutely lowering blood pressure, including diazoxide, nitroprusside, intravenous methyldopa, intramuscular reserpine, and trimethaphan.

20. AMA Committee on Hypertension. The treatment of malignant hypertension and hypertensive emergencies. JAMA 1974; 228:1673–9.
   A complete review of the various agents available for the treatment of malignant or accelerated hypertension.

21. Case DB, Atlas SA, Sullivan PA, Laragh JH. Acute and chronic treatment of severe and malignant hypertension with the oral angiotensin-converting enzyme inhibitor captopril. Circulation 1981; 64:765–71.
   In 20 patients with severe or malignant hypertension, captopril, alone or in combination with other drugs, was effective in acute and long-term management.

CONGENITAL HEART DISEASE IN THE ADULT

Atrial septal defect (ASD) is one of the most common congenital heart abnormalities detected in adulthood. It is generally one of three types: (1) an ostium secundum defect, (2) an ostium primum defect (endocardial cushion defect, incomplete AV canal defect), or (3) a sinus venosus defect. In contrast, a *patent foramen ovale* is a potential rather than an actual defect, is generally an incidental finding at cardiac catheterization, and is usually benign. However, it may allow passage of paradoxical emboli from the right to the left atrium. In addition, it may be the site of right-to-left shunting of blood when there is either obstruction to blood flow at the right atrial or ventricular level or severe pulmonary hypertension.

Regardless of its exact anatomic location in the interatrial septum, the physiologic consequence of an ASD is shunting of blood from one atrium to the other. The magnitude and direction of such shunting are determined by the size of the ASD and the relative distensibility of the two ventricles. During infancy, there may be minimal shunting of blood, since both ventricles are hypertrophied and noncompliant. In most adults with an ASD, the right ventricle is more compliant than the left; as a result, left atrial blood is shunted to the right atrium, causing an increase in pulmonic blood flow. Eventually, if the right ventricle fails or its compliance is reduced, the left-to-right shunt diminishes in magnitude and may even be replaced by a right-to-left shunt.

Anomalies of pulmonary venous drainage may coexist with an ASD, in which case one or more pulmonary veins enter the right atrium or a systemic vein. With partial anomalous venous return, some or all of the veins from the right lung drain into the superior vena cava or the right atrium. Occasionally, the anomalous veins may drain into the inferior vena cava, in which case abnormalities of the right lung often coexist. The consequences of anomalous pulmonary venous drainage coexisting with an ASD depend on the number of veins involved and the magnitude of the additional left-to-right shunt. The possibility of this abnormality should be considered in the evaluation of the patient with an ASD.

The most common type of ASD is an ostium secundum defect. It occurs in females 1½ to 3 times more often than in males. These defects can be familial and can recur through successive generations. The mode of inheritance is uncertain, being variously described as autosomal dominant or recessive. Autosomal dominant inheritance with familial occurrence is recognized in patients with ASDs and the Holt-Oram syndrome (ASD in association with a hypoplastic thumb, an accessory phalanx, and/or abnormalities of the forearm). In addition, mitral valve prolapse can occur in association with a secundum ASD. Spontaneous closure of an atrial septal defect is very uncommon.

An ASD can go undetected clinically for years, since in many patients it produces no symptoms and is accompanied by only subtle abnormalities on physical examination. The diagnosis may be suspected initially on the basis of a routine chest x-ray that demonstrates prominent proximal pulmonary arteries and a peripheral pulmonary vascular pattern of "shunt vascularity" (i.e., the small pulmonary arteries are unusually well visualized in the periphery of both lungs). Some patients with ASDs are troubled by recurrent pulmonary infections due to greatly augmented pulmonic blood flow. Bacterial endocarditis is rare in the patient with an otherwise uncomplicated ASD, probably due to the absence of "jet" lesions and turbulent blood flow. However, endocarditis does occur in those with ostium primum defects, primarily because of the coexisting cleft mitral valve.

On physical examination, the patient with an uncomplicated ASD has equal A and V waves in the jugular venous pulse. On palpation of the precordium, a prominent right ventricular impulse may be felt in patients whose shunts are at least 2 : 1 in magnitude. Characteristically, this impulse is forceful and of short duration. Presystolic right ventricular distention may be palpable. In addition, a pulmonary artery impulse may be palpable in the second left intercostal space, and a systolic thrill—indicative of a large shunt or coexisting pulmonic stenosis—may also be palpable in this location. On auscultation, the S_1 is often "split," with the second component being pronounced. If the pulmonary artery is dilated, an ejection click may be audible. The typical murmur of an ASD begins immediately after the S_1 and is ejection in quality, reaching a peak in midsystole and ending well before the S_2. The rapid ejection of a large right ventricular stroke volume into a dilated pulmonary artery accounts for the murmur. The flow of blood across the ASD itself does not produce a murmur. The systolic ejection murmur is typically soft and is often labeled an "innocent murmur." When the murmur is loud, there may be associated pulmonic stenosis or an unusually large left-to-right shunt. Wide radiation of the murmur suggests coexisting peripheral pulmonary artery stenosis. Apart from these systolic murmurs, there may be a diastolic rumble resulting from the large blood flow across the tricuspid valve (i.e., a murmur of "relative" tricuspid stenosis).

One of the classic physical findings in the patient with an ASD is wide and fixed splitting of the S_2; that is, the aortic and pulmonic components of the S_2 are widely split during inspiration and demonstrate no change in splitting with expiration. The wide splitting is caused by a delay in pulmonic valve closure, resulting from an increased duration of right ventricular ejection. The splitting is fixed because phasic changes in systemic venous return during respiration are associated with reciprocal changes in the volume of shunted blood from the left to the right atrium. Although fixed splitting of the S_2 is the typical finding in the patient with an ASD, it is not invariably present. Since shunting of blood from the left to the right atrium occurs predominantly during diastole, the duration of diastole is an important determinant of shunt volume and, therefore, of the degree to which the splitting of the S_2 is fixed. Thus, as heart rate increases, diastole is shortened, and the left-to-right shunt per beat decreases. As a result, right ventricular stroke volume is diminished, and the splitting of the S_2 is lessened. Bradycardia produces the opposite result. With atrial fibrillation, the splitting of the S_2 varies inversely with the duration of the preceding cardiac cycle. Finally, the patient's postural position at the time of auscultation is a determinant of the degree to which the S_2 exhibits fixed splitting.

With the development of pulmonary hypertension, the physical findings in the patient with an ASD are substantially altered. The jugular venous pulse may demonstrate prominent A waves (due to enhanced right atrial contraction) or V waves (due to the development of tricuspid regurgitation). The patient may have cyanosis because of right-to-left shunting. On precordial palpation, the right ventricular thrusting impulse may become more sustained and less dynamic, and the pulmonary artery impulse may be easily palpable. On auscultation, the S_2, particularly the pulmonic component, increases appreciably in intensity. The splitting of the S_2 may become narrow, and in fact, as pulmonary artery pressure and resistance approach systemic levels, the S_2 may become single. As the left-to-right shunt becomes balanced or begins to reverse, the systolic murmur may disappear. At the same time, a holosystolic murmur of tricuspid regurgitation may appear. A diastolic decrescendo murmur of pulmonic regurgitation may be present in the patient with severe pulmonary hypertension, and a systolic ejection click may be audible. If the right ventricle fails, a gallop sound may be present.

The ECG in the patient with a secundum ASD demonstrates a rightward frontal QRS axis and an incomplete right bundle branch block pattern. In older patients, the QRS axis may be normal because of the leftward axis shift with age. In striking contrast, the patient with an ostium primum ASD has left axis deviation and an incomplete right bundle branch block pattern. *Indeed, the combined presence of left axis deviation and a right bundle branch block pattern in a young patient with no other reason for this electrocardiographic pattern and with other findings consistent with an atrial septal defect suggests an ostium primum ASD.* The patient with a sinus venosus–type ASD typically has a normal or rightward QRS axis but a P wave axis to the left of +15 degrees. The patient with an ASD usually remains in sinus rhythm during the first three decades of life. In later adult years, however, the incidence of atrial arrhythmias increases, with atrial fibrillation being the most common rhythm disturbance. The P–R interval is usually normal or only slightly prolonged. Finally, ventricular preexcitation has been reported in patients with ASDs, and complete right bundle branch block can occur in those with uncomplicated ASDs. With the development of pulmonary hypertension, electrocardiographic evidence of right ventricular hypertrophy, complete right bundle branch block, and right axis deviation increases in frequency.

The presence of an ASD is confirmed by cardiac catheterization when a distinct increase in oxygen saturation is demonstrated in the right atrium. Although venous catheterization usually allows one to cross the defect with a catheter, this does not help to distinguish an ASD from a patent foramen ovale. The presence and degree of pulmonary hypertension is assessed by measuring the pulmonary arterial pressure. Contrast angiography is essential in the patient with an ostium primum ASD to evaluate the interventricular septum and mitral valve. In addition, it usually demonstrates a "swan-neck" deformity of the left ventricular outflow tract. Echocardiography may reveal "paradoxical septal motion" and an enlarged right ventricular chamber. Two-dimensional echocardiography may be particularly useful for assessing the interventricular septum, tricuspid, and mitral valves.

Prolonged survival of the patient with an ASD is not uncommon, and some persons are in their 70s or 80s when the ASD is discovered. In large part, survival depends on whether pulmonary hypertension develops during adulthood, since it markedly shortens longevity. Death in the patient with an ASD is most commonly caused by right ventricular failure or arrhythmias. Left ventricular dysfunction, when it occurs, is often secondary to right ventricular dysfunction (rather than to an intrinsic abnormality of left ventricular function).

An ASD with a left-to-right shunt of 1.5:1.0 or greater should be closed surgically (by direct suture or by means of a patch) even in an asymptomatic patient. This is performed to prevent the development of pulmonary hypertension and right ventricular dysfunction from chronic volume overload. Such surgery should be performed even in patients over the age of 60 years, and closure of the ASD in these individuals can improve both symptoms and survival. The operative mortality is less than 1 percent for an uncomplicated secundum ASD but is somewhat higher for an ostium primum ASD. In the uncommon patient who has developed severe pulmonary hypertension due to irreversible pulmonary vascular disease, closure of the ASD should not be performed.

Postoperatively, a faint end-systolic ejection murmur, probably due to dilatation of the pulmonary artery, may be present in many patients after successful repair of a secundum ASD. However, the tricuspid diastolic murmur should disappear. A small, residual left-to-right atrial shunt—often impossible to detect clinically and of no hemodynamic consequence—is present in about 7 percent of patients. A murmur of mitral regurgitation is present in the patient with an ostium primum defect because of the associated cleft in the mitral valve. Postoperatively, the ECG may not return completely to normal in the patient with a secundum ASD, but the mean QRS frontal axis may become normal. With an ostium primum defect, the QRS axis usually does not change. Although supraventricular arrhythmias (paroxysmal atrial tachycardia, atrial flutter-fibrillation) can occur postoperatively, junctional and ventricular arrhythmias are uncommon. Sinus node dysfunction is particularly common after repair of a sinus venosus defect, and complete heart block occasionally occurs following the repair of an ostium primum ASD. Hemodynamic abnormalities may persist after repair of an ostium primum defect, particularly mitral regurgitation, even when a mitral valvuloplasty is performed at the time of ASD closure. Since this may necessitate later surgery, long-term follow-up is mandatory. Antibiotic prophylaxis against endocarditis is unnecessary after repair of a secundum ASD (in the absence of mitral valve prolapse) but should be continued following the repair of an ostium primum defect.

1. Dexter L. Atrial septal defect. Br Heart J 1956; 18:209–25.
   A thorough review of the hemodynamic findings in 60 patients with ASDs.
2. Dalen JE, Haynes FW, Dexter L. Life expectancy with atrial septal defect: influence of complicating pulmonary vascular diseases. JAMA 1967; 200:442–6.
   The data presented in this study show that those patients with ASD and pulmonary vascular disease have a very poor prognosis. Therefore, all ASDs without pulmonary vascular disease should be surgically corrected.
3. Rodstein M, Zeman FD, Gerber IE. Atrial septal defect in the aged. Circulation 1961; 23:665–74.
   The clinical findings in 18 elderly patients with ASDs are reviewed.
4. Nasrallah AT, Hall RJ, Garcia E, Leachman RD, Cooley DA. Surgical repair of atrial septal defect in patients over 60 years of age. Circulation 1976; 53:329–31.
   This study demonstrates that surgical repair of secundum ASDs in patients older than 60 is safe, has low morbidity, and generally causes symptomatic improvement.
5. Markman P, Howitt G, Wade EG. Atrial septal defect in the middle aged and elderly. Q J Med 1965; 34:409–26.
   A review of the findings in 67 patients, aged 40–69, with ASDs.
6. Bonow RO, Borer JS, Rosing DR, Bacharach SL, Green MV, Kent KM. Left ventricular functional reserve in adult patients with atrial septal defect: pre and postoperative studies. Circulation 1981; 63:1315–22.
   Left ventricular dysfunction appears to be due to abnormal systolic-diastolic relations of the interventricular septum in patients with ASDs.
7. Adams CW. A reappraisal of life expectancy with atrial shunts of the secundum type. Chest 1965; 48:357–75.
   A massive review of over 2,500 patients with secundum ASDs.
8. Bedford DE. The anatomical type of atrial septal defect: their incidence and clinical diagnosis. Am J Cardiol 1960; 6:568–74.
   This paper emphasizes the importance of the standard ECG in allowing one to differentiate an ostium primum defect from other types of ASD.
9. Aygen MM, Braunwald E. The splitting of the second heart sound in normal subjects and in patients with congenital heart disease. Circulation 1962; 25:328–45.
   The phonocardiograms in 350 patients (normal individuals and patients with congenital heart disease) are reviewed to evaluate the splitting of S_2.
10. Barritt DW, Davies DH, Jacob G. Heart sounds and pressures in atrial septal defect. Br Heart J 1965; 27:90–8.
    A detailed phonocardiographic and hemodynamic study of 23 patients with uncomplicated secundum ASDs.
11. Cayler GC. Spontaneous functional closure of symptomatic atrial septal defects. N Engl J Med 1967; 276:65–73.

The spontaneous functional closures of large symptomatic ASDs in 3 infants are presented.

12. Craig RJ, Selzer A. Natural history and prognosis of atrial septal defect. Circulation 1968; 37:805–15.
The clinical courses in 128 adults with ASDs were evaluated in this study. In this group, pulmonary hypertension developed in 18 (14%).

13. McNamara DG, Latson LA. Long-term follow-up of patients with malformations for which definitive surgical repair has been available for 25 years or more. Am J Cardiol 1982; 50:560–8.
A detailed summary of physical findings, electrocardiographic and radiographic abnormalities in patients following ASD closure.

14. Gall JC Jr, Stern AM, Cohen MM, Adams MS, Davidson RT. Holt-Oram syndrome: clinical and genetic study of a large family. Am J Hum Genet 1966; 18:187–200.
An extensive and detailed analysis of a pedigree with this syndrome, emphasizing the wide variability in clinical expression.

15. Gotsman MS, Astley R, Parsons CG. Partial anomalous pulmonary venous drainage in association with atrial septal defect. Br Heart J 1965; 27:566–71.
The cardiac catheterization findings in 11 children with ASDs and partial anomalous pulmonary venous return are described, and various angiographic techniques of demonstrating the anomalous venous drainage are outlined.

16. Pryor R, Woodwark GM, Blount SG Jr. Electrocardiographic changes in atrial septal defects: ostium secundum defect versus ostium primum (endocardial cushion) defect. Am Heart J 1959; 58:689–700.
The ECGs of 100 patients with secundum ASDs and 33 patients with primum ASDs are reviewed and their differences discussed.

17. Somerville J. Ostium primum defect: factors causing deterioration in the natural history. Br Heart J 1965; 27:413–9.
Of 122 patients with ostium primum ASDs, 27 showed evidence of hemodynamic decompensation. Such deterioration was usually temporally related to the appearance of various tachyarrhythmias.

18. Leachman RD, Cokkinos DV, Cooley DA. Association of ostium secundum atrial septal defects with mitral valve prolapse. Am J Cardiol 1976; 38:167–9.
Severe mitral valve prolapse was observed in 16 of 92 patients with secundum ASDs.

19. St John Sutton MG, Tajik AJ, McGoon DC. Atrial septal defect in patients ages 60 years or older: operative results and long-term postoperative follow-up. Circulation 1981; 64:402–9.
A review of 66 patients aged 60 years or older at the time of secundum ASD closure. Surgery resulted in marked symptomatic improvement and improved late survival.

20. Liberthson RR, Boucher CA, Strauss HW, Dinsmore RE, McKusick KA, Pohost GM. Right ventricular function in adult atrial septal defect: preoperative and postoperative assessment and clinical implications. Am J Cardiol 1981; 47:56–60.
This study suggests that right ventricular dysfunction in patients with ASDs can be prevented by early closure.

21. Goldfaden DM, Jones M, Morrow AG. Long-term results of repair of incomplete persistent atrioventricular canal. J Thorac Cardiovasc Surg 1981; 82:669–73.
Of 39 patients followed for >10 years after ASD repair, 34 (88%) were alive 13 years post-operatively, but only 20 (52%) were free of complications).

22. Brandenburg RO Jr, Holmes DR Jr, Brandenburg RO, McGoon DC. Clinical follow-up study of paroxysmal supraventricular tachyarrhythmias after operative repair of a secundum type atrial septal defect in adults. Am J Cardiol 1983; 51:273–6.
Of 16 adult patients with ASD and preoperative paroxysmal atrial fibrillation, 14 (88%) continued to have frequent paroxysms of atrial fibrillation postoperatively.

VENTRICULAR SEPTAL DEFECT

Ventricular septal defects (VSDs) account for about 30 percent of all congenital cardiac abnormalities in full-term, live births. Because of the prominent physical findings associated with them, most VSDs are detected before adulthood. Anatomically, a VSD may lie above or below the crista supraventricularis (the muscular ridge separating the main portion of the right ventricle from the infundibular portion). Those positioned above this ridge are termed *supracristal,* whereas those lying below are termed *infracristal.* A supracristal defect lies immediately beneath the pulmonary orifice, so that the pulmonic valve forms part of the superior margin of the defect. Viewed from the left ventricle, a supracristal VSD is located just below the commissure that joins the left and right aortic cusps. An infracristal defect may be located in the membranous or muscular septum. Infracristal VSDs that are located in the region of the membranous septum are most common. When viewed from the left ventricle, they are located immediately beneath the aortic valve, adjacent to the commissure joining the right and noncoronary cusps.

A VSD that is present at birth may close spontaneously during the first years of life, a period in which the growth rate of the heart is rapid. Spontaneous closure is estimated to occur in 25 to 40 percent of VSDs. If a VSD does not close completely, its relative size may diminish substantially during the first 2 years of life. In addition, septal muscle may contract around the defect, further reducing its size, in which case the defect may remain anatomically patent but functionally unimportant, since the left-to-right shunt is small.

Congenital VSDs occur with similar frequency in males and females. Familial occurrence has been described but is uncommon. The presence of a VSD usually is discovered in early infancy, primarily because of the loud murmur it produces. This murmur first appears as the high neonatal pulmonary vascular resistance falls to normal, thus allowing left-to-right shunting through the defect. In addition, a VSD can be acquired as a result of acute myocardial infarction or trauma (blunt or sharp) to the chest.

In the patient with a large VSD, mortality is highest in early childhood, with most deaths resulting from left ventricular failure or severe pulmonary hypertension with associated right ventricular failure. In those who survive to adolescence and adulthood, symptoms of biventricular congestive heart failure (dyspnea, orthopnea, and peripheral edema) are often present. In addition, the patient may have poor growth and development as well as frequent pulmonary infections. Finally, bacterial endocarditis is a major risk in the patient with a VSD. It is especially likely to occur in the patient in whom a high velocity "jet" of shunted blood causes a traumatic lesion on the right ventricular endocardium.

The physiologic consequences of a VSD depend on its size and the degree of elevation of pulmonary arterial pressure and resistance. A small VSD causes little or no functional disturbance, since the intracardiac shunt is negligible. With a larger VSD (i.e., a defect through which a 2:1 or greater shunt exists), several hemodynamic problems can develop, including volume overload of the left ventricle as well as a substantial elevation of pulmonary arterial pressure and resistance. If the VSD is very large, systolic pressures in the two ventricles are equal, and the magnitude of blood flow to the pulmonary and systemic circulations is determined by the vascular resistances in each bed. Therefore, as resistance in the pulmonary bed rises, left-to-right shunting is reduced; as the pulmonary vascular resistance equals or exceeds systemic, the shunt becomes balanced and finally reversed (i.e., right-to-left [Eisenmenger syndrome]).

Pressure overload of the right ventricle ensues, and the pulmonary vasculature resembles that described under Eisenmenger Syndrome (see p. 168).

The classic murmur of a VSD is holosystolic and is loudest along the lower left sternal border; it is usually accompanied by a thrill. When the VSD is located below the crista supraventricularis, the murmur and thrill are maximal in the third and fourth intercostal spaces to the left of the sternum. In contrast, when the defect is located above the crista supraventricularis, the accompanying murmur and thrill are maximal in the second left intercostal space and may radiate to the neck. Small VSDs produce prominent, high-frequency, early systolic murmurs. As the size of the defect increases, the murmur remains loud, harsh, and holosystolic, provided there is a substantial pressure difference between the left and right ventricles throughout systole. As pulmonary hypertension develops and the pressure gradient between the left and right ventricles diminishes, the systolic murmur and thrill become progressively softer, ultimately disappearing completely.

Apart from the murmur produced by the shunt, flow into a dilated pulmonary artery can produce an ejection sound as well as a short, soft systolic ejection murmur maximal at the second left intercostal space. The murmur of pulmonic insufficiency (a high-frequency diastolic decrescendo murmur best heard in the second left intercostal space) is audible in some patients with pulmonary hypertension. A short diastolic apical rumble (due to augmented antegrade flow through the mitral valve) may be audible if the left-to-right shunt is large (at least 2:1). When sizable left-to-right shunts occur with little or no pulmonary hypertension, the left ventricular impulse is dynamic and displaced laterally, and the right ventricular impulse is unimpressive. However, with the development of pulmonary hypertension, a heaving right ventricular impulse and a pulsation over the pulmonary trunk become palpable. Pulmonic valve closure also may be palpated.

In the patient with a VSD, the presence of clubbing and either intermittent or continuous cyanosis is suggestive of marked pulmonary hypertension. The patient with pulmonary hypertension and a balanced shunt may have cyanosis only with exercise or emotional upset. A large VSD with concomitant pulmonary hypertension is associated with an elevated jugular venous pressure. Prominent V waves are present in the jugular venous pulse in the patient in whom right ventricular failure develops. A prominent A wave is not present in the patient with a large VSD, even though pulmonary hypertension and right ventricular failure may be severe.

The ECG is a helpful guide to the hemodynamic impairment caused by a VSD. A large left-to-right shunt produces electrocardiographic evidence of left atrial enlargement, as well as left ventricular hypertrophy with strain. The QRS axis is generally directed downward. Once severe pulmonary hypertension develops, a rightward shift in axis occurs, and the ECG demonstrates right ventricular hypertrophy and right atrial enlargement. A small VSD is associated with a normal chest radiograph, whereas a large VSD with persistent left-to-right shunting is associated with left ventricular enlargement and "shunt vascularity." When severe pulmonary hypertension develops, the chest radiograph reveals marked enlargement of the main pulmonary trunk and proximal pulmonary arteries as well as rapid tapering of the pulmonary vasculature, so that the peripheral pulmonary arterial radicals appear small and the distal lung fields oligemic.

The diagnosis of a VSD is confirmed by cardiac catheterization, which reveals an increase in oxygen saturation at the right ventricular level. The site, size, and number of VSDs, as well as the presence or absence of associated lesions, are demonstrated by contrast angiography. The size of the shunt can be assessed qualitatively (by angiography) or quantitatively (by measuring the increase in oxygen saturation at the right ventricular level or the magnitude of recirculation by indicator dilution).

In 5 to 10 percent of patients with a VSD, aortic valvular regurgitation occurs concomitantly. Although the VSD in these individuals can be supra- or infracristal, it is more commonly the latter and is located immediately beneath the right coronary and noncoronary aortic cusps. The aortic regurgitation usually develops years after birth and is thought to result from a congenital abnormality in aortic leaflet support. On physical examination, these patients have murmurs of both a VSD and aortic regurgitation, closely mimicking a true continuous murmur.

The definitive treatment of a VSD entails its surgical closure, usually with a patch, if the left-to-right shunt is greater than 1.5:1.0. Such closure is preferably accomplished before the age of 2 years. The infant with a small VSD and no hemodynamic sequelae may be treated expectantly, since these defects may close spontaneously. The likelihood of spontaneous closure falls markedly with age. If a VSD is not treated surgically, antibiotic prophylaxis for endocarditis is mandatory. In early infancy, a large VSD can lead to congestive heart failure and respiratory distress, and palliative banding of the pulmonary artery to diminish pulmonary blood flow may be necessary until surgical closure of the defect is feasible. In this situation, systemic arterial vasodilators, such as hydralazine or nitroprusside, may be lifesaving, since they reduce systemic vascular resistance relative to pulmonary vascular resistance and, as a result, diminish pulmonary blood flow.

Most patients are improved symptomatically following VSD closure, even though the hemodynamic result may not be perfect. A faint pulmonary systolic murmur may persist. A residual VSD (usually small and of no hemodynamic consequence) is present in up to 25 percent of patients. A widely split S_2 is common and is due to right bundle branch block. The patient's age and pulmonary vascular resistance at the time of surgery are important in predicting which patients may have progressive pulmonary hypertension postoperatively; progressive pulmonary vascular obstructive disease seldom develops in patients operated on before 2 years of age, whereas the results in older patients with a moderate to severe increase in pulmonary vascular resistance are less predictable.

The radiographic findings postoperatively depend on preoperative hemodynamics and the results of surgery. Patients with a large defect and high pulmonary blood flow usually show a marked early decrease in heart size and pulmonary arterial plethora, but some patients continue to have at least mild enlargement of both ventricles. An initial decrease in heart size after operation followed by late cardiomegaly generally signifies progressive pulmonary vascular obstructive disease. The electrocardiographic evidence of atrial and ventricular hypertrophy generally regresses after VSD closure. Right bundle branch block occurs frequently (in 44–100% of patients) when the repair is performed by a right ventricular approach and somewhat less frequently following repair performed through the tricuspid valve by way of an atriotomy. Such right bundle branch block can be produced by a proximal lesion in the right bundle branch, a distal injury to the peripheral Purkinje fibers, or both. Right bundle branch block can occur early or late postoperatively. In a small percentage of patients, such right bundle branch block occurs with left anterior hemiblock. Complete heart block, once a common problem, now occurs in less than 2 percent of patients. If complete heart block persists beyond 3 to 4 weeks, a permanent pacemaker should be inserted. Supraventricular and ventricular arrhythmias can also occur, and late sudden death following VSD repair occurs rarely.

The risk of endocarditis decreases dramatically after complete closure of a VSD. However, if even a small VSD persists, this risk is not reduced (and may even be increased). Therefore, endocarditis prophylaxis should be continued in all patients following VSD repair.

1. Mitchell SC, Korones SB, Berendes HW. Congenital heart disease in 56,109 births: incidence and natural history. Circulation 1971; 43:323–32.
   Of these 56,000 births, 457 had some kind of congenital heart disease, and VSD was by far the most common. Of infants with VSD who survived more than 6 months, spontaneous closure occurred in 35%.
2. Hoffman JIE. Natural history of congenital heart disease: problems in its assessment with special reference to ventricular septal defects. Circulation 1968; 37:97–125.
   There is clearly a high incidence (perhaps 50%) of spontaneous closure of VSDs during childhood.
3. Perloff JK, Lindgren KM. Adult survival in congenital heart disease. Part III: Common and uncommon defects with exceptional adult survival. Geriatrics 1974; 29:93–102.
   The patient with an isolated VSD is usually discovered in childhood. By the time he reaches adulthood, the defect has either closed spontaneously or been surgically repaired.
4. Corone P, Doyon F, Gaudeau S, Guerin F, Vernant P, Ducam H, Rumeau-Rouquette C, Gaudeul P. Natural history of ventricular septal defect: a study involving 790 cases. Circulation 1977; 55:908–15.
   A 25-year study of 790 patients with VSDs who were not operated on. Of the patients who reach 1 year of age, only those with large shunts require surgical closure.
5. Campbell M. Natural history of ventricular septal defect. Br Heart J 1971; 33:246–57.
   VSD and PDA are the only 2 congenital cardiac defects that may close spontaneously. This paper describes the natural history of medically treated VSDs.
6. Evans JR, Rowe RD, Keith JD. Spontaneous closure of ventricular septal defects. Circulation 1960; 22:1044–54.
   The fact that spontaneous closure of VSDs occurs is emphasized in this report. Such spontaneous closure appears to be common with small VSDs and may rarely occur with lesions large enough to produce congestive heart failure.
7. Glancy DL, Roberts WC. Complete spontaneous closure of ventricular septal defect: necropsy study of 5 subjects. Am J Med 1967; 43:846–53.
   Five patients who had evidence of spontaneous closure of their VSDs at necropsy are reviewed, and it is speculated that spontaneous closure is a common occurrence in early childhood.
8. Somerville J, Brandao A, Ross DN. Aortic regurgitation with ventricular septal defect: surgical management and clinical features. Circulation 1970; 41:317–30.
   Of 20 patients with VSDs and aortic regurgitation who underwent surgical correction, 18 survived the surgery, and 17 of these had a long-term satisfactory result.
9. Graham AF, Stinson EB, Daily PO, Harrison DC. Ventricular septal defects after myocardial infarction: early operative treatment. JAMA 1973; 225:708–11.
   Twelve patients who had VSDs in association with acute anterior myocardial infarction are described. In most, successful early operative closure was accomplished, and 6 of the 12 lived at least 6 months.
10. Hoffman JIE, Rudolph AM. Increasing pulmonary vascular resistance during infancy in association with ventricular septal defect. Pediatrics 1966; 38:220–30.
    Three infants who had large VSDs and who developed substantial increases in pulmonary vascular resistance during the first 2 years of life are described.
11. Hunt CE, Formanek G, Levine MA, Castaneda A, Moller JH. Banding of the pulmonary artery: results in 111 children. Circulation 1971; 43:395–406.

The overall mortality for banding in patients with isolated VSD is 10%. Mortality is highest in those under 3 months of age and lowest in those older than 1 year.

12. Bloomfield DK. The natural history of ventricular septal defect in patients surviving infancy. Circulation 1964; 29:914–55.
    A comprehensive review that attempts to define the natural history of uncomplicated VSDs.

13. Leatham A, Segal B. Auscultatory and phonocardiographic signs of ventricular septal defect with left to right shunt. Circulation 1962; 25:318–27.
    A detailed review of the auscultatory findings in patients with small and large VSDs.

14. Frenckner BP, Olin CL, Bomfim V, Bjarke B, Wallgren CG, Bjork VO. Detachment of the septal tricuspid leaflet during transatrial closure of the isolated ventricular septal defect. J Thorac Cardiovasc Surg 1981; 82:773–8.
    A review of the transatrial technique of closing VSDs in 151 patients.

15. Karpawich PP, Duff DF, Mullins CE, Cooley DA, McNamara DG. Ventricular septal defect with associated aortic valve insufficiency. J Thorac Cardiovasc Surg 1981; 82:182–9.
    This report suggests that repair of the prolapsed aortic valve at the time of VSD closure leads to a more satisfactory late result.

16. Sutherland GR, Godman MJ, Smallhorn JF. Ventricular septal defects: Two dimensional echocardiographic and morphologic correlations. Br Heart J 1982; 47:316–28.
    In this study of 280 infants and children with VSDs, two dimensional echocardiography was quite good at identifying membranous defects, but its ability to identify muscular defects was quite limited.

17. Whitman V, Ellis NG. Pulmonary hemodynamics after repair of left to right shunt lesions associated with pulmonary artery hypertension. Prog Cardiovasc Dis 1975; 17:467–73.
    This review indicates that mild to moderate pulmonary hypertension due to a large shunt usually regresses but does not disappear postoperatively. Surgical closure of VSDs before 2 years of age is recommended.

18. Griffiths SP, Turi GK, Ellis K, Krongrad E, Swift LH, Gersony WM, Bowman FO Jr, Malm JR. Muscular ventricular septal defects repaired with left ventriculotomy. Am J Cardiol 1981; 48:877–86.
    A description of the technique for closure of single or multiple VSDs in the muscular septum via the left ventricle.

19. Beekman RH, Rocchini AP, Rosenthal A. Hemodynamic effects of hydralazine in infants with a large ventricular septal defect. Circulation 1981; 65:523–8.
    Systemic arterial vasodilators may be life-saving in the emergency management of large VSDs.

20. McNamara DG, Latson LA. Long-term follow-up of patients with malformations for which definitive surgical repair has been available for 25 years or more. Am J Cardiol 1982; 50:560–8.
    A detailed review of the late effects of VSD repair. Although most of these patients live a normal life, many have residua or sequelae that require close observation or treatment.

21. Vetter VL, Horowitz LN. Electrophysiologic residua and sequelae of surgery for congenital heart defects. Am J Cardiol 1982; 50:588–604.
    The etiology and incidence of right bundle branch block and complete heart block following VSD closure are discussed.

22. Elliott LP, Bargeron LM Jr, Bream PR, Soto B, Curry GC. Axial cineangiography in congenital heart disease. Section II. Specific lesions. Circulation 1977; 56:1084–93.
    A description of the optimal angiographic delineation of VSDs and other lesions.

23. Schrire V, Vogelpoel L, Beck W, Nellen M, Swanepael A. Ventricular septal defect: the clinical spectrum. Br Heart J 1965; 27:813–28.
    This study, which was based on a series of 160 patients, provides an extremely useful clinical approach to the assessment of VSDs.

24. Soto B, Becker AE, Moulaert AJ, Lie JT, Anderson RH. Classification of ventricular septal defects. Br Heart J 1980; 43:332–43.

A review of the pathological findings in 220 hearts and a proposed comprehensive new classification for VSDs.

PATENT DUCTUS ARTERIOSUS

Patent ductus arteriosus (PDA) is an arterial channel that connects the left (or, rarely, the right) pulmonary artery to the aorta just distal to the left subclavian artery. Embryologically, the ductus consists of the distal portion of the sixth left thoracic arch. During fetal life, it allows blood from the pulmonary artery to bypass the lungs and enter the descending aorta. The ductus arteriosus ordinarily closes during the last weeks of intrauterine life or the several weeks after birth. Such closure is believed to be induced by an increase in the oxygenation of fetal blood, but prostaglandins may also play a role in the closure of the ductus. Persistent hypoxemia and maternal rubella have been implicated as possible etiologic factors in persistent patency of the ductus after birth. Infants born at a high altitude and premature infants have a higher incidence of a persistently patent ductus arteriosus.

Shortly after an infant's birth, pulmonary arterial pressure and resistance decrease, and systemic vascular resistance increases (due to occlusion of the umbilical cord). As a result, the direction of blood flow through the ductus is reversed, and blood moves from the aorta to the pulmonary artery. With normal pulmonary arterial pressure, the flow through the ductus occurs during both systole and diastole, resulting in a continuous murmur. This "runoff" occurs during all phases of the cardiac cycle, resulting in a wide systemic pulse pressure and a relatively low diastolic arterial pressure. With large shunts through the ductus, the left ventricular stroke volume is markedly increased; in fact, the work of the left ventricle may be augmented to such an extent that congestive heart failure ensues. Pulmonary arterial hypertension and pulmonary vascular obstruction can develop in association with a PDA. If pulmonary vascular resistance equals or exceeds systemic vascular resistance, the direction of the shunt is reversed.

An isolated PDA occurs three times more often in females than in males. A small PDA ordinarily is well tolerated, and symptoms may be absent or may not become evident until childhood or early adult life. However, with a large shunt through the ductus, left ventricular failure develops.

On physical examination, bounding peripheral pulses with a widened pulse pressure are present. A systolic or systolic and diastolic thrill is palpable in the suprasternal notch and second left intercostal space. The left ventricular impulse is displaced laterally, reflecting left ventricular dilatation. On auscultation, a normal S_1 may be followed by an aortic ejection sound at the apex and left sternal border. The S_2, often obscured by the murmur, is narrowly split. As pulmonary arterial pressure rises, the pulmonic component may become accentuated. An S_3 occasionally is heard. The characteristic "machinery murmur" is heard best in the second left intercostal space, with radiation to the anterior chest, neck, and back. The murmur begins after the S_1, persists through the S_2, and fades gradually during diastole. It begins softly and increases in intensity, reaching its peak at or immediately after the S_2; from that point, it gradually wanes until its termination. (See Table 1 for the causes of continuous murmurs other than a PDA.) When a large shunt is present, an apical mid-diastolic murmur (due to increased flow across the mitral valve) may be noted, and a systolic murmur (due to increased flow across the aortic valve) may also be present.

With increasing pulmonary hypertension, the diastolic component of the murmur may disappear, and the systolic component becomes shorter and softer until it may disappear as well. At this point, only an ejection click is audible. When severe pulmonary hypertension develops, the diastolic decrescendo murmur of pulmonic regurgitation may be present.

It is important to distinguish a PDA from an aortopulmonary septal defect. Although patients with a PDA frequently survive to adulthood without surgery, those with an aortopulmonary septal defect rarely do so. In the latter condition, the defect (and consequently the shunt) is large, and severe pulmonary hypertension usually develops early. The distinction between these two entities is best made at cardiac catheterization.

On the ECG, left ventricular hypertrophy and left atrial enlargement usually are obvious when there is a large left-to-right shunt through a PDA. If present, right ventricular hypertrophy indicates a substantial increase in pulmonary arterial pressure. The chest x-ray demonstrates left ventricular and left atrial enlargement, as well as a prominent main pulmonary artery; there is a filling in of the angle between the main pulmonary artery and the aortic knob. Chest fluoroscopy ordinarily reveals a pulsating aortic arch, increased pulmonary vascular markings, and increased pulsations in the hilar shadows. With pulmonary hypertension, right ventricular enlargement may also be noted. At the time of cardiac catheterization, there is an increase in oxygen saturation at the level of the pulmonary artery, with the highest saturation in the left pulmonary artery. The peripheral systemic arterial saturation is normal unless the shunt is bidirectional. In addition, one may be able to pass a catheter from the pulmonary artery through the ductus into the descending aorta, thus proving the patency of the ductus arteriosus.

A PDA may be associated with several different cardiac abnormalities, including ventricular septal defect, coarctation of the aorta, aortic stenosis, and pulmonic stenosis. In some patients, the ductus arteriosus may be the primary source of blood flow to the lungs (e.g., in pulmonary atresia), or it may be the primary source of blood flow to the distal aorta (e.g., in complete interruption of the aortic arch). If these conditions are not recognized preoperatively and the ductus is ligated, the outcome is likely to be catastrophic.

A PDA rarely closes spontaneously after early infancy. The potential complications include bacterial endarteritis, congestive heart failure, and severe pulmonary hypertension. Pulmonary vascular obstruction can develop relatively late in the adult. A reversal of flow (i.e., right-to-left shunting) through a PDA can cause differential cyanosis (cyanosis of the lower but not of the upper extremities). If present, this implies that the patient is probably inoperable. Rupture of a PDA is a rare complication and is usually associated with the development of an aneurysm or calcification. The life expectancy of the patient with a PDA who does not have surgical closure depends on the size of the shunt but averages about 40 years. However, a small shunt through a PDA is compatible with a normal life expectancy.

In the past, the medical treatment of a PDA has centered on potential complications, including antibiotic prophylaxis against bacterial endarteritis and measures to treat congestive heart failure if it develops. More recently, inhibitors of prostaglandin synthesis (e.g., indomethacin) have been used successfully to induce closure in premature infants. Conversely, prostaglandin E has been used to prevent closure of the ductus in patients in whom its presence is essential for survival.

In 1938, Gross performed the first surgical correction of a PDA. Surgical closure is ordinarily a simple procedure and is accomplished by simple ligation or division of the ductus. Elective surgery is advised for all patients over 1 year of age in whom a substantial shunt is present. Surgical therapy carries a very small mortality (approximately 0.5%) and is generally highly successful. In older patients and in those with aneurysmal dilatation or calcification of the ductus, surgical resection (rather than simple ligation) may require cardiopulmonary bypass. Once severe pulmonary hypertension and pulmonary vascular obstructive disease develop, surgery is contraindicated. It may also be contraindicated in patients in whom inoperable associated anomalies are present, since the ductus then serves as the essential pathway connecting the pulmonary and arterial systems.

The repair of a PDA in the absence of pulmonary vascular obstructive disease or left ventricular dysfunction is probably the only cardiac operation (with the possible exception of repair of an uncomplicated secundum atrial septal defect in childhood) that can be considered truly "curative," that is, it produces completely normal cardiac structure and function. The physical examination of the patient after surgical closure of a PDA should be completely normal. However, a faint systolic murmur, probably related to persistent dilatation of the main pulmonary artery, occurs in about 20 percent of patients postoperatively. Recanalization of a ligated rather than a divided ductus has been observed rarely.

Electrocardiographic evidence of left ventricular hypertrophy usually regresses promptly after surgery. If right ventricular hypertrophy is present preoperatively, its persistence beyond several months is an ominous sign of pulmonary vascular obstructive disease. There is no increased incidence of arrhythmias in patients following successful repair of a PDA. The chest x-ray usually shows a measurable decrease in heart size within days to weeks. If there was marked cardiomegaly preoperatively, it may require a year to subside. The main pulmonary artery and aorta may remain prominent despite successful repair, but the caliber of the peripheral pulmonary vessels should decrease promptly.

Approximately 10 percent of the patients with PDAs have substantially elevated pulmonary arterial pressures preoperatively. Those with a large left-to-right shunt and only mildly elevated pulmonary vascular resistance rarely develop pulmonary vascular obstructive disease, particularly if operated on before 2 years of age. However, even a moderately elevated pulmonary vascular resistance preoperatively can persist and progress. This finding has led to the recommendation that all PDAs be ligated before the patient reaches the age of 2 years, if possible.

The risk of bacterial endarteritis after successful repair of a PDA appears to be the same as that of the general population. Therefore, routine prophylaxis for bacterial endarteritis is generally discontinued 6 months postoperatively if there is no evidence of a residual shunt or associated cardiac abnormalities.

1. Gross RE, Hubbard JP. Surgical ligation of a patent ductus arteriosus. JAMA 1939; 112:729–31.
   The initial report of successful surgical closure of a PDA.
2. Boyer NH. Patent ductus arteriosus. Ann Thorac Surg 1967; 4:570–3.
   The historical aspects relevant to PDA are reviewed in this report.
3. Coggin CJ, Parker KR, Keith JD. Natural history of isolated patent ductus arteriosus and the effect of surgical correction: twenty years' experience at the Hospital for Sick Children, Toronto. Can Med Assoc J 1970; 102:718–20.
   The clinical course and findings in 744 children with PDA are reviewed. It is concluded that operative ligation is best performed between 6 and 12 months of age.
4. Campbell M. Patent ductus arteriosus: some notes on prognosis and on pulmonary hypertension. Br Heart J 1955; 17:511–33.
   The clinical findings and clinical courses in 160 patients with PDA are described.

5. Morrow AG, Clark WD. Closure of the calcified patent ductus. J Thorac Cardiovasc Surg 1966; 51:534–8.
   A surgical technique for closing a large calcified patent ductus is described. Such closure can be technically hazardous and, therefore, should probably be performed on cardiopulmonary bypass.

6. White PD, Mazurkie SJ, Boschetti AE. Patency of the ductus arteriosus at 90. N Engl J Med 1969; 280:146–7.
   A case report of a very elderly man with a PDA.

7. Heymann M, Rudolph A, Silverman NH. Closure of the ductus arteriosus in premature infants by inhibition of prostaglandin synthesis. N Engl J Med 1976; 295:530–3.
   Five premature infants are described in whom it was possible to close the ductus by the administration of indomethacin.

8. Kitterman JA, Edmunds LH Jr, Gregory GA, Heymann MA, Tooley WH, Rudolph AM. Patent ductus arteriosus in premature infants: incidence, relation to pulmonary disease and management. N Engl J Med 1972; 287:473–7.
   Among premature infants, PDAs are common, occurring in 15% of infants weighing less than 1,750 grams.

9. Heymann M, Berman W, Rudolph A, Whitman V. Dilatation of the ductus arteriosus by prostaglandin E_1 in aortic arch abnormalities. Circulation 1979; 59:169–73.
   A demonstration that prostaglandin E_1 can dilate the ductus arteriosus in at least some infants with aortic arch abnormalities.

10. Friedman WF, Hirschklau MJ, Printz MP, Pitlick PT, Kirkpatrick SE. Pharmacologic closure of patent ductus arteriosus in the premature infant. N Engl J Med 1976; 295:526–9.
    Six consecutive premature infants in whom indomethacin administration resulted in closure of a PDA are described.

11. Nadas AS. Patent ductus revisited. N Engl J Med 1976; 295:563–5.
    An editorial commenting on the usefulness of prostaglandin synthesis inhibition in producing closure of a PDA.

12. Freed MD, Heymann MA, Lewis AB, Roehl SL, Kensey RC. Prostaglandin E_1 in infants with ductus arteriosus–dependent congenital heart disease. Circulation 1981; 64:899–905.
    A report of 492 infants treated with PGE_1; 80% showed clinical improvement.

13. John S, Muralidharan S, Jairaj PS, Mani GK, Babuthaman MD, Krishnaswamy S, Sukumar IP, Cherian G. The adult ductus: review of surgical experience with 131 patients. J Thorac Cardiovasc Surg 1981; 82:314–9.
    This report discusses the findings, surgical management, and generally favorable outcome following surgery for a PDA in a large group of adults.

14. McNamara DG, Latson LA. Long-term follow-up of patients with malformations for which definitive surgical repair has been available for 25 years or more. Am J Cardiol 1982; 50:560–8.
    The clinical, hemodynamic, radiographic, and electrocardiographic alterations that occur following surgery for PDA are detailed.

15. Baylen B, Meyer RA, Korfhagen J, Benzing G III, Bubb ME, Kaplan S. Left ventricular performance in the critically ill premature infant with patent ductus arteriosus and pulmonary disease. Circulation 1977; 55:182–8.
    In the premature infant with a PDA and pulmonary disease, the echocardiographic assessment of left ventricular size and function may be helpful in determining the need for surgical closure.

16. Campbell M. Natural history of persistent ductus arteriosus. Br Heart J 1968; 30:4–13.
    A review of the literature dealing with the natural history of PDA in a group of unoperated patients.

Table 1. Differential diagnosis of continuous murmurs

Location	Underlying disease entity
First to second left intercostal spaces (and under left clavicle)	Patent ductus arteriosus
Second to fourth intercostal spaces	Aortopulmonary septal defect
Usually best heard in the second to third left intercostal spaces; occasionally may be heard best at the right of the sternum in the same area	Surgical shunts, e.g., aortopulmonary anastomoses
Usually heard best along the lower left sternal border, although it may be audible over the entire precordium	Rupture of sinus of Valsalva aneurysm
Audible over the left precordium	Coronary arteriovenous fistulae
May be audible anywhere that they occur	Arteriovenous fistulae

Source: Adapted from JT Willerson, CA Sanders (Eds). Clinical Cardiology. New York: Grune & Stratton, 1977.

ANOMALOUS PULMONARY VENOUS CONNECTION

The four pulmonary veins generally open separately into the left atrium. The term *anomalous pulmonary venous connection* implies that all four (in total anomalous connection) or one or more (in partial anomalous connection) pulmonary veins drain into a site other than the left atrium. *Total anomalous pulmonary venous connection (TAPVC)* accounts for 1 to 3 percent of all cases of congenital heart disease. The four anomalously connecting pulmonary veins emerge individually from the lungs and usually unite before entering the right atrium or one of the veins that drains into it. It is caused by agenesis of the common pulmonary vein (a temporary outgrowth of the left atrium) with persistence and enlargement of anastomotic vessels between the pulmonary and systemic venous beds. In this condition, the pulmonary veins may connect to a systemic vein within the thorax (*supradiaphragmatic*) or abdomen (*subdiaphragmatic*). Supradiaphragmatic venous connections most commonly involve the left innominate vein, coronary sinus, right superior vena cava, right atrium, and azygos vein; alternatively, a subdiaphragmatic connection enters the diaphragm through the esophageal hiatus and terminates in the portal vein or its tributaries.

An obstruction to pulmonary venous return, with resultant pulmonary venous hypertension, is invariably present in patients with subdiaphragmatic TAPVC, and it occurs in 50 percent of patients with a supradiaphragmatic connection. In fact, in most patients, the main determinant of pulmonary pressure and resistance is less related to increased pulmonary blood flow and pulmonary arteriolar vascular obstruction than to the presence and severity of pulmonary *venous* obstruction. In the patient with TAPVC, an interatrial communication (either an atrial septal defect [ASD] or a patent foramen ovale) is essential so that blood from the pulmonary veins can reach the left heart. Systemic cardiac output is limited to the volume of blood passing from the right to the left atrium; the larger this communication, the more effective the interchange between the atria. In the patient with a large interatrial communication, the magnitude of shunting is determined by (1) the relative compliance of the right and left ventricles and (2) the relative opposition to blood flow presented by the pulmonary and systemic vascular beds. Thus, the most favorable arrangement is a combination of no pulmonary obstruction, low pulmonary vascular resistance, little or no pulmonary hypertension, and a large ASD.

TAPVC, particularly of the subdiaphragmatic type, affects males more frequently than females. This is in contrast to ASD, with which there is a female predominance. There is 75- to 90-percent mortality during the first year of life. Those who survive the first year usually have a supradiaphragmatic connection, low pulmonary vascular resistance and pressure, no pulmonary venous obstruction, and a large ASD. An occasional patient with these features survives to adulthood without surgical therapy. The patient without pulmonary hypertension and with a large interatrial communication most often has dyspnea, particularly during feeding. In addition, he may have frequent respiratory infections, congestive heart failure, and physical underdevelopment.

On physical examination, cyanosis is often mild or undetectable (even though arterial oxygen desaturation is inevitable); such cyanosis may be intermittent or occur only with exertion. Severe cyanosis is uncommon in patients who survive to adulthood, since it implies severe pulmonary hypertension, high pulmonary vascular resistance, and a small interatrial communication. When TAPVC occurs without pulmonary hypertension and with a sizable interatrial communication, the clinical findings (apart from cyanosis) and auscultatory signs resemble those of a secundum ASD with a large left-to-right shunt: wide, fixed splitting of the S_2; a diastolic flow murmur across the tricuspid valve; and a systolic ejection murmur due to increased flow across the pulmonic valve. Some patients may also have a continuous murmur along the upper left sternal border. In patients with severe pulmonary hypertension, flow murmurs are less marked or even absent, and the pulmonic component of the S_2 is accentuated.

The ECG of the patient with a large left-to-right shunt without severe pulmonary hypertension resembles that of an uncomplicated ostium secundum ASD. The mean frontal QRS axis is directed rightward, and a pattern of incomplete or complete right bundle branch block is evident. *In a patient with the clinical and auscultatory features of a secundum ASD with a large left-to-right shunt and cyanosis, the presence of a leftward frontal QRS axis should suggest a common atrium (single atrium) rather than TAPVC.* The chest x-ray of the patient with a large left-to-right shunt without pulmonary hypertension also resembles that of an uncomplicated secundum ASD: the lung fields are plethoric, and the right atrium, right ventricle, and main pulmonary arterial segments are enlarged. In addition, the specific site of anomalous connection may alter the cardiac silhouette. Thus, in the patient with TAPVC to the left brachiocephalic vein, the superior vena cava on the right, the left brachiocephalic vein superiorly, and the vertical vein on the left distort the cardiac silhouette so that it resembles a snowman, figure eight, or cottage loaf. Alternatively, the upper right cardiac border may be prominent when the anomalous connection is to the right superior vena cava.

Echocardiography demonstrates marked enlargement of the right ventricle and a small left atrium. Occasionally, an echo-free space (representing the common pulmonary venous chamber) can be seen behind the left atrium. At cardiac catheterization, arterial oxygen desaturation is invariable, ranging from mild to severe. A variation in oxygen saturation in the venous circulation may serve to localize the site of entry of the anomalous veins. Indicator dilution studies are invaluable in the diagnosis of this condition, and selective angiography should be performed to define the drainage pathways of the pulmonary veins.

The drainage from both lungs must be outlined clearly to exclude a mixed type of anomalous venous drainage. Pulmonary venous obstruction may be detected by noting a gradient between the pulmonary capillary wedge and right atrial pressures.

Balloon atrial septostomy can provide dramatic palliation for the infant in whom a small interatrial communication limits blood flow from the right to the left atrium. Definitive surgical repair of TAPVC entails the creation of an anastomosis between the common pulmonary venous channel and left atrium as well as the closing of the interatrial defect and the anomalous venous pathway. If pulmonary vascular disease is not present, the results of the operation are generally good in patients older than 1 year. Normal hemodynamics and cardiac function have been demonstrated after total surgical correction of TAPVC.

Partial anomalous pulmonary venous connection (PAPVC) implies that one or more (but not all) of the pulmonary veins are connected to the right atrium or its venous tributaries. The right lung is involved 10 times more frequently than the left, with the usual connection being between the veins of the right upper and middle lobe and the superior vena cava. An ASD invariably accompanies PAPVC, and in 80 to 90 percent of cases it is of the sinus venosus type. Rarely, venous drainage of the right lung occurs into the inferior vena cava. Although this anomaly is usually not associated with an interatrial communication, it is often accompanied by hypoplasia of the right lung, dextroposition of the heart, pulmonary parenchymal abnormalities, and an anomalous arterial blood supply to the lower lobe of the right lung from the abdominal aorta or its main branches. This complex has been designated the *scimitar syndrome* because of the characteristic x-ray finding of a crescent-like shadow in the right lower lung field produced by the anomalous venous channel.

The usual patient with PAPVC is not cyanosed, and the physical findings are similar to those of an ASD. A leftward P wave axis in association with a rightward QRS axis in a patient with the clinical features of an ASD should suggest a sinus venosus defect, and by implication, PAPVC to the superior vena cava. In the absence of other associated anomalies, including ventricular septal defect, tetralogy of Fallot, and a variety of complex anomalies (all of which occur in 20% of cases), the physiologic disturbance caused by PAPVC is determined by the number of anomalous veins, their site of connection, the presence and size of an accompanying ASD, and the state of the pulmonary vascular bed.

The diagnosis of PAPVC may not be suspected clinically and may be made only at the time of cardiac catheterization or surgery. At catheterization, connection to the coronary sinus, azygos vein, or superior vena cava may be identified by a careful oximetric analysis. Selective angiography and indicator dilution curves may also prove valuable. Surgical reimplantation of the anomalous pulmonary venous connection into the left atrium and closure of the interatrial communication are usually curative unless obliterative pulmonary vascular disease has developed.

Total Anomalous Pulmonary Venous Connection

1. Edwards JE, Helmholz HF, Burchell HB, DuShane JW, Bruwer A, Swan HJC, Toscano-Barboza E, Wood EH, Burroughs JT, Kirklin JW. Symposium on total anomalous pulmonary venous connection. Proc Staff Meet Mayo Clin 1956; 31:151–188.
   An early detailed review of the anatomic, clinical, radiographic, and hemodynamic findings in this condition, as well as a report of surgical correction of this anomaly in 3 cases.
2. Levin B, Borden CW. Anomalous pulmonary venous drainage into the left vertical vein. Radiology 1954; 63:317–24.

The striking radiologic features of this condition are described. The cardiac silhou-ette is said to resemble a "figure of 8" on the posteroanterior projection.

3. Bonham Carter RE, Capriles M, Noe Y. Total anomalous pulmonary venous drainage: a clinical and anatomical study of 75 children. Br Heart J 1969; 31:45–51.
   In this series, more than 75% of patients with TAPVC died before 1 year of age. This paper emphasizes both the importance and difficulty of early diagnosis.

4. Gathman GE, Nadas AS. Total anomalous pulmonary venous connection: clinical and physiologic observations of 75 pediatric patients. Circulation 1970; 42:143–154.
   A comprehensive review of the findings on physical examination and at cardiac catheterization. Surgical correction before 1 year of age is recommended.

5. Duff DF, Nihill MR, McNamara DG. Infradiaphragmatic total anomalous pulmo-nary venous return: review of clinical and pathological findings and results of op-eration in 28 cases. Br Heart J 1977; 39:619–26.
   In this series, only 9 patients were considered operable, and only 3 were long-term survivors. More than one-third had additional complex lesions.

6. Clarke DR, Stark J, DeLeval M, Pincott JR, Taylor JFN. Total anomalous pulmo-nary venous drainage in infancy. Br Heart J 1977; 39:436–44.
   A review of 39 infants operated on for TAPVC; 14 were under 1 month of age at the time of operation. Of the 39, 14 (36%) died during or shortly after surgery.

7. Joffe HS, O'Donovan TG, Glaun BP, Chesler E, Schrire V. Subdiaphragmatic total anomalous pulmonary venous drainage: report of a successful surgical correction. Am Heart J 1971; 81:250–4.
   A case report and review of 6 cases of surgical correction of subdiaphragmatic TAPVC.

8. Delisle G, Ando M, Calder AL, Zuberbuhler JR, Rochenmacher S, Alday LE, Man-gini O, Van Praagh S, Van Praagh R. Total anomalous pulmonary venous connec-tion: report of 93 autopsied cases with emphasis on diagnostic and surgical consid-erations. Am Heart J 1976; 91:99–122.
   An excellent review of a large autopsy series of patients with this anomaly. The or-der of frequency of various types of TAPVC was: left innominate ("snowman"), 26%; subdiaphragmatic, 24%; coronary sinus, 18%; right superior vena cava, 15%; right atrium, 8%, and mixed, 5%.

9. El-Said G, Mullins CE, McNamara DG. Management of total anomalous pulmo-nary venous return. Circulation 1972; 45:1240–50.
   A review of 35 cases of this anomaly. The authors recommend palliative therapy with balloon atrial septostomy for most patients in the first 6 months of life.

10. Behrendt DM, Aberdeen E, Waterston DJ, Bonham-Carter RE. Total anomalous pulmonary venous drainage in infants: clinical and hemodynamic findings, meth-ods, and results of operation in 37 cases. Circulation 1972; 46:347–56.
    Survival was closely related to the degree of pulmonary hypertension, which was dependent on the type of anomaly and the presence of pulmonary venous obstruc-tion. The best survival was in patients with supracardiac drainage who were oper-ated on between 3 and 12 months of age.

11. Mathew R, Thilenius OG, Replogle RL, Arcilla RA. Cardiac function in total anomalous pulmonary venous return before and after surgery. Circulation 1977; 55:361–370.
    Cardiac performance was evaluated in 12 patients with this syndrome. Right ven-tricular volume was increased, and left atrial and left ventricular volumes were reduced preoperatively. Following surgery, cardiac function returned to normal.

12. Newfeld EA, Wilson A, Paul MH, Reisch JS. Pulmonary vascular disease in total anomalous pulmonary venous drainage. Circulation 1980; 61:103–9.
    A detailed histopathologic analysis of lung specimens in 40 patients with this anomaly. Patients with pulmonary venous obstruction died earlier and had a greater degree of pulmonary vascular disease than those with unobstructed venous drainage.

13. Turley K, Tucker WY, Ullyot DJ, Ebert PA. Total anomalous pulmonary venous connection in infancy: influence of age and type of lesions. Am J Cardiol 1980; 45:92–7.

A study of 22 infants with this syndrome who underwent surgical correction in the first year of life. Nineteen (87%) patients survived surgery, but 2 died later due to intimal fibroplasia of the pulmonary veins proximal to the site of atrial anastomosis. The strongest determinants of survival were type of lesion, pulmonary venous obstruction, and depressed left ventricular function, rather than age at time of operation.

14. Katz NM, Kirklin JW, Pacifico AD. Concepts and practices in surgery for total anomalous pulmonary venous connection. Ann Thorac Surg 1978; 25:479–87.
An excellent review of the surgical approach to TAPVC. The authors recommend definitive repair between 6 and 12 months of age.

Partial Anomalous Pulmonary Venous Connection

15. Swan HJC, Kirklin JW, Becu LM, Wood EH. Anomalous connections of right pulmonary veins to superior vena cava with interatrial communications: hemodynamic data in eight cases. Circulation 1957; 16:54–66.
An excellent early review of the value of cardiac catheterization in detecting and defining PAPVC. The value of careful oximetry and indicator dilution studies is emphasized.

16. Schumacker HB Jr, Judd D. Partial anomalous pulmonary venous return with reference to drainage into the inferior vena cava and to an intact atrial septum. J Cardiovasc Surg 1964; 5:271–8.
A review of the findings in PAPVC. While an interatrial communication is present in 91% of patients when drainage occurs into the superior vena cava, it occurs in only 5% of patients with drainage into the inferior vena cava.

17. Kalke BR, Carlson RG, Ferlic RM, Sellers RD, Lillehei CW. Partial anomalous pulmonary venous connections. Am J Cardiol 1967; 20:91–101.
A review of 57 patients treated surgically. The clinical findings and surgical approach are reviewed.

18. Kuiper-Oosterwal CH, Moulaert A. The scimitar syndrome in infancy and childhood. Eur J Cardiol 1973; 1:55–61.
Nine children with the scimitar syndrome are presented. The prognosis and indications for surgical correction are related to the magnitude of the left-to-right shunt.

19. Saalouke MG, Shapiro SR, Perry LW, Scott LP. Isolated partial anomalous pulmonary venous drainage associated with pulmonary vascular obstructive disease. Am J Cardiol 1977; 39:439–44.
Five patients with PAPVC and intact atrial septum are described.

20. Mascarenhas E, Javier RP, Samet P. Partial anomalous pulmonary venous connection and drainage. Am J Cardiol 1973; 31:512–8.
The clinical, diagnostic, and pathophysiologic features of 5 different types of PAPVC are discussed. The value and interpretation of indicator dilution curves in this anomaly are also discussed.

21. Davia JE, Cheitlin MD, Bedynek JL. Sinus venosus atrial septal defect: analysis of fifty cases. Am Heart J 1973; 85:177–85.
A review of 50 patients who underwent surgery; 23 (46%) had a P wave axis less than − 30°, and 43 (86%) had partial anomalous pulmonary venous connections.

22. Friedli B, Guerin R, Davignon A, Fouron JC, Stanley P. Surgical treatment of partial anomalous pulmonary venous drainage: a long-term follow-up study. Circulation 1972; 45:159–70.
A clinical, hemodynamic, and angiographic review of 14 cases 1 to 9 years after surgery. The surgical result was generally good except when the anomalous vein drained high into the superior vena cava.

23. Dickinson DF, Galloway RW, Massey R, Sankey R, Arnold R. Scimitar syndrome in infancy: role of embolization of systemic arterial supply to right lung. Br Heart J 1982; 47:468–72.
A discussion of the "scimitar syndrome" and the possible value of embolization of the systemic arterial supply to the hypoplastic right lung.

EISENMENGER SYNDROME

The term *Eisenmenger complex* refers specifically to the triad of a ventricular septal defect (VSD), severe pulmonary vascular disease, and resultant right-to-left shunting of blood. The term *Eisenmenger syndrome* is used to describe any communication between the systemic and pulmonary circulations that produces pulmonary vascular disease of sufficient severity to cause right-to-left shunting. The characteristic pathologic alterations that occur in the pulmonary vasculature as a result of a large left-to-right shunt and that ultimately lead to a reversal in the direction of the shunt include (in order of increasing severity) medial hypertrophy, intimal thickening, prominence of the elastic membrane, plexiform lesions in the arterioles, and necrotizing arteritis. These changes cause marked luminal narrowing and eventual obliteration of the pulmonary arterioles, with thrombosis in situ, resulting in an increase in pulmonary vascular resistance to levels similar or even greater than systemic vascular resistance.

The Eisenmenger syndrome occurs with equal frequency in both sexes. Its occurrence is related to the site, size, and duration of the left-to-right intracardiac shunt. The Eisenmenger syndrome is a distinctly uncommon complication in the patient with an atrial septal defect (ASD), whereas it is more common in the patient with a VSD or patent ductus arteriosus (PDA). Since the syndrome is uncommon before 2 years of age, surgical closure of left-to-right shunts is recommended before this age to prevent its occurrence. The syndrome occurs more frequently and earlier in patients with left-to-right shunts who live at high altitudes.

Patients with the Eisenmenger syndrome complain most often of easy fatigability, dyspnea on exertion, and hemoptysis. Hemoptysis is uncommon in young children as well as adults, but its occurrence is generally regarded as an ominous event. Such hemoptysis is usually caused by the rupture of the thin-walled, fragile, and dilated plexiform lesions or small aneurysms of the pulmonary arterioles. Although syncope occasionally occurs in patients with the Eisenmenger syndrome, it is uncommon, since exercise is usually accompanied by an increase in right-to-left shunting (and cyanosis) but not by right ventricular failure or a fall in systemic output. Some patients with the Eisenmenger syndrome complain of chest pain that resembles angina pectoris. Similar to patients with other kinds of right-to-left shunting, those with the Eisenmenger syndrome tolerate systemic vasodilatation poorly, since it increases the magnitude of right-to-left shunting, thus diminishing pulmonary blood flow and exaggerating systemic desaturation. As a result, hot weather, hot baths, and fever are poorly tolerated.

On physical examination, central cyanosis and clubbing are usually present. Differential cyanosis (i.e., blue, clubbed toenails in association with pink lips and fingernails) is characteristic of the patient with the Eisenmenger syndrome and a PDA. The jugular venous pressure is usually elevated, and a prominent A wave is present in the patient with an ASD or PDA but not in the patient with a VSD. A right ventricular impulse and a pulmonary arterial impulse are palpable, and the pulmonic valve closure sound is markedly accentuated. In the patient with the Eisenmenger syndrome and a VSD, the S_2 is usually single and loud. In contrast, persistent splitting of the S_2, with accentuation of pulmonic valve closure, is present in the patient with the Eisenmenger syndrome and an ASD or PDA. A systolic ejection click that does not diminish (or diminishes minimally) with inspiration is often present, originating within the dilated main pulmonary arterial trunk. A right ventricular S_3 and

S_4 may be present. In an occasional patient, no murmur is audible, and the correct diagnosis may be missed if the clinical, electrocardiographic, and radiographic features of severe pulmonary hypertension are not appreciated. There is frequently a trivial ejection systolic murmur, best heard in the pulmonic area. A holosystolic murmur along the left sternal border that increases with inspiration is caused by tricuspid regurgitation, which may result from right ventricular failure. A high-pitched diastolic decrescendo murmur of pulmonary valvular incompetence is audible in about 50 percent of patients.

The ECG usually demonstrates right axis deviation, right ventricular hypertrophy, and right atrial enlargement. The rhythm may be sinus, although supraventricular rhythm disturbances sometimes occur, including atrial flutter, atrial fibrillation, or atrial tachycardia. The chest x-ray ordinarily demonstrates a prominent main pulmonary trunk and proximal pulmonary arteries, as well as enlargement of the right atrium and ventricle. The peripheral pulmonary arteries taper rapidly, so that the marked proximal enlargement stands in sharp contrast to peripheral oligemia.

At cardiac catheterization, the Eisenmenger syndrome is documented by demonstrating a marked increase in pulmonary vascular resistance (to at least 80% of systemic vascular resistance). It is important to appreciate that a marked increase in pulmonary arterial *pressure* may occur due to a large left-to-right shunt *without* an increase in pulmonary vascular *resistance;* such a patient may still be suitable for surgical correction. In addition, the patient with the Eisenmenger syndrome has systemic arterial desaturation and polycythemia. The left atrial pressure (measured as pulmonary capillary wedge pressure) ordinarily is normal. It may be possible to pass a catheter directly through a PDA or an ASD, thus confirming the presence of these defects. Selective angiography may help to demonstrate the site of the defect as well as the characteristic changes in the pulmonary arterial vascular system, but angiography in patients with severe pulmonary hypertension carries an increased mortality.

Although children with the Eisenmenger syndrome can reach young adulthood, the overall life expectancy is severely shortened; most individuals do not survive past the fourth decade. Death is caused by congestive heart failure, brain abscess, pulmonary infection, pulmonary thromboses and infarction, bacterial endocarditis, ventricular arrhythmias, or (rarely) severe hemoptysis. Pregnancy is especially dangerous for the patient with the Eisenmenger syndrome: maternal mortality is estimated at 30 to 70 percent and tends to occur at the time of delivery or during the puerperium. Fetal mortality is also markedly increased. Even those women who were asymptomatic before pregnancy are at increased risk. As a result, it is recommended that pregnancies in women with the Eisenmenger syndrome be terminated.

The medical therapy of the patient with the Eisenmenger syndrome is directed toward prevention and treatment of complications. Digitalis, diuretics, and salt restriction should be utilized for the treatment of ventricular failure. Phlebotomy with appropriate volume replacement is performed in patients with severe polycythemia. As noted, pregnancy should be avoided. Once pulmonary vascular resistance approaches systemic vascular resistance, surgical correction of the shunt is contraindicated, since such attempted repair carries a high mortality. In addition, even if the patient survives the operation, there is little change in the degree of pulmonary vascular obstructive disease. Recently, complete heart-lung transplantation has been performed successfully in patients with the Eisenmenger syndrome. This operation would seem to afford some hope for patients with this otherwise fatal condition.

At least three other disease entities require mention in the differential diagnosis of apparent Eisenmenger syndrome: primary pulmonary hypertension, idiopathic dilatation of the pulmonary artery, and recurrent pulmonary embolism. Primary pulmonary hypertension is caused by intrinsic, obstructive disease in the small terminal arteries and arterioles of the pulmonary vascular bed. Its etiology is unknown. On microscopic examination of the lungs, medial hypertrophy, cellular intimal proliferation, cellular fibrous vascular occlusion, and necrotizing arteritis are evident, and microscopic in situ thrombi are usually present. Thus, the pathologic characteristics of this disease entity may be indistinguishable from those of patients with the Eisenmenger syndrome, except, of course, that there is no abnormal communication between the systemic and pulmonary circulations. Irrespective of how pulmonary hypertension is initiated, it is propagated through changes that progressively increase resistance to flow through the lungs. Eventually, pulmonary arterial pressure and resistance rise to levels equal to or above those in the systemic circulation. (Primary pulmonary hypertension is discussed in detail on p. 329).

Idiopathic dilatation of the pulmonary artery is characterized by a congenital dilatation of the pulmonary trunk (and occasionally of its main branches) without associated anatomic or physiologic abnormalities. It is a completely benign entity, but its radiographic appearance can be mistaken for severe pulmonary hypertension. (This condition is discussed in detail on p. 195).

Recurrent pulmonary embolism eventually may cause marked enlargement of the main pulmonary trunk and its proximal branches, and there may be evidence of pulmonary hypertension on physical examination, the ECG, and the chest x-ray. In addition, there may be other clinical manifestations that suggest pulmonary embolism, such as peripheral venous disease. It may be difficult to distinguish clinically primary from secondary pulmonary hypertension due to recurrent pulmonary emboli.

1. Perloff JK. Auscultatory and phonocardiographic manifestations of pulmonary hypertension. Prog Cardiovasc Dis 1967; 9:303–40.
   A detailed and thorough review of the auscultatory manifestations of pulmonary arterial hypertension. Includes 120 references.
2. Elliott LP, Schiebler GL. A roentgenologic-electrocardiographic approach to cyanotic forms of heart disease. Pediatr Clin North Am 1971; 18:1133–61.
   A detailed discussion of the usefulness of combined radiographic and electrocardiographic findings in facilitating proper recognition of various types of congenital heart disease.
3. Wood P. The Eisenmenger syndrome. Br Med J 1958; 2:701–9, 755–62.
   An elegant and complete review of the clinical features of this syndrome.
4. Hirschfeld S, Meyer R, Schwartz DC, Korfhagen J, Kaplan S. The echocardiographic assessment of pulmonary artery pressure and pulmonary vascular resistance. Circulation 1975; 52:642–50.
   Marked elevation of the right ventricular preejection period–right ventricular ejection time ratio indicates the presence of pulmonary hypertension.
5. Clarkson PM, Fraye RL, DuShane JW, Burchell HB, Wood EH, Wiedman WH. Prognosis for patients with ventricular septal defect and severe pulmonary vascular obstructive disease. Circulation 1968; 38:129–35.
   This report evaluated 58 patients, 3 to 57 years of age, who had ventricular septal defects and a marked increase in pulmonary vascular resistance; 46 (80%) were alive 5 years or longer after diagnostic catheterization. The most common causes of death were "sudden" or "unknown."
6. Young D, Mark H. Fate of the patient with the Eisenmenger syndrome. Am J Cardiol 1971; 28:658–69.
   A review of the clinical features and courses of 57 patients with Eisenmenger syndrome who were treated conservatively.
7. Heath D, Edwards JE. The pathology of hypertensive pulmonary vascular disease. Circulation 1958; 18:533–47.

The histologic features occurring in pulmonary arteries and arterioles as a consequence of chronically elevated pulmonary arterial pressure are described in detail.

8. Jones AM, Howitt G. Eisenmenger syndrome in pregnancy. Br Med J 1965;1:1627–31.
   Pregnancy carries an extremely high mortality in patients with the Eisenmenger syndrome.
9. Fischbein CA, Rosenthal A, Fischer EG, Nadas AS, Welch K. Risk factors for brain abscess in patients with congenital heart disease. Am J Cardiol 1974; 34:97–102.
   Brain abscess in patients with congenital heart disease is rare prior to 2 years of age. Morbidity and mortality of brain abscess are inversely related to oxygen saturation levels.
10. Pitts JA, Crosby WM, Basta LL. Eisenmenger's syndrome in pregnancy. Am Heart J 1977; 93:321–6.
    Of 7 patients with Eisenmenger syndrome who were carried through pregnancy, 5 died, emphasizing the inadvisability of pregnancy in these individuals.
11. Haroutunian LM, Neill CA. Pulmonary complications of congenital heart disease: hemoptysis. Am Heart J 1972; 84:540–59.
    This review delineates the major pulmonary complications encountered in patients with congenital heart disease and resultant pulmonary vascular obstruction. In these patients, hemoptysis is a rare but major complication.
12. Rosenthal A, Nathan DG, Marty AT, Button LN, Miettinen OS, Nadas AS. Acute hemodynamic effects of red cell volume reduction in polycythemia of cyanotic congenital heart disease. Circulation 1970; 42:297–307.
    Acute reduction in red cell volume without significant alterations in blood volume in 22 patients with severe polycythemia secondary to cyanotic congenital heart disease substantially improved hemodynamics and oxygen delivery.
13. Reitz BA, Wallwork JL, Hunt SA, Pennock JL, Billingham ME, Oyer PE, Stinson EB, Shumway NE. Heart-lung transplantation: successful therapy for patients with pulmonary vascular disease. N Engl J Med 1982; 306:557–64.
    The initial report of this procedure in humans in three patients with severe pulmonary hypertension.
14. Cartmill TB, DuShane JW, McGoon DC. Results of repair of ventricular septal defect. J Thorac Cardiovasc Surg 1966; 52:486–501.
    An important study of 447 patients with VSDs that clearly relates early and late postoperative mortality to the level of pulmonary vascular resistance rather than pulmonary artery pressure.
15. Brammell HL, Vogel JHK, Pryor R, Blount SG. The Eisenmenger syndrome. Am J Cardiol 1971; 28:679–92.
    In 91 patients with this syndrome, management (medical or surgical) was predicated on the reactivity of the pulmonary vascular bed to tolazoline, a potent vasodilator.
16. Friedli B, Kidd BSL, Mustard TW, Keith JD. Ventricular septal defect with increased pulmonary vascular resistance. Am J Cardiol 1974; 33:403–9.
    This paper describes the experience of 57 children who underwent VSD closure in the presence of increased pulmonary vascular resistance. Operative mortality was high (18 [32%] died) and long-term survival was poor.

EBSTEIN'S ANOMALY

Ebstein's anomaly is a congenital malformation of the tricuspid valve in which the septal and posterior leaflets are abnormally attached to the anulus. Although the anterior leaflet arises from its normal position on the anulus fibrosus, it is structurally abnormal. The effective tricuspid valve orifice is displaced downward into the right ventricle, and the functional right ventricle is, therefore, substantially reduced in size. In addition, there are abnormalities of the atrioventricular sulcus, the tricuspid valve leaflet tissue, and the structure and internal morphology of the right ventricle. The right atrium is dilated, consisting of a normal atrium plus the "atrialized" portion of the right ventricle. Although the malformed tricuspid valve is usually incompetent, it can occasionally be stenotic or even imperforate. In most patients with Ebstein's anomaly, a patent foramen ovale or true atrial septal defect (ASD) is also present, thus allowing the right atrium to decompress into the left atrium, with resultant right-to-left shunting. Rarely, Ebstein's anomaly affects a *left-sided* AV valve when this valve is, in fact, the tricuspid valve, as occurs with ventricular inversion (i.e., corrected transposition of the great vessels).

A wide spectrum of symptoms and signs can occur in the patient with Ebstein's anomaly, depending on the degree of anatomic derangement and the presence of associated abnormalities. On the one extreme, some patients are totally asymptomatic, and the diagnosis is made in the patient's seventh or eighth decade. On the other extreme, the anomaly can cause death in infancy due to severe heart failure. Approximately one-third of patients have minimal or no symptoms for many years, whereas the remainder become markedly symptomatic due to congestive heart failure and systemic arterial desaturation. In these individuals, dyspnea on exertion, fatigue, generalized weakness, and cyanosis are common. A minority of patients complain of pedal edema or palpitations. Some patients are acyanotic at rest but become cyanosed during exercise. The majority of patients with Ebstein's anomaly reach early adulthood, and some lead an active life into middle age and beyond.

The physical development of the patient with Ebstein's anomaly is generally normal. Cyanosis and digital clubbing of variable degree may be present. The arterial and jugular venous pulses are usually normal, even in the presence of severe cardiac failure and tricuspid regurgitation (since right ventricular function is sufficiently impaired to prevent the appearance of a prominent V wave). Similarly, a prominent A wave is not seen in this condition. The precordium is typically *not* overactive, in contrast to that of patients with left-to-right shunting. A systolic thrill (due to tricuspid regurgitation) is rarely palpable at the lower left sternal border. On auscultation, there may be a *multiplicity of sounds and murmurs,* all emanating from the right heart, none of which are diagnostic. The S_1 is typically widely split; the second component originates from the malformed tricuspid valve, which closes relatively late. The S_2 is widely and persistently split (but not fixed) due to right bundle branch block and delayed pulmonic valve closure. The intensity of the pulmonic component of the S_2 may be normal or soft, the latter resulting from low pulmonary arterial pressure in the presence of an associated right-to-left shunt. A right-sided S_3 and S_4 may be heard, and there is often summation of these sounds. A murmur of tricuspid regurgitation is almost invariably audible. Diastolic and presystolic murmurs, which may be "scratchy," are occasionally audible. Typically, all these murmurs increase in intensity with inspiration.

The ECG is generally helpful in the diagnosis of Ebstein's anomaly. Normal sinus rhythm is usually present, although supraventricular arrhythmias are not uncommon. Ventricular preexcitation (classically Wolff-Parkinson-White type B) occurs in an occasional patient. The P wave is typically tall and peaked but may be normal, and the P–R interval is frequently prolonged. The large P wave and P–R prolongation are due to right atrial enlargement. The mean frontal QRS axis is normal or displaced rightward (in contrast to congenital tricuspid atresia, in which the QRS axis is displaced leftward). A right bundle branch block pattern is usually present. The QRS complex may be unusually prolonged, splintered, and of low voltage. Electrocardiographic evidence of right ventricular hypertrophy is not seen. The chest x-ray usually demonstrates an enlarged heart, with most of the cardiomegaly due to an enlarged right atrium, but occasionally it may be normal. The globular-shaped heart on chest x-ray may closely resemble the picture usually associated with a large pericardial effusion. The right ventricular outflow tract may be dilated, but the aorta is small. In cyanosed patients, pulmonary vascularity is reduced. Indeed, *the finding of increased pulmonary vascularity should suggest a diagnosis other than isolated Ebstein's anomaly.*

The M-mode echocardiogram can provide useful information in the patient suspected of having Ebstein's anomaly. The tricuspid and mitral valves are frequently visualized simultaneously because of the abnormal leftward displacement of the tricuspid valve. Indeed, the tricuspid valve often is imaged to the left of the midclavicular line, a finding that is strongly suggestive of Ebstein's anomaly. In addition, a delay in tricuspid valve closure (to more than 65 msec after mitral valve closure) is almost diagnostic of this anomaly. Since the delay in tricuspid valve closure is due to its mechanical derangement, patients with the greatest delay are likely to have the most severe form of the anomaly. Two-dimensional echocardiography allows an accurate evaluation of the anatomic relationships among the tricuspid valve, the right atrium, and the right ventricle, and it also allows an assessment of right ventricular function. It may even be possible to obtain a semiquantitative impression of the magnitude of the right-to-left shunt and of tricuspid regurgitation by performing a peripheral venous injection of saline or indocyanine green during echocardiography.

A definitive diagnosis of Ebstein's anomaly can be made at cardiac catheterization. With present techniques and equipment, this procedure is not associated with a particularly increased mortality. Right atrial pressure is moderately elevated. Right ventricular systolic pressure is generally normal, diastolic pressure is elevated, and there is usually no gradient across the tricuspid valve. Pulmonary arterial pressure is normal or low. In the patient with a right-to-left shunt at the atrial level, systemic arterial desaturation is present. Such shunting is demonstrable by the early appearance of indicator at the systemic arterial sampling site following the injection of indocyanine green into the superior or inferior vena cava. *The diagnosis of Ebstein's anomaly is most readily made by recording the intracardiac pressure and electrogram simultaneously with an electrode catheter: when this catheter is pulled from the right ventricle to the right atrium, right ventricular electrical potentials continue to be recorded after the pressure contour has changed from right ventricular to right atrial in form.* The atrial pressure that is recorded coincident with the ventricular electrical potential results from the atrialized portion of the ventricle. In the presence of severe tricuspid regurgitation, this change in waveform may be difficult to detect, since the waveform in the right atrium and ventricle may be similar. Right ventricular angiography in the anteroposterior projection (and lateral projection, if possible) is usually diagnostic, except in mild cases. By angiography, the anterior leaflet of the tricuspid valve is large and "sail-like" and is displaced to the left of the spine (in the anteroposterior projection) and anteriorly (in the lateral projection). Some patients with severe tricuspid regurgitation appear to have three chambers on the right side of the heart, a so-called trilobed angiographic appearance, consisting of the right atrium, the atrialized portion of the right ventricle, and the outflow portion of the right ventricle.

The management of the patient with Ebstein's anomaly depends on its severity. The acyanotic patient with minimal tricuspid regurgitation who is asymptomatic should be treated conservatively, whereas the symptomatic patient with marked tricuspid regurgitation, right heart failure, and cyanosis may benefit from surgery. Milder degrees of heart failure may benefit from conventional medical therapy, and arrhythmias should be treated in the usual manner. Bacterial endocarditis is unusual in this condition. Death, when it occurs, is usually due to congestive heart failure or arrhythmias. Although surgical therapy is associated with a high mortality, it can lead to marked symptomatic improvement. The Glenn procedure (superior vena cava–right pulmonary artery anastomosis) has been performed in an attempt to increase pulmonary blood flow and has been modestly successful. Tricuspid valve replacement with closure of the ASD or patent foramen ovale has been advocated by others. Most recently, a plastic repair procedure, including plication of the free wall of the atrialized portion of the right ventricle, right atrial reduction, and posterior tricuspid annuloplasty, has been suggested as the procedure of choice. However, long-term follow-up after this operation is not yet available.

1. Mayer FE, Nadas AS, Ongley PA. Ebstein's anomaly: presentation of ten cases. Circulation 1957; 16:1057–69.
   The complete histories, physical findings, noninvasive and invasive results, and clinical courses of 10 patients with Ebstein's anomaly are presented.

2. Yim BJB, Yu PN. Value of an electrode catheter in diagnosis of Ebstein's disease. Circulation 1958; 17:543–8.
   Various features of Ebstein's anomaly are reviewed, and the value of simultaneous electrocardiographic and pressure recordings in the right ventricle and right atrium is emphasized.

3. Schiebler GL, Adams P Jr, Anderson RC, Amplatz K, Lester RG. Clinical study of 23 cases of Ebstein's anomaly of the tricuspid valve. Circulation 1959; 19:165–87.
   Clinical findings in 23 patients with this problem are presented, and the diagnostic and surgical aspects are reviewed. Of these 23 cases, 6 had the electrocardiographic pattern of Wolff-Parkinson-White syndrome.

4. Adams JCL, Hudson R. Case of Ebstein's anomaly surviving to the age of seventy-nine. Br Heart J 1956; 18:129–32.
   A woman surviving to 79 years of age with Ebstein's anomaly is described; this is one of the longest survivals recorded.

5. Hernandez FA, Rochkind R, Cooper HR. The intracavitary electrocardiogram in the diagnosis of Ebstein's anomaly. Am J Cardiol 1958; 1:181–90.
   The cardiac catheterization findings in 3 patients for whom simultaneous electrocardiographic and pressure recordings were obtained are reported.

6. Genton E, Blount SG Jr. The spectrum of Ebstein's anomaly. Am Heart J 1967; 73:395–425.
   The findings in 17 patients with Ebstein's anomaly are described in great detail, and a thorough bibliography of 92 references is provided.

7. Vacca JB, Bussmann DW, Mudd JG. Ebstein's anomaly: complete review of 108 cases. Am J Cardiol 1958; 2:210–26.
   A complete review of the Ebstein's literature and a report of 3 new cases of the abnormality are included in this report. Includes 71 references.

8. Barnard CN, Schrire V. Surgical correction of Ebstein's malformation with prosthetic tricuspid valve. Surgery 1963; 54:302–8.
   The initial report of successful tricuspid valve replacement in 2 patients with this anomaly.

9. Anderson KR, Zuberbuhler JR, Anderson RH, Becker AE, Lie JT. Morphologic spectrum of Ebstein's anomaly of the heart. Mayo Clin Proc 1979; 54:174–80.
   A detailed discussion of the pathologic findings in patients with left- and right-sided Ebstein's anomaly.

10. Danielson GK, Maloney JD, Devloo RAE. Surgical repair of Ebstein's anomaly. Mayo Clin Proc 1979; 54:185–92.
    A description of the plication of the free wall of the atrialized portion of the right ventricle, posterior tricuspid annuloplasty, and right atrial reduction performed successfully in 16 patients.

11. Seward JB, Tajik AJ, Feist DJ, Smith HC. Ebstein's anomaly in an 85-year-old man. Mayo Clin Proc 1979; 54:193–6.
    This is the longest reported survival of a patient with Ebstein's anomaly.
12. Gussenhoven WJ, Spitaels SEC, Bom N, Becker AE. Echocardiographic criteria for Ebstein's anomaly of tricuspid valve. Br Heart J 1980; 43:31–7.
    In this study, 2-dimensional echocardiography permitted a reliable visualization of the septal origin of the tricuspid valve and, therefore, was very useful in the diagnosis of Ebstein's anomaly. In contrast, M-mode echocardiography was not nearly as reliable.
13. Ng R, Somerville J, Ross D. Ebstein's anomaly: late results of surgical correction. Eur J Cardiol 1979; 9:39–52.
    The long-term (2–9 year) follow-up of 10 severely disabled patients with Ebstein's anomaly who underwent surgical therapy.
14. Kastor JA, Goldreyer BN, Josephson ME, Perloff JK, Scharf DL, Manchester JH, Shelburne JC, Hirschfeld JW Jr. Electrophysiologic characteristics of Ebstein's anomaly of the tricuspid valve. Circulation 1975; 52:987–95.
    Detailed electrophysiologic studies of 5 patients with Ebstein's anomaly were performed, demonstrating a normal position of the bundle of His but prolonged intra-right atrial and infranodal conduction.
15. Watson H. Electrode catheters and the diagnosis of Ebstein's anomaly of the tricuspid valve. Br Heart J 1966; 28:161–71.
    A detailed description, with examples, of the simultaneous recording of an electrical and pressure signal to establish a diagnosis of Ebstein's anomaly.
16. Kumar AE, Flyer DC, Miettinen OS, Nadas AS. Ebstein's anomaly: clinical profile and natural history. Am J Cardiol 1971; 28:84–95.
    A description and discussion of 55 patients with Ebstein's anomaly. Prognosis tended to be poor in the presence of complicating cardiac lesions, marked cyanosis, and extreme cardiomegaly.
17. Daniel W, Rathsack P, Walpurger G, Kahle A, Gisbertz R, Schmitz J, Lichtlen PR. Value of M-mode echocardiography for non-invasive diagnosis of Ebstein's anomaly. Br Heart J 1980:43:38–44.
    In this study, a tricuspid valve closure delay $\geq$ 0.065 seconds on M-mode echocardiography was considered to be diagnostic of Ebstein's anomaly, in that it did not occur in any patients without this anomaly. Of the 11 patients with Ebstein's, such tricuspid valve closure delay was demonstrable in 9.
18. Kambe T, Ichimiya S, Toguchi M, Hibi N, Fukui Y, Nishimura K, Sakamoto N, Hojo Y. Apex and subxiphoid approaches to Ebstein's anomaly using cross-sectional echocardiography. Am Heart J 1980; 100:53–8.
    A detailed description of various 2-dimensional echocardiographic views in the diagnosis of Ebstein's anomaly.
19. Cabin HS, Roberts WC. Ebstein's anomaly of the tricuspid valve and prolapse of the mitral valve. Am Heart J 1981; 101:177–80.
    Of 5 adult patients with Ebstein's anomaly who came to postmortem, 3 had mitral valve prolapse.
20. Charles RG, Barnard CN, Beck W. Tricuspid valve replacement for Ebstein's anomaly: a 19-year review of the first case. Br Heart J 1981; 46:578–80.
    The first published case of tricuspid valve replacement for Ebstein's anomaly is reviewed 19 years after operation.

COARCTATION OF THE AORTA

Coarctation of the aorta is a narrowing of the aortic lumen that usually is located in the region of the ligamentum arteriosus, although rarely it occurs higher in the aortic arch, in the descending thoracic aorta, or even in the abdominal aorta. It can be *preductal* (the so-called infantile type) or *postductal* (the so-called adult type). A preductal coarctation is a relatively long, constricted segment of aorta proximal to the ductus arteriosus, whereas the postductal type is a localized narrowing at or distal to the ductus arteriosus. Alternatively, coarctation of the aorta can be classified according to which ventricle supplies blood to the lower half of the body: in almost all adults with coarctation, the left ventricle supplies the entire systemic circulation; in some infants with coarctation, the left ventricle supplies the upper half of the body, but the lower half is supplied by the right ventricle through a patent ductus arteriosus. If the condition is left uncorrected, these infants usually do not live beyond 1 year of age.

Regardless of the exact type of coarctation, the major hemodynamic problem created by this abnormality is the maintenance of adequate blood flow to those organs distal to the obstruction, particularly the kidneys. Adequate renal blood flow is accomplished by an elevation of systemic arterial pressure proximal to the coarctation and by the development of collateral channels that connect vessels proximal and distal to the obstruction. Coarctation of the aorta often coexists with a patent ductus arteriosus or with various aortic valve abnormalities, most commonly a bicuspid aortic valve. Other less frequently associated intracardiac abnormalities include ventricular septal defect, congenital mitral regurgitation, and endocardial fibroelastosis. Coarctation of the aorta is a frequent finding in patients with Turner's syndrome. Finally, aneurysms of the circle of Willis occur frequently in those with coarctation, and rupture of these aneurysms is a well-recognized cause of death in these patients.

Most children and young adults with coarctation of the aorta are asymptomatic. Twice as many males as females are affected. The diagnosis is often made during a routine physical examination, when systemic arterial hypertension is observed in the upper extremities, with absent or diminished femoral arterial pulses. The hypertension is chiefly systolic. When symptoms are present, they are usually referable to hypertension: headache, epistaxis, dizziness, and palpitations. Occasionally, diminished blood flow to the lower extremities causes intermittent claudication. Symptoms of congestive heart failure may be the initial complaint in a small percentage of patients with coarctation.

On physical examination, the patient with coarctation may be well developed in the arms, shoulders, and chest, and systolic arterial pressure is higher in the arms than in the legs. The diastolic pressures are usually similar. Thus, a widened pulse pressure is present in the upper extremities. In comparison to the radial or brachial pulses, the femoral pulses are weak and delayed. A systolic thrill may be palpable in the suprasternal notch, and left ventricular enlargement may be present. A systolic ejection click often is audible, and increased prominence of the aortic closure sound is noted. A characteristic rough systolic ejection murmur may be audible along the left sternal border and in the back, particularly over the area of the coarcted segment. In addition, a continuous murmur may be heard over the back or in the interscapular or subscapular areas, indicating increased blood flow through collateral channels. In about 30 percent of patients with aortic coarctation, a systolic murmur of an associated bicuspid aortic valve is audible at the base. A murmur of aortic regurgitation may be present in some patients.

The ECG may demonstrate evidence of left ventricular hypertrophy. Although heart size by chest x-ray may be normal, left ventricular enlargement is often noted. Notching of the ribs, due to increased collateral flow through the intercostal arteries, develops along the posterior third through eighth ribs. Such notching is usually symmetrical but rarely may be unilateral. The anterior ribs do not demonstrate notching, since the anterior intercostal arteries are not located in costal grooves. Notching of the ribs rarely develops prior to age 4. The coarctation itself may be visible as an indentation in the aorta, and one may see prestenotic and poststenotic aortic dilatation. Together, these abnormalities produce a characteristic pattern on the lateral wall of the aorta (the so-called reversed E sign) that may be visible on a standard chest x-ray. In addition, a dilated left subclavian artery may be visible. Aortography outlines the site and extent of obstruction as well as the collateral circulation. True coarctation must be differentiated from pseudocoarctation, an anomaly of the aortic arch characterized by kinking at or just beyond the ligamentum arteriosum. The absence of narrowing of the aortic lumen at the site of the localized external deformity distinguishes pseudocoarctation from true coarctation. It is important to document the presence and severity of a pressure gradient at the site of coarctation before surgical correction is performed.

The patient with coarctation is at risk of developing a cerebrovascular accident, congestive heart failure, and hypertensive encephalopathy. In addition, bacterial endarteritis can occur. Aortic dissection and rupture are potential complications, particularly during pregnancy.

The medical treatment of coarctation of the aorta is directed toward control of blood pressure and treatment of complications. Coarctation with a substantial pressure gradient between the proximal and distal portions of the aorta should be treated surgically, either by resection of the coarctation and reanastomosis or by aortoplasty using a dacron patch or flap from the left subclavian artery. Elective surgery should be performed at 4 to 5 years of age, since earlier surgical therapy is likely to result in restenosis of the aortic lumen and later repair may be associated with persistent hypertension. Such hypertension may persist after surgical correction for a variety of reasons, including inadequate relief of the coarctation, progressive aortic regurgitation, or long-standing activation of the renin-angiotensin system, with resultant fluid retention. An exercise-induced increase in arm systolic blood pressure to greater than 200 mm Hg or an exercise-induced arm-leg systolic blood pressure gradient in excess of 35 mm Hg suggests persistent coarctation, constituting an indication for recatheterization and possible further surgery. Additional problems related to surgical correction include possible brain or spinal cord injury, renal damage, mesenteric arteritis, and late aneurysm formation. Older patients face additional technical hazards associated with an atherosclerotic aorta.

Symptoms, Diagnosis, Natural History, and Prognosis

1. Fraser RS, Stobey J, Rossall RE, Dvorkin J, Taylor RF. Coarctation of the aorta in adults. Can Med Assoc J 1976; 115:415–7.

   Of 36 adults with coarctation, 12 had aortic stenosis or insufficiency.

2. Reifenstein GH, Levine SA, Gross RE. Coarctation of the aorta: a review of 104 autopsied cases of the "adult type" 2 years of age or older. Am Heart J 1947, 33:146–68.

   Of these 104 cases, rupture of the aorta or an intracranial vascular catastrophe accounted for one-third of all deaths.

3. Campbell M. Natural history of coarctation of the aorta. Br Heart J 1970; 32:633–40.

   Of those patients with coarctation who survived the first 1–2 years of life and were then treated medically, mortality was substantial: 25% were dead by age 20, 50% by age 32, and 75% by age 46.

4. Freed MD, Keane JF, van Praagh R, Castaneda AR, Bernhard WF, Nadas AS. Coarctation of the aorta with congenital mitral regurgitation. Circulation 1974, 49:1175–84.

   Among 861 infants and children with coarctation of the aorta, 18 (2%) had congenital mitral regurgitation.

5. Goodwin JF. Pregnancy and coarctation of the aorta. Lancet 1958; 1:16–20.
   The risks for the pregnant patient with aortic coarctation are reviewed. If the blood pressure is adequately controlled, pregnancy does not offer a prohibitive risk.
6. Figley MM. Accessory roentgen signs of coarctation of the aorta. Radiology 1954; 62:671–87.
   Of 75 patients with coarctation of the aorta, 58 (77%) had rib notching.
7. Amsterdam EA, Albers WH, Christlieb A, Morgan CL, Nadas AS, Hickler RB. Plasma renin activity in children with coarctation of the aorta. Am J Cardiol 1969; 23:396–9.
   In 16 children (ages 2–13) with coarctation, the associated hypertension was not associated with increased activity of the renin-angiotensin system.
8. Boone ML, Swenson BE, Felson B. Rib notching: its many causes. AJR 1964; 91:1075–88.
   A complete review of this differential diagnosis.
9. Lavin N, Mehta S, Liberson M, Pouget JM. Pseudocoarctation of the aorta. Am J Cardiol 1969; 24:584–90.
   The patient with pseudocoarctation is generally asymptomatic, and surgical correction is generally not warranted.
10. Tawes RL, Berry CL, Aberdeen E. Congenital bicuspid aortic valves associated with coarctation of the aorta in children. Br Heart J 1969; 31:127–8.
    In this study, congenitally bicuspid aortic valves were found in 27% of children dying with coarctation of the aorta.
11. Alpert BS, Bain HH, Balfe JW, Kidd BSL, Olley PM. Role of the renin-angiotensin-aldosterone system in hypertensive children with coarctation of the aorta. Am J Cardiol 1979; 43:828–34.
    The renin and aldosterone responses of patients with coarctation suggest that their hypertension resembles a one-kidney Goldblatt model.

Therapy and Postoperative Assessment

12. Rathi L, Keith JD. Postoperative blood pressures in coarctation of the aorta. Br Heart J 1964; 26:671–8.
    In this series of 150 patients operated on for coarctation of the aorta, most became normotensive at some point following coarctectomy.
13. Nanton MA, Olley PM. Residual hypertension after coarctectomy in children. Am J Cardiol 1976; 37:769–72.
    Although coarctectomy in 190 children 1–15 years of age produced a reduction in blood pressure in the majority, 46 (24%) remained hypertensive.
14. Taylor SH, Donald KW. Circulatory studies at rest and during exercise in coarctation of the aorta before and after operation. Br Heart J 1960; 22:117–39.
    Following successful repair of a coarctation, there is a large reduction in left ventricular work at rest and during exercise.
15. Morris GC Jr, Cooley DA, DeBakey ME, Crawford ES. Coarctation of the aorta with particular emphasis upon improved techniques of surgical repair. J Thorac Cardiovasc Surg 1960; 40:705–22.
    A discussion of the various early surgical approaches for coarctation.
16. Schuster SR, Gross RE. Surgery for coarctation of the aorta: a review of 500 cases. J Thorac Cardiovasc Surg 1962; 43:54–70.
    In general, repair of coarctation induced a substantial fall in blood pressure.
17. Maron BJ, Humphries JO, Rowe RD, Mellits ED. Prognosis of surgically corrected coarctation of the aorta: a 20-year postoperative appraisal. Circulation 1973; 47:119–26.
    Of 248 patients operated for coarctation, long-term follow-up eventually revealed cardiovascular disease in 193 (78%). Importantly, 99 (40%) had a persistently elevated blood pressure.
18. Liberthson RR, Pennington DG, Jacobs ML, Daggett WM. Coarctation of the aorta: review of 234 patients and clarification of management problems. Am J Cardiol 1979; 43:835–40.
    This large study recommends elective surgical correction of coarctation at the age of 4 years.

19. Connor TM, Baker WP. A comparison of coarctation resection and patch angio-plasty using postexercise blood pressure measurements. Circulation 1981; 64:567–72.
    This study suggests that a dacron patch is preferable to simple resection of the coarcted segment.

20. Hamilton DI, Medici D, Oyonarte M, Dickinson DF. Aortoplasty with the left sub-clavian flap in older children. J Thorac Cardiovasc Surg 1981; 82:103–6.
    A description of the technique of aortoplasty in 10 patients with coarctation of the aorta.

21. Simon AB, Zloto AE. Coarctation of the aorta: longitudinal assessment of oper-ated patients. Circulation 1974; 50:456–64.
    Of 190 patients over age 2 operated on for coarctation of the aorta and followed long-term, 11 died, and most of the remaining 179 required medical follow-up for associated or related abnormalities, such as coexistent aortic or mitral valve dis-ease.

22. Connor TM. Evaluation of persistent coarctation of aorta after surgery with blood pressure measurement and exercise testing. Am J Cardiol 1979; 43:74–8.
    An exercise-induced arm:leg systolic blood pressure gradient greater than 35 mm Hg after repair of coarctation is an indication for recatheterization.

23. Freed MD, Rocchini A, Rosenthal A, Nadas AS, Castaneda AR. Exercise-induced hypertension after surgical repair of coarctation of the aorta. Am J Cardiol 1979; 43:253–8.
    This study suggests that an exercise-induced arm systolic blood pressure greater than 200 mm Hg is an indication for recatheterization.

24. Beekman RH, Rocchini AP, Behrendt DM, Rosenthal A. Reoperation for coarcta-tion of the aorta. Am J Cardiol 1981; 48:1108–14.
    A report of 21 patients requiring reoperation for coarctation of the aorta. The inci-dence of reoperation is increased in patients who are younger than 3 years at the time of initial repair.

CORRECTED TRANSPOSITION OF THE GREAT VESSELS

Uncorrected transposition (so-called d-transposition) of the great vessels is one of the two most common forms of congenital heart disease that cause cyanosis. In this condition, the aorta arises anterior to the pulmonary artery and origi-nates from the right ventricle, whereas the pulmonary artery comes from the left ventricle. As a result, unoxygenated, mixed venous blood enters the aorta, the pulmonary artery is subjected to systemic arterial pressure, and oblitera-tive pulmonary vascular disease and death occur at a young age. Recent at-tempts at early surgical correction have been somewhat successful in allowing infants with uncorrected transposition of the great vessels to reach adulthood. Without surgical correction, 90 percent die within the first year.

In the patient with *corrected* transposition (so-called l-transposition) of the great vessels, the aorta and pulmonary artery are arranged in a manner iden-tical to uncorrected transposition (i.e., the aorta is anterior to the pulmonary artery), but the ventricles are also reversed. Thus, venous blood enters a right-sided ventricle with the morphologic and anatomic features of a left ventricle, from which it is propelled into the pulmonary artery. Similarly, pulmonary ve-nous blood enters a left-sided ventricle that morphologically resembles a right ventricle and is then ejected into the aorta. The AV valves are also reversed: the valve connecting the right atrium with the right-sided ventricle is bicuspid (anatomically similar to the mitral valve), whereas the valve connecting the left atrium with the left-sided ventricle is tricuspid. Thus, despite the transposed great vessels, the intracardiac movement of blood is normal.

Only a small percentage of patients with corrected transposition have no other cardiac abnormalities. Most of them have an associated abnormality, such as ventricular septal defect, single ventricle, regurgitation into the left atrium through the left-sided AV valve (frequently due to an Ebstein-type malformation of the valve), or pulmonic or subpulmonic stenosis. In addition, the AV conducting system is abnormal in all patients: the His bundle is longer than normal, and the bundle branches are inverted, following the appropriate morphologic ventricle. These anatomic derangements of the conduction system result in a disturbance of AV conduction in some patients.

Corrected transposition of the great vessels is more common in men than women. The patient with a totally corrected transposition and no other cardiac abnormality is generally asymptomatic. On physical examination, the S_1 may be reduced in intensity. The S_2 is generally single (because of the posterior position of the pulmonary trunk, making pulmonic valve closure virtually inaudible). If associated defects are present, the physical examination may reveal the appropriate murmurs.

On the ECG, roughly 75 percent of patients with corrected transposition have disturbances of AV conduction, including P–R interval prolongation, second degree AV block, and even complete heart block due to the abnormal course of the conduction system. Paroxysmal tachycardia or the Wolff-Parkinson-White syndrome may be present. *The characteristic electrocardiographic finding is a reversal of the initial forces of ventricular activation, resulting in the absence of Q waves in lead I and the left precordial leads and the presence of Q waves in the right precordial leads.* The chest x-ray may suggest the correct diagnosis because of the appearance of the heart, which resembles an egg on a stalk. Because of the rotation of the great vessels, the ascending aortic convexity (normally on the right) is absent, as is the pulmonary arterial segment and aortic knuckle on the left. The left cardiac border has a "humped" appearance due to the convex systemic ventricle.

At cardiac catheterization, angiographic studies are used to delineate the abnormal position of the pulmonary artery, which lies medial and to the right of the ascending aorta in the frontal projection and posterior to it in the lateral projection. Angiography may also demonstrate inversion of the ventricles. The coronary arteries have a course appropriate to their ventricles, that is, the anterior descending and circumflex arteries supply the morphologic left ventricle, and the right coronary artery supplies the morphologic right ventricle.

In the patient with uncomplicated corrected transposition of the great vessels, there is no circulatory derangement, and no treatment is required. If symptomatic AV block complicates corrected transposition, pacemaker insertion is indicated. Antiarrhythmic agents may be necessary in the treatment of recurrent supraventricular tachyarrhythmias. If coexisting intracardiac defects are present, congestive heart failure may occur, and surgical treatment of these associated abnormalitites may be indicated.

1. Schiebler GL, Edwards JE, Burchell HB, DuShane JW, Ongley PA, Wood EH. Congenital corrected transposition of the great vessels: a study of 33 cases. Pediatrics 1961; 27:851–88.
   A morphologic and anatomic review of 33 cases of congenitally corrected transposition of the great vessels.
2. Cumming GR. Congenital corrected transposition of the great vessels without associated intracardiac anomalies: a clinical, hemodynamic, and angiographic study. Am J Cardiol 1962; 10:605–14.
   This paper describes 2 patients with corrected transposition of the great vessels

without associated anomalies. In such individuals, heart block often develops in early adulthood.

3. Rotem CE, Hultgren HN. Corrected transposition of the great vessels without associated defects. Am Heart J 1965; 70:305–18.
   This paper describes 2 patients with complete AV block and corrected transposition of the great vessels without intracardiac shunting.

4. Selden R, Schaeffer RA, Kennedy BJ, Neill WA. Corrected transposition of the great arteries simulating coronary heart disease in adults. Chest 1976; 69:188–91.
   Two adult patients with chest pain and dyspnea initially thought to have coronary artery disease were ultimately shown to have normal coronary arteries and corrected transposition of the great vessels. The authors speculate that angina pectoris resulted from inadequate coronary reserve of the systemic ventricle (which was supplied by the right coronary artery).

5. Lieberson AD, Schumacher RR, Childress RH, Genovese PD. Corrected transposition of the great vessels in a 73-year-old man. Circulation 1969; 39:96–100.
   The patient described herein is a 73-year-old man with corrected transposition and associated mitral and aortic regurgitation. Although corrected transposition is theoretically compatible with a normal life span, few patients with this lesion survive past 40 years of age because of associated congenital defects or the subsequent development of AV valvular insufficiency or heart block.

6. Waldo AL, Pacifico AD, Bargeron LM Jr, James TN, Kirklin JW. Electrophysiological delineation of the specialized AV conduction system in patients with corrected transposition of the great vessels and ventricular septal defect. Circulation 1975; 52:435–41.
   A detailed study of the AV conduction system in 4 patients with these abnormalities.

7. Van Mierop LHS, Alley RD, Kausel HW, Stranahan A. Ebstein's malformation of the left atrioventricular valve in corrected transposition, with subpulmonary stenosis and ventricular septal defect. Am J Cardiol 1961; 8:270–4.
   One of the earliest case reports showing the association of Ebstein's anomaly in a patient with corrected transposition.

8. Jaffe RB. Systemic atrioventricular valve regurgitation in corrected transposition of the great vessels. Am J Cardiol 1976; 37:395–402.
   Most patients with corrected transposition have an associated VSD or AV valvular regurgitation.

9. Bjarke BB, Kidd BSL. Congenitally corrected transposition of the great arteries: a clinical study of 101 cases. Acta Paediatr Scand 1976; 65:153–60.
   The anatomy, clinical features, and natural history of 101 patients with this entity are presented. Only 1 had no associated cardiac lesion. Of the 101, 87 had VSDs.

10. Friedberg DZ, Nadas AS. Clinical profile of patients with congenital corrected transposition of the great arteries: a study of 60 cases. N Eng J Med 1970; 282:1053–9.
    These authors noted the following associated anomalies in patients with corrected transposition of the great vessels: single ventricle in 42%, VSD in 54%, pulmonic stenosis in 45%, and left AV valve regurgitation in 23%.

11. Hagler DJ, Tajik AJ, Seward JB, Edwards WD, Mair DD, Ritter DG. Atrioventricular and ventriculoarterial discordance (corrected transposition of the great arteries): wide-angle two dimensional echocardiographic assessment of ventricular morphology. Mayo Clin Proc 1981; 56:591–600.
    An elegant, well-illustrated discussion of the value of two-dimensional echocardiography in the diagnosis of corrected transposition of the great arteries in 27 patients.

12. Elliott LP, Amplatz K, Edwards JE. Coronary arterial patterns in transposition complexes: anatomic and angiographic studies. Am J Cardiol 1966; 17:362–78.
    A detailed review of this subject, based on 115 pathology specimens and 17 angiographic studies.

13. Stanger P, Rudolph AM, Edwards JE. Cardiac malpositions: an overview based on study of 65 necropsy specimens. Circulation 1977; 56:159–72.
    A comprehensive, scholarly review of the nomenclature applied to cardiac malpositions, including the transposition complexes.

14. Graham TP Jr, Parrish MD, Boucek RJ Jr, Boerth RC, Breitweser JA, Thompson S, Robertson RM, Morgan JR, Friesinger GC. Assessment of ventricular size and function in congenitally corrected transposition of the great arteries. Am J Cardiol 1983; 51:244–51.

In children, systemic and pulmonary ventricular pump function is usually normal. After childhood, systemic ventricular dysfunction is common and may reflect the inability of the anatomic right ventricle to function as the systemic pumping chamber.

TETRALOGY OF FALLOT

Tetralogy of Fallot is the most common cause of cyanosis in patients with congenital heart disease who survive infancy. It is comprised of four distinct anatomic lesions: right ventricular outflow tract obstruction, ventricular septal defect (VSD), dextraposition of the aorta (i.e., an aorta that "overrides" the VSD), and right ventricular hypertrophy. Although the right ventricular outflow tract obstruction is usually infundibular in location, it can occur at the level of the pulmonic valve in up to one-third of cases, and rarely it can involve both sites. The VSD is typically large and *nonrestrictive,* so that pressures in the left and right ventricles are equal. When the VSD is smaller and *restrictive* (so that there is a difference in left and right ventricular pressures), the entity is designated *pulmonary stenosis with VSD.* Thus, the term *tetralogy of Fallot* is reserved for a large, nonrestrictive VSD with right ventricular outflow tract obstruction that offers a resistance near, at, or above systemic levels. When this resistance is lower than systemic, the shunt is predominantly or entirely left-to-right (so-called *acyanotic tetralogy of Fallot*). When the resistance equals systemic, the shunt is bidirectional. Finally, when this resistance exceeds systemic, the shunt becomes right-to-left, with resultant central cyanosis. When a large VSD is associated with complete pulmonary stenosis, so that blood flow to the lungs is entirely through collaterals from the systemic circulation, the entity is termed *pulmonary atresia with VSD.*

Males and females are equally affected by tetralogy of Fallot. The patient most commonly complains of dyspnea on exertion and a variable degree of exercise intolerance. Cyanosis usually develops within the first few months of life, and slow growth and development are noted. The patient with severe right ventricular outflow obstruction often has episodes of severe cyanosis that are sometimes associated with loss of consciousness or convulsions. These episodes, termed *anoxic spells,* are believed to result from additional right ventricular outflow obstruction induced by reactive spasm in the infundibulum or pulmonary arterial tree associated with emotional lability. The additional right ventricular outflow obstruction increases right-to-left shunting, producing more cyanosis and loss of consciousness or convulsions. Patients with this entity (particularly young children) commonly squat in an attempt to increase systemic oxygenation, since squatting increases systemic vascular resistance, thereby decreasing the magnitude of right-to-left shunting and encouraging the flow of blood from the right ventricle to the pulmonary artery. In addition, squatting reduces venous return from the legs and minimizes the effects of orthostatic hypotension.

On physical examination, cyanosis and clubbing are generally present in patients with tetralogy of Fallot. A right ventricular lift with no clear left ventricular impulse is ordinarily present. A systolic ejection click is often audible; this can be detected in patients with pulmonary valvular stenosis, in whom it diminishes or disappears completely with inspiration. In some patients with severe right ventricular outflow obstruction, a hypoplastic pulmonary trunk, and a relatively large aortic root, the click may originate in the aortic root. The S_2 is ordinarily single, representing aortic valve closure; pulmonic valve closure is rarely audible but, when present, is soft and markedly delayed. A systolic ejection murmur of varying intensity is best heard in the third and fourth left intercostal spaces. The intensity of the murmur is proportional to the magnitude of blood flow through the right ventricular outflow tract: the more severe the obstruction (and the greater the right-to-left shunting and degree of cyanosis), the softer the murmur; the milder the obstruction, the louder the murmur. Pulmonary blood flow, the intensity of the murmur, and the degree of cyanosis are influenced in a predictable manner by agents that increase or decrease systemic vascular resistance: systemic vasodilatation is detrimental, whereas systemic vasoconstriction can be beneficial. An early diastolic murmur of aortic regurgitation or a continuous murmur of a patent ductus arteriosus may be heard, since these lesions are not uncommonly associated with tetralogy of Fallot. A continuous murmur, representing blood flow through enlarged bronchial collaterals, is often heard over the back, particularly in patients with pulmonary atresia.

The ECG discloses right axis deviation and right ventricular hypertrophy. There is typically a large monophasic R wave in V1 with an abrupt transition to an RS complex in V2 and V3, with normal progression to Rs complexes in V5 and V6. The characteristic chest x-ray shows a relatively normal sized heart with a right ventricular contour, a concavity in the region of the main pulmonary artery, and decreased pulmonary vascularity, or *oligemia*. The radiographic appearance of the heart has been termed *coeur en sabot,* or *boot-shaped heart.* The aortic arch is right-sided in 25 to 30 percent of cases. In general, the likelihood of a right-sided arch increases with the severity of right ventricular outflow obstruction and is particularly common in patients with pulmonary atresia.

The anoxic spells that occur in patients with tetralogy of Fallot typically develop during early childhood and are rare after the fifth year of life. Treatment should be instituted immediately when they occur, consisting of oxygen administration, the correction of acid-base and electrolyte disturbances, administration of morphine, and placing the patient in the knee-chest position to increase systemic vascular resistance. Morphine is given because of its sedative effect and because it relaxes the right ventricular infundibulum. Beta-blocking agents such as propranolol also have been used to decrease right ventricular infundibular obstruction.

Patients with cyanotic congenital heart disease (particularly those with tetralogy of Fallot) are at risk for the development of a brain abscess. The most frequently involved causative organism is the alpha streptococcus, and the most common site for abscess development in the brain is the right parieto-occipital region. The treatment consists of intense antibiotic therapy and surgical drainage. Other potential complications of tetralogy of Fallot are bacterial endocarditis, polycythemia, and the eventual development of right ventricular or biventricular failure.

Infants with tetralogy of Fallot who are severely cyanotic at birth, with markedly reduced pulmonary blood flow and severe systemic arterial desaturation, rarely survive the first year of life without surgery. Conversely, most patients with tetralogy of Fallot have only moderately severe obstruction to right ventricular outflow, and systemic arterial desaturation is less severe. As children, their exercise tolerance is poor, and they squat frequently. Without some form of surgery, either palliative or corrective, they rarely survive beyond the third decade of life. Death usually results from cerebrovascular accidents, brain abscess, endocarditis, anoxia, or pulmonary hemorrhage.

The surgical treatment of tetralogy of Fallot consists of either a palliative procedure (to increase pulmonary blood flow) or a definitive procedure (to correct the malformation completely). The palliative procedure consists of the creation of a shunt from a systemic to a pulmonary artery. The Blalock-Taussig procedure anastomoses the left subclavian artery to the side of the left pulmonary artery (in a patient with a left-sided aortic arch). The Waterston procedure is a side-to-side anastomosis of the ascending aorta and the right pulmonary artery, whereas the Potts procedure is an anastomosis of the aorta and the main pulmonary artery. Of these, the Blalock-Taussig procedure is preferred, since the other two procedures can lead to an excessively large shunt. The Blalock-Taussig anastomosis often provides considerable clinical and hemodynamic benefit for several years. The operative mortality for this procedure varies, depending on the clinical status and size of the patient, but it is less than 5 percent in centers where the staff is experienced in caring for such patients. Complications of such shunting include thrombosis (with resultant systemic desaturation), endocarditis, pulmonary arterial hypertension (when the shunt is too large), localized hemorrhagic pulmonary edema, and underdevelopment of the right or left arm (when the corresponding subclavian artery is used for the shunt).

Complete repair of tetralogy of Fallot requires cardiopulmonary bypass. An accurate preoperative delineation of anatomy is imperative, including an angiographic assessment of the right ventricular outflow tract, the left ventricle and VSD, the aortic root, and the coronary arteries. It is particularly important to determine the presence or absence of associated anomalies, such as aortic regurgitation, coronary arterial abnormalities, multiple VSDs, patent ductus arteriosus, and a hypoplastic, stenosed, or absent left or right pulmonary artery. In addition, one must distinguish tetralogy of Fallot from other entities, particularly double outlet right ventricle, pulmonary atresia with VSD, and pulmonary stenosis with intact ventricular septum. Two-dimensional echocardiography, used in conjunction with cardiac catheterization, may help to elucidate the underlying anatomy and physiology. The major contraindications to complete repair of tetralogy of Fallot are hypoplasia of the pulmonary arteries and small size of the patient. Presently, if the child's anatomy is suitable, the procedure is performed routinely in patients under 3 years of age and in many centers under 1 year of age, with an operative mortality less than 10 percent. Propranolol has been shown to postpone the need for surgical correction by approximately 13 months in most patients, thus obviating the need for an early shunt procedure followed by later definitive correction with its attendant risks. Complete repair of tetralogy of Fallot entails resection of the infundibular stenosis, relief of the pulmonary valvular stenosis (if present) by open valvotomy, and placement of a patch over the VSD. It is occasionally necessary to place a patch to enlarge the outflow tract or pulmonary valve ring, but this is generally avoided if possible.

The long-term results following total correction of tetralogy of Fallot are generally extremely good, but certain electrophysiologic and hemodynamic derangements can occur. With present surgical techniques, right bundle branch block occurs in 60 to 100 percent of cases, bifascicular block (right bundle branch block and left anterior hemiblock) in 7 to 25 percent, and permanent complete heart block in 1 to 2 percent. In addition, 2 to 3 percent of patients die suddenly. Postoperative hemodynamic derangements include right or left ventricular failure (due to inadequate closure of the VSD), incomplete relief of right ventricular outflow tract obstruction, and excessive enlargement of the outflow tract, with resultant pulmonary regurgitation. These conditions may necessitate surgical repair or placement of a prosthetic pulmonic valve. Following complete repair with a satisfactory technical result, there may still be subtle evidence of right or left ventricular dysfunction (demonstrable by exercise or afterload stress), particularly when operative correction is performed in adolescents or adults. Even when the physical examination suggests a good technical result following complete repair, long-term antibiotic prophylaxis is recommended because of the risk of endocarditis due to a small residual VSD.

1. Reduto LA, Berger HJ, Johnstone DE, Hellenbrand W, Wackers FJT, Whittemore R, Cohen LS, Gottschalk A, Zaret BL. Radionuclide assessment of right and left ventricular exercise reserve after total correction of tetralogy of Fallot. Am J Cardiol 1980; 45:1013–8.
   This study suggests that right ventricular function may appear normal at rest but is abnormal during exercise in most patients following surgical correction of tetralogy. Conversely, left ventricular function appears to be normal both at rest and during exercise.
2. Ruzyllo W, Nihill MR, Mullins CE, McNamara DG. Hemodynamic evaluation of 221 patients after intracardiac repair of tetralogy of Fallot. Am J Cardiol 1974; 34:565–76.
   Following intracardiac repair of tetralogy of Fallot, 221 patients were studied. The results suggest that total correction provides acceptable hemodynamic results even in children younger than age 4 if right ventricular outflow obstruction is relieved without producing or aggravating pulmonary insufficiency.
3. Reid JM, Coleman EN, Barclay RS, Stevenson JG. Blalock-Taussig anastomosis in 126 patients with Fallot's tetralogy. Thorax 1973; 28:269–72.
   The long-term results of Blalock-Taussig anastomosis in 126 patients with Fallot's tetralogy are reviewed; operative mortality was 10%, and overall mortality was 38%. In the long-term survivors, complications were few.
4. Cole RB, Muster AJ, Fixler DE, Paul MH. Long-term results of aortopulmonary anastomosis for tetralogy of Fallot. Circulation 1971; 43:263–71.
   A review of 340 patients with tetralogy of Fallot undergoing aortopulmonary anastomosis is presented. There were 30 operative deaths and 52 late medical deaths, most of which were related to anastomotic channels that were made or eventually became too large.
5. Waldhausen JA, Friedman S, Tyers GFO, Rashkind WJ, Petry E, Miller WW. Ascending aorta–right pulmonary artery anastomosis: clinical experience with 35 patients with cyanotic congenital heart disease. Circulation 1968; 38:463–7.
   Of the 35 patients in this report undergoing this palliative procedure, 3 died in the immediate postoperative period; the other 32 did well.
6. Fellows KE, Smith J, Keane JF. Preoperative angiocardiography in infants with Tetrad of Fallot. Am J Cardiol 1981; 47:1279–85.
   A detailed description of the optimal angiographic techniques in patients with tetralogy of Fallot.
7. Soto B, Pacifico AD, Ceballos R, Bargeron LM. Tetralogy of Fallot: an angiographic-pathologic correlative study. Circulation 1981; 64:558–66.
   A detailed discussion of the cineangiographic findings in patients with tetralogy of Fallot.
8. Hagler DJ, Tajik AJ, Seward JB, Mair DD, Ritter DG. Wide-angle two-dimensional echocardiographic profiles of conotruncal abnormalities. Mayo Clin Proc 1980; 55:73–82.
   A description in 150 patients of the value of two-dimensional echocardiography for distinguishing tetralogy of Fallot from persistent truncus arteriosus or pulmonary atresia with VSD.
9. Edwards WD: Double-outlet right ventricle and tetralogy of Fallot. J Thorac Cardiovasc Surg 1981; 82:418–22.
   A description of the morphology of tetralogy of Fallot and double outlet right ventricle and of the relationship between the two.
10. Dabizzi RP, Caprioli G, Aiazzi L, Castelli C, Baldrighi G, Parenzan L, Baldrighi

V. Distribution and anomalies of coronary arteries in tetralogy of Fallot. Circulation 1980; 61:95–102.
Of 119 patients with tetralogy, 11 had angiographically demonstrable anomalies of the coronary arteries.

11. Capelli H, Ross D, Somerville J. Aortic regurgitation in Tetrad of Fallot and pulmonary atresia. Am J Cardiol 1982; 49:1979–83.
The authors discuss this association and recommend routine retrograde ascending aortography in all adolescents or adults with tetralogy or pulmonary atresia with VSD.

12. Garson A Jr, Gillette PC, McNamara DG. Propranolol: the preferred palliation for tetralogy of Fallot. Am J Cardiol 1981; 47:1098–1104.
Propranolol is effective in preventing hypoxemic spells in 80% of infants and can enable operation to be postponed for 13 months.

13. Castaneda AR, Freed MD, Williams RG, Norwood WI. Repair of tetralogy of Fallot in infancy: early and late results. J Thorac Cardiovasc Surg 1977; 74:372–81.
Of 41 consecutive children less than 1 year of age undergoing primary repair of tetralogy of Fallot, 3 (7.5%) died during or soon after surgery.

14. Poirier RA, McGoon DC, Danielson GK, Wallace RB, Ritter DG, Moodie DS, Wiltse CG. Late results after repair of tetralogy of Fallot. J Thorac Cardiovasc Surg 1977; 73:900–8.
This study of 311 patients undergoing complete repair of tetralogy emphasizes the importance of relieving right ventricular outflow tract obstruction.

15. Daily PO, Stinson EB, Griepp RB, Shumway NE. Tetralogy of Fallot: choice of surgical procedure. J Thorac Cardiovasc Surg 1978; 75:338–45.
A statistical analysis to determine the most effective surgical management of patients with tetralogy of Fallot at different ages. Even for infants under 2 years of age, these authors recommend complete correction unless the patient has hypoplastic pulmonary arteries.

16. Kirklin JW, Blackstone EH, Pacifico AD, Brown RN, Bargeron LM Jr. Routine primary repair vs two-stage repair of tetralogy of Fallot. Circulation 1979; 60:373–86.
Except for very small infants, primary repair of tetralogy of Fallot without a transannular patch is safer than a staged procedure with an initial Blalock-Taussig or Waterston shunt.

17. Fuster V, McGoon DC, Kennedy MA, Ritter DG, Kirklin JW. Long-term evaluation (12 to 22 years) of open heart surgery for tetralogy of Fallot. Am J Cardiol 1980; 46:635–42.
The largest series of its kind (475 patients), this study emphasizes the good long-term results following complete repair of tetralogy of Fallot.

18. Vetter VL, Horowitz LN. Electrophysiologic residua and sequelae of surgery for congenital heart defects. Am J Cardiol 1982; 50:588–604.
A detailed discussion of the effects of surgery on the conduction system in patients with tetralogy of Fallot.

19. Cairns JA, Dobell ARC, Gibbons JE, Tessler I. Prognosis of right bundle branch block and left anterior hemiblock after intracardiac repair of tetralogy of Fallot. Am Heart J 1975; 90:549–54.
This report suggests that the combination of right bundle branch block and left anterior hemiblock has a benign prognosis in patients who have undergone complete repair of tetralogy provided that they have not had transient periods of complete heart block.

20. Ebert PA. Second operations for pulmonary stenosis or insufficiency after repair of tetralogy of Fallot. Am J Cardiol 1982; 50:637–40.
This paper describes 24 patients with previous complete repair of tetralogy of Fallot who required subsequent operative procedures for either residual pulmonary stenosis or valvular incompetence.

21. Graham TP, Cordell D, Atwood GF, Boucek RJ Jr, Boerth RC, Bender HW, Nelson JH, Vaughn WK. Right ventricular volume characteristics before and after palliative and reparative operation in tetralogy of Fallot. Circulation 1976; 54:417–23.
Right heart volume data were obtained in 63 patients with tetralogy of Fallot, and alterations that occur after palliative and total surgical correction are reported.

22. James FW, Kaplan S, Schwartz DC, Chou TC, Sandker MJ, Naylor V. Response to exercise in patients after total surgical correction of tetralogy of Fallot. Circulation 1976; 54:671–9.

    Heart rate, blood pressure, work capacity, and electrocardiographic changes during upright bicycle exercise were evaluated in 43 asymptomatic patients after total surgical correction of tetralogy of Fallot. These patients had a reduced work capacity, and 10 of the 43 developed arrhythmias with exercise.

23. Borow KM, Green LH, Castaneda AR, Keane JF. Left ventricular function after repair of tetralogy of Fallot and its relationship to age at surgery. Circulation 1980; 61:1150–8.

    Left ventricular dysfunction may be unmasked by afterload stress in older patients but not in those repaired during infancy. These findings raise the possibility that early definitive repair may preserve left ventricular function.

TRUNCUS ARTERIOSUS

Truncus arteriosus is an uncommon congenital anomaly in which a single great vessel exits the base of the heart through a single semilunar valve. This valve is located directly above a ventricular septal defect (VSD) and receives blood from both ventricles. Thus, the truncus gives rise to the systemic, pulmonary, and coronary arteries. Although the truncal semilunar valve is usually tricuspid, it may have from two to six cusps. Regurgitation and stenosis of this valve are each seen in 10 to 15 percent of patients. In addition, a right-sided aortic arch is present in 25 percent. Truncus arteriosus occurs with equal frequency in males and females.

Anatomically, there are four types of truncus arteriosus. In type 1, a short pulmonary trunk emerges from the truncus arteriosus and gives rise to the right and left pulmonary arteries. In type 2, the right and left pulmonary arteries arise directly from the posterior wall of the truncus. In type 3, both pulmonary arteries originate from the lateral walls of the truncus. In type 4, the pulmonary arteries are completely absent, and the arterial supply to the lungs occurs through bronchial collaterals. This type of truncus is more correctly termed a solitary aortic trunk with pulmonary agenesis and is anatomically and physiologically similar to pulmonary atresia with VSD (so-called pseudotruncus arteriosus).

Since the truncal valve overrides a large VSD, the pressures in the left and right ventricles are equal. As a result, the physiologic consequences of truncus arteriosus depend on the presence and size of the pulmonary arteries as well as the resistance to flow through the lungs. Thus, truncus arteriosus may be associated with (1) *increased pulmonary blood flow and minimal cyanosis,* (2) *decreased pulmonary blood flow* and *marked cyanosis,* or (3) *near normal pulmonary blood flow and moderate cyanosis.* Most infants with truncus have an increased pulmonary blood flow (due to a low pulmonary vascular resistance) with minimal or mild cyanosis, and the arterial oxygen saturation may be normal. These infants usually die within 6 months of severe congestive heart failure. With prolonged survival, the pulmonary vascular resistance gradually rises, pulmonary blood flow falls, cyanosis increases, and volume overload of the left ventricle is partially relieved. When pulmonary vascular resistance rises to very high levels, flow to the lungs is markedly reduced, the arterial oxygen saturation is low, and cyanosis with diminished pulmonary blood flow is present. Less commonly, truncus arteriosus can occur in childhood with small or absent pulmonary arteries, decreased pulmonary blood flow, and early, severe cyanosis. *The relatively few individuals who survive infancy and reach childhood or even adulthood are those in whom pulmonary blood flow is adequate but not excessive.*

On physical examination, the patient with truncus arteriosus is underdeveloped and cyanosed, and there is evidence of heart failure. The child with marked pulmonary plethora may be acyanotic at rest but cyanotic during crying or feeding. When truncus arteriosus is associated with large pulmonary arteries, a precordial bulge due to cardiac enlargement is common. The dynamic left ventricular impulse reflects the hypertrophy and dilatation of volume overload. Since the right ventricle ejects at systemic pressures, a right ventricular impulse is virtually always noted. When separate pulmonary arteries arise directly from the truncus, there is no systolic impulse in the second left intercostal space. However, when the truncus gives rise to a short main pulmonary artery, this vessel may dilate and produce a palpable impulse in the second left intercostal space.

In the patient with truncus arteriosus and enlarged pulmonary arteries, the S_1 is normal and is ordinarily followed by a systolic ejection click originating from the dilated solitary trunk. Systolic murmurs are common and, as a rule, are ejection in timing. When the VSD is moderate or large in size and the left ventricular output is large, a conspicuous murmur is generated. However, when a rising pulmonary vascular resistance causes pulmonary blood flow and left ventricular stroke volume to diminish, this murmur shortens and becomes softer. Occasionally, no murmur is audible, particularly in the patient with increased pulmonary blood flow and a very large VSD. In this circumstance, flow from the left ventricle into the truncus presumably occurs with relatively little turbulence, so that the interventricular communication is silent. When a murmur is present, it is often preferentially transmitted to the second right intercostal space, since the truncus follows the same course as the aorta. The S_2 is loud, since the semilunar valve of the large solitary truncus is positioned near the chest wall, and the cusps close at systemic pressure. The truncus has only one valve, and as a result, the S_2 lacks splitting. A diastolic murmur may originate from two sources. In the patient with large pulmonary arteries and increased pulmonary blood flow, an apical mid-diastolic murmur results from increased antegrade flow across the mitral valve. A loud S_3 may accompany the "flow rumble." A high-frequency, early diastolic murmur, maximal along the left sternal border, is sometimes present and is due to incompetence of the truncal valve.

The ECG ordinarily reflects volume overload of the left ventricle and pressure overload of the right ventricle. Sinus rhythm is usually present. Evidence of right atrial enlargement may be apparent. The mean QRS axis ordinarily is directed inferiorly and to the right. A rightward shift in mean QRS axis is present when pulmonary blood flow is reduced, and a leftward shift is likely when pulmonary blood flow is large. However, marked axis deviation to either the right or left is unusual.

When the truncus arteriosus coexists with large pulmonary arteries and increased pulmonary blood flow, the radiographic pulmonary vascular pattern is plethoric. *The combination of increased pulmonary blood flow and cyanosis is an important clue in the clinical recognition of truncus arteriosus.* The usual radiographic findings include gross cardiomegaly with left or combined ventricular enlargement, left atrial enlargement, a small or absent main pulmonary arterial segment, and pulmonary plethora. The pulmonary arterial segment is flat or concave when separate pulmonary arterial branches arise from the truncus. This concavity is especially apparent in the right anterior oblique projection. Occasionally, a large left pulmonary artery creates a relatively high shadow as it emerges from the cardiac silhouette and curves upward and to the left; this sign is termed a *left hilar comma*. A short, dilated main pulmonary artery may originate from the truncus and form a convex shadow. The truncus itself may produce a conspicuous rightward shadow in young adults and older children; the ascending portion may sweep to the right, forming a convex upper border that resembles a dilated ascending aorta. The sweep may continue upward, so that the level of the arch appears high. As pulmonary vascular resistance increases, pulmonary blood flow falls, and the radiologic evidence of plethora diminishes; in fact, the peripheral pulmonary lung fields may appear oligemic. With type 4 truncus arteriosus (common aortic trunk with absent pulmonary arteries), the chest x-ray is indistinguishable from that seen with pulmonary atresia and VSD.

By echocardiography, one sees a large truncal root overriding the VSD, mitral valve–truncal root continuity, and a large right ventricle. The size of the left atrium provides a good index of pulmonary blood flow. Differentiation of truncus arteriosus from tetralogy of Fallot rests on the demonstration of a pulmonic valve in the latter condition.

In the absence of surgery, early death due to heart failure or the early development of pulmonary vascular obstructive disease with systemic desaturation is the rule. In infants and young children with a large left-to-right shunt, surgical banding of one or both pulmonary arteries has been employed to reduce pulmonary blood flow. Corrective surgery is preferred before 1 to 2 years of age if the patient is free of severe pulmonary vascular obstructive disease. Surgical correction of this anomaly entails closure of the VSD, excision of the pulmonary arteries from the truncus, and insertion of a valve-containing conduit from the right ventricle to the pulmonary arteries. Corrective surgery can be performed in the patient with at least one adequate pulmonary artery and a low distal pressure and resistance. Conversely, a high pulmonary vascular resistance may render the patient inoperable. Associated truncal valvular regurgitation or stenosis necessitating valve replacement greatly increases the surgical mortality.

1. Anderson RC, Obata W, Lillehei CW. Truncus arteriosus: clinical study of 14 cases. Circulation 1957; 16:586–98.
   The clinical findings in 14 patients with type I truncus arteriosus are reviewed.
2. Campbell M, Deuchar DC. Continuous murmurs in cyanotic congenital heart disease. Br Heart J 1961; 23:173–93.
   A detailed review of causes of continuous murmurs in patients with cyanotic congenital heart disease.
3. Collett RW, Edwards JE. Persistent truncus arteriosus: a classification according to anatomic types. Surg Clin North Am 1949; 29:1245–70.
   An early anatomic classification of the different types of truncus arteriosus.
4. Tandon R, Hauck AJ, Nadas AS. Persistent truncus arteriosus: a clinical, hemodynamic, and autopsy study of 19 cases. Circulation 1963; 28:1050–60.
   Clinical and postmortem data in 19 patients with this abnormality are presented.
5. Taussig HB. Clinical and pathological findings in cases of truncus arteriosus in infancy. Am J Med 1947; 2:26–34.
   The clinical findings in 2 patients with truncus arteriosus are described.
6. van Praagh R, van Praagh S. The anatomy of common aorticopulmonary trunk (truncus arteriosus communis) and its embryologic implications: a study of 57 necropsy cases. Am J Cardiol 1965; 16:406–25.
   A study of 57 necropsy cases with truncus arteriosus and a detailed description of the findings.
7. Victorica BE, Elliott LP. The roentgenologic findings and approach to persistent truncus arteriosus in infancy. AJR 1968; 104:440–51.

A review of the radiographic findings in 14 patients with persistent truncus arteriosus.

8. Victorica BE, Gessner IH, Schiebler GL. Phonocardiographic findings in persistent truncus arteriosus. Br Heart J 1968; 30:812–6.
The auscultatory findings in 13 patients with truncus arteriosus are described.
9. Rothko K, Moore GW, Hutchins GM. Truncus arteriosus malformation: a spectrum including fourth and sixth aortic arch interruptions. Am Heart J 1980; 99:17–24.
A necropsy study of 19 patients with this anomaly, including a detailed discussion of the possible embryology of this condition.
10. Smallhorn JF, Anderson RH, Macartney FJ. Two dimensional echocardiographic assessment of communications between ascending aorta and pulmonary trunk or individual pulmonary arteries. Br Heart J 1982; 47:563–72.
This study documents the value of two-dimensional echocardiography in distinguishing truncus arteriosus from aortopulmonary window and anomalous origin of the left or right pulmonary artery from the aorta.
11. Bailey LL, Petry EL, Doroshow RW, Jacobson JG, Wareham EE. Biologic reconstruction of the right ventricular outflow tract: preliminary experimental analysis and clinical application in a neonate with type I truncus arteriosus. J Thorac Cardiovasc Surg 1981; 82:779–84.
A detailed account of a preliminary canine study of a technique for reconstructing the right ventricular outflow tract and its application to a neonate with type I truncus arteriosus.
12. Barron JV, Sahn DJ, Attie F, Valdes-Cruz LM, Grenadier E, Allen HD, Lima CO, Goldberg SJ. Two-dimensional echocardiographic study of right ventricular outflow and great artery anatomy in pulmonary atresia with ventricular septal defects and in truncus arteriosus. Am Heart J 1983; 105:281–6.
This article identifies specific echocardiographic criteria for diagnosing truncus arteriosus.

CONGENITAL COMPLETE HEART BLOCK

Complete heart block is one of the two most commonly encountered congenital arrhythmias. Anatomically, it can be caused by (1) a total absence of the AV node, (2) the replacement of AV junctional tissue with fibrotic scar, or (3) the separation of the His bundle from the AV junction by fibrous bands, with a resultant disruption of the normal conduction pathway. On occasion, congenital complete heart block is associated with an infection in utero or with an ongoing generalized inflammatory process in the mother, most often systemic lupus erythematosus. Although most patients with this entity have a morphologically normal heart, some have additional congenital abnormalities, most commonly corrected transposition of the great vessels, atrial septal defect, or ventricular septal defect.

Since most patients with congenital complete heart block have a resting heart rate above 40 beats per minute, this entity is ordinarily well tolerated at rest. However, during exercise, heart rate and cardiac output increase only modestly, so that most of these patients have a diminished exercise capacity. In addition, some give a history of Stokes-Adams attacks, and an occasional patient develops symptoms of congestive heart failure. Finally, a rare individual with congenital complete heart block dies suddenly. The mechanism of sudden death is not well understood. During exercise, many of these patients have an abundance of complex ventricular ectopic activity, suggesting the possibility that sudden death may be due to ventricular tachyarrhythmias. Electrocardiographically, the patient with congenital complete heart block demonstrates a junctional or, at times, a ventricular pacemaker, usually at a rate of 50 to 60 beats per minute. Such a patient with an adequate escape mechanism usually has no symptoms and, as a result, requires no therapy. In contrast, the patient in whom severe bradycardia leads to symptoms—Stokes-Adams attacks, pulmonary or peripheral venous congestion, or severe limitation of exercise capacity—requires placement of a permanent pacemaker. After pacemaker implantation, a variety of problems may be anticipated that are related to the growth of the patient, including the fragility of the lead system in a physically active young patient and the limited lifespan of the pulse generator. In general, patients with congenital complete heart block who survive infancy have an excellent prognosis.

1. Gerlis LM, Anderson RH, Becker AE. Complete heart block as a consequence of atrionodal discontinuity. Br Heart J 1975; 37:345–56.
   In a 2-year-old child with complete heart block, detailed studies of the AV junction showed discontinuity of the atrial tissue and the more peripheral parts of the atrioventricular conduction tissue.
2. James TN, McKone RC, Hudspeth AS. DeSubitaneis mortibus: X. Familial congenital heart block. Circulation 1975; 51:379–88.
   A report of congenital complete heart block developing in 2 siblings (not twins).
3. Pahlajani DB, Miller RA, Serrato M. Patterns of atrioventricular conduction in children. Am Heart J 1975; 90:165–71.
   His bundle electrogram studies were obtained in 20 children to establish normal conduction patterns.
4. DuBrow IW, Fisher EA, Amat-y-Leon F, Denes P, Wu D, Rosen K, Hastreiter AR. Comparison of cardiac refractory periods in children and adults. Circulation 1975; 51:485–91.
   This study evaluated atrial and AV nodal effective and functional refractory periods in 40 children, demonstrating that refractory periods are shorter in children than in adults.
5. Ayers CR, Boineau JP, Spach MS. Congenital complete heart block in children. Am Heart J 1966; 72:381–90.
   A thorough review of the etiology, symptoms, signs, and complications of congenital complete heart block.
6. Carter JB, Blieden LC, Edwards JE. Congenital heart block: anatomic correlations and review of the literature. Arch Pathol Lab Med 1974; 97:51–7.
   The postmortem evaluation of the conduction system in a patient with congenital heart block is discussed, and 28 other cases from the literature are reviewed.
7. James TN. Cardiac conduction system: fetal and postnatal development. Am J Cardiol 1970; 25:213–26.
   A thorough review of the histologic and gross anatomic development of the cardiac conduction system.
8. Lev M. Pathogenesis of congenital atrioventricular block. Prog Cardiovasc Dis 1972; 15:145–57.
   A detailed discussion of the anatomic bases of this disease.
9. Stephensen O, Cleland WP, Hallidie-Smith K. Congenital complete heart block and persistent ductus arteriosus associated with maternal systemic lupus erythematosus. Br Heart J 1981; 46:104–6.
   A woman with SLE who had 2 children, both of whom had congenital complete heart block and PDA, is described.
10. Campbell M, Emanuel R. Six cases of congenital complete heart block followed for 34–40 years. Br Heart J 1967; 29:577–87.
    These 6 patients were not treated with permanent pacemaker insertion. During very long-term follow-up, none developed symptoms referable to heart block.
11. Benrey J, Gillette PC, Nasrallah AT, Hallman GL. Permanent pacemaker implantation in infants, children, and adolescents: long-term follow-up. Circulation 1976; 53:245–8.
    Of 24 children requiring pacemaker placement, 18 are alive and well an average of 5 years after implantation. Death occurred in the remaining 6, 5 of whom had complex congenital heart defects.

12. Garcia OL, Mehta AV, Pickoff AS, Tamer DF, Ferrer PL, Wolff GS, Gelband H. Left isomerism and complete atrioventricular block: a report of six cases. Am J Cardiol 1981; 48:1103–7.

    In 6 patients, left isomerism (polysplenia syndrome or double left-sidedness syndrome) occurred in association with congenital heart block.

13. Karpawich PP, Gillette PC, Garson A Jr, Hesslein PS, Porter C, McNamara DG. Congenital complete atrioventricular block: clinical and electrophysiologic predictors of need for pacemaker insertion. Am J Cardiol 1981; 48:1098–1102.

    In this study, heart rate at rest, surface electrocardiographic morphology, intracardiac electrophysiologic data, and response to exercise were compared in patients with and without syncope. Only a persistent resting heart rate less than 50 beats/min was strongly associated with syncope.

14. Winkler RB, Freed MD, Nadas AS. Exercise-induced ventricular ectopy in children and young adults with complete heart block. Am Heart J 1980; 99:87–92.

    In this series, 68% of patients with congenital complete heart block developed ventricular ectopy during exercise.

15. Reid JM, Coleman EN, Doig W. Complete congenital heart block: report of 35 cases. Br Heart J 1982; 48:236–9.

    This report emphasizes the need for long-term follow-up of patients with congenital complete heart block. In this group of patients, many required permanent pacing before age 50.

16. Walker WJ, Cooley DA, McNamara DG, Moser RH. Corrected transposition of the great vessels, atrioventricular heart block, and ventricular septal defect. Circulation 1958; 17:249–54.

    An early description of the association between AV block and corrected transposition of the great vessels.

17. Anderson RH, Wenick ACG, Losekoot TG, Becker AE. Congenitally complete heart block: developmental aspects. Circulation 1977; 56:90–101.

    Of the 3 cases described in this report, 2 had no communication between the atrial and conducting tissues, and the other had a discontinuity of the penetrating atrioventricular bundle.

18. McCue CM, Mantakas ME, Tingelstad JB, Ruddy S. Congenital heart block in newborns of mothers with connective tissue disease. Circulation 1977; 56:82–90.

    Of 22 children with congenital complete heart block, 14 were born of mothers with connective tissue disease, primarily systemic lupus erythematosus.

19. Chameides L, Truex RC, Vetter V, Rashkind WJ, Galioto FM Jr, Noonan JA. Association of maternal systemic lupus erythematosus with congenital complete heart block. N Engl J Med 1977; 297:1204–7.

    Six infants with congenital complete heart block, all of whose mothers had SLE, are described.

CARDIAC MALPOSITION

An abnormal anatomic position of either the entire heart or the atria or ventricles separately constitutes a *cardiac malposition.* Although this subject is rampant with problems of nomenclature and semantics, a uniform system of classification is now available to minimize the confusion. Normally, the major part of the heart lies to the left of midline. The terms *levocardia* (left-sided heart), *dextrocardia* (right-sided heart), and *mesocardia* (midline heart) indicate cardiac position only and imply nothing about cardiac structure or the interconnections of the atria, ventricles, and great vessels. *Cardiac displacement* describes a shifting of the heart within the thorax by extracardiac factors; this is also referred to as *dextroposition, mesoposition, or levoposition,* depending on the direction of the shift. The visceroatrial *situs* (or body configuration) is determined by the position of certain asymmetric thoracoabdominal structures.

Hence, *situs solitus* is the normal arrangement of viscera and atria: the anatomic left atrium is on the left, the right atrium on the right; the trilobed lung with an eparterial bronchus is on the right, while the bilobed lung with the hyparterial bronchus is on the left; the major lobe of the liver and the venae cavae are on the right; and the stomach and spleen are on the left. In contrast, *situs inversus* is a mirror image of normal. *Situs ambiguus*, or *visceral heterotaxy*, refers to an anatomically uncertain, indeterminate body configuration that occurs in conjunction with the polysplenia and asplenia syndromes. Finally, *transposition* is used to describe the heart whose aorta arises from the morphologic right ventricle and pulmonary artery from the morphologic left ventricle. *Any heart other than a left-sided heart in a situs solitus individual represents a cardiac malposition.*

In describing an anatomic cardiac complex, three segments must be considered: (1) the total body configuration *(situs),* including the atria; (2) the ventricular positions and connections to the atria; and (3) the position of the great arteries and connections to the ventricles. First, one must determine the situs. This can usually be accomplished with a routine x-ray of the chest and abdomen. Although the left atrium cannot be distinguished from the right atrium on x-ray, the venae cavae drain into the right atrium, and the atria invariably follow the corresponding visceral situs. Second, one must define the ventricular positions and connections to the atria, or *bulboventricular loop.* This generally requires contrast angiography, although the direction in which the septum is depolarized may provide a clue to the presence or absence of ventricular inversion. The morphologic features of each ventricle are distinctive and can be identified angiographically. Specifically, the morphologic right ventricle is equipped with a tricuspid valve, is highly trabeculated, and contains the septal band of a single papillary muscle. Its infundibulum lies anterior and superior to the outlet of the left ventricle. The morphologic right ventricle generally connects with whichever of the two great arteries is the more anterior. It is smooth-walled, contains an outlet that lies posterior to the infundibulum, and is equipped with a bicuspid mitral valve. The anterior leaflet of the mitral valve is in continuity with elements of the left ventricular semilunar valve. Normally, the primitive cardiac tube bends to the right (a so-called *d-bulboventricular loop*), which brings the morphologic right ventricle to the right of the anatomic left ventricle. Conversely, an *l-loop* brings the morphologic right ventricle to the left side relative to the morphologic left ventricle. A d-loop is normal in situs solitus, whereas an l-loop is normal in situs inversus. With ventricular inversion, there is an l-loop in situs solitus and a d-loop in situs inversus.

Finally, the anatomy of the great arteries can be defined in terms of their lateral interrelationships and ventricular attachments. Normally-attached great arteries are characterized by the pulmonary artery arising from the morphologic right ventricle and the aorta from the morphologic left ventricle. In this situation, the pulmonic valve is more cephalad than the aortic. In transposition of the great arteries, the origin of the aorta usually lies anterior to that of the pulmonary artery and arises from the infundibulum. The latter interrelationships of the great arteries are best described using "d" and "l" terms. With "d"-related great arteries, the ascending aorta sweeps toward the right and lies to the right of the main pulmonary artery. With "l"-related great arteries, the ascending aorta sweeps to the left and lies to the left of the main pulmonary artery. These lateral relationships apply to normally related great arteries, to transposed great arteries, and to situations in which both great arteries arise from one ventricle (double-outlet right ventricle or double-outlet left ventricle). In addition, there are transpositions in which the aorta lies directly in front of the pulmonary artery, a situation that has been designated "anterotransposition," or "a-trans." The "d," "l," or "a" descriptions of the aortic–pulmonary arterial interrelationships should not be confused with the d- or l-loop designation of the ventricular interrelationships.

Employing segmental sets composed of descriptive units of visceroatrial situs–bulboventricular loop–great artery relationships greatly simplifies expression of the type of cardiac anatomy in patients with complex congenital heart disease and cardiac malposition. Once the positional and morphologic relationships are understood and the presence or absence of associated abnormalities has been established, the principles of medical and surgical treatment can be applied to these cardiac malpositions in the same manner as with normally located hearts.

Although the presence of a cardiac malposition frequently implies a complex congenital cardiac abnormality that may or may not be surgically correctable, *mirror-image dextrocardia* (situs inversus/l-loop/l-normal), a relatively common condition, is usually an incidental finding on a chest x-ray or during a physical examination and is generally benign. About 90 percent of patients with this condition have hearts that are otherwise normal. Conversely, among patients with known congenital heart disease, situs inversus occurs in about 1 percent, a higher frequency than in the general population. If a congenital defect is present, it is most likely to be corrected transposition of the great vessels. In patients with mirror-image dextrocardia, life expectancy is normal. Left-handedness is said to occur in approximately 40 percent of these individuals. The ECG is helpful in identifying mirror-image dextrocardia, since the P wave is negative in standard lead I. If the left and right arm leads are reversed and the precordial electrodes are positioned across the right side of the chest, the resulting ECG should be normal. If these patients develop coronary artery disease and angina pectoris, their pain may have an unusual location and radiation.

In contradistinction to patients with mirror-image dextrocardia, patients with *isolated dextrocardia without situs inversus* almost invariably have additional cardiac malformations, most commonly corrected transposition of the great vessels, pulmonic stenosis, ventricular septal defect, or atrial septal defect. These entities can occur singly or in combination. Longevity is determined by the nature of the underlying cardiac anomaly.

1. Wilkinson JL, Acerete F. Terminological pitfalls in congenital heart disease. Br Heart J 1973; 35:1166–77.
   This review presents a simplified system of basic nomenclature for congenitally abnormal hearts. Previous ambiguous terminology is discussed and clarified.
2. De La Cruz MV, Berrazueta JR, Arteaga M, Attie F, Soni J. Rules for diagnosis of arterioventricular discordances and spatial identification of ventricles: crossed great arteries and transposition of the great arteries. Br Heart J 1976; 38:341–54.
   This paper presents rules for the diagnosis of arterioventricular discordances and the spatial position of the ventricles based on cineangiography and the position of catheters.
3. Shinebourne EA, Macartney FJ, Anderson RH. Sequential chamber localization—logical approach to diagnosis in congenital heart disease. Br Heart J 1976; 38:327–40.
   A nomenclature for congenital heart disease that is based on sequential chamber localization is described. Controversial topics are discussed with regard to previous definitions.
4. van Praagh R, van Praagh S, Vlad P, Keith JD. Diagnosis of the anatomic types of congenital dextrocardia. Am J Cardiol 1965; 15:234–47.
   This review describes a clinical approach to the elucidation of complex congenital cardiac abnormalities using clinical, electrocardiographic, and angiographic findings.

5. van Praagh R, van Praagh S, Vlad P, Keith JD. Anatomic types of congenital dex-
    trocardia. Am J CArdiol 1964; 13:510–31.
    *A detailed review of 51 autopsied cases of dextrocardia. The embryological basis
    for dextrocardia is described in detail.*
6. van Mierop LHS, Eisen S, Schiebler GL. The radiographic appearance of the
    tracheobronchial tree as an indicator of visceral situs. Am J Cardiol 1970; 26:432–
    5.
    *An excellent review of the importance of an anteroposterior chest x-ray for deter-
    mining visceroatrial situs.*
7. Stanger P, Rudolph AM, Edwards JE. Cardiac malpositions: an overview based on
    study of 65 necropsy specimens. Circulation 1977; 56:159–72.
    *This classic article elucidates the segmental approach to a description of cardiac
    malpositions.*
8. van Praagh R. Terminology of congenital heart disease: glossary and commen-
    tary. Circulation 1977; 56:139–43.
    *This editorial complements the classic article by Stanger and his associates (ref.
    no. 7), providing a glossary of the terms used as well as an abbreviated approach
    to the segmental description of cardiac malpositions.*
9. Bharati S, Lev M. The course of the conduction system in dextrocardia. Circula-
    tion 1978; 57:163–71.
    *A detailed description of the conduction system in 5 patients with dextrocardia. A
    majority of these patients have anatomic derangements of the conducting system.*
10. Hartline JV, Zelkowitz PS. Kartagener's syndrome in childhood. Am J Dis Child
    1971; 121:349–52.
    *A report of 3 cases of this syndrome. The authors suggest that vigorous medical
    management may prevent bronchiectasis.*
11. Holmes LB, Blennerhassett JB, Austen KF. A reappraisal of Kartagener's syn-
    drome. Am J Med Sci 1968; 255:13–28.
    *Of the 13 cases with Kartagener's syndrome presented in this report, 10 had mirror-
    image dextrocardia, and the remaining 3 had complex congenital cardiac anoma-
    lies.*
12. Miller RD, Divertie MB. Kartagener's syndrome. Chest 1972; 62:130–5.
    *This paper describes the clinical findings in 19 patients with this syndrome, one of
    whom lived to 72 years.*
13. Adams R, Churchill ED. Situs inversus, sinusitis, bronchiectasis: a report of five
    cases including frequency statistics. J Thorac Surg 1937; 7:206–17.
    *These authors estimate that the incidence of situs inversus is 1:8,000 and that
    bronchiectasis coexists in 12% to 23%.*

IDIOPATHIC DILATATION OF THE PULMONARY ARTERY

Idiopathic dilatation of the pulmonary artery is a relatively uncommon congenital defect found in asymptomatic and otherwise normal individuals. It is usually characterized by a congenital dilatation of the main pulmonary trunk, but
on occasion it may also involve the main branches. It is probably the result of a
developmental defect in pulmonary arterial elastic tissue. Although idiopathic
dilatation of the pulmonary artery is usually benign, it can be aggravated by
either pulmonic regurgitation or progressive dilatation and aneurysm formation. Its clinical importance lies in its recognition and distinction from other
conditions, such as atrial septal defect, pulmonic stenosis, and severe pulmonary hypertension.

Idiopathic dilatation of the pulmonary artery is generally first detected as an
isolated finding on a routine chest x-ray, or it may become clinically manifest
when a murmur is heard during a routine physical examination. The patient's
physical appearance and arterial and jugular venous pulses are normal. Ex-

amination of the precordium frequently shows a visible and palpable systolic impulse in the second left intercostal space, particularly during held expiration. A pulmonary ejection click and the pulmonic component of the S_2 may also be palpable. The left ventricular impulse is normal, and there is no evidence of a right ventricular impulse. *Indeed, the presence of a right ventricular impulse is incompatible with a diagnosis of idiopathic dilatation of the pulmonary artery, since this condition causes neither pressure nor volume overload of the right ventricle.* Similarly, a thrill is not present.

On auscultation, the S_1 is normal and is characteristically followed by a pulmonic ejection click, maximal in the second left interspace, which generally increases on expiration and may disappear on inspiration. A short, end-systolic ejection murmur, maximal in the second left interspace, occurs as blood is ejected into the dilated pulmonary trunk. In addition, a decrescendo diastolic murmur of pulmonic regurgitation may be present due to dilatation of the pulmonic valve ring. The S_2 may be entirely normal. However, the pulmonic component of the S_2 is frequently accentuated, since the dilated main pulmonary artery is especially close to the anterior chest wall. In some patients, the S_2 may be widely split, suggesting a diagnosis of an atrial septal defect or mild pulmonic stenosis; this delay in the pulmonic component of the S_2 is thought to be due to delayed elastic recoil of the dilated pulmonary trunk. Although there is some disagreement, it seems that the splitting of the S_2 may at times be *wide* and *fixed*.

The patient with idiopathic dilatation of the pulmonary artery has a totally normal ECG. Even minor abnormalities, such as upright T waves in the right precordial leads or incomplete right bundle branch block, should suggest an alternative diagnosis. On the chest x-ray, dilatation of the main pulmonary artery is obvious, and it may occasionally involve the left or right pulmonary arteries. At the same time, the distal pulmonary arteries and lung fields appear normal, so that there is no evidence of increased or decreased pulmonary blood flow.

It is obvious that the patient with idiopathic dilatation of the pulmonary artery requires no specific therapy for this condition. If there is associated pulmonic regurgitation, antibiotic prophylaxis for bacterial endocarditis should be considered.

1. Greene DG, Baldwin ED, Baldwin JS, Himmelstein A, Roh CE, Cournand A. Pure congenital pulmonary stenosis and idiopathic congenital dilatation of the pulmonary artery. Am J Med 1949; 6:24–40.
   A review of the clinical findings in 8 patients with idiopathic dilatation of the pulmonary artery and a comparison with the findings in isolated pulmonic stenosis.
2. Goetz RH, Nellen M. Idiopathic dilatation of the pulmonary artery. S Afr Med J 1953; 27:360–7.
   A report of 4 cases and a review of the literature. The importance of cardiac catheterization in differentiating this entity from pulmonic stenosis is emphasized.
3. Kaplan BM, Schlichter JG, Graham G, Miller G. Idiopathic congenital dilatation of the pulmonary artery. J Lab Clin Med 1953; 41:697–707.
   Six patients with this disease are described in detail.
4. Leatham A, Vogelpoel L. The early systolic sound in dilatation of the pulmonary artery. Br Heart J 1954; 16:21–33.
   A phonocardiographic study of 50 patients with idiopathic or secondary dilatation of the pulmonary artery, emphasizing the association between radiographic dilatation of the pulmonary artery and the presence of a pulmonic ejection click.
5. Deshmukh M, Guvenc S, Bentivoglio L, Goldberg H. Idiopathic dilatation of the pulmonary artery. Circulation 1960; 21:710–6.
   Thirteen patients with idiopathic dilatation of the pulmonary artery are described, and their clinical, radiographic, electrocardiographic, and hemodynamic features are elaborated.

6. Brayshaw JR, Perloff JK. Congenital pulmonary insufficiency complicating idiopathic dilatation of the pulmonary artery. Am J Cardiol 1962; 10:282–6.
   A description of a 10-year-old boy who had pulmonic regurgitation and idiopathic dilatation of the pulmonary artery.
7. Schrire V, Vogelpoel L. The role of the dilated pulmonary artery in abnormal splitting of the second heart sound. Am Heart J 1962; 63:501–7.
   A discussion of wide (but not fixed) splitting of S_2 in 6 patients with idiopathic dilatation of the pulmonary artery.
8. Karnegis JN, Wang Y. The phonocardiogram in idiopathic dil tation of the pulmonary artery. Am J Cardiol 1964; 14:75–8.
   A hemodynamic and phonocardiographic study of 8 patients, 6 of whom appeared to have fixed, wide splitting of S_2.
9. Shaver JA, Nadolny RA, O'Toole JD, Thompson ME, Reddy PS, Leon DF, Curtiss EI. Sound pressure correlates of the second heart sound. Circulation 1974; 49:316–25.
   A detailed hemodynamic-phonocardiographic study of the factors that influence the degree of splitting of S_2.

ANOMALOUS ORIGIN OF THE CORONARY ARTERIES

Three anomalies involving the origin of the coronary arteries are of clinical significance in adults: (1) origin of one coronary artery from the pulmonary artery, (2) origin of both coronary arteries from the right sinus of Valsalva, and (3) origin of both coronary arteries from the left sinus of Valsalva. *Anomalous origin of one or more coronary arteries from the pulmonary artery* is a life-threatening congenital abnormality. When *both coronary arteries* arise from the pulmonary artery, death usually occurs soon after birth. Conversely, the patient with origin of *only the right coronary artery* from the pulmonary artery is usually asymptomatic as long as right ventricular oxygen demand is normal, but these individuals tolerate pulmonary hypertension poorly. In general, this anomaly is an incidental finding at autopsy in patients who have died of other causes.

Anomalous origin of the *left coronary artery* from the pulmonary artery is usually detected in infancy. Infants with this anomaly appear normal at birth, but within 1 to 2 months they have evidence of myocardial ischemia and congestive heart failure. Approximately 80 to 90 percent die within the first year of life; the remaining 10 to 20 percent may reach adulthood, largely as a result of effective intercoronary collaterals. Those individuals reaching adulthood may come to medical attention because of symptoms of myocardial ischemia or left ventricular failure, a murmur of mitral regurgitation (caused by dysfunction of the papillary muscle supplied by the anomalous coronary artery), or sudden death.

On physical examination, the patient with anomalous origin of the left coronary artery from the pulmonary artery usually has a holosystolic murmur of mitral regurgitation, which radiates to the axilla and back, since the anterolateral papillary muscle is often involved. In addition, a continuous or diastolic murmur may be audible over the precordium, reflecting retrograde flow through the intercoronary anastomoses that connect the right and left coronary arteries. An S_3 is often audible (due to left ventricular dysfunction).

The ECG may demonstrate left atrial enlargement and left ventricular hypertrophy. There may be electrocardiographic evidence of anterolateral ischemia or infarction. The chest x-ray usually shows enlargement of the left atrium and left ventricle as well as pulmonary vascular redistribution, and M-mode and two-dimensional echocardiography confirm the presence of left atrial and left ventricular enlargement.

At cardiac catheterization, selective injection of contrast material into the right coronary artery usually opacifies the entire coronary arterial system. The right coronary artery is markedly dilated and tortuous, and there are extensive collateral vessels that connect the distal right coronary artery to the left circumflex and left anterior descending coronary arteries. If opacification of the left coronary artery is optimal, one may visualize the emptying of contrast material from the left main coronary artery into the pulmonary artery. The left ventriculogram demonstrates mitral regurgitation and left ventricular dysfunction.

Once the origin of the left coronary artery is shown to be from the pulmonary artery, surgical correction is indicated. If there is adequate collateral flow from the right to the left coronary artery, ligation of the anomalous left coronary artery is sufficient. Alternatively, the left main coronary artery can be detached from the pulmonary artery and anastomosed to the ascending aorta. However, such a transposition may be technically impossible, in which case a segment of saphenous vein can be interposed from the ascending aorta to the ligated left coronary artery.

The incidence of one or more coronary arteries arising aberrantly from the aorta is 0.6 to 1.2 percent. In the normal individual, the right coronary artery arises from the right (or anterior) sinus of Valsalva, and the left coronary artery arises from the left sinus of Valsalva. In an occasional patient, the left circumflex coronary artery may arise anomalously from the right sinus of Valsalva or the proximal portion of the right coronary artery, after which it courses posterior to both the aorta and right ventricular infundibulum and supplies its normal area of distribution. This anomaly has not been reported to cause angina pectoris, myocardial infarction, or other clinical problems; it is usually an incidental finding at cardiac catheterization or autopsy.

A less common but potentially serious anomaly is *origin of the left main coronary artery from the right sinus of Valsalva*. If the left main coronary artery courses *anterior* to the right ventricular outflow tract and supplies its normal area of distribution, the condition is benign. In contrast, if it courses *between the aorta and the right ventricular outflow tract* to supply its normal area of distribution, the outlook is different. This anomaly has been reported in young, otherwise healthy men who die suddenly during or immediately following vigorous physical exertion. Approximately 30 percent of patients found to have this anomaly have sudden death; others present with angina or myocardial infarction, and occasionally it is an incidental finding in older individuals who are asymptomatic. Although the exact mechanism of sudden death is unclear, it is believed to be related to either extrinsic compression of the left main coronary artery during physical exertion or a distortion of the vessel orifice, with resultant global ischemia and ventricular fibrillation. Since this anomaly can cause sudden death, its presence is an indication for surgical correction, particularly in young patients, either by reimplantation of the vessel or by saphenous vein grafting. Finally, an anomalous left main coronary artery may rarely course *posterior* to the aorta. This entity is exceedingly rare and not well documented. However, myocardial infarction (in the absence of atherosclerosis) has been reported with this entity, so that its presence may be an indication for surgical correction, particularly in the symptomatic patient.

The *right coronary artery may arise aberrantly from the left sinus of Valsalva*, after which it courses between the aorta and the right ventricular outflow tract to supply its normal area of distribution. A small number of patients with this anomaly have been reported to have angina pectoris, myocardial infarction, or varying degrees of "heart block," but sudden death has not been reported. If this anomaly is discovered in association with symptoms or signs of myocardial ischemia, it should be corrected surgically.

1. Perloff JK. Anomalous origin of the left coronary artery from the pulmonary artery. In: The clinical recognition of congenital heart disease. Philadelphia: Saunders, 1970: 450–8.
   A superb, succinct review of the clinical findings in this anomaly.
2. Burchell HB, Brown AL Jr. Anomalous origin of coronary artery from pulmonary artery masquerading as mitral insufficiency. Am Heart J 1962; 63:388–93.
   A case report of a 14-year-old boy presenting with gross mitral insufficiency and a left coronary artery arising from the pulmonary artery.
3. Cooley DA, Hallman GL, Bloodwell RD. Definitive surgical treatment of anomalous origin of left coronary artery from pulmonary artery: indications and results. J Thorac Cardiovasc Surg 1966; 52:798–808.
   The first report of successful definitive repair of this anomaly with the use of autologous saphenous vein grafting in 2 patients, aged 4 and 5 years.
4. Harthorne JW, Scannell JG, Dinsmore RE. Anomalous origin of the left coronary artery: remediable cause of sudden death in adults. N Engl J Med 1966; 275:660–3.
   This article reports the successful surgical ligation of an anomalous left coronary artery originating from the pulmonary artery in an 18-year-old athlete.
5. Likar I, Criley JM, Lewis KB. Anomalous left coronary artery arising from the pulmonary artery in an adult: a review of the therapeutic problem. Circulation 1966; 33:727–32.
   The report of a 29-year-old woman with this anomaly in whom surgical ligation was performed.
6. Roche AHG. Anomalous origin of the left coronary artery from the pulmonary artery in the adult: a report of uneventful ligation in two cases. Am J Cardiol 1967; 20:561–5.
   Two cases of anomalous origin of the left coronary artery from the pulmonary artery in adults aged 24 and 47 years are reported. Both were symptomatically improved more than 1 year after surgical ligation.
7. Flamm MD, Stinson EB, Hultgren HN, Shumway NE, Hancock EW. Anomalous origin of the left coronary artery from the pulmonary artery. Circulation 1968; 38:113–23.
   Two cases of anomalous origin of the left coronary artery from the pulmonary artery in asymptomatic patients aged 15 and 27 years are reviewed. During exercise, both showed evidence of marked myocardial ischemia, which improved following ligation of the vessel.
8. Summer GL, Hendrix GH. Surgical ligation of an anomalous left coronary artery arising from the pulmonary artery in an adult. Am Heart J 1969; 76:812–5.
   A report of a patient treated in this manner and a review of the literature. This approach seems feasible if there is good retrograde filling of the left coronary artery via collaterals from the right coronary artery.
9. Laborde F, Marchand M, Leca F, Jareau MM, Dequirot A, Hazan E. Surgical treatment of anomalous origin of the left coronary artery in infancy and childhood: early and late results in 20 consecutive cases. J Thorac Cardiovasc Surg 1981; 82:423–8.
   The results of surgery to correct anomalous origin of the left coronary artery from the pulmonary artery are presented. Among the 20 patients, there were 6 operative deaths. In patients under 1 year of age, 80% died postoperatively, usually due to poor left ventricular function. However, there was marked symptomatic improvement in the survivors.
10. Cheitlin MD, DeCastro CM, McAllister HA. Sudden death as a complication of anomalous left coronary origin from the anterior sinus of Valsalva: a not-so-minor congenital anomaly. Circulation 1974; 50:780–7.
    A review of 33 patients in whom both coronary arteries arose from the right sinus of Valsalva and of 18 patients in whom both coronary arteries arose from the left sinus of Valsalva. In the former group, 9 (27%) died suddenly, while none died suddenly in the latter group.

11. Liberthson RR, Dinsmore RE, Bharati S, Rubenstein JJ, Caulfield J, Wheeler EO, Harthorne JW, Lev M. Aberrant coronary artery origin from the aorta: diagnosis and clinical significance. Circulation 1974; 50:774–9.
    Twenty-one cases of anomalous coronary artery origin from the aorta are discussed. Aberrant origin of the circumflex alone from the right coronary artery or sinus occurred in 11; aberrant origin of the left anterior descending and circumflex from the right coronary artery or sinus occurred in 6; aberrant origin of the right coronary artery from the left coronary artery or sinus occurred in 4.

12. Liberthson RR, Dinsmore RE, Fallon JT. Aberrant coronary artery origin from the aorta: report of 18 patients, review of literature and delineation of natural history and management. Circulation 1979; 59:748–54.
    A report of 9 patients whose right coronary artery and 9 whose left coronary artery arose aberrantly and passed between the aorta and right ventricular infundibulum. Sudden death occurred in none of the former and 3 of the latter group.

13. Jokl E, McClellan JT, Williams WC, Gouze FJ, Bartholomew RD. Congenital anomaly of the left coronary artery in young athletes. Cardiologia 1966; 49:253–8.
    A report of a 16-year-old boy who died during exercise. He was found to have an anomalous origin of the left coronary artery from the right coronary sinus, with passage of the vessel between the aorta and right ventricular outflow tract.

14. Cohen LS, Shaw LD. Fatal myocardial infarction in an 11-year-old boy associated with a unique coronary artery anomaly. Am J Cardiol 1967; 19:420–3.
    This article describes a fatal myocardial infarction in an 11-year-old boy that was associated with anomalous origin of the left coronary artery from the right coronary sinus with passage between the aorta and right ventricular outflow tract.

15. Benson PA, Lack AR. Anomalous aortic origin of the left coronary artery: report of two cases. Arch Path 1968; 86:214–6.
    Postmortem findings in two 13-year-old boys who died suddenly during exercise. Both had anomalous origin of the left coronary artery from the right coronary sinus with passage of the vessel between the aorta and right ventricular outflow tract.

16. Moodie DS, Gill C, Loop FD, Sheldon WC. Anomalous left main coronary artery originating from the right sinus of Valsalva. J Thorac Cardiovasc Surg 1980; 80:198–205.
    A report of 4 cases and review of the literature on anomalous origin of the left main coronary artery from the right sinus of Valsalva with passage between the aorta and pulmonary artery. Although most patients with this anomaly are symptomatic, it is occasionally an incidental finding.

17. Mustafa I, Gula G, Radley-Smith R, Durrer S, Yacoub M. Anomalous origin of the left coronary artery from the anterior aortic sinus: a potential cause of sudden death. Anatomic characterization and surgical treatment. J Thorac Cardiovasc Surg 1981; 82:297–300.
    Two patients with anomalous origin of the left coronary artery from the right coronary sinus had symptoms of myocardial ischemia during exercise. Both became asymptomatic following surgical correction of the anomaly. A possible mechanism for myocardial ischemia is discussed.

18. Murphy DA, Roy DL, Sohal M, Chandler BM. Anomalous origin of left main coronary artery from anterior sinus of Valsalva with myocardial infarction. J Thorac Cardiovasc Surg 1978; 75: 282–5.
    This is the first report of myocardial infarction associated with anomalous origin of the left coronary artery when this vessel passes posterior to the aorta rather than between the aorta and pulmonary arterial trunk.

19. Thompson SI, Vieweg WVR, Alpert JS, Hagan AD. Anomalous origin of the right coronary artery from the left sinus of Valsalva with associated chest pain: report of two cases. Cathet Cardiovasc Diagn 1976; 2:397–402.
    Two cases of angina associated with anomalous origin of the right coronary artery from the left coronary sinus are presented. In both, the vessel passed between the aorta and the right ventricular outflow tract.

20. Benge W, Martins JB, Funk DC. Morbidity associated with anomalous origin of the right coronary artery from the left sinus of Valsalva. Am Heart J 1980; 99:96–100.

A case report of a 25-year-old patient with anomalous origin of the right coronary artery from the left sinus of Valsalva who developed syncope and complete heart block in association with an acute inferior myocardial infarction. There was no evidence of coronary atherosclerosis.

21. Mintz GS, Iskandrian AS, Bemis CE, Mundth ED, Owens JS. Myocardial ischemia in anomalous origin of the right coronary artery from the pulmonary trunk: proof of a coronary steal. Am J Cardiol 1983; 51:610–2.

    A 47-year-old man with this abnormality is described; during exercise, he developed scintigraphic evidence of myocardial ischemia.

22. Bloomfield P, Erhlich C, Folland ED, Bianco JA, Tow DE, Parisi AF. Anomalous right coronary artery: a surgically correctable cause of angina pectoris. Am J Cardiol 1983; 51:1235–7.

    This report describes a 65-year-old man who had anomalous origin of the right coronary artery from the left sinus of Valsalva. Because of this anomaly, he developed severe angina that eventually required bypass grafting.

VALVULAR HEART DISEASE

Obstruction to left ventricular outflow can be subvalvular, valvular, or supravalvular. *Subvalvular* stenosis results from the abnormal proliferation of myocardium directly below the aortic valve; the resultant obstruction can be fixed (discrete anatomic stenosis) or variable (obstructive hypertrophic cardiomyopathy, discussed on p. 117). *Supravalvular* stenosis is caused by a localized, segmental, hourglass-shaped narrowing immediately above the aortic sinuses; it sometimes occurs in conjunction with mental retardation and hypercalcemia. *Valvular* aortic stenosis can be caused by (1) calcification and progressive narrowing of a congenitally deformed valve (most often one with an abnormal number of cusps), (2) atherosclerotic damage of the valve, or (3) gradual narrowing of a valve damaged by rheumatic fever. About 2 percent of infants are born with a bicuspid aortic valve. During childhood and early adult life, the contact between the cusps is abnormal, resulting in focal fibrous thickening and eventually dystrophic calcification. In contrast, rheumatic deformation usually occurs in an anatomically normal aortic valve. As part of the rheumatic process, the patient almost always has concomitant mitral valve involvement.

The patient with aortic stenosis may complain of one of several symptoms. Angina pectoris or myocardial infarction occurs in 35 to 50 percent of patients with aortic stenosis. Although many of these patients have underlying arteriosclerotic heart disease, some have symptoms of left ventricular ischemia without demonstrable coronary artery disease. Because of an elevated left ventricular wall tension, myocardial oxygen requirements are increased in patients with aortic stenosis; at the same time, subendocardial blood flow may be diminished. As a result, even in the patient with normal coronary arteries, an imbalance between coronary blood flow and the metabolic demands of the hypertrophied left ventricle can occur.

Syncope or near-syncope occurs in some patients with severe aortic stenosis. Although complete heart block is intermittently present in some patients, most syncopal episodes are not initiated by heart block or an arrhythmia. Instead, left ventricular baroreceptors are activated by an increased left ventricular cavitary pressure, causing peripheral vasodilatation. Because of the obstruction to left ventricular outflow, cardiac output cannot increase; as a result, cerebral perfusion falls, leading to dizziness or syncope.

Many patients with aortic stenosis complain of symptoms of left ventricular failure, which are attributable to an increased left ventricular filling pressure. Left ventricular systolic function may remain normal in many of these patients, but left ventricular filling pressures are elevated because of an increased wall tension during diastole. In turn, this increase in left ventricular filling pressure is transmitted to the left atrium and pulmonary capillary bed, resulting in dyspnea on exertion, paroxysmal nocturnal dyspnea, and orthopnea. Eventually, right ventricular failure may ensue, causing peripheral edema, abdominal tenderness due to hepatomegaly, and ascites. Finally, approximately 3 to 5 percent of patients with aortic stenosis die suddenly without prior symptoms. The mechanism of sudden death is unknown, but it may result from the extreme intolerance of these patients to complete heart block or atrial tachyarrhythmias.

On physical examination of the adult patient with severe aortic stenosis, the carotid arterial pulse has a delayed upstroke, a relatively low volume, and at times, a palpable anacrotic shoulder; in addition, a shudder or bruit may be present. On precordial palpation, a systolic thrill may be present in the second right intercostal space, and the point of maximal intensity (PMI) may or may not be displaced laterally. The auscultatory findings include (1) a well-preserved S_1 with a diminished or inaudible aortic component of the S_2 (since a heavily calcified, immobile aortic valve produces little sound on closure), (2) an early systolic ejection click, (3) an S_4, and (4) a harsh, crescendo-decrescendo systolic murmur at the second right intercostal space and along the left sternal border, radiating to the carotids. Although the murmur is often audible at the apex, it is usually not transmitted to the axilla.

The chest x-ray of the patient with aortic stenosis typically demonstrates a normal cardiac silhouette. The left ventricle is concentrically hypertrophied, but marked left ventricular dilatation does not occur unless long-standing congestive heart failure is present or additional valvular or coronary disease exists. Aortic valve calcification may be visible on oblique or lateral projections or, more frequently, by fluoroscopy. In the patient with valvular aortic stenosis, the ascending aorta is dilated. If left ventricular failure is present, pulmonary vascular redistribution will appear on the chest x-ray. The ECG usually demonstrates normal sinus rhythm and left ventricular hypertrophy. If aortic valve calcification is extensive, the conduction system may be damaged, leading to left bundle branch block or even advanced AV block.

In the patient with calcific aortic stenosis, the echocardiogram demonstrates concentric left ventricular hypertrophy. The M-mode echocardiogram may show thickened aortic valve leaflets. Although two-dimensional echocardiography has been used in an attempt to estimate the size of the aortic valve orifice, such assessments are frequently misleading. An alternative echocardiographic approach entails a noninvasive estimation of left ventricular systolic pressure from the relationship of left ventricular wall thickness and cavity radius (based on Laplace's law). Systemic arterial pressure is determined with a blood pressure cuff, and the gradient across the aortic valve is the difference between the noninvasively calculated left ventricular systolic pressure and the cuff-determined systemic arterial pressure. Although this technique appears to be useful in children, it is not generally reliable in adults.

Systolic time intervals, obtained from an external recording of the carotid pulse, phonocardiogram, and ECG, may be helpful in the diagnosis of aortic stenosis. If the patient has significant left ventricular outflow tract obstruction, the left ventricular ejection time is usually prolonged, the carotid upstroke is slowed, the time interval from the beginning of the QRS complex to the peak of the crescendo-decrescendo murmur (so-called Q to peak murmur) is prolonged, and the maximal rate of rise of the carotid pressure is diminished. Like the echocardiogram, the systolic time intervals are helpful in the noninvasive assessment of the patient with possible aortic stenosis, but they are not diagnostic, since systemic arterial hypertension, intrinsic carotid disease, and other valvular or myocardial abnormalities can markedly alter them.

Although the noninvasive findings that have been enumerated may provide information that is consistent with aortic stenosis, none makes the diagnosis with certainty. With the simultaneous recording of left ventricular and systemic arterial pressures during catheterization, one can determine the presence and severity of aortic stenosis. Although the normal aortic valve area is 2.6 to 3.5 cm^2, hemodynamically significant aortic stenosis does not occur until the valve area is reduced to approximately 1.0 cm^2. Severe aortic stenosis is present with a valve area less than 0.7 cm^2.

The patient with a bicuspid valve at birth ordinarily has no symptoms of aortic stenosis for many years, even though auscultation may reveal an ejection click and a systolic ejection murmur at the aortic area and along the left sternal border due to turbulent blood flow through the abnormally shaped aortic valve. After many years, however, the bicuspid valve calcifies and narrows. When symptoms appear (angina pectoris or myocardial infarction, syncope or near-syncope, and symptoms of left ventricular failure), diagnostic catheterization should be performed, and if significant aortic stenosis is demonstrated, valve replacement should follow. The outlook for the patient with symptomatic aortic stenosis without surgery is poor: with the appearance of angina pectoris, the average life expectancy is 4 years; with syncope or near-syncope, it is 3 years; and with symptoms of left ventricular failure, it is only 2 years. Clearly, therefore, once these symptoms develop in a patient with aortic stenosis, valve replacement should be performed without delay. Prior to the development of symptoms, the patient with aortic sclerosis should receive antibiotics as prophylaxis against endocarditis before a surgical procedure or dental manipulation.

Several types of prosthetic valves have been shown to be effective in the aortic position. The longest experience has been accrued with the Starr-Edwards caged-ball prosthesis, with which the 5-year life expectancy for operative survivors is about 80 percent, and the 10-year survival is approximately 60 percent. All patients with caged-ball prosthetic valves require chronic anticoagulation. Thromboembolic episodes are reported to occur in 7 to 9 percent of these patients over a 5-year period. The Starr-Edwards valve has proved to be extremely durable. Tilting disc valve prostheses, particularly the Björk-Shiley valve, provide a relatively larger orifice than caged-ball prostheses, are durable, but also require long-term anticoagulant therapy because of the risk of systemic embolization. Recently, glutaraldehyde-preserved porcine heterografts (bioprostheses) have been used extensively in the aortic position. Their advantage is that long-term anticoagulation is not required. There is a comparable incidence of paravalvular leakage and bacterial endocarditis with mechanical and porcine heterograft prostheses and a lower incidence of hemolysis with bioprostheses. However, the porcine bioprostheses are less durable than the mechanical prostheses, particularly in children and adolescents, in whom an alarming incidence of stenosis and calcification has been reported.

Clinical Manifestations and Natural History

1. Bergeron J, Abelmann WH, Vazquez-Milan H, Ellis LB. Aortic stenosis: clinical manifestations and course of the disease. Arch Intern Med 1954; 94:911–24.
   A detailed clinical review of 100 patients with aortic stenosis, demonstrating that the prognosis is guarded when symptoms appear.
2. Bertrand ME, Lablanche JM, Tilmant PY, Thieuleux FP, Delforge MR, Carre AG. Coronary sinus blood flow at rest and during isometric exercise in patients with aortic valve disease: mechanism of angina pectoris in presence of normal coronary arteries. Am J Cardiol 1981; 47:199–205.
   In 46 patients with aortic valve disease and normal coronary arteries, coronary sinus blood flow at rest and during exercise was similar in those with and without angina. Underperfusion of the subendocardium is suggested as a causative factor of angina in these patients.
3. Fallen EL, Elliott WC, Gorlin R. Mechanisms of angina in aortic stenosis. Circulation 1967; 36:480–8.
   Angina pectoris in patients with aortic stenosis is due not only to increased energy demands but also to an impaired coronary vascular reserve.
4. Fifer MA, Gunther S, Grossman W, Mirsky I, Carabello B, Barry WH. Myocardial contractile function in aortic stenosis as determined from the rate of stress development during isovolumic systole. Am J Cardiol 1979; 44:1318–25.
   This study suggests that contractile function at the myocardial fiber level may be normal in aortic stenosis, even in the presence of left ventricular failure.
5. Forman R, Firth BG, Barnard MS. Prognostic significance of preoperative left ventricular ejection fraction and valve lesion in patients with aortic valve replacement. Am J Cardiol 1980; 45:1120–5.

This study of 229 patients with aortic valve replacement indicates that the 3-year survival is good, despite a depressed preoperative left ventricular ejection fraction in patients with aortic stenosis but not in those with aortic regurgitation.

6. Frank S, Johnson A, Ross J Jr. Natural history of valvular aortic stenosis. Br Heart J 1973; 35:41–6.
   Another study confirming that significant aortic valve stenosis with symptoms portends an extremely poor prognosis.

7. Glancy DL, Freed TA, O'Brien KP, Epstein SE. Calcium in the aortic valve: roentgenologic and hemodynamic correlations in 148 patients. Ann Intern Med 1969; 71:245–50.
   In general, the extent of aortic valve calcification correlates with the severity of aortic stenosis in adult patients over age 35.

8. Graboys TB, Cohn PF. The prevalence of angina pectoris and abnormal coronary arteriograms in severe aortic valvular disease. Am Heart J 1977; 93:683–6.
   It is unusual for the patient with aortic valve disease without angina pectoris to have significant arteriosclerotic coronary artery disease.

9. Johnson AM. Aortic stenosis, sudden death and the left ventricular baroceptors. Br Heart J 1971; 33:1.
   Inferential evidence suggests that stimulation of left ventricular baroreceptors leads to peripheral vasodilatation.

10. Johnson LL, Sciacca RR, Ellis K, Weiss MB, Cannon PJ. Reduced left ventricular myocardial blood flow per unit mass in aortic stenosis. Circulation 1978; 57:582–90.
    Myocardial blood flow per unit mass is significantly lower in patients with aortic stenosis than in those without it.

11. Perloff JK. Clinical recognition of aortic stenosis: the physical signs and differential diagnosis of the various forms of obstruction to left ventricular outflow. Prog Cardiovasc Dis 1968; 10:323–52.
    A detailed description of the physical examination in patients with subvalvular, valvular, and supravalvular aortic stenosis.

12. Roberts WC. The congenitally bicuspid aortic valve: a study of 85 autopsy cases. Am J Cardiol 1970; 26:72–83.
    A large necropsy study demonstrating that bicuspid aortic valve is the most frequent congenital malformation of the heart or great vessels.

13. Rapaport E. Natural history of aortic and mitral valve disease. Am J Cardiol 1975; 35:221–33.
    A review of a large series of patients with stenosis or regurgitation of the aortic or mitral valves.

14. Roberts WC. Anatomically isolated aortic valvular disease: the case against its being a rheumatic etiology. Am J Med 1970; 49:151–9.
    Anatomically isolated aortic valve disease is almost always of nonrheumatic etiology and is most frequently the result of a congenital malformation.

15. Schwartz LS, Goldfischer J, Sprague GJ, Schwartz SP. Syncope and sudden death in aortic stenosis. Am J Cardiol 1969; 23:647–58.
    Syncope in patients with aortic stenosis is not initiated by heart block or atrial tachyarrhythmias.

16. Spann JF, Bove AA, Natarajan G, Kreulen T. Ventricular performance, pump function and compensatory mechanisms in patients with aortic stenosis. Circulation 1980; 62:576–82.
    This study suggests that the end-systolic pressure-volume relationship or the relationship between peak systolic wall stress and end-diastolic volume may be used to distinguish depressed left ventricular function due to excess afterload from that due to intrinsic depression of contractility.

17. Takeda J, Warren R, Holzman D. Prognosis of aortic stenosis. Arch Surg 1963; 87:931–6.
    Of 65 patients with aortic stenosis who were followed medically, the mean life expectancy following the onset of angina was 4.4 years; of syncope, 3.8 years; and of congestive heart failure, 2.8 years.

18. Wagner S, Selzer A. Patterns of progression of aortic stenosis: a longitudinal hemodynamic study. Circulation 1982; 65:709–12.

There is wide variability in the rate at which aortic stenosis progresses. Those with severe calcific aortic stenosis tend to progress more rapidly than other patients.

Diagnosis

19. Bennett DH, Evans DW, Raj MVJ. Echocardiographic left ventricular dimensions in pressure and volume overload: their use in assessing aortic stenosis. Br Heart J 1975; 37:971–7.
    In patients with good left ventricular function, systolic intraventricular pressure can be estimated from the echocardiographic measurement of wall thickness and left ventricular dimension.

20. Blackwood RA, Bloom KR, Williams CM. Aortic stenosis in children: experience with echocardiographic prediction of severity. Circulation 1978; 57:263–8.
    From a combination of the Laplace relationship, wall stress studies, and left ventricular wall thickness, a simple formula has been developed to predict left ventricular pressure by echo; the results correlate closely with those obtained at catheterization.

21. Bonner AJ Jr, Sacks HN, Tavel ME. Assessing the severity of aortic stenosis by phonocardiography and external carotid pulse recordings. Circulation 1973; 48:247–52.
    If the ejection time is markedly prolonged, the maximum rate of arterial pulse rise diminished, and the peaking of the systolic ejection murmur late, severe aortic stenosis is likely to be present.

22. DeMaria AN, Bommer W, Joye J, Lee G, Bouteller J, Mason DT. Value and limitations of cross-sectional echocardiography of the aortic valve in the diagnosis and quantification of valvular aortic stenosis. Circulation 1980; 62:304–12.
    Although two-dimensional echo is a sensitive method of detecting valvular aortic stenosis, it cannot distinguish critical from non-critical stenosis.

23. DePace N, Ren JF, Iskandrian AS, Kotler MN, Hakki AH, Segal BL. Correlation of echocardiographic wall stress and left ventricular pressure and function in aortic stenosis. Circulation 1983; 67:854–9.
    M-mode echocardiography is not reliable in assessing the severity of aortic stenosis in adults; such an assessment requires a precise measurement of the pressure gradient and flow by catheterization.

Therapy

24. Edmunds LH, Wagner HR, Heymann MA. Aortic valvulotomy in neonates. Circulation 1980; 61:421–7.
    Aortic valvulotomy is the procedure of choice in neonates with severe, life-threatening aortic stenosis.

25. Thompson R, Yacoub M, Ahmed M, Seabra-Gomes R, Rickards A, Towers M. Infuence of preoperative left ventricular function on results of homograft replacement of the aortic valve for aortic stenosis. Am J Cardiol 1979; 43:929–38.
    In this study of 103 patients, a depressed left ventricular ejection fraction preoperatively was found not to increase the risk of aortic valve replacement for aortic stenosis. Improvement in ejection fraction occurred in the majority of patients.

Subvalvular and Supravalvular Stenosis

26. Katz NM, Buckley MJ, Liberthson RR. Discrete membranous subaortic stenosis: report of 31 patients, review of the literataure, and delineation of management. Circulation 1977; 56:1034–8.
    Presentation, management, and long-term postoperative follow-up of patients with this disease are discussed.

27. Krueger SK, French JW, Forker AD, Caudill CC, Popp RL. Echocardiography in discrete subaortic stenosis. Circulation 1979; 59:506–13.
    Using M-mode echocardiography, one can differentiate subaortic from aortic stenosis.

28. Sung CS, Price EC, Cooley DA. Discrete subaortic stenosis in adults. Am J Cardiol 1978; 42:283–90.
    A thorough review of a large series of patients with this disorder.

29. Flaker G, Teske D, Kilman J, Hosier D, Wooley C. Supravalvular aortic stenosis: a 20-year clinical perspective and experience with patch aortoplasty. Am J Cardiol 1983; 51:256–60.
Of 16 patients with supravalvular stenosis who underwent patch aortoplasty, 3 died in the perioperative period; of the remainder, 10 were asymptomatic during long-term (1–12 year) follow-up.

CHRONIC AORTIC REGURGITATION

Chronic aortic regurgitation can be caused by numerous disease processes and can appear in conjunction with a number of systemic diseases. *Congenital* aortic regurgitation can occur in association with discrete subvalvular or supravalvular aortic stenosis or with a bicuspid aortic valve. Aortic regurgitation can be *acquired* through several disease processes: (1) *rheumatic* scarring and contracture of the aortic valve, usually accompanied by some mitral valve involvement; (2) *acute bacterial endocarditis* involving a previously normal aortic valve, leading to leaflet destruction and resultant regurgitation; (3) *syphilitic* involvement of the aortic root, causing dilatation and valve incompetence; (4) systemic arterial *hypertension* sufficiently severe and prolonged to produce a dilated aortic root, leading to aortic valve leakage; (5) blunt or sharp *trauma* to the chest, damaging the aortic cusps; and (6) a *dissecting aneurysm* of the aorta extending into the aortic valve and causing regurgitation. In addition, aortic regurgitation can occur in association with Marfan's syndrome (see p. 369), Ehlers-Danlos syndrome, osteogenesis imperfecta, rheumatoid arthritis, ankylosing spondylitis, Reiter's syndrome, and psoriasis. Finally, it can occur in conjunction with several other cardiac defects, specifically ventricular septal defect, coarctation of the aorta, tetralogy of Fallot, and a ruptured sinus of Valsalva aneurysm.

Early in the course of chronic aortic regurgitation, the patient may have symptoms attributable to an augmented stroke volume: a forceful heart beat and prominent arterial pulsations in the neck. As the disease progresses, the patient eventually notes symptoms of left ventricular failure (dyspnea on exertion and eventually at rest, orthopnea, and paroxysmal nocturnal dyspnea). In turn, if left ventricular failure is allowed to continue, right ventricular dilatation and failure eventually develop, with peripheral edema and abdominal tenderness and swelling due to hepatomegaly and ascites. In an occasional patient, right-sided decompensation may predominate because of a shift of the interventricular septum and a resultant decrease in right ventricular cavity size (the Bernheim effect). In addition to symptoms of left ventricular decompensation, the patient may complain of angina pectoris (due to a relative imbalance of myocardial oxygen supply and demand). Although dizziness, syncope, and sudden death occasionally occur in the patient with chronic aortic regurgitation, they are distinctly less common than with aortic stenosis.

The physical examination of the extremities in the patient with long-standing aortic regurgitation may reveal the following: (1) a widened pulse pressure, due to a lowering of diastolic pressure and an increase in systolic pressure; (2) bounding peripheral arterial pulsations with a rapid upstroke and an equally rapid downstroke, resulting in a so-called water-hammer quality; (3) visible capillary pulsations in the nail beds (Quincke's pulses); and (4) a systolic pressure in the leg that exceeds that in the arm by more than 15 to 20 mm Hg (Hill's sign). Precordial inspection reveals a forceful apical impulse displaced downward and to the left, and palpation may reveal a diastolic thrill at the left sternal border and a palpable S_3 at the apex. On auscultation, the S_1 is normal in intensity, whereas the S_2 is clearly diminished. A high-pitched, decrescendo murmur begins immediately after the S_2 and extends through part or all of diastole. *A systolic ejection murmur along the left sternal border (due to increased forward blood flow across the aortic valve) is a usual finding in chronic aortic regurgitation and does not necessarily imply an associated stenosis of the valve.* An S_3 is often audible. In the left lateral decubitus position, a low-pitched diastolic rumble (indistinguishable from the murmur of mitral stenosis except for the absence of an opening snap), the so-called Austin Flint murmur, may be audible.

The chest x-ray in the patient with long-standing aortic regurgitation demonstrates dilatation of the aortic root. In contrast to many patients with aortic stenosis, those with symptomatic aortic regurgitation always have left ventricular dilatation. Severe aortic regurgitation causes marked left ventricular enlargement, pulmonary vascular redistribution, and eventually right ventricular enlargement. As in most patients with aortic stenosis, the ECG demonstrates left ventricular hypertrophy. On M-mode echocardiography, the left ventricular chamber at end-diastole is dilated, and its diameter at end-systole may be normal or enlarged. High-frequency vibrations of the anterior mitral valve leaflet are frequently present, and vibrations of the same frequency are visible on the interventricular septum in some patients. If the regurgitation is severe, the mitral valve may close prematurely because of the rapid increase in left ventricular pressure during early diastole.

Although the presence of aortic regurgitation is easily demonstrable by physical examination and noninvasive testing, its severity is accurately assessed only by cardiac catheterization. On the aortic root angiogram, contrast material regurgitates into the left ventricle, and the severity of regurgitation can be estimated by analyzing the breadth of the regurgitant stream, the density and amount of left ventricular opacification, and the rapidity with which the contrast medium is cleared. In addition, its severity can be assessed by calculating the regurgitant volume (or regurgitant fraction) from the difference between the *total* (angiographic) left ventricular output and the *net forward* output (by the Fick or indicator dilution method). Hemodynamically, the systemic arterial pulse pressure is characteristically widened. In the patient with severe aortic regurgitation, the left ventricular end-diastolic pressure is abnormally high and may be identical to the aortic diastolic pressure. If left ventricular failure has occurred, the pulmonary capillary wedge pressure is elevated.

As with aortic stenosis, the patient with chronic aortic regurgitation usually has an extended asymptomatic period (i.e., about 10 years) after the valve becomes incompetent. As the valve becomes more incompetent, the left ventricle dilates and hypertrophies to provide a greater total stroke volume and to maintain the forward stroke volume and cardiac output. Ultimately, left ventricular failure develops, either because the limits of left ventricular compensation are exceeded or because of intrinsic left ventricular dysfunction. As a result, there is an increased pressure in the pulmonary capillaries as well as a decreased cardiac output.

The asymptomatic patient with chronic aortic regurgitation requires antibiotic prophylaxis before general surgical or dental procedures. The patient whose symptoms are related to aortic regurgitation should undergo aortic valve replacement. Medical therapy with digitalis, diuretics, and vasodilators should be reserved for the symptomatic patient with chronic aortic regurgitation (1) when the degree of regurgitation is mild and out of proportion to the degree of left ventricular dysfunction, (2) when the patient refuses surgical therapy, and

(3) when the patient has a contraindication to surgery, such as disseminated malignant disease. The management of the asymptomatic patient with aortic regurgitation is controversial, since left ventricular dysfunction may be present and persist following surgery in some of these individuals. Although it is agreed that aortic valve replacement should be performed before the left ventricle is *irreversibly* damaged, the best method of detecting early irreversible left ventricular dysfunction is in dispute. Once left ventricular ejection fraction or cardiac output is depressed *at rest,* postoperative survival is reduced. Recently, echocardiography and radionuclide ventriculography at rest have been used in an attempt at further stratifying asymptomatic patients with aortic regurgitation into high- and low-risk subgroups. At present, severe left ventricular dysfunction at rest due to chronic aortic regurgitation, even in the absence of symptoms, is an indication for surgery at our institution. Since left ventricular dysfunction provoked by exercise or afterload stress appears to precede the appearance of abnormalities at rest, it may represent an intermediate stage in the natural history of chronic aortic regurgitation. Patients with stress-induced abnormalities of left ventricular function but normal resting function should be followed closely with noninvasive techniques and offered surgery if cardiac dilatation or a decrease in ventricular performance occurs.

Clinical Manifestations and Course

1. Abdulla AM, Frank MJ, Erdin RA, Canedo MI. Clinical significance and hemodynamic correlates of the third heart sound gallop in aortic regurgitation: a guide to optimal timing of cardiac catheterization. Circulation 1981; 64:464–71.
   An S_3 gallop in patients with chronic aortic regurgitation reflects left ventricular dysfunction rather than a more severe degree of regurgitation.

2. Bland EF, Wheeler EO. Severe aortic regurgitation in young people: a long-term perspective with references to prognosis and prosthesis. N Engl J Med 1957; 256:667–72.
   A sizable minority of young patients with aortic regurgitation remain asymptomatic for as long as 20 to 25 years.

3. Goldschlager N, Pfeifer J, Cohn K, Popper R, Selzer A. The natural history of aortic regurgitation: A clinical and hemodynamic study. Am J Med 1973; 54:577–88.
   In 126 patients with chronic aortic regurgitation, the clinical course was long and protracted.

4. Kumpuris AG, Quinones MA, Waggoner AD, Kanon DJ, Nelson JG, Miller RR. Importance of preoperative hypertrophy, wall stress and end-systolic dimension as echocardiographic predictors of normalization of left ventricular dilatation after valve replacement in chronic aortic insufficiency. Am J Cardiol 1982; 49:1091–1100.
   Inadequate hypertrophy in chronic aortic regurgitation leads to progressive increases in wall stress, with resultant dilatation and ultimately irreversible cardiac failure.

5. Rapaport E. Natural history of aortic and mitral valve disease. Am J Cardiol 1975; 35:221–7.
   A review of a large series of patients with stenosis or regurgitation of the aortic or mitral valves.

6. Reicheck N, Shelburne JC, Perloff JK. Clinical aspects of rheumatic valvular disease. Prog Cardiovasc Dis 1973; 15:491–537.
   The clinical findings in patients with rheumatic aortic and/or mitral valve disease.

7. Roberts WC, Morrow AG, McIntosh CL, Jones M, Epstein SE. Congenitally bicuspid aortic valve causing severe, pure aortic regurgitation without superimposed infective endocarditis. Am J Cardiol 1981; 47:206–9.
   A report of 13 patients who required aortic valve replacement for this condition.

8. Rotman M, Morris JJ Jr, Behar VS, Peter RH, Kong Y. Aortic valve disease: comparison of types and their medical and surgical management. Am J Med 1971; 51:241–57.

A concise review of 158 patients with aortic stenosis, aortic regurgitation, or mixed aortic valve disease, detailing their prognosis with medical management and the optimal timing of surgical intervention.

9. Sabbah HN, Khaja F, Anbe DT, Stein PD. The aortic closure sound in pure aortic insufficiency. Circulation 1977; 56:859–63.
   Intracardiac phonocardiography clearly demonstrates that S_2 in aortic regurgitation is reduced.

10. Segal J, Harvey WP, Hufnagel C. A clinical study of 100 cases of severe aortic insufficiency. Am J Med 1956; 21:200–10.
    Patients with aortic regurgitation often remain asymptomatic for many years, until congestive heart failure or angina pectoris finally appears.

11. Spagnuolo M, Kloth H, Taranta A, Doyle E, Pasternack B. Natural history of rheumatic aortic regurgitation: criteria predictive of death, congestive heart failure, and angina in young patients. Circulation 1970; 44:368–80.
    Moderate or marked left ventricular enlargement, electrocardiographic evidence of left ventricular hypertrophy, and an abnormally wide pulse pressure in the patient with aortic regurgitation are indications of impending death or symptoms.

Diagnosis and Assessment of Severity

12. Bolen JL, Holloway EL, Zener JC, Harrison DC, Alderman EL. Evaluation of left ventricular function in patients with aortic regurgitation using afterload stress. Circulation 1976; 53:132–8.
    Left ventricular dysfunction induced by an increase in afterload may represent early evidence of irreversible myocardial damage.

13. Borer JS, Bacharach SL, Green MV, Kent KM, Henry WL, Rosing DR, Seides SF, Johnston GS, Epstein SE. Exercise-induced left ventricular dysfunction in symptomatic and asymptomatic patients with aortic regurgitation: assessment with radionuclide cineangiography. Am J Cardiol 1978; 42:351–7.
    The radionuclide assessment of left ventricular function during exercise may be valuable in sequentially following left ventricular function in patients with aortic regurgitation before the onset of symptoms.

14. Botvinick EH, Schiller NB, Wickramasekaran R, Klausner SC, Gertz E. Echocardiographic demonstration of early mitral valve closure in severe aortic insufficiency: its clinical implications. Circulation 1975; 51:836–47.
    Early closure of the anterior leaflet of the mitral valve is a reliable sign of torrential aortic regurgitation that often requires immediate aortic valve replacement.

15. Cope GD, Kisslo JA, Johnson ML, Myers S. Diastolic vibration of the interventricular septum in aortic insufficiency. Circulation 1975; 51:589–93.
    One of several echocardiographic features in patients with aortic regurgitation.

16. Dehmer GJ, Firth BG, Hillis LD, Corbett JR, Lewis SE, Parkey RW, Willerson JT. Alterations in left ventricular volumes and ejection fraction at rest and during exercise in patients with aortic regurgitation. Am J Cardiol 1981; 48:17–27.
    Abnormal alterations in left ventricular volumes occur during exercise in patients with aortic regurgitation and may be helpful in the early detection of left ventricular dysfunction.

17. Firth BG, Dehmer GJ, Nicod P, Willerson JT, Hillis LD. Effect of increasing heart rate in patients with aortic regurgitation: effect of incremental atrial pacing on scintigraphic, hemodynamic and thermodilution measurements. Am J Cardiol 1982; 49:1860–7.
    Incremental atrial pacing produces a decremental reduction in left ventricular end-diastolic and end-systolic volumes, as well as in the regurgitant volume per stroke, but no change in the regurgitant volume per minute, forward cardiac output, or mean femoral arterial and pulmonary capillary wedge pressures.

18. Nicod P, Corbett JR, Firth BG, Dehmer GJ, Izquierdo C, Markham RV, Hillis LD, Willerson JT, Lewis SE. Radionuclide techniques for valvular regurgitant index: comparison in patients with normal and depressed ventricular function. J Nucl Med 1982; 23:763–9.
    Although radionuclide techniques are specific (97%), they are relatively insensitive for detecting valvular regurgitation, particularly in patients with a depressed (<

0.35) left ventricular ejection fraction; furthermore, they do not consistently differentiate among mild, moderate, and severe regurgitation.

19. Schuler G, von Olshausen K, Schwarz F, Mehmel H, Hofman M, Hermann HJ, Lange D, Kubler W. Noninvasive assessment of myocardial contractility in asymptomatic patients with severe aortic regurgitation and normal left ventricular ejection fraction at rest. Am J Cardiol 1982; 50:45–52.
    This radionuclide study in 14 asymptomatic patients with chronic aortic regurgitation suggests that afterload stress (with methoxamine) and bicycle exercise may both uncover an abnormal contractile state in certain asymptomatic individuals with aortic regurgitation.

20. Winsberg F, Gabor GE, Hernberg JG, Weiss B. Fluttering of the mitral valve in aortic insufficiency. Circulation 1970; 41:225–9.
    Fluttering of the anterior leaflet of the mitral valve is a specific echocardiographic sign of aortic regurgitation.

21. Skorton DJ, Child JS, Perloff JK. Accuracy of the echocardiographic diagnosis of aortic regurgitation. Am J Med 1980; 69:377–82.
    Diastolic fluttering of the anterior mitral leaflet is a reliable sign of severe chronic aortic regurgitation except when concomitant mitral stenosis is present.

Therapy

22. Bonow RO, Rosing DR, Kent KM, Epstein SE. Timing of operation for chronic aortic regurgitation. Am J Cardiol 1982; 50:325–336.
    The authors recommend surgery for all symptomatic patients as well as for those with left ventricular dysfunction at rest even, if symptoms and deterioration in exercise tolerance have not developed.

23. Borer JS, Rosing DR, Kent KM, Bacharach SL, Green MV, McIntosh CJ, Morrow AG, Epstein SE. Left ventricular function at rest and during exercise after aortic valve replacement in patients with aortic regurgitation. Am J Cardiol 1979; 44:1297–1305.
    Aortic valve replacement can improve but usually does not normalize left ventricular function during exercise in symptomatic patients with aortic regurgitation.

24. Forman R, Firth BG, Barnard MS. Prognostic significance of preoperative left ventricular ejection fraction and valve lesion in patients with aortic valve replacement. Am J Cardiol 1980; 45:1120–5.
    This study of 229 patients with isolated aortic valve replacement indicates that the 3-year survival rate is good in patients with aortic stenosis, despite a depressed preoperative left ventricular ejection fraction, but that survival rate is poor in patients with aortic regurgitation and a depressed preoperative ejection fraction.

25. Gaasch WH, Andrias CW, Levine HJ. Chronic aortic regurgitation: the effect of aortic valve replacement on left ventricular volume, mass, and function. Circulation 1978; 58:825–36.
    After aortic valve replacement, patients with chronic aortic regurgitation had a normalization of left ventricular volumes and a reduction of left ventricular muscle mass.

26. Greenberg BH, DeMots H, Murphy E, Rahimtoola S. Beneficial effects of hydralazine on rest and exercise hemodynamics in patients with chronic severe aortic insufficiency. Circulation 1980; 62:49–55.
    In 10 patients with chronic, severe aortic regurgitation, hydralazine produced symptomatic and hemodynamic improvement at rest and during exercise.

27. Henry WL, Bonow RO, Rosing DR, Epstein SE. Observations on the optimum time for operative intervention for aortic regurgitation: II. Serial echocardiographic evaluation of asymptomatic patients. Circulation 1980; 61:484–492.
    This study suggests that a left ventricular end-systolic dimension > 55 mm should serve as an indication for aortic valve replacement, even in asymptomatic patients with aortic regurgitation.

28. O'Rourke RA, Crawford MH. Timing of valve replacement in patients with chronic aortic regurgitation. Circulation 1980; 61:493–5.
    This editorial points out the potential pitfalls and limitations of M-mode echocardiographic measurements in defining when to operate on the asymptomatic patient with chronic aortic regurgitation.

29. Greenberg BH, Rahimtoola SH. Long-term vasodilator therapy in aortic insufficiency: evidence for regression of left ventricular dilatation and hypertrophy and
improvement in systolic pump function. Ann Intern Med 1980; 93:440–2.

*In a 54-year-old woman with severe aortic regurgitation, long-term hydralazine
therapy induced hemodynamic improvement and a recovery of left ventricular systolic performance.*

30. Carroll JD, Gaasch WH, Zile MR, Levine HJ. Serial changes in left ventricular
function after correction of chronic aortic regurgitation: dependence on early
changes in preload and subsequent regression of hypertrophy. Am J Cardiol 1983;
51:476–82.

*After valve replacement for chronic aortic regurgitation, some patients have a de-
crease in left ventricular preload, a regression of hypertrophy, and evidence of clinical and hemodynamic improvement; others have persistent left ventricular hypertrophy and dysfunction and little (or no) improvement.*

ACUTE AORTIC REGURGITATION

Acute aortic regurgitation is most commonly caused by bacterial endocarditis,
a dissection of the ascending aorta involving the aortic valve, or trauma. The
left ventricle is confronted with an overwhelming blood volume during diastole, resulting in extreme elevations of left ventricular diastolic pressure,
which may approach or equal aortic diastolic pressure.

The patient with acute aortic regurgitation usually has symptoms of left ventricular decompensation: dyspnea, orthopnea, and paroxysmal nocturnal dyspnea. These symptoms often begin abruptly and progress rapidly to pulmonary
edema. Although angina pectoris occasionally is present in the patient with
acute aortic regurgitation, it is usually overshadowed by symptoms of left ventricular failure. Syncope (or near-syncope) is not a clinical characteristic of
acute aortic regurgitation.

On physical examination, many of the signs of chronic aortic regurgitation
are absent, since they have had insufficient time to develop. Most of the peripheral manifestations of chronic aortic regurgitation (widened pulse pressure,
water-hammer pulses, Duroziez's sign, Quincke's pulses, Hill's sign) are not
present, since they are indicative of a greatly increased left ventricular stroke
volume. The patient usually has sinus tachycardia. Cardiomegaly is not prominent, and as a result, the point of maximal impulse is not displaced laterally.
Left ventricular dilatation during diastole, the primary compensatory mechanism of the left ventricle with chronic aortic regurgitation, has not had sufficient time to become manifest. On auscultation, the S_1 may be unusually quiet,
since the mitral valve often closes prematurely and the mitral component of the
S_1 occurs early. The S_2 is also diminished. A loud S_3 is audible but may be obscured by the decrescendo diastolic murmur of aortic regurgitation. This murmur may be relatively low-pitched and may end partway through diastole, reflecting the equalization of diastolic pressure between the left ventricle and the
aorta. An Austin Flint murmur (a short diastolic rumble at the apex) is almost
always audible. Examination of the lung fields usually reveals rales at both
bases.

In the patient with acute aortic regurgitation, the chest x-ray usually does
not demonstrate marked left ventricular enlargement, since weeks to months
are required for the development of left ventricular dilatation. Pulmonary vascular redistribution is usually present. Similarly, the ECG usually shows only
sinus tachycardia. Left ventricular hypertrophy, a characteristic electrocardi-

ographic manifestation of chronic aortic regurgitation, is usually absent. The M-mode echocardiogram is extremely helpful in the assessment of acute aortic regurgitation. First, if the regurgitation is due to aortic valve endocarditis, vegetations may be visualized on the aortic valve leaflets. Second, the left ventricular end-diastolic volume usually is not increased, and the left ventricular end-systolic volume is normal. Third, the anterior leaflet of the mitral valve and the left ventricular septal endocardium may demonstrate high-frequency vibrations during diastole, indicative of aortic regurgitation. Fourth, because of the rapid increase in left ventricular pressure during early diastole, the mitral valve may close prematurely. In the absence of other cardiac defects, the extent of early closure correlates with the elevation of left ventricular end-diastolic pressure.

Acute aortic regurgitation is often a life-threatening condition. If the etiology is *infective endocarditis,* systemic antibiotics should be commenced as soon as appropriate blood samples have been obtained for culture. When instituted early, they may be curative. However, because of the subtle physical findings in acute aortic regurgitation, the diagnosis is frequently made late in the course of the disease, at a time when it has already caused hemodynamic decompensation. If the patient is sufficiently stable to tolerate cardiac catheterization, it should be performed to exclude endocarditic involvement of other valves. If congestive heart failure develops, it should be treated initially with digitalis, diuretics, and vasodilator therapy. If the patient has rapidly progressive cardiac dilatation or hemodynamic and symptomatic deterioration despite medical therapy, aortic valve replacement should be performed expediently. In addition, major systemic embolization or conduction disturbances (usually AV block) are indications for early aortic valve replacement. Recent studies have demonstrated that prosthetic valve replacement can be performed in this setting with a low risk of endocarditis developing on the prosthesis. Indeed, a delay in operation in the patient who is deteriorating causes a greater mortality than early surgery after limited antibiotic therapy. If acute aortic regurgitation is due to *aortic dissection* or *trauma,* the patient should be stabilized medically, cardiac catheterization should be performed to define the severity of regurgitation and the presence of associated abnormalities, and aortic valve replacement should be performed immediately.

Clinical Manifestations and Course

1. Goldschlager N, Pfiefer J, Cohn K, Popper R, Selzer A. The natural history of aortic regurgitation: a clinical and hemodynamic study. Am J Med 1973; 54: 577–88.
   The sudden development of severe aortic regurgitation, such as may occur with valve perforation in infective endocarditis, is often a catastrophic event.
2. Rees JR, Epstein EJ, Criley JM, Ross RS. Hemodynamic effects of severe aortic regurgitation. Br Heart J 1964; 26:412–21.
   In 8 patients with severe aortic regurgitation, left ventricular and central aortic pressures were the same at end diastole.
3. Tompsett R, Lubash GD. Aortic valve perforation in bacterial endocarditis. Circulation 1961; 23:662–4.
   Ten patients are described who acutely worsened during therapy for aortic valve endocarditis; at postmortem examination, they were found to have perforation or rupture of an aortic valve cusp.
4. Wigle ED, Labrosse CJ. Sudden, severe aortic insufficiency. Circulation 1965; 32:708–20.
   Fourteen cases of acute severe aortic regurgitation are described, with catheterization data included.

Diagnosis and Assessment of Severity

5. Botvinick EH, Schiller NB, Wickramasekaran R, Klausner SC, Gertz E. Echocardiographic demonstration of early mitral valve closure in severe aortic insufficiency: its clinical implications. Circulation 1975; 51:836–47.
Early mitral valve closure is a simple, noninvasive indicator of the need for immediate aortic valve replacement.

6. Mann T, McLaurin L, Grossman W, Craige E. Assessing the hemodynamic severity of acute aortic regurgitation due to infective endocarditis. N Engl J Med 1975; 293:108–113.
Early mitral valve closure correlates with the degree of elevation of the left ventricular end-diastolic pressure.

7. Meadows WR, Van Praagh S, Indreika M, Sharp JT. Premature mitral valve closure: a hemodynamic explanation for absence of the first heart sound in aortic insufficiency. Circulation 1963; 28:251–8.
Premature mitral valve closure occurs only in patients with severe aortic regurgitation and, therefore, implies a bad prognosis.

8. Winsberg F, Gabor GE, Hernberg JG, Weiss B. Fluttering of the mitral valve in aortic insufficiency. Circulation 1970; 41:225–9.
Fluttering of the anterior leaflet of the mitral valve is virtually a specific echocardiographic sign of aortic regurgitation.

Therapy

9. Crosby IK, Carrell R, Reed WA. Operative management of valvular complications of bacterial endocarditis. J Thorac Cardiovasc Surg 1972; 64:235–46.
When forced by hemodynamic deterioration, valve replacement can be performed safely even in the setting of infective endocarditis.

10. Lewis BS, Agathangelou NE, Colsen PR, Antunes M, Kinsley RH. Cardiac operation during active infective endocarditis: results of aortic, mitral and double valve replacement in 94 patients. J Thorac Cardiovasc Surg 1982; 84:579–84.
In this large series of patients treated surgically for infective endocarditis, there was an acceptable operative mortality and good long-term results following emergent or semi-emergent surgery.

11. Wilson WR, Danielson GK, Giuliani ER, Washington JA II, Jaumin PM, Geraci JE. Valve replacement in patients with active infective endocarditis. Circulation 1978; 58:585–88.
The hemodynamic status of patients with infective endocarditis, rather than the activity of the infection or the length of preoperative antimicrobial therapy, should be the determining factor in the timing of cardiac valve replacement.

12. Richardson JV, Karp RB, Kirklin JW, Dismukes WE. Treatment of infective endocarditis: a 10-year comparative analysis. Circulation 1978; 58:589–97.
Early valve replacement is recommended for patients with infective endocarditis and moderate or severe heart failure.

13. Wise JR Jr, Bentall HH, Cleland WP, Goodwin JF, Hallidie-Smith KA, Oakley CM. Urgent aortic valve replacement for acute aortic regurgitation due to infective endocarditis. Lancet 1971; 2:115–21.
Acute aortic regurgitation differs from chronic aortic regurgitation and, therefore, may be difficult to recognize clinically.

AORTIC VALVE SURGERY

The indications for surgical intervention in the patient with aortic stenosis or regurgitation have been reviewed in the discussions of these valvular abnormalities. In brief, the patient with aortic stenosis should undergo aortic valve replacement when any of the triad of symptoms attributable to that disorder develops: syncope, angina pectoris, or congestive heart failure. The *onset* of symptoms is an indication for immediate surgical intervention. Similarly, surgical therapy of the patient with chronic aortic regurgitation is indicated once the patient is symptomatic. In addition, valve replacement is generally recommended before irreversible left ventricular dysfunction occurs, even in the absence of symptoms, since such dysfunction may not improve following valve replacement. Thus, left ventricular dysfunction at rest (as indicated by a depressed left ventricular ejection fraction), even without symptoms, probably constitutes an indication for aortic valve replacement in the patient with moderate or severe aortic regurgitation. Finally, since exercise- or afterload-induced alterations in left ventricular volumes or ejection fraction appear to precede left ventricular dysfunction at rest, they should alert one to the possibility of early left ventricular dysfunction.

Aortic valve replacement is performed on cardiopulmonary bypass via a median sternotomy, using systemic and topical hypothermia (25–28°C) as well as cardioplegic arrest of the heart. The aortic valve is exposed by an aortotomy a few centimeters above the valve. The valve is excised, the anulus measured, and a prosthetic valve inserted and sutured in position. Care must be taken with a heavily calcified valve to retrieve all calcium debris. Since the cardiac conduction system is immediately adjacent to the commissure between the right and noncoronary cusps, care must also be taken to avoid damaging this tissue.

Several different kinds of prosthetic valves have been used in the aortic position. The caged-ball valve (most commonly the Starr-Edwards valve) has the longest proven record of durability of any artificial valve. The original Starr-Edwards valve, developed in 1960 (Model 1000), was composed of a Silastic ball and metal struts. In many patients, swelling, grooving, and cracking of the Silastic ball eventually developed, a condition known as ball variance. As a result, the ball was improved in 1965 (Model 1200–1260) and subsequently has presented no problems of variance. Because of thromboembolic problems, a new model (Model 2300–2320) was introduced in 1968, in which the metal struts were covered with cloth. From 1968 to 1972, modifications were made on this prosthesis to eliminate occasional ball sticking and cloth tearing, which included the incorporation of a non-cloth-covered "track" on the inside of the struts. Recently, the manufacturers have reverted to only the non-cloth-covered model 1200-1260 aortic prosthesis, since recent studies suggest that cloth-covering of the struts, with or without a track, confers little or no advantage. Since 1972, the Starr-Edwards caged-ball prosthesis has enjoyed wide popularity. It is extremely durable and has been used so extensively that most of its technical pitfalls have been eliminated. Its major disadvantages center (1) on the relatively high incidence of thromboembolic complications, (2) on the chronic low-grade hemolysis that occurs in patients with this valve in the aortic position, and (3) on the degree of obstruction it causes when it is placed in a small aortic root.

The tilting disc prosthesis, of which the prototype is the Bjork-Shiley valve, was introduced in 1969. In general, it has excellent structural characteristics, and it is less obstructive than the Starr-Edwards valve for any given external diameter. Its long-term durability appears to be satisfactory. Hemolysis is not a problem with this prosthesis, but thrombosis and embolic complications make long-term anticoagulant therapy mandatory. Recently, the St. Jude prosthesis, a tilting-disc valve with two leaflets, and the Medtronic (Hall-Kaster) valve have been used in the aortic position. Although both have excellent hemodynamic characteristics, they are liable to thrombosis and embolic phenomena and, therefore, require anticoagulation.

The porcine heterograft prosthesis offers several advantages over the Starr-Edwards and tilting-disc prostheses but also has certain disadvantages. Thromboembolic complications occur rarely in the patient with a porcine prosthesis in the aortic position, so that these patients do not require anticoagulation. Similarly, hemolysis does not occur in the patient with a normally functioning porcine heterograft. Its disadvantages center (1) on its lack of durability and (2) on its relatively poor hemodynamic function. After 10 years, approximately 50 percent of these prostheses may require replacement because of degeneration. In children and adolescents, stenosis and calcification of this prosthesis may occur within 1 to 2 years. For a given external diameter, the porcine heterograft prosthesis is more obstructive than a tilting-disc valve.

In some surgical centers, the bovine pericardial xenograft (Ionescu-Shiley valve) is preferred to the porcine prosthesis. At others, unstented "fresh" homograft aortic valves are used. Although the hemodynamic characteristics and durability of these valves appear superior to the porcine bioprosthesis, problems of procurement and the skill required for their insertion limit their widespread use.

In summary, in the choice of a prosthetic aortic valve, one should consider durability, hemodynamic function, and thromboembolic potential. The caged-ball Starr-Edwards valve is durable and has good hemodynamic function, but its thromboembolic potential is great. The disc prostheses have reasonable durability and excellent hemodynamic characteristics, but they also pose a thromboembolic risk. The porcine heterograft is less durable than these mechanical prostheses and offers only marginal hemodynamic improvement in the patient with a small aortic root, but its thromboembolic potential is low, and therefore, long-term anticoagulation ordinarily is not required.

The operative mortality for aortic valve replacement is 3 to 10 percent. In general, operative risk depends on the patient's preoperative functional class, left ventricular function, presence of coronary artery disease, and extent of left ventricular hypertrophy. Once the patient survives the perioperative period, the long-term outlook is good: 50 to 75 percent are free of symptoms, and most of the remainder are improved. The 5-year survival rate is around 80 percent.

General

1. Bonchek LI. Current status of cardiac valve replacement: selection of a prosthesis and indications for operation. Am Heart J 1981; 101:96–106.
   An excellent review of the advantages and disadvantages of currently available prosthetic heart valves.
2. Copeland JG, Griepp RB, Stinson EB, Shumway NE. Long-term follow-up after isolated aortic valve replacement. J Thorac Cardiovasc Surg 1977; 74:875–89.
   In a large group of patients undergoing aortic valve replacement only, perioperative mortality was 7% to 8%, and the linear attrition rate thereafter was 2.7% per year.
3. Copeland JG, Griepp RB, Stinson EB, Shumway NE. Isolated aortic valve replacement in patients older than 65 years. JAMA 1977; 237:1578–81.
   Even in elderly patients, aortic valve replacement can be performed with an acceptable risk, and overall outlook is good.
4. Croke RP, Pifarre R, Sullivan H, Gunnar R, Loeb H. Reversal of advanced left ventricular dysfunction following aortic valve replacement for aortic stenosis. Ann Thorac Surg 1977; 24:38–43.
   A small series emphasizing the point that patients with aortic stenosis and severely compromised left ventricular ejection fraction often show a marked improvement in this variable following aortic valve replacement.
5. Roberts WC. Choosing a substitute cardiac valve: type, size, surgeon. Am J Cardiol 1976; 38:633–44.
   An excellent review of the advantages and disadvantages of the various kinds of prosthetic valves.
6. Smith N, McAnulty JH, Rahimtoola SH. Severe aortic stenosis with impaired left

ventricular function and clinical heart failure: results of valve replacement. Circulation 1978; 58:255–64.
This study suggests that all patients with aortic stenosis and congestive heart failure should be offered aortic valve replacement, regardless of left ventricular ejection fraction.

7. Jamieson WRE, Dooner J, Munro AI, Janusz MT, Burgess JJ, Miyagishima RR, Gerein AN, Allen P. Cardiac valve replacement in the elderly: a review of 320 consecutive cases. Circulation 1981; 64(Suppl II):177–183.
Of 190 patients aged 65 years and older, 9 (5%) died in surgery for aortic valve replacement; long-term results were good.

8. Kennedy JW, Doces J, Stewart DK. Left ventricular function before and following aortic valve replacement. Circulation 1977; 56:944–50.
Left ventricular dilatation, hypertrophy, and reduced systolic function are largely reversible after successful aortic valve replacement.

9. Kloster FE. Diagnosis and management of complications of prosthetic heart valves. Am J Cardiol 1975; 35:872–85.
A superb review of commonly encountered problems after valve replacement, including hemolytic anemia, thrombotic problems, and systemic embolization.

10. Kugler JD, Campbell E, Vargo TA, McNamara DG, Hallman GL, Cooley DA. Results of aortic valvotomy in infants with isolated aortic valvular stenosis. J Thorac Cardiovasc Surg 1979; 78:553–8.
A report of 52 infants (aged 2 days to 10 months) who were treated by this technique. One patient required aortic valve replacement 17 years later.

11. McKay R, Ross DN. Technique for the relief of discrete subaortic stenosis. J Thorac Cardiovasc Surg 1982; 84:917–20.
The technique of enucleation of discrete subaortic stenosis is described.

12. Miller DC, Stinson EB, Oyer PE, Rossiter SJ, Reitz BA, Shumway NE. Surgical implications and results of combined aortic valve replacement and myocardial revascularization. Am J Cardiol 1979; 43:494–501.
All patients undergoing cardiac catheterization for aortic valve disease should undergo coronary arteriography, even in the absence of angina pectoris.

13. Newfeld EA, Muster AJ, Paul MH, Idriss FS, Riker WL. Discrete subvalvular aortic stenosis in childhood: study of 51 patients. Am J Cardiol 1976; 38:53–61.
A detailed description of the pathophysiology and therapy of children with subvalvular aortic stenosis.

14. Rahimtoola SH. Valve replacement should not be performed in all asymptomatic patients with severe aortic incompetence. J Thorac Cardiovasc Surg 1980; 79:163–72.
This editorial concludes that aortic valve replacement is not indicated in the asymptomatic patient with aortic regurgitation if left ventricular systolic pump function is normal, but is indicated if resting left ventricular systolic pump function is impaired.

15. Richardson JV, Kouchoukos NT, Wright JO, Karp RB. Combined aortic valve replacement and myocardial revascularization: results in 220 patients. Circulation 1979; 59:75–81.
Combined valve replacement and coronary bypass should be performed in all patients in whom aortic valve disease and coronary artery disease coexist.

Porcine Heterografts and Homografts

16. Angell WW, Angell JD. Porcine valves. Prog Cardiovasc Dis 1980; 23:141–166.
An excellent review of porcine bioprostheses, including their advantages, complications, and a comparison with mechanical prostheses.

17. Ashraf M, Bloor CM. Structural alterations of the porcine heterograft after various durations of implantation. Am J Cardiol 1978; 41:1185–90.
A detailed study of morphologic changes in porcine heterografts removed 2 months to 2 years after implantation.

18. Cohn LH, Mudge GH, Pratter F, Collins JJ Jr. Five to eight-year follow-up of patients undergoing porcine heart-valve replacement. N Engl J Med 1981; 304:258–62.
In this group of 128 patients with aortic or mitral porcine prostheses, the probability of prosthetic dysfunction before 6 years was very low.

19. Lakier JB, Khaja F, Magilligan DJ Jr, Goldstein S. Porcine xenograft valves: long-term (60–89 month) follow-up. Circulation 1980; 62:313–8.
    Porcine xenograft failures increase in frequency 48 months after insertion. The incidence of valve failures is especially high in young persons.

20. Ferrans VJ, Spray TL, Billingham ME, Roberts WC. Structural changes in glutaraldehyde-treated porcine heterografts used as substitute cardiac valves. Am J Cardiol 1978; 41:1159–84.
    By electron microscopy, porcine valves undergo certain morphologic changes that may limit their durability.

21. Ishihara T, Ferrans VJ, Boyce SW, Jones M, Roberts WC. Structure and classification of cuspal tears and perforations in porcine bioprosthetic cardiac valves implanted in patients. Am J Cardiol 1981; 48:665–78.
    An excellent review of the degenerative changes that may occur in porcine bioprostheses.

22. Levine FH, Carter JE, Buckley MJ, Daggett WM, Akins CW, Austen WG. Hemodynamic evaluation of Hancock and Carpentier-Edwards bioprostheses. Circulation 1981; 64(Suppl II):192–5.
    This study suggests that in both the aortic and mitral positions, Carpentier-Edwards porcine bioprostheses are less obstructive than Hancock porcine prostheses.

23. Morris DC, King SB III, Douglas JS Jr, Wickliffe CW, Jones EL. Hemodynamic results of aortic valvular replacement with the porcine xenograft valve. Circulation 1977; 56:841–4.
    Although the hemodynamics of the larger porcine heterografts are comparable to other available prostheses, the very small orifice areas for the 19-mm and 21-mm prostheses render their use inadvisable.

24. Rothkopf M, Davidson T, Lipscomb K, Narahara K, Hillis LD, Willerson JT, Estrera A, Platt M, Mills L. Hemodynamic evaluation of the Carpentier-Edwards bioprosthesis in the aortic position. Am J Cardiol 1979; 44:209–14.
    This study in 17 patients suggests that for the same anulus, the Carpentier-Edwards bioprosthesis has a similar orifice area to that reported for the Hancock bioprosthesis.

25. Williams DB, Danielson GK, McGoon DC, Puga FJ, Mair DD, Edwards WD. Porcine heterograft valve replacement in children. J Thorac Cardiovasc Surg 1982; 84:446–50.
    In 49 patients under the age of 18 years, bioprosthetic valve dysfunction occurred in 20 (40%) by 5 years. The authors recommend using mechanical rather than bioprosthetic valves in this age group.

26. Levine FH, Buckley MJ, Austen WG. Hemodynamic evaluation of the Hancock-modified orifice bioprosthesis in the aortic position. Circulation 1978; 58(Suppl I):33–5.
    Recent modification of the Hancock bioprosthesis produces a larger effective orifice area for any given anulus diameter.

27. Thompson R, Yacoub M, Ahmed M, Somerville W, Towers M. The use of "fresh" unstented homograft valves for replacement of the aortic valve: analysis of 8 years experience. J Thoracic Cardiovasc Surg 1980; 79:896–903.
    Experience with 679 patients who underwent aortic valve replacement with "fresh" unstented homograft valves. Actuarial survival was 87% at 5 years and 81% at 8 years, with a low incidence of late valve failure.

28. Ionescu MI, Tandon AP, Mary DAS, Abid A. Heart valve replacement with the Ionescu-Shiley pericardial xenograft. J Thorac Cardiovasc Surg 1977; 73:31–42.
    After 30 months, this prosthesis was still functioning satisfactorily in a large series of patients.

Disc Prostheses

29. Bjork VO, Henze A, Holmgren A. Five years' experience with the Bjork-Shiley tilting-disc valve in isolated aortic valvular disease. J Thorac Cardiovasc Surg 1974; 68:393–404.
    Of 470 patients with this prosthesis in the aortic position, valvular function at 5 years was generally satisfactory.

30. Bjork VO, Henze A. Ten years' experience with the Bjork-Shiley tilting disc valve. J Thorac Cardiovasc Surg 1979; 78:331–42.

A detailed discussion of experience with 1,800 patients who received a Bjork-Shiley prosthesis, including a consideration of recent modifications to the prosthesis.

31. Karp RB, Cyrus RJ, Blackstone EH, Kirklin JW, Kouchoukos NT, Pacifico AD. The Bjork-Shiley valve: intermediate-term follow-up. J Thorac Cardiovasc Surg 1981; 81:602–14.

    After a mean follow-up of 38 months, the authors conclude that the Bjork-Shiley valve is durable and effective but is associated with problems of thrombosis and thromboembolism.

32. Nicoloff DM, Emery RW, Arom KV, Northrup WF III, Jorgensen CR, Wang Y, Lindsay WG. Clinical and hemodynamic results with the St. Jude medical cardiac valve prosthesis: a three year experience. J Thorac Cardiovasc Surg 1981; 82:674–83.

    This study in 232 patients followed for 3 years suggests that the St. Jude prosthesis has excellent hemodynamic characteristics and is a viable alternative in the surgical therapy of valvular heart disease.

33. Wright JO, Hiratzka LF, Brandt B III, Doty DB. Thrombosis of the Bjork-Shiley prosthesis: illustrative cases and review of the literature. J Thorac Cardiovasc Surg 1982; 84:138–44.

    This review highlights the problem of thrombosis of the Bjork-Shiley valve in both the aortic and mitral positions.

34. Yoganathan AP, Corcoran WH, Harrison EC, Carl JR. The Bjork-Shiley aortic prosthesis: flow characteristics, thrombus formation, and tissue overgrowth. Circulation 1978; 58:70–6.

    Thrombus formation and tissue overgrowth are reported in 9 patients with Bjork-Shiley valves in the aortic position.

35. Beaudet RL, Gagnon RM, Poirier N, David A. Clinical and hemodynamic evaluation of a new pivoting disc valvular prosthesis (Hall-Kaster). abstract. Circulation 1980; 62 (Suppl III):236.

    A report of the Hall-Kaster valve in 120 patients.

36. Silver MD. Wear in Bjork-Shiley heart valve prostheses recovered at necropsy or operation. J Thorac Cardiovasc Surg 1980; 79:693–9.

    Thirteen Bjork-Shiley valves in situ for up to 27 months showed evidence of only minor wear that was unlikely to affect valve function during the normal lifetime of an individual.

Ball-in-Cage Prostheses

37. Starr A, Grunkemeier GL, Lambert LE, Thomas DR, Sugimura S, Lefrak EA. Aortic valve replacement: a ten-year follow-up of non-cloth-covered vs. cloth-covered caged-ball prostheses. Circulation 1977; 56(Suppl II):133–9.

    A detailed analysis of the Portland, Oregon, experience with the Starr-Edwards valve, confirming its durability.

MITRAL STENOSIS

Mitral stenosis occasionally occurs as an isolated congenital lesion. Rarely, the symptoms and clinical characteristics of mitral stenosis can be mimicked by an atrial tumor (myxoma) or thrombus that partially occludes the valve orifice. In most patients, mitral stenosis is the result of previous rheumatic carditis. The mitral valve apparatus is affected by the rheumatic process in several ways: (1) the valve leaflets contract and become scarred, (2) the valve leaflets commonly fuse together at the level of the commissures, and (3) the chordae tendineae shorten and become fused. In many patients the leaflets calcify, thus contributing to their rigidity and immobility.

The patient with mitral stenosis may note symptoms of pulmonary vascular congestion and a reduced cardiac output. When the stenosis is mild, the patient may note dyspnea only with vigorous physical exertion. Such exertion increases heart rate, shortens the diastolic filling period, and therefore increases left atrial pressure, leading to pulmonary congestion. As the stenosis becomes more severe, the patient notes dyspnea on minimal exertion and finally even at rest, orthopnea, and paroxysmal nocturnal dyspnea. At the same time, the patient may note generalized fatigue because exertion does not increase cardiac output.

In response to an elevated pulmonary capillary pressure, the pulmonary arterial pressure rises, eventually leading to pulmonary hypertension. Right ventricular dilatation and failure develop, and the patient may complain of peripheral edema as well as abdominal tenderness and swelling (due to hepatomegaly and the accumulation of ascitic fluid). In patients with severe pulmonary hypertension, angina pectoris or syncope occasionally occurs, probably related to hypoxia, hypotension, and a reduced cardiac output.

As mitral stenosis becomes severe, episodes of recurrent arterial embolization may occur. Thrombus formation in the left atrium is especially likely in the patient with mitral stenosis and atrial fibrillation, and portions of a left atrial thrombus may be dislodged and travel to the systemic circulation. As a result, the patient with mitral stenosis may note the sudden onset of (1) a neurologic deficit (due to embolization of an artery supplying the brain), (2) chest pain due to a myocardial infarction (caused by embolization of a coronary artery), or (3) abdominal or flank pain (due to embolization of a splanchnic or renal artery).

On physical examination, the carotid upstroke is normal but small in volume. In the patient with pulmonary hypertension and right-sided congestion, jugular venous distention, hepatomegaly, and ankle edema may be present. Palpation of the precordium reveals a quiet and nondisplaced cardiac apex as well as a right ventricular lift along the midsternal and lower left sternal border. On auscultation, the S_1 is loud, as is the pulmonic component of the S_2. The S_2 is followed closely by the opening snap of the mitral valve. The time delay from the aortic component of the S_2 to the opening snap provides a rough indication of the severity of stenosis: a short A2–OS interval (0.04–0.07 sec) is characteristic of severe mitral stenosis, whereas a relatively long interval (0.09–0.12 sec) signifies mild stenosis. The opening snap is followed by a low-pitched diastolic rumble most easily audible at the apex with the patient in the left lateral decubitus position. In the patient with severe mitral stenosis, the murmur is long and occupies most of diastole. However, when cardiac output is low and the flow across the valve is markedly reduced, the murmur may be soft. As pulmonary hypertension develops, a murmur of pulmonic regurgitation (Graham Steell murmur) may become audible in the second left intercostal space. Finally, as right ventricular dilatation and failure develop, the holosystolic murmur of tricuspid regurgitation may be audible at the lower left sternal border, along with a right ventricular S_3.

The chest x-ray in the patient with mitral stenosis usually demonstrates enlargement of the left atrium and the left atrial appendage. Pulmonary vascular redistribution is almost inevitably present. Once pulmonary hypertension develops, the main pulmonary artery and the right ventricle become enlarged. Finally, one may occasionally see mitral valve calcification on the routine chest x-ray. In adults with mitral stenosis, the ECG shows atrial fibrillation in about two-thirds of cases. In the patient with mitral stenosis who is still in sinus rhythm, there is evidence of left atrial enlargement. As pulmonary hypertension develops, right axis deviation and right ventricular hypertrophy become manifest. The M-mode echocardiogram demonstrates a deformed and scarred mitral apparatus. The rate of diastolic closure of both mitral leaflets is reduced, and the posterior leaflet usually moves in the same direction as the anterior leaflet. If pulmonary hypertension is present, the right ventricle may be abnormally large, and the interventricular septum may move paradoxically with systole. In addition, the slowing of left atrial emptying typical of mitral stenosis alters the motion of the posterior aortic wall and may be used to quantitate the severity of stenosis. With two-dimensional echocardiography, the mitral valve orifice can be visualized directly.

At the time of catheterization, there is a pressure gradient between the left atrium (usually measured as the pulmonary capillary wedge pressure) and the left ventricle during diastole. From this pressure gradient and the cardiac output, one can calculate a mitral valve area. Although the normal mitral valve has an area of 4 to 5 cm^2, symptoms due to mitral stenosis seldom appear until the valve area falls below 1.5 cm^2. Severe mitral stenosis is present when the mitral valve area is 1 cm^2 or below; stenosis is moderate with an area of 1.0 to 1.5 cm^2 and mild with an area of 1.5 to 2.0 cm^2. The pulmonary arterial and right ventricular pressures may be elevated, with an associated elevation in pulmonary arteriolar resistance.

Symptoms attributable to mitral stenosis do not usually develop until about 20 years following the initial rheumatic injury, even though the murmur of mitral stenosis is clearly audible for the last 5 to 10 of these years. Then, over a 5- to 10-year period, the patient gradually becomes more symptomatic. Mitral stenosis occasionally may develop more rapidly, however, particularly when rheumatic fever occurs in infancy. Without surgical correction of the stenosis, severe congestive heart failure eventually develops and is the most common cause of death. Less common causes of death include catastrophic systemic arterial embolization, infective endocarditis, and pulmonary infection.

The asymptomatic patient with signs of mitral stenosis and normal sinus rhythm requires no therapy but should receive antibiotic prophylaxis for infective endocarditis during periods of high risk. Once atrial fibrillation develops, the patient should receive digitalis (for control of the ventricular rate) and anticoagulants. If symptoms of congestive heart failure appear, diuretics and salt restriction should be instituted. Once the patient is symptomatic despite digitalis and diuretics, mitral valve surgery should be considered. In the patient without mitral valve calcification, immobility of the valve, and concomitant mitral regurgitation, a commissurotomy (either "closed" or—more common today—"open") can usually be performed. If commissurotomy is not feasible, mitral valve replacement is the procedure of choice.

After commissurotomy or mitral valve replacement, the patient often remains in atrial fibrillation. As a result, continued digitalization is required to control the ventricular rate, and anticoagulation is recommended. Following mitral valve commissurotomy, the patient ordinarily has marked symptomatic improvement for several years (often as many as 10–15 years), then begins to have symptoms of recurrent stenosis. Despite more than 20 years of experience with a wide variety of prosthetic heart valves, it is now widely appreciated that no prosthesis is ideal, particularly in children and young adults. The use of mechanical prostheses (particularly in the mitral position) mandates lifelong anticoagulant therapy, which may be difficult to achieve. Conversely, the use of porcine heterograft or pericardial xenograft prostheses is associated with an alarming incidence of valve dysfunction due to stenosis and calcification of the leaflets in young patients. For this reason, every attempt should be made to perform a commissurotomy rather than a valve replacement, especially in younger patients with mitral stenosis.

Etiology, Clinical Characteristics, and Natural History

  1. Collins-Nakai RL, Rosenthal A, Casteneda AR, Bernhard WF, Nadas AS. Congenital mitral stenosis: a review of 20 years' experience. Circulation 1977; 56:1039–47.

A review of the clinical course, hemodynamic findings, treatment, and prognosis of 38 children with congenital mitral stenosis.

2. Dubin AA, March HW, Cohn K, Selzer A. Longitudinal hemodynamic and clinical study of mitral stenosis. Circulation 1971; 44:381–9.
   Of those patients with mitral stenosis, some demonstrate steadily increasing disability, whereas others have a distinctly more gradual course.

3. McHenry MM. Systemic arterial embolism in patients with mitral stenosis and minimal dyspnea. Am J Cardiol 1966; 18:169–74.
   Fourteen patients with mitral stenosis and systemic arterial embolization without symptoms of congestive heart failure are described. Mitral valve surgery was successful in preventing recurrent embolization.

4. Oakley C, Yusuf R, Hollman A. Coronary embolism and angina in mitral stenosis. Br Heart J 1961; 23:357–69.
   Embolic rather than thrombotic coronary occlusion may be the most common cause of ischemic cardiac pain in patients with mitral stenosis.

5. Olesen KH. The natural history of 271 patients with mitral stenosis under medical treatment. Br Heart J 1962; 24:349–57.
   The poor long-term outlook of patients with mitral stenosis treated medically is stressed.

6. Rowe JC, Bland EF, Sprague HB, White PD. The course of mitral stenosis without surgery: ten and twenty-year perspectives. Ann Intern Med 1960; 57:741–9.
   A study of 250 patients with mitral stenosis who were not operated on; after 10 years, 100 (40%) had died, and after 20 years 200 (80%) were dead.

7. Wroblewski E, James F, Spann JF, Bove AA. Right ventricular performance in mitral stenosis. Am J Cardiol 1981; 47:51–5.
   When pressure overload is not extreme, right ventricular function is normal in patients with mitral stenosis. However, left ventricular performance appears to be diminished in mitral stenosis for reasons that are not understood.

8. Gash AK, Carabello BA, Cepin D, Spann JF. Left ventricular ejection performance and systolic muscle function in patients with mitral stenosis. Circulation 1983; 67:148–54.
   Patients with mitral stenosis have reduced left ventricular ejection fractions because of reduced preload; left ventricular muscle function is generally normal.

Diagnosis

9. Amplatz K. The roentgenographic diagnosis of mitral and aortic valvular disease. Am Heart J 1962; 64:556–66.
   A thorough discussion of the findings on chest x-ray and cineangiography of patients with mitral valve disease.

10. Chen JTT, Behar VS, Morris JJ Jr, McIntosh HD, Lester RG. Correlation of roentgen findings with hemodynamic data in pure mitral stenosis. AJR 1968; 102:280–92.
    A carefully performed correlative study between findings on chest x-ray and at cardiac catheterization in patients with mitral stenosis.

11. Duchak JM Jr, Chang S, Feigenbaum H. The posterior mitral valve echo and the echocardiographic diagnosis of mitral stenosis. Am J Cardiol 1972; 29:628–32.
    In true mitral stenosis, the anterior and posterior mitral valve leaflets move concordantly during diastole.

12. Egeblad H, Berning J, Saunamaki K, Jacobsen JR, Wennevold A. Assessment of rheumatic mitral valve disease: value of echocardiography in patients clinically suspected of predominant stenosis. Br Heart J 1983; 49:38–44.
    In patients with pure mitral stenosis, mitral valve orifice area by 2-dimensional echo and cardiac catheterization correspond closely. However, when there is concomitant aortic or mitral regurgitation, echocardiography is less reliable.

13. Hugenholtz PG, Ryan TJ, Stein SW, Abelmann WH. The spectrum of pure mitral stenosis: hemodynamic studies in relation to clinical disability. Am J Cardiol 1962; 10:773–84.
    A detailed examination of catheterization hemodynamics in 44 patients with pure mitral stenosis.

14. Leo T, Hultgren H. Phonocardiographic characteristics of tight mitral stenosis. Medicine 1959; 38:85–101.

A detailed description of the classic phonocardiographic findings in 20 patients with mitral stenosis.

15. Levisman JA, Abbasi AS, Pearce ML. Posterior mitral leaflet motion in mitral stenosis. Circulation 1975; 51:511–4.
    Although most patients with mitral stenosis demonstrate anterior movement of the posterior mitral valve leaflet during diastole, a small number continue to have posterior movement of this leaflet.

16. Martin RP, Rakowski H, Kleiman JH, Beaver W, London E, Popp RL. Reliability and reproducibility of two dimensional echocardiographic measurement of the stenotic mitral valve orifice area. Am J Cardiol 1979; 43:560–8.
    With the proper care in obtaining two-dimensional echocardiographic images, there is a good correlation between echocardiographic and hemodynamic measurements of mitral valve area in patients with mitral stenosis.

17. Nanda NC, Gramiak R, Shah PM, deWeese JA. Mitral commisurotomy versus replacement: preoperative evaluation by echocardiography. Circulation 1975; 51:263–7.
    Echocardiographic assessment of mitral valve calcification and mobility is valuable in planning the surgical approach in patients with pure or predominant mitral stenosis.

18. Nichol PM, Gilbert BW, Kisslo JA. Two-dimensional echocardiographic assessment of mitral stenosis. Circulation 1977; 55:120–8.
    With this technique, the stenotic mitral valve can be visualized directly.

19. Strunk BL, London EJ, Fitzgerald J, Popp RL, Barry WH. The assessment of mitral stenosis and prosthetic mitral valve obstruction using the posterior aortic wall echocardiogram. Circulation 1977; 55:885–91.
    A useful echocardiographic method of gauging the severity of mitral stenosis by estimating the rapidity of left atrial emptying during early diastole.

20. Wann LS, Weyman AE, Feigenbaum H, Dillon JC, Johnston KW, Eggleton RC. Determination of mitral valve area by cross-sectional echocardiography. Ann Intern Med 1978; 88:337–41.
    In both stenosis and regurgitation, two-dimensional echocardiography in experienced hands appears to be a reliable method for measuring mitral valve area.

Therapy

21. Cohn LH, Sanders JH, Collins JJ Jr. Actuarial comparison of Hancock porcine and prosthetic disc valves for isolated mitral valve replacement. Circulation 1976; 54(Suppl III):60–3.
    The porcine valve offers a reduced risk of thromboembolism when compared to a prosthetic disc valve.

22. Ellis LB, Harken DE. Closed valvuloplasty for mitral stenosis: a 12-year follow up study of 1,571 patients. N Engl J Med 1964; 270:643–50.
    The overall survival of patients with mitral stenosis is clearly better when treated surgically than medically.

23. Macmanus Q, Grunkemeier G, Thomas D, Lambert LE, Starr A. The Starr-Edwards Model 6000 valve: a fifteen-year follow-up of the first successful mitral prosthesis. Circulation 1977; 56:623–5.
    Despite a high rate of thromboembolism, this original Starr-Edwards valve has proved to be durable.

24. Zener JC, Hancock EW, Shumway NE, Harrison DC. Regression of extreme pulmonary hypertension after mitral valve surgery. Am J Cardiol 1972; 30:820–6.
    In patients with mitral stenosis, even extreme pulmonary hypertension and increased pulmonary vascular resistance regress if surgery adequately decompresses the left atrium.

CHRONIC MITRAL REGURGITATION

Chronic mitral regurgitation can occur as a result of certain congenital diseases, including Marfan's syndrome, the Ehlers-Danlos syndrome, endocardial fibroelastosis, idiopathic hypertrophic subaortic stenosis, endocardial cushion defect, and anomalous origin of a coronary artery from the pulmonary artery. However, in the adult patient, mitral regurgitation is usually acquired. It can result from rheumatic involvement of the mitral valve, in which case it tends to occur in association with some degree of valvular stenosis. In the United States, the most common cause of *isolated severe* mitral regurgitation is myxomatous degeneration of the valve. Mitral regurgitation can also occur in patients with coronary artery disease due to papillary muscle rupture or dysfunction. In addition, it can result from mitral valve endocarditis, rupture of the chordae tendineae, or left ventricular dilatation with stretching of the mitral valve anulus. Finally, it occasionally occurs in patients with blunt or sharp cardiac trauma or in association with a heavily calcified mitral anulus fibrosus.

The patient with chronic mitral regurgitation usually notes symptoms of pulmonary vascular congestion. Early in the course of the disease, the patient may have dyspnea only with exertion. As the regurgitation becomes more severe, the patient notes dyspnea with less exertion, and orthopnea and paroxysmal nocturnal dyspnea appear. In response to an elevated pulmonary capillary pressure, the pulmonary arterial pressure increases, eventually leading to pulmonary hypertension. In response to this, the right ventricle may eventually dilate and fail, as a result of which peripheral edema and abdominal tenderness develop (the latter due to hepatomegaly), and ascitic fluid accumulates. Angina pectoris or syncope may occur, probably due to systemic hypoxemia, hypotension, and a reduced cardiac output.

An occasional patient with chronic mitral regurgitation may complain primarily of fatigue, which is caused by a low cardiac output and—importantly—by the failure of output to increase appropriately during exertion. Patients with all sorts of mitral valve disease sometimes complain of atypical chest pain. Recurrent episodes of peripheral arterial embolization occur in some patients with chronic mitral regurgitation and atrial fibrillation, although such episodes occur more commonly in patients with mitral stenosis. As a result of such embolization, the patient may note the sudden onset of a neurologic deficit, chest pain (due to coronary artery involvement), or abdominal discomfort (due to embolization of a splanchnic artery).

The physical examination of the patient with chronic mitral regurgitation reveals a brisk but low-volume carotid upstroke. The pulse may be regular or irregularly irregular due to atrial fibrillation. The incidence of atrial fibrillation increases with age. If right ventricular failure has occurred, the patient may have jugular venous distention, hepatomegaly, and peripheral edema. On palpation of the precordium, the point of maximal impulse is displaced downward and to the left. A systolic thrill or an S_3 may be palpable at the apex. On auscultation, the S_1 is usually diminished in intensity. The S_2 is widely split; if pulmonary hypertension is present, the P_2 may be especially loud. A holosystolic murmur is often loudest at the apex and radiates to the axilla; it may also be audible in the back and over the entire precordium. At times, it radiates up the vertebral column and may be heard on top of the head. If the regurgitation is severe, an S_3 is usually easily audible at the apex, and a short diastolic rumble (due to increased flow across a nonstenotic mitral valve) may be audible. In the patient with mitral regurgitation due to posterior papillary muscle dysfunction or rupture, the murmur may radiate medially rather than to the axilla, thus resembling a left ventricular outflow tract murmur.

The chest x-ray in the patient with chronic mitral regurgitation reveals an enlarged left atrium and ventricle. In addition, one may see pulmonary vascular redistribution and calcification of the mitral anulus. The ECG shows sinus rhythm or atrial fibrillation. If the patient is in sinus rhythm, the P wave morphology usually suggests left atrial enlargement. Left ventricular hypertrophy is usually present. The M-mode echocardiogram demonstrates an enlarged left ventricle with symmetric contraction. The left atrium is almost always enlarged and in some patients is huge.

At the time of cardiac catheterization, the left atrial (pulmonary capillary wedge) pressure is elevated and may demonstrate a large regurgitant wave. The pulmonary arterial and right ventricular pressures may be elevated. The left ventriculogram demonstrates regurgitation of contrast material from the left ventricle into the left atrium. The cardiac output may be normal or depressed; with minimal to moderate exertion, it may not increase appropriately, signifying reduced myocardial reserve.

As with mitral stenosis, the patient with chronic mitral regurgitation has a long asymptomatic period between the episode of rheumatic fever and the onset of cardiac symptoms, sometimes 15 to 30 years. The murmur of mitral regurgitation is audible during this period. Finally, fatigue or symptoms of left ventricular failure occur, and the patient's symptoms gradually worsen over a 5- to 10-year period.

All patients with chronic mitral regurgitation, even those who are asymptomatic, should receive antibiotic prophylaxis at the time of surgical procedures or dental manipulations. If atrial fibrillation develops, the patient should receive anticoagulants as well as digitalis to control the heart rate. In the minimally symptomatic patient with chronic mitral regurgitation, digitalis and diuretics are probably sufficient to induce symptomatic relief. If symptoms are not readily controlled by digitalis and diuretics, if there is evidence of rapidly progressive left ventricular dilatation, or if there is a deterioration in left ventricular performance, mitral valve surgery should be performed. This entails either an annuloplasty and plastic reparative procedure of the mitral valve (with or without the use of a ring to support the anulus) or valve replacement. Because of the inherent problems associated with the use of any prosthetic valve, particularly in young patients and especially in the mitral position, a reparative procedure should be performed if at all possible.

Clinical and Hemodynamic Features

1. Bentivoglio L, Uricchio J, Goldberg H. Clinical and hemodynamic features of advanced rheumatic mitral regurgitation. Am J Med 1961; 30:372–81.
   Patients with chronic mitral regurgitation remain asymptomatic for many years, then complain of dyspnea or fatigue.
2. Braunwald E. Mitral regurgitation: physiological, clinical, and surgical considerations. N Engl J Med 1969; 281:425–33.
   An elegant discussion of the effects of mitral regurgitation on left ventricular function.
3. Ellis LB, Ramirez A. The clinical course of patients with severe "rheumatic" mitral insufficiency. Am Heart J 1969; 78:406–18.
   Many patients with mitral regurgitation remain totally asymptomatic for many years.
4. Fuchs RM, Heuser RR, Yin FCP, Brinker JA. Limitations of pulmonary wedge V waves in diagnosing mitral regurgitation. Am J Cardiol 1982; 49:849–54.
   Mitral regurgitation is the most common cause of large V waves, but they are neither sensitive nor specific for severe regurgitation.

5. Grossman M, Knott AP Jr, Jacoby WJ Jr. Calcified anulus fibrosus with mitral insufficiency in the Marfan syndrome. Arch Intern Med 1968; 121:561–3.
    A young woman (age 21) is reported with the Marfan syndrome, massive calcification of the mitral anulus, and severe mitral regurgitation.

6. Korn D, DeSanctis RW, Sell S. Massive calcification of the mitral anulus: a clinicopathological study of 14 cases. N Engl J Med 1962; 267:900–9.
    The original description of a heavily calcified mitral anulus.

7. Merendino KA, Hessel EA II. The "murmur on top of the head" in acquired mitral insufficiency. JAMA 1967; 199:892–6.
    Seven patients whose murmur of mitral regurgitation radiated to the cranium are described; in 5, the mitral regurgitation was due to ruptured chordae tendineae of the anterior mitral valve leaflet.

8. Movitt ER, Gerstl B. Pure mitral insufficiency of rheumatic origin in adults. Ann Intern Med 1953; 38:981–1001.
    A thorough discussion of the diagnostic features of pure, isolated mitral regurgitation.

9. Perloff JK, Roberts WC. The mitral apparatus: functional anatomy of mitral regurgitation. Circulation 1972; 46:227–39.
    An anatomic analysis of the mitral valve apparatus in normal patients and those with regurgitation.

10. Priest EA, Finlayson JK, Short DS. The x-ray manifestations in the heart and lungs of mitral regurgitation. Prog Cardiovasc Dis 1962; 5:219–29.
    Patients with mitral regurgitation usually have enlargement of both left atrium and ventricle, and the left atrium can be gigantic.

11. Selzer A, Katayama F. Mitral regurgitation: clinical patterns, pathophysiology, and natural history. Medicine 1972; 51:337–66.
    An extensive review of acute and chronic mitral regurgitation.

12. Shillingford JP. The estimation of severity of mitral incompetence. Prog Cardiovasc Dis 1962; 5:248–63.
    An accurate assessment of the magnitude of mitral regurgitation can be difficult; it should involve a careful analysis of the physical examination, ECG, left ventriculography, and hemodynamic findings at catheterization.

13. Talner NS, Stern AM, Sloan HE Jr. Congenital mitral insufficiency. Circulation 1961; 23:339–49.
    Ten patients with congenital mitral regurgitation are discussed, including their hemodynamic findings.

14. Waller BF, Morrow AG, Maron BJ, Del Negro AA, Kent KM, McGrath FJ, Wallace RB, McIntosh CL, Roberts WC. Etiology of clinically isolated, severe, chronic, pure mitral regurgitation: analysis of 97 patients over 30 years of age having mitral valve replacement. Am Heart J 1982; 104:276–88.
    In these 97 patients with pure mitral regurgitation, the etiology was mitral valve prolapse in 60 (62%), papillary muscle dysfunction in 29 (30%), endocarditis in 5 (5%), and rheumatic in 3 (3%).

Therapy

15. Boucher CA, Bingham JB, Osbakken MD, Okada RD, Strauss HW, Block PC, Levine FH, Phillips HR, Pohost GM. Early changes in left ventricular size and function after correction of left ventricular volume overload. Am J Cardiol 1981; 47:991–1004.
    Removal of chronic left ventricular volume overload due to aortic or mitral regurgitation produces an early decrease in ejection fraction and end-diastolic volume, and the reduction in ejection fraction persists in patients with mitral regurgitation.

16. Cohn LH, Sanders JH, Collins JJ Jr. Actuarial comparison of Hancock porcine and prosthetic disc valves for isolated mitral valve replacement. Circulation 1976; 54(Suppl III):60–3.
    The porcine valve offers a reduced risk of thromboembolism when compared to a prosthetic disc valve.

17. Gann D, Colin C, Hildner FJ, Samet P, Yahr WZ, Byrd C, Greenberg JJ. Mitral valve replacement in medically unresponsive congestive heart failure due to papillary muscle dysfunction. Circulation 1977; 56(Suppl II):101–4.

For patients with severe congestive heart failure due to papillary muscle dysfunction, mitral valve replacement can be performed successfully and with an acceptable risk.

18. Goodman DJ, Rossen RM, Holloway EL, Alderman EL, Harrison DC. Effect of nitroprusside on left ventricular dynamics in mitral regurgitation. Circulation 1974; 50:1025–32.
In 14 patients with chronic mitral regurgitation, nitroprusside caused a decrease in left-sided filling pressures and an increase in cardiac output.

19. Greenberg BH, Massie BM, Brundage BH, Botvinick EH, Parmley WW, Chatterjee K. Beneficial effects of hydralazine in severe mitral regurgitation. Circulation 1978; 58:273–9.
Reduction of afterload with hydralazine decreases the amount of regurgitation and increases cardiac output.

20. Harshaw CW, Grossman W, Munro AB, McLaurin LP. Reduced systemic vascular resistance as therapy for severe mitral regurgitation of valvular origin. Ann Intern Med 1975, 83:312–6.
In 7 patients, nitroprusside caused a reduction in left atrial and left ventricular filling pressures and a substantial increase in cardiac output.

21. Lappas DG, Ohtaka M, Fahmy NR, Buckley MJ. Systemic and pulmonary effects of nitroprusside during mitral valve replacement in patients with mitral regurgitation. Circulation 1978; 58(Suppl I):18–22.
The intraoperative infusion of nitroprusside increases cardiac output and reduces mitral regurgitation in patients undergoing valve replacement.

22. Macmanus Q, Grunkemeier G, Thomas D, Lambert LE, Starr A. The Starr-Edwards Model 6000 valve: a fifteen year follow-up of the first successful mitral prosthesis. Circulation 1977; 56:623–5.
Despite a high rate of thromboembolism, the original Starr-Edwards valve has been durable.

23. Phillips HR, Levine FH, Carter JE, Boucher CA, Osbakken MD, Okada RD, Akins CW, Daggett WM, Buckley MJ, Pohost GM. Mitral valve replacement for isolated mitral regurgitation: analysis of clinical course and late postoperative left ventricular ejection fraction. Am J Cardiol 1981; 48:647–54.
In addition to age, only preoperative left ventricular ejection fraction predicts survival in patients undergoing mitral valve replacement for mitral regurgitation. However, in most patients, there is a postoperative decrease in ejection fraction.

24. Salomon NW, Stinson EB, Griepp RB, Shumway NE. Mitral valve replacement: long-term evaluation of prosthesis-related mortality and morbidity. Circulation 1977; 56(Suppl II):94–101.
A review of a large series of mitral valve replacements with various prosthetic valves, documenting the lower incidence of thromboembolic complications with porcine heterografts.

25. Schuler G, Peterson KL, Johnson A, Francis G, Dennish G, Utley J, Daily PO, Ashburn W, Ross J Jr. Temporal response of left ventricular performance to mitral valve surgery. Circulation 1979; 59:1218–31.
In this study, patients with a left ventricular end-systolic dimension greater than 5.0 cm or an end-diastolic dimension greater than 7.0 cm on M-mode echocardiography showed evidence of persistent left ventricular dysfunction following valve replacement.

26. Yoran C, Yellin EL, Becker RM, Gabbay S, Frater RWM, Sonnenblick EH. Mechanism of reduction of mitral regurgitation with vasodilator therapy. Am J Cardiol 1979; 43:773–7.
Reduction of left ventricular volume (with a concomitant reduction in the size of the mitral regurgitant orifice) rather than a mere reduction in afterload may explain the acute beneficial effects of vasodilators in patients with mitral regurgitation.

27. Huikuri HV, Ikaheimo MJ, Linnaluoto MMK, Takkunen JT. Left ventricular response to isometric exercise and its value in predicting the change in ventricular function after mitral valve replacement for mitral regurgitation. Am J Cardiol 1983; 51:1110–5.
Isometric exercise-induced changes in left ventricular function appear to predict the results of mitral valve replacement in patients with mitral regurgitation.

ACUTE MITRAL REGURGITATION

Acute mitral regurgitation is often a life-threatening event that leads to pulmonary vascular congestion and pulmonary edema. It is generally due to (1) rupture of the chordae tendineae, (2) rupture of a papillary muscle, or (3) acute bacterial endocarditis (most often staphylococcal), leading to mitral valve damage with rapidly progressive regurgitation. Rupture of the chordae tendineae can occur in association with several conditions that affect the mitral valve, including myxomatous degeneration, rheumatic carditis, blunt or sharp trauma to the chest, bacterial endocarditis, or one of several connective tissue disorders, but it does not occur as a result of myocardial ischemia or infarction. Conversely, rupture of a papillary muscle almost invariably results from myocardial infarction. Myocardial ischemia in the absence of infarction may cause transient papillary muscle dysfunction with resultant mitral regurgitation.

The patient with acute mitral regurgitation complains of severe dyspnea, orthopnea, and paroxysmal nocturnal dyspnea, and he often can recall the exact time at which these symptoms appeared. If the regurgitation is due to a ruptured papillary muscle, the patient may complain of the symptoms of a myocardial infarction: chest pain, diaphoresis, nausea, and vomiting. On physical examination, the patient is tachypneic and dyspneic and often prefers the upright to the supine posture. The peripheral pulse is regular and rapid. There is a loud, rough systolic murmur at the apex; at times it is holosystolic, and at other times it diminishes in amplitude in late systole. *If the posterior papillary muscle or its chordae tendineae are involved, the resultant murmur may radiate to the base, in which case it may be confused with the murmur of aortic stenosis.* The intensity of the murmur bears no relationship to the magnitude of regurgitation; thus, severe mitral regurgitation may be accompanied by a loud or a faint murmur. Both an S_3 and S_4 are frequently audible. If the magnitude of the regurgitation is large, a diastolic flow rumble across the mitral valve may be audible. Examination of the lungs generally reveals moist inspiratory rales. Peripheral edema is unusual.

The chest x-ray generally demonstrates only mild cardiomegaly without left atrial enlargement. There is usually pulmonary vascular redistribution or even pulmonary edema. The ECG usually demonstrates sinus rhythm (rather than atrial fibrillation). A flail mitral valve leaflet (due to a ruptured papillary muscle or chordae tendineae) may be visible on M-mode or two-dimensional echocardiography. The left ventricle is modestly enlarged at end-diastole, whereas the end-systolic dimension is often normal; as a result, the ejection fraction may be high. If the acute mitral regurgitation is due to rupture of a papillary muscle, the echocardiogram may demonstrate an akinetic septal or posterior wall.

At the time of cardiac catheterization, there is angiographic evidence of mitral regurgitation. The left atrial chamber is usually normal in size or only minimally enlarged. The mean pulmonary capillary wedge pressure (which is equal to left atrial pressure) is elevated, with especially prominent regurgitant waves. In most instances, the regurgitant waves are more than twice the height of the mean pulmonary capillary wedge pressure. If the regurgitation is severe, the regurgitant waves may be transmitted to the main pulmonary artery and, therefore, may appear on the pulmonary arterial pressure trace.

Since the patient with acute severe mitral regurgitation tolerates the condition poorly, he usually requires immediate valve replacement. If the risk of valve replacement is prohibitive (as in the patient with myocardial infarction and papillary muscle rupture), hemodynamic stability may be obtained temporarily by intra-aortic balloon counterpulsation and afterload reduction with an agent such as sodium nitroprusside. If possible, the patient should be stabilized and maintained on medical therapy for 3 to 6 weeks, after which mitral valve replacement can be performed, at least on a semielective basis. However, it may not be possible to stabilize the patient medically, and emergency valve replacement may be mandatory, in which case the operative mortality is high.

Clinical Characteristics and Diagnosis

1. Breneman GM, Drake EH. Ruptured papillary muscle following myocardial infarction with long survival: report of two cases. Circulation 1962; 25:862–8.
   Two patients with ruptured papillary muscle and prolonged survival are discussed.
2. DeBusk RF, Harrison DC. The clincal spectrum of papillary muscle disease. N Engl J Med 1969; 281:1458–67.
   A thorough discussion of papillary muscle dysfunction and rupture.
3. Child JS, Skorton DJ, Taylor RD, Krivokapich J, Abbasi AS, Wong M, Shah PD. M-mode and cross-sectional echocardiographic features of flail posterior mitral leaflets. Am J Cardiol 1979; 44:1383–90.
   A succinct review of the M-mode and two-dimensional echocardiographic findings associated with a flail posterior mitral leaflet.
4. Marchand P, Barlow JB, DuPlessis LA, Webster I. Mitral regurgitation with rupture of normal chordae tendineae. Br Heart J 1966, 28:746–58.
   In 6 patients, severe chordal rupture occurred in histologically normal chordae because of severe tension placed on them by anular dilatation.
5. Meister SG, Helfant RH. Rapid bedside differentiation of ruptured interventricular septum from acute mitral insufficiency. N Engl J Med 1972; 287:1024–5.
   Bedside catheterization of the right heart allows one to separate a ruptured papillary muscle, with resultant mitral regurgitation, from a ruptured interventricular septum.
6. Mintz GS, Kotler MN, Segal BL, Parry WR. Two-dimensional echocardiographic recognition of ruptured chordae tendineae. Circulation 1978; 57:244–50.
   Two-dimensional echo can identify flail mitral and tricuspid valves and is useful in distinguishing ruptured chordae from valvular prolapse.
7. Mintz GS, Kotler MN, Parry WR, Segal BL. Statistical comparison of M-mode and two dimensional echocardiographic diagnosis of flail mitral leaflets. Am J Cardiol 1980; 45:253–9.
   Two dimensional echocardiography is distinctly superior to M-mode echocardiography in the diagnosis of flail mitral valve leaflets.
8. Ronan JA Jr, Steelman RB, DeLeon AC Jr, Waters TJ, Perloff JK, Harvey WP. The clinical diagnosis of acute severe mitral insufficiency. Am J Cardiol 1971; 27:284–90.
   The differences between acute and chronic mitral regurgitation are discussed.
9. Selzer A, Kelly JJ Jr, Vannitamby M, Walker P, Gerbode F, Kerth WJ. The syndrome of mitral insufficiency due to isolated rupture of the chordae tendineae. Am J Med 1967; 43:822–36.
   Rupture of the chordae tendineae can result in trivial or massive mitral regurgitation, depending on how many chordae are involved.
10. Sweatmen T, Selzer A, Kamagaki M, Cohn K. Echocardiographic diagnosis of mitral regurgitation due to ruptured chordae tendineae. Circulation 1972; 46:580–6.
    In many patients with ruptured chordae, one can visualize the flail leaflet and chordae by M-mode echocardiography.

Therapy

11. Austen WG, Sokol DM, DeSanctis RW, Sanders CA. Surgical treatment of papillary muscle rupture complicating myocardial infarction. N Engl J Med 1968; 278:1137–41.
    Mitral valve replacement was performed in 5 patients 14 days to 14 months after papillary muscle rupture; 4 of them survived.
12. DeBusk RF, Kleiger RE, Ebnother CL, Daily PO, Harrison DC. Successful early operation for papillary muscle rupture. Chest 1970; 58:175–8.

A report of a patient in whom early surgical intervention (within 36 hours of myo-cardial infarction) successfully alleviated mitral regurgitation.

MITRAL VALVE PROLAPSE SYNDROME

Mitral valve prolapse syndrome (also called the midsystolic click-murmur syndrome, Barlow's syndrome, billowing mitral valve syndrome, and the floppy valve syndrome) is common but extremely variable in its clinical and morphologic manifestations. It is the most prevalent valvular abnormality, affecting 5 to 10 percent of the general population. On the one extreme is the asymptomatic patient with only auscultatory, echocardiographic, or angiographic evidence of prolapse, whereas on the other is the patient with severe mitral regurgitation or life-threatening arrhythmias.

The etiology and pathogenic mechanism of the mitral valve prolapse syndrome are diverse. It is most commonly due to myxomatous degeneration or proliferation of the mitral valve, anulus, and chordae tendineae, with resultant redundancy and abnormality of the valve leaflets. The posterior leaflet may be involved alone, or both the posterior and anterior leaflets may be involved. Prolapse of only the anterior leaflet is rare, however. In addition, the mitral valve prolapse syndrome can occur in the absence of myxomatous degeneration; it has been reported in patients with Marfan's syndrome (90% of cases), rheumatic endocarditis, coronary artery disease, congestive cardiomyopathy, myocarditis, idiopathic hypertrophic subaortic stenosis, following mitral valve surgery, secundum atrial septal defect, trauma, left ventricular aneurysm, and a variety of connective tissue disorders.

Most patients with the mitral valve prolapse syndrome are asymptomatic. Those with symptoms may complain of palpitations, chest discomfort, or fatigue. The palpitations may be due to atrial or ventricular tachyarrhythmias. Although the chest pain may be typical of angina, it is usually somewhat atypical and may last for hours or days. Syncope and presyncope occur occasionally, and sudden death has been reported rarely. Many of the symptoms in patients with the mitral valve prolapse syndrome may be due to autonomic nervous system dysfunction with resultant postural hypotension and sinus tachycardia.

The physical examination often reveals an asthenic body habitus. The thorax may show a loss of normal thoracic kyphosis (so-called straight back), a pectus excavatum, and scoliosis. On cardiac examination, the point of maximal impulse is usually not displaced laterally. On auscultation, a high-frequency click (or combination of clicks) occurs in midsystole. At a given time, this click may be absent, single, or multiple and may be heard in mid-, late, or even early systole. The click is frequently (but not invariably) followed by a late systolic murmur. Any maneuver that decreases left ventricular volume (reduction of impedance to left ventricular outflow, reduction in venous return, or an augmentation of contractility) results in an earlier occurrence of prolapse during systole, so that the click and murmur move closer to the S_1. In contrast, any maneuver that increases left ventricular cavitary size (increase in impedance to left ventricular ejection, increase in venous return, or decrease in contractility) moves the click toward the S_2 and delays the murmur's onset. In most patients with mitral valve prolapse, the mitral regurgitation is trivial, but an occasional patient may have severe mitral regurgitation and require valve replacement. *Indeed, myxomatous degeneration of the mitral valve is the most common cause of isolated severe mitral regurgitation.*

The chest x-ray usually demonstrates a heart of normal size and configuration. There may be thoracic bony abnormalities. The ECG may demonstrate many abnormalities. Most commonly, S–T and T wave flattening or inversion is seen in the inferior leads. The Q–T interval may be prolonged. Paroxysmal supraventricular tachycardia is the most common *sustained* tachyarrhythmia in patients with the mitral valve prolapse syndrome, probably related to the high incidence of left-sided AV bypass tracts in patients with this condition. Specifically, 60 percent of patients with the mitral valve prolapse syndrome and supraventricular tachycardia have such a bypass tract, whereas only 20 percent of those with supraventricular tachycardia without mitral valve prolapse have a bypass tract. A wide variety of ventricular and supraventricular arrhythmias have been described in patients with this syndrome. *Indeed, the mitral value prolapse syndrome should be considered in patients with otherwise unexplained tachyarrhythmias.* Ventricular premature beats occur commonly. Serious ventricular arrhythmias are more frequent in patients with S–T and T wave abnormalities on the resting ECG. Finally, conduction disturbances may occur in patients with mitral valve prolapse, including first degree AV block, right or left bundle branch block, and (rarely) second or third degree AV block.

On M-mode echocardiography, late systolic prolapse of one or both mitral valve leaflets can be directly visualized as posterior movement interrupting the normal anterior motion. In addition, one may see exaggerated mitral leaflet mobility, producing diastolic contact with the interventricular septum. Two-dimensional echocardiography allows for the direct visualization of the prolapsing mitral valve leaflets. In many patients with auscultatory or echocardiographic evidence of mitral valve prolapse, the left ventricular cineangiogram does not demonstrate any abnormality of the mitral valve; rather, it may show only late systolic mitral regurgitation. Although gross mitral valve prolapse may be readily evident on the left ventricular cineangiogram, subtle evidence of prolapse is difficult to detect. Therefore, the diagnosis of prolapse can be made by phonocardiography alone, echocardiography alone, or a combination of the two. Certain physical and pharmacologic interventions are designed either to enhance or to diminish the severity of prolapse: prompt standing, inhalation of amyl nitrite, and the straining phase of the Valsalva maneuver cause a reduction in left ventricular size, and the click and murmur move earlier in systole; conversely, leg raising, squatting, and maximal isometric exercise delay the click and the onset of the murmur.

Most patients with prolapse are not limited by symptoms and do not have progressive disease. However, the patient with mitral valve prolapse may have one of four serious complications: (1) infective endocarditis, (2) rupture of the chordae tendineae, (3) progressive severe mitral regurgitation, or (4) intractable arrhythmias and even sudden death. One of these serious complications occurs in 10 to 15 percent of patients with prolapse, most commonly in those with an easily audible late systolic murmur. All patients with mitral valve prolapse are at risk of infective endocarditis. Therefore, antibiotic prophylaxis is advisable in the patient with a typical systolic murmur and characteristic echocardiographic features. Opinions are divided as to whether patients with only a nonejection click or minor echocardiographic abnormalities should receive prophylaxis. Spontaneous rupture of the chordae tendineae may suddenly worsen mitral regurgitation in the patient with a previous click-murmur, changing trivial mitral regurgitation to that which may be hemodynamically severe. An occasional patient with mitral valve prolapse has the slow, progressive worsening of mitral regurgitation that finally requires valve replacement. Finally, a rare patient with prolapse dies suddenly, presumably as a consequence of ventricular arrhythmias. Propranolol is useful in patients with frequent ventricular premature beats or supraventricular tachycardia, and if necessary, quinidine or procainamide may be added. In addition, propranolol is often effective in the treatment of chest pain in these patients. Asymptomatic patients (or those whose principal complaint is anxiety) with no evidence of arrhythmias or ECG abnormalities should be reassured about their prognosis and seen every 2 to 3 years. Conversely, patients with a long systolic murmur should be followed more closely and treated appropriately if signs or symptoms of cardiac decompensation occur.

Clinical and Echocardiographic Characteristics

1. Barlow JB, Bosman CK, Pocock WA, Marchand P. Late systolic murmurs and non-ejection (mid-late) systolic clicks: an analysis of 90 patients. Br Heart J 1968; 30:203–18.
   The late systolic murmur denotes mitral regurgitation, whereas the nonejection clicks result from unequal lengths of the chordae tendineae.
2. Barlow JB, Pocock WA. The problem of non-ejection systolic clicks and associated mitral systolic murmurs: emphasis on the billowing mitral leaflet syndrome. Am Heart J 1975; 90:636–55.
   A superb overview of this syndrome.
3. Cabeen WR Jr, Reza MJ, Kovick RB, Stern MS. Mitral valve prolapse and conduction defects in Ehlers Danlos syndrome. Arch Intern Med 1977; 137:1227–31.
   A case of type 3 Ehlers-Danlos syndrome with associated mitral valve prolapse and bifascicular block is described.
4. Criley JM, Lewis KB, Humphries JO, Ross RS. Prolapse of the mitral valve: clinical and cine-angiocardiographic findings. Br Heart J 1966; 28:488–96.
   One of the early studies attempting to correlate the phonocardiographic and angiographic features of mitral prolapse.
5. DeMaria AN, King JF, Bogren HG, Lies JE, Mason DT. The variable spectrum of echocardiographic manifestations of the mitral valve prolapse syndrome. Circulation 1974; 50:33–41.
   The echocardiographic findings of mitral valve prolapse are quite variable and often occur in the absence of classical auscultatory findings.
6. Devereux RB, Perloff JK, Reichek N, Josephson ME. Mitral valve prolapse. Circulation 1976; 54:3–14.
   A concise yet adequately detailed review of valve prolapse.
7. Gaffney FA, Karlsson ES, Campbell W, Schutte JE, Nixon JV, Willerson JT, Blomqvist CG. Autonomic dysfunction in women with mitral valve prolapse syndrome. Circulation 1979; 59:894–901.
   This study suggests decreased parasympathetic and increased alpha-adrenergic tone and responsiveness in women with mitral valve prolapse.
8. Hutter AM Jr, Dinsmore RE, Willerson JT, DeSanctis RW. Early systolic clicks due to mitral valve prolapse. Circulation 1971; 44:516–22.
   The click due to mitral valve prolapse may be early rather than midsystolic in some patients.
9. Jeresaty RM. Mitral valve prolapse-click syndrome. Prog Cardiovasc Dis 1973; 15:623–52.
   An in-depth review of mitral valve prolapse, including a summary of 100 patients seen by the author.
10. Josephson ME, Horowitz LN, Kastor JA. Paroxysmal supraventricular tachycardia in patients with mitral valve prolapse. Circulation 1978; 57:111–5.
    There is a high incidence of atrioventricular bypass tracts in patients with mitral valve prolapse. They are always left-sided.
11. Kerber RE, Isaeff DM, Hancock EW. Echocardiographic patterns in patients with the syndrome of systolic click and late systolic murmur. N Engl J Med 1971; 284:691–3.
    Detailed echocardiographic studies of 10 patients with mitral valve prolapse support the cineangiographic observation that this syndrome results from systolic prolapse of one or both mitral valve leaflets into the left atrium.

12. Lesch M. Mitral valve prolapse: a clinical spectrum. N Engl J Med 1976;
    294:1117–8.
    *Serious complications (i.e., death, bacterial endocarditis) are very rare in patients
    with mitral valve prolapse.*

13. Markiewicz W, Stoner J, London E, Hunt SA, Popp RL. Mitral valve prolapse in
    100 presumably healthy young females. Circulation 1976; 53:464–73.
    *Of 100 healthy coeds, 21 were found to have pansystolic or late systolic prolapse by
    echocardiography.*

14. McLaren MJ, Hawkins DM, Lachman AS, Lakier JB, Pocock WA, Barlow JB.
    Non-ejection systolic clicks and mitral systolic murmurs in black school children
    in Soweto Johannesburg. Br Heart J 1976; 38:718–24.
    *In this study of more than 12,000 schoolchildren in Johannesburg, a nonejection
    click and/or late systolic murmur were present in 14 of every 1,000 children stud-
    ied.*

15. Morganroth J, Jones RH, Chen CC, Naito M. Two dimensional echocardiography
    in mitral, aortic and tricuspid valve prolapse: the clinical problem, cardiac nu-
    clear imaging considerations and a proposed standard for diagnosis. Am J Cardiol
    1980; 46:1164–77.
    *Primary myxomatous degeneration is not confined to the mitral valve. Two-dimen-
    sional echocardiography has detected tricuspid valve prolapse in up to 50% and
    aortic valve prolapse in 20% of patients with idiopathic mitral valve prolapse.*

16. Pocock WA, Barlow JB. Etiology and electrocardiographic features of the billow-
    ing posterior mitral leaflet syndrome: analysis of a further 130 patients with a
    late systolic murmur or non-ejection systolic click. Am J Med 1971; 51:731–9.
    *Of 130 patients with prolapse, no cause could be found in 80, but in 23 a familial
    occurrence was noted, and in 18 prolapse was associated with some form of congen-
    ital heart disease.*

17. Popp RL, Brown OR, Silverman JF, Harrison DC. Echocardiographic abnormali-
    ties in the mitral valve prolapse syndrome. Circulation 1974; 49:428–33.
    *Echocardiographic evidence of mitral valve prolapse may be unassociated with
    auscultatory findings.*

18. Procacci PM, Savran SV, Schreiter SL, Bryson AL. Prevalence of clinical mitral
    valve prolapse in 1,169 young women. N Engl J Med 1976; 294:1086–8.
    Mitral valve prolapse is present in over 6% of otherwise healthy young women.

19. Reid JVO. Mid-systolic clicks. S Afr Med J 1961; 35:353–5.
    The original clinical description of mitral valve prolapse.

20. Salomon J, Shah PM, Heinle RA. Thoracic skeletal abnormalities in idiopathic
    mitral valve prolapse. Am J Cardiol 1975; 36:32–6.
    *In 24 patients with prolapse, pectus excavatum was present in 62%, "straight back"
    in 17%, and severe scoliosis in 8%; in sum, 18 of the 24 (75%) had a definite tho-
    racic skeletal deformity.*

21. Schreiber TL, Feigenbaum H, Weyman AE. Effect of atrial septal defect repair on
    left ventricular geometry and degree of mitral valve prolapse. Circulation 1980;
    61:888–96.
    *Atrial septal defect closure leads to normalization of left ventricular geometry and
    is associated with a decrease in the degree of prolapse in those with this entity.*

22. Shell WE, Walton JA, Clifford ME, Willis PW III. The familial occurrence of the
    syndrome of mid-late systolic click and late systolic murmur. Circulation 1969;
    39:327–37.
    Four families in which prolapse was present in numerous members are described.

23. Smith ER, Fraser DB, Purdy JW, Anderson RN. Angiographic diagnosis of mitral
    valve prolapse: correlation with echocardiography. Am J Cardiol 1977; 40:165–70.
    *Some end-systolic bulging of one or more scallops of the mitral valve into the left
    atrium is a common angiographic finding and does not necessarily reflect mitral
    valve prolapse.*

24. Winkle RA, Goodman DJ, Popp RL. Simultaneous echocardiographic-phonocar-
    diographic recordings at rest and during amyl nitrite administration in patients
    with mitral valve prolapse. Circulation 1975; 51:522–9.
    *Detailed studies in 21 patients demonstrate that amyl nitrite administration causes
    earlier prolapse of the mitral valve and that a decrease in left ventricular volume is
    a reasonable explanation for the earlier onset of prolapse.*

25. Wei JY, Bulkley BH, Schaeffer AH, Greene HL, Reid PR. Mitral valve prolapse syndrome and recurrent ventricular tachyarrhythmias. Ann Intern Med 1978; 89:6–9.
   Refractory ventricular arrhythmias may be associated with the mitral valve prolapse syndrome.
26. Winkle RA, Lopes MG, Fitzgerald JW, Goodman DJ, Schroeder JS, Harrison DC. Arrhythmias in patients with mitral valve prolapse. Circulation 1975; 52:73–81.
   Atrial and ventricular arrhythmias are common in patients with prolapse, but there is a poor correlation between symptoms and electrocardiographic abnormalities.

Potential Complications and Prognosis

27. Bissett GS III, Schwartz DC, Meyer RA, James FW, Kaplan S. Clinical spectrum and long-term follow-up of isolated mitral valve prolapse in 119 children. Circulation 1980; 62:423–9.
   In this series, only 2 patients required antiarrhythmic therapy, and none progressed to severe mitral regurgitation.
28. Clemens JD, Horwitz RI, Jaffe CC, Feinstein AR, Stanton BF. A controlled evaluation of the risk of bacterial endocarditis in persons with mitral valve prolapse. N Engl J Med 1982; 307:776–81.
   In this study, 25% of patients with endocarditis had mitral valve prolapse, emphasizing that those with mitral valve prolapse and a murmur have a higher risk of endocarditis than those without a murmur.
29. Corrigall D, Bolen J, Hancock EW, Popp RL. Mitral valve prolapse and infective endocarditis. Am J Med 1977; 63:215–22.
   Mitral valve prolapse is the basis for endocarditis in about one-third of cases.
30. Goodman D, Kimbiris D, Linhart JW. Chordae tendineae rupture complicating the systolic click–late systolic murmur syndrome. Am J Cardiol 1974; 33:681–4.
   One of the well-recognized complications of mitral valve prolapse.
31. Jeresaty RM. Sudden death in the mitral valve prolapse–click syndrome. Am J Cardiol 1976; 37:317–8.
   Twelve patients with prolapse and sudden death are described, and their common features are discussed.
32. Mills P, Rose J, Hollingsworth J, Amara I, Craige E. Long-term prognosis of mitral valve prolapse. N Engl J Med 1977; 297:13–8.
   The long-term prognosis of patients with prolapse is generally good, although a small percentage has serious complications.
33. Shappell SD, Marshall CE, Brown RE, Bruce TA. Sudden death and the familial occurrence of mid-systolic click, late systolic murmur syndrome. Circulation 1973; 48:1128–34.
   A patient with mitral valve prolapse and sudden death is described, and several members of his family are discussed.
34. Walsh PN, Kansu TA, Corbett JJ, Savino PJ, Goldburgh WP, Schatz NJ. Platelets, thromboembolism and mitral valve prolapse. Circulation 1981; 63:552–9.
   The incidence of platelet coagulant hyperactivity in patients with mitral valve prolapse was 76% compared with 6% in control patients, which may explain the purported association of thromboembolism and mitral valve prolapse.
35. Grenadier E, Alpan G, Keidar S, Palant A. The prevalence of ruptured chordae tendineae in the mitral valve prolapse syndrome. Am Heart J 1983; 105:603–10.
   Of 134 consecutive patients with the mitral valve prolapse syndrome, 15(11%) had echocardiographic evidence of ruptured chordae tendineae.

Therapy

36. Winkle RA, Lopes MG, Goodman DJ, Fitzgerald JW, Schroeder JS, Harrison DC. Propranolol for patients with mitral valve prolapse. Am Heart J 1977; 93:422–7.
   Although propranolol is not uniformly effective in patients with mitral valve prolapse, it results in symptomatic improvement in more than one-third.
37. Yacoub M, Halim M, Radley-Smith R, McKay R, Nijveld A, Towers M. Surgical treatment of mitral regurgitation caused by floppy valves: repair versus replacement. Circulation 1981; 64(Suppl II):210–6.

In patients with prolapse, mitral valve repair was safer and more successful than valve replacement.

MITRAL VALVE SURGERY

Surgical correction of mitral *stenosis* is indicated primarily for the patient with moderate or severe stenosis who has symptoms despite digitalis and diuretic therapy. Such a patient usually complains of dyspnea, orthopnea, paroxysmal nocturnal dyspnea, or fatigue. Surgical correction of mitral *regurgitation* is indicated for the symptomatic patient with moderate or severe mitral regurgitation. In addition, it may be recommended for an occasional patient with severe mitral regurgitation who is asymptomatic or minimally symptomatic but who has a rapidly progressive increase in heart size. Finally, mitral valve surgery should be considered for the patient with mitral valve disease and repeated systemic arterial embolization despite adequate anticoagulation.

Mitral stenosis can be treated surgically by (1) closed commissurotomy, (2) open commissurotomy, or (3) mitral valve replacement. Pure mitral stenosis is preferably treated by commissurotomy. Three features mitigate against a commissurotomy in the patient with mitral stenosis: (1) associated mitral regurgitation, (2) mitral valve calcification, and (3) the absence of pliability and mobility of the mitral valve leaflets. Thus, if the stenotic mitral valve is regurgitant, calcified, and/or relatively immobile, commissurotomy is likely to be unsuccessful. If a commissurotomy is feasible, it can be performed by either the closed or the open technique. Closed commissurotomy was developed in the 1920s but was first popularized and used extensively in the 1940s and 1950s. This procedure is performed through a left thoracotomy without cardiopulmonary bypass. The surgeon places a purse-string suture around the left atrial appendage. A small incision is made in the appendage, through which the surgeon quickly inserts a finger, and the purse-string suture is tightened to prevent blood loss around the finger. Subsequently, *without the benefit of direct visualization*, the surgeon passes a finger through the mitral valve orifice, manually "fractures" the scarred and stenotic valve, and withdraws his finger, after which the purse-string suture around the left atrial appendage is tied.

The major advantage of the closed commissurotomy is that cardiopulmonary bypass is not required. In experienced hands, its morbidity and mortality are less than those for valve replacement. Its disadvantages are (1) that the surgeon may dislodge a thrombus from the left atrium and produce systemic arterial embolization, (2) that the success of the procedure depends heavily on the experience and expertise of the surgeon, and (3) that it is not possible to assess visually whether insufficient or excessive dilatation of the stenotic valve has been achieved.

With the advent of cardiopulmonary bypass, the closed commissurotomy has given way in many instances to the open commissurotomy. To accomplish this procedure, the patient is placed on cardiopulmonary bypass, and the left atrium is opened. Under direct vision, thrombus is removed from the left atrium, and the mitral valve leaflets are separated and fractured so as to relieve the stenosis. Following open commissurotomy, the left atrial appendage usually is resected, and the pericardium is closed. Today, mitral valve commissurotomy, either closed or open, carries a low mortality (1–3%). The long-term outlook for the patient following commissurotomy is reasonably good; on the average, a repeat surgical procedure on the mitral valve is not needed for 8 to 10 years.

If the patient has predominant mitral regurgitation, surgical treatment consists of either (1) a plastic procedure on the mitral valve and annuloplasty (with or without a ring prosthesis to buttress the anulus) or (2) mitral valve replacement. A plastic procedure on the valve combined with an annuloplasty is the preferred treatment, since the native valve leaflets are retained in situ.

Mitral valve replacement is indicated in the patient with mitral stenosis whose valve is not suitable for commissurotomy, in the patient with mitral regurgitation whose valve is not suitable for a plastic repair procedure and annuloplasty, and in the patient with severe mixed mitral stenosis and regurgitation. As is the case in the aortic position, mitral valve replacement can be performed using either (1) a mechanical prosthesis or (2) a bioprosthesis. The mechanical prostheses are of two main types, namely, the caged-ball valve and the tilting-disc valve. The Starr-Edwards prosthesis is the prototype caged-ball valve and has a record of durability unsurpassed by other prostheses. Although early models were subject to ball variance and a high incidence of thromboembolism, more recent models have not displayed ball variance, and with the use of oral anticoagulants the incidence of systemic embolization has fallen to 2 to 3 percent per year. However, this prosthesis is somewhat obstructive and is associated with a higher incidence of hemolysis than other prostheses. In addition, in the patient with a small left ventricle, there may be insufficient room to accommodate the large cage. For this reason, tilting-disc valves (such as the Bjork-Shiley valve), which are less obstructive and protrude less into the left ventricular cavity, have become popular in the mitral position, even though the Bjork-Shiley valve also mandates long-term anticoagulant therapy. If anticoagulant therapy is not well maintained, this prosthesis is subject to sudden thrombotic occlusion, which is catastrophic. Other tilting-disc valves, including the St. Jude Medical valve (which has two tilting leaflets), appear to be subject to similar advantages and disadvantages as the Bjork-Shiley prosthesis.

Bioprostheses (including porcine bioprostheses and pericardial xenograft prostheses) have as their major advantage a low incidence of thromboembolic phenomena. However, they tend to be more obstructive than the tilting-disc valves, and they are considerably less durable than the mechanical prostheses. Within 10 years of their placement, as many as 50 percent may require replacement. Valvular insufficiency develops with time and is usually a slowly progressive phenomenon, but sudden and catastrophic valvular insufficiency can occur on occasion. In addition, these prostheses may become stenotic and calcify, particularly in children. Indeed, severe stenosis and calcification may occur within 1 year of implantation in children. Therefore, the use of bioprostheses in children and young adults is a calculated risk and is not recommended as a routine practice. Although the bioprostheses are associated with a lower incidence of thromboemboli than the mechanical prostheses, a finite risk of this complication remains. Therefore, anticoagulant therapy is recommended in patients with atrial fibrillation or a markedly enlarged left atrium.

Mitral valve replacement carries an overall operative and postoperative mortality of 5 to 8 percent. Following valve replacement, many patients remain in atrial fibrillation and are noted to have persistent left atrial enlargement. The patient may continue to require digitalis for the control of the ventricular response in atrial fibrillation. If atrial fibrillation and an enlarged left atrium were present for several years preoperatively, they probably will remain postoperatively despite mitral valve surgery.

General

1. Bonchek LI. Current status of cardiac valve replacement: selection of a prosthesis and indications for operation. Am Heart J 1981; 101:96–106.

   An excellent review of the current status of prosthetic valve replacement and plastic procedures on the mitral valve.

2. Dalby AJ, Firth BG, Forman R. Preoperative factors affecting the outcome of isolated mitral valve replacement: a 10-year review. Am J Cardiol 1981; 47:826–34.

   This study of 545 patients with mitral valve disease suggests that patients with a large cardiothoracic ratio, large left atrium, or poor hemodynamics have a reduced operative survival. They should be managed with great care in the perioperative period, since their survival is good if they survive this period.

3. Fowler NO, Van Der Bel-Kahn JM. Indications for surgical replacement of the mitral valve: with particular reference to common and uncommon causes of mitral regurgitation. Am J Cardiol 1979; 44:148–57.

   A succinct review of the indications for mitral valve replacement.

Commissurotomy and Annuloplasty

4. Carpentier A, Deloche A, Dauptain J, Soyer R, Blondeau P, Piwnica A, DuBost C. A new reconstructive operation for correction of mitral and tricuspid insufficiency. J Thorac Cardiovasc Surg 1971; 61:1–13.

   The initial description by Carpentier et al. of their technique of mitral valve reconstruction and ring annuloplasty.

5. Carpentier A, Chauvaud S, Fabiani JN, Deloche A, Relland J, Lessana A, d'Allaines C, Blondeau P, Piwnica A, DuBost C. Reconstructive surgery of mitral valve incompetence: ten-year appraisal. J Thorac Cardiovasc Surg 1980; 79:338–48.

   An excellent review of 551 patients with mitral regurgitation treated by mitral valve reconstruction and plication incorporating a prosthetic anular ring.

6. Commerford PJ, Hastie T, Beck W. Closed mitral valvotomy: actuarial analysis of results in 654 patients over 12 years and analysis of preoperative predictors of long-term survival. Ann Thorac Surg 1982; 33:473–9.

   The operative mortality in this large series of young patients (mean age 33 years) was less than 3%. At 12 years, the survival was 78%; 47% of patients had not required reoperation. The usual clinical indicators of suitability for closed valvotomy were successful in predicting improved survival.

7. Duran CG, Pomar JL, Revuelta JM, Gallo I, Poveda J, Ochoteco A, Ubago JL. Conservative operation for mitral insufficiency: critical analysis supported by postoperation hemodynamic studies of 72 patients. J Thorac Cardiovasc Surg 1980; 79:326–37.

   A comparison of annuloplasty using a flexible ring or Hancock valve replacement reveals a lower operative mortality for the former and a comparable postoperative course.

8. Ellis LB, Singh JB, Morales DD, Harken DE. Fifteen to twenty-year study of one thousand patients undergoing closed mitral valvuloplasty. Circulation 1973; 48:357–64.

   Those patients who did not fare well with closed commissurotomy usually had mitral valve calcification.

9. Gross RI, Cunningham JN, Snively SL, Catinella FP, Nathan IM, Adams PX, Spencer FC. Long-term results of open radical commissurotomy: ten year follow-up study of 202 patients. Am J Cardiol 1981; 47:821–5.

   In this large series, the operative mortality was 1.7% and the long-term mortality 2.5%.

10. Heger JJ, Wann LS, Weyman AE, Dillon JC, Feigenbaum H. Long-term changes in mitral valve area after successful mitral commissurotomy. Circulation 1979; 59:443–8.

    Of 18 patients with closed mitral commissurotomy studied 10–14 years postoperatively, 13 had no diminution in mitral valve area, whereas the other 5 had only a mild decrease.

11. Magilligan DJ, Lam CR, Lewis JW Jr, Davila JC. Mitral valve: the third time around. Circulation 1978; 58(Suppl I):36–8.
    A report of 28 patients who had mitral valve surgery 3 times; the average length of time after the initial closed commissurotomy was 5.7 years, and after the second operation (open commissurotomy or valve replacement) it was 7.4 years.

12. Nanda NC, Gramiak R, Shah PM, DeWeese JA. Mitral commissurotomy versus replacement: preoperative evaluation by echocardiography. Circulation 1975; 51:263–7.
    M-mode echocardiographic assessment of mitral valve calcification and mobility is helpful in planning the surgical approach in patients with mitral stenosis.

13. Smith WM, Neutze JM, Barratt-Boyes BG, Lowe JB. Open mitral valvotomy: effect of pre-operative factors on result. J Thorac Cardiovasc Surg 1981; 82:738–51.
    The operative mortality in 154 patients undergoing open commissurotomy was less than 1%. Associated mitral regurgitation, valvular calcification, previous operation, atrial fibrillation, marked symptoms, subvalvular fusion, and an inadequate commissurotomy were associated with an unfavorable long-term result.

Tissue Valve Replacement

14. Cevese PG, Gallucci V, Morea M, Dalla Volta S, Fasoli G, Casarotto D. Heart valve replacement with the Hancock bioprosthesis: analysis of long-term results. Circulation 1977; 56(Suppl II):111–6.
    Of 336 patients in whom isolated mitral valve replacement with the porcine heterograft was performed, 23(7%) died in surgery.

15. Curcio CA, Commerford PJ, Rose AG, Stevens JE, Barnard MS. Calcification of glutaraldehyde-preserved porcine xenografts in young patients. J Thorac Cardiovasc Surg 1981; 81:621–5.
    Severe stenosis of a porcine xenograft occurred in 11 of 54 patients under the age of 16 years an average of 21 months after insertion.

16. Ferrans VJ, Spray TL, Billingham ME, Roberts WC. Structural changes in glutaraldehyde-treated porcine heterografts used as substitute cardiac valves. Am J Cardiol 1978; 41:1159–84.
    An elegant study of the gross and microscopic changes that occur in porcine heterografts.

17. Frater RWM, Gabbay S, Shore D, Factor S, Strom J. Reproducible replacement of elongated or ruptured mitral valve chordae. Ann Thorac Surg 1983; 35:14–28.
    A report of replacement of ruptured chordae with tanned xenograft pericardium in 11 patients. Valvular competence was good more than 3 years postoperatively.

18. Geha AS, Hammond GL, Laks H, Stansel HC, Glenn WML. Factors affecting performance and thromboembolism after porcine xenograft cardiac valve replacement. J Thorac Cardiovasc Surg 1982; 83:377–84.
    There is a high incidence (23%) of relatively early valve failure in children and young adults. Thromboembolism occurs mainly in those with atrial fibrillation who are not on anticoagulants.

19. Hetzer R, Hill JD, Kerth WJ, Ansbro J, Adappa MG, Rodvien R, Kamm B, Gerbode F. Thromboembolic complications after mitral valve replacement with Hancock xenograft. J Thorac Cardiovasc Surg 1978; 75–651–8.
    Thromboemboli occurred in 9 of 126 patients. All were in atrial fibrillation, and 7 of 9 emboli occurred in the first 3 months postoperatively.

20. Human DG, Joffe HS, Fraser CB, Barnard CN. Mitral valve replacement in children. J Thorac Cardiovasc Surg 1982; 83:873–7.
    In children under 12, the operative mortality was less than 2%; however, porcine heterograft valves had a much higher complication rate than mechanical valves in this age group. By 5 years, fewer than 10% of porcine bioprostheses were still functioning satisfactorily.

21. Ionescu MI, Tandon AP, Mary DAS, Abid A. Heart valve replacement with the Ionescu-Shiley pericardial xenograft. J Thorac Cardiovasc Surg 1977; 73:31–42.
    In this group of patients, the incidence of systemic embolism was 2.48 episodes per 100 patient years when the prosthesis was used in the mitral position without anticoagulant therapy. After 30 months of follow-up, structural integrity of the prostheses was good.

22. Lurie AJ, Miller RR, Maxwell KS, Grehl TM, Vismara LA, Hurley EJ, Mason DT. Hemodynamic assessment of the glutaraldehyde-preserved porcine heterograft in the aortic and mitral positions. Circulation 1977; 56(Suppl II):104–110.
   Of 14 patients receiving mitral porcine heterografts, the average valve area was 1.84 cm²; only 2 patients had regurgitation.

23. Oyer PE, Stinson EB, Reitz BA, Miller DC, Rossiter SJ, Shumway NE. Long-term evaluation of the porcine xenograft bioprosthesis. J Thorac Cardiovasc Surg 1979; 78:343–50.
   In this study of Hancock prostheses in the mitral position followed for 5 years, 92% were free of embolism, and 93% were free of dysfunction.

24. Rose AG, Forman R, Bowen RM. Calcification of glutaraldehyde-fixed porcine xenograft. Thorax 1978; 33:111–4.
   The initial report of calcification of a porcine bioprosthesis. It occurred 12 months after implantation in a 14-year-old patient.

25. Thandroyen FT, Whitton IN, Pirie D, Rogers MA, Mitha AS. Severe calcification of glutaraldehyde-preserved porcine xenografts in children, Am J Cardiol 1980; 45:690–6.
   A report of 4 cases of calcification of porcine bioprostheses in the mitral position after 17–25 months. All four patients were aged 13 to 15 years.

26. Williams DB, Danielson GK, McGoon DC, Puga FJ, Mair DD, Edwards WD. Porcine heterograft valve replacement in children. J Thorac Cardiovasc Surg 1982; 84:446–50.
   In 49 patients under the age of 18 followed for 5 years, only half were free of complications. Therefore, the authors advise against the use of porcine heterografts in children.

Mechanical Valve Replacement

27. Barnhorst DA, Oxman HA, Connolly DC, Pluth JR, Danielson GK, Wallace RB, McGoon DC. Isolated replacement of the mitral valve with the Starr-Edwards prosthesis. J Thorac Cardiovasc Surg 1976; 71:230–7.
   A review of 657 patients receiving a Starr-Edwards mitral prosthesis from 1961 to 1972; 59(9%) died in surgery.

28.. Bjork VO, Book K, Cernigliaro C, Holmgren A. The Bjork Shiley tilting disc valve in isolated mitral lesions. Scand J Thorac Cardiovasc Surg 1973; 7:131–148.
   An early report by Bjork's group of the satisfactory results of mitral valve replacement with the Bjork-Shiley valve.

29. Copans H, Lakier JB, Kinsley RH, Colsen PR, Fritz VU, Barlow JB. Thrombosed Bjork-Shiley mitral prostheses. Circulation 1980; 61:169–74.
   During a 4½ year period, 18 of 224 patients died suddenly due to sudden thrombotic occlusion of a Bjork-Shiley mitral prosthesis. Poor anticoagulant control appeared to be the major predisposing factor to this complication.

30. Forman R, Beck W, Barnard CN. Results after mitral valve replacement with cloth-covered Starr-Edwards prostheses (Models 6300, 6310/6320, and 6400). Br Heart J 1978; 40:612–6.
   In this series of 332 patients treated with cloth-covered Starr-Edwards prostheses, the operative mortality was 8%; 53 patients had thromboembolic events in the first 3 years, and valve thrombosis occurred in 4 patients despite adequate anticoagulant therapy.

31. Horstkotte D, Haerten K, Herzer JA, Seipel L, Bircks W, Loogen F. Preliminary results in mitral valve replacement with the St. Jude medical prosthesis: comparison with the Bjork-Shiley valve. Circulation 1981; 64 (Suppl II):203–9.
   In prostheses with equal anular diameters (29 mm), the calculated effective orifice is larger with the St. Jude than the Bjork-Shiley prosthesis.

32. Macmanus Q, Grunkemeier GL, Lambert LE, Teply JF, Harlan BJ, Starr A. Year of operation as a risk factor in the late results of valve replacement. J Thorac Cardiovasc Surg 1980; 80:834–41.
   This study of the non-cloth-covered Starr-Edwards prosthesis suggests that the 5-year embolus-free rate is approximately 80–90% for valves implanted within the last 10 years. This is similar to the embolus-free rate with other prostheses.

33. Miller DC, Oyer PE, Stinson EB, Reitz BA, Jamieson SW, Baumgartner WA, Mitchell RS, Shumway NE. 10 to 15 year reassessment of the performance char-

acteristics of the Starr-Edwards model 6120 mitral valve prosthesis. J Thorac Cardiovasc Surg 1983; 85:1–20.

An excellent report of 509 patients followed for 10–15 years, with a detailed analysis of the rates of thromboembolism, anticoagulant hemorrhage, reoperation rate, and valve-related morbidity and mortality.

34. Nicoloff DM, Emery RW, Arom KV, Northrup WF III, Jorgensen CR, Wang Y, Lindsay WG. Clinical and hemodynamic results with the St. Jude medical cardiac valve prosthesis: a three year experience. J Thorac Cardiovasc Surg 1981; 82:674–83.

    In 232 patients with aortic or mitral valve prostheses, the incidence of thromboemboli was 3 per 1,000 patient months for the mitral position; 2 patients developed valvular thrombosis, but the hemodynamic characteristics of the valve were good.

35. Sala A, Schoevaerdts JC, Jaumin P, Ponlot R, Chalant CH. Review of 387 isolated mitral valve replacements by the model 6120 Starr-Edwards prosthesis. J Thorac Cardiovasc Surg 1982; 84:744–50.

    In this large series, the operative mortality was 6%, the 5-year survival 78%, and the 10-year survival 72% following mitral valve replacement with the non-cloth-covered Starr-Edwards valve.

36. Salomon NW, Stinson EB, Griepp RB, Shumway NE. Mitral valve replacement: long-term evaluation of prosthesis-related mortality and morbidity. Circulation 1977; 56(Suppl II)94–101.

    With the Starr-Edwards ball-in-cage prosthesis, thromboembolic problems are substantial, whereas they are less of a problem with the porcine heterograft.

37. Starr A, Grunkemeier G, Lambert L, Okies JE, Thomas D. Mitral valve replacement: a 10-year follow-up of non-cloth-covered vs. cloth-covered caged-ball prostheses. Circulation 1976; 54(Suppl III):47–56.

    A thorough review of 290 patients who received one of the early models of the Starr-Edwards prosthesis in the mitral position.

VALVULAR PULMONIC STENOSIS

Obstruction to right ventricular outflow can be supravalvular, subvalvular, or valvular. *Supravalvular* pulmonic stenosis results from narrowing of the pulmonary trunk, its bifurcation, or its primary or peripheral branches. Although pulmonary arterial stenosis occurs as an isolated congenital lesion, it frequently coexists with other cardiac abnormalities, including valvular pulmonic stenosis, atrial septal defect, ventricular septal defect (VSD), patent ductus arteriosus, and tetralogy of Fallot. *Subvalvular* pulmonic stenosis can be infundibular or subinfundibular; in either case, it is usually associated with a VSD and is uncommon as an isolated anomaly. *Valvular* pulmonic stenosis is a congenital lesion in the vast majority of patients. In fact, isolated valvular pulmonic stenosis is now recognized as one of the more common congenital cardiac abnormalities, constituting 10 to 12 percent of cases of congenital heart disease. When it is acquired, it is most likely due to rheumatic scarring, bacterial endocarditis, or trauma to the valve. It may occur with a VSD or an intact ventricular septum.

The adult patient with valvular pulmonic stenosis is often asymptomatic. Eventually, he may complain of dyspnea on exertion or easy fatigability; less often, he may report anterior chest pain or syncope with exertion. Eventually, if right ventricular failure develops, the patient may complain of peripheral edema and abdominal swelling. If the foramen ovale is patent, intermittent or even continuous shunting of blood from the right to the left atrium may occur, resulting in cyanosis and clubbing.

On physical examination, jugular venous distention, ankle edema, and hepatomegaly are observed if right ventricular failure is present. Examination of the neck veins reveals a prominent a wave; if tricuspid regurgitation is present, a prominent V wave may be noted. On cardiac examination, the point of maximal impulse is usually not displaced laterally. A right ventricular lift may be palpable at the left sternal border, and there may be a systolic thrill at the pulmonic area (second left intercostal space). On auscultation, the S_1 is normal, and the S_2 is widely split but moves with respiration; the pulmonic component is soft and markedly delayed. A harsh, crescendo-decrescendo systolic murmur is audible along the left sternal border and is loudest at the pulmonic area. An ejection click may be audible at the pulmonic area; typically, it softens or disappears with inspiration. If the murmur radiates widely into the lung fields, additional pulmonary arterial branch stenosis should be suspected. The auscultatory signs of valvular pulmonic stenosis may give some indication of its severity. As the stenosis becomes more severe, the crescendo-decrescendo systolic murmur peaks later in systole, and the ejection click moves closer to the S_1. In fact, if the stenosis is severe, the ejection click blends with the S_1 and becomes inaudible as a separate sound.

The chest x-ray demonstrates several abnormalities in the patient with pulmonic stenosis. The pulmonary vascular markings may be diminished, and the main pulmonary artery is dilated and appears unusually large. The right ventricle may also be enlarged. Cardiomegaly ranges from mild to massive; in fact, pulmonic stenosis with an intact ventricular septum is recognized as one of the causes of marked cardiomegaly. The ECG demonstrates right axis deviation, right ventricular hypertrophy, and, in some cases, right atrial enlargement. An incomplete or complete right bundle branch block may be present. The M-mode echocardiogram may demonstrate right ventricular enlargement and hypertrophy, with "paradoxical motion" of the interventricular septum during systole. Two-dimensional echocardiography may allow for direct visualization of the pulmonic valve.

At the time of cardiac catheterization, there is a pressure gradient between the right ventricle and the pulmonary artery. The pulmonary arterial pressure is normal or low, whereas the right ventricular systolic pressure is elevated. If the right ventricular systolic pressure is 30 to 50 mm Hg, the patient is said to have mild stenosis; if it is 50 to 100 mm Hg, moderate stenosis is present; and if it is greater than 100 mm Hg, severe stenosis is present.

In the adult patient with valvular pulmonic stenosis, the long-term outlook is good. Specifically, the patient with mild or moderate pulmonic stenosis may remain asymptomatic for his entire life and, therefore, may never require surgery. Although some patients with severe stenosis have done well for many years, there is a legitimate concern that they eventually may develop right ventricular failure. Operative repair of valvular pulmonic stenosis appears warranted (1) if the patient has symptoms attributable to the stenosis, (2) if the patient is intermittently cyanotic, or (3) if the patient has a right ventricular systolic pressure greater than 100 mm Hg, even without symptoms. If surgical intervention is necessary, a pulmonary valvotomy generally suffices, but pulmonic valve replacement may rarely be necessary.

Clinical Characteristics

1. Bassingthwaighte JB, Parkin TW, DuShane JW, Wood EH, Burchell HB. The electrocardiographic and hemodynamic findings in pulmonary stenosis with intact ventricular septum. Circulation 1963; 28:893–905.

   A study correlating electrocardiographic and catheterization data in 53 patients with valvular pulmonic stenosis.

2. Blount SG Jr, Komesu S, McCord MC. Asymptomatic isolated valvular pulmonary stenosis: diagnosis by clinical methods. N Engl J Med 1953; 248:5–11.
   Isolated valvular pulmonic stenosis is one of the more common forms of congenital heart disease seen in the adult.

3. Blount SG Jr, Vigoda PS, Swan H. Isolated infundibular stenosis. Am Heart J 1959; 57:684–700.
   Infundibular stenosis comprises only 3% of all cases of pulmonary stenosis with intact ventricular septum.

4. D'Cruz IA, Agustsson MH, Bicoff JP, Weinberg M Jr, Arcilla RA. Stenotic lesions of the pulmonary arteries: clinical and hemodynamic findings in 84 cases. Am J Cardiol 1964; 13:441–50.
   Of these 84 cases, 32 were unilateral, and 52 were bilateral.

5. Delaney TB, Nadas AS. Peripheral pulmonic stenosis. Am J Cardiol 1964; 13:451–61.
   A detailed discussion of the physical findings, natural history, and therapy of 17 patients with this entity.

6. Franch RH, Gay BB Jr. Congenital stenosis of the pulmonary artery branches: a classification, with postmortem findings in two cases. Am J Med 1963; 35:512–29.
   The diagnosis of isolated stenosis of the pulmonary arterial branches should be considered in a patient with right ventricular preponderance and an atypical holosystolic or continuous murmur easily audible over the lung fields.

7. Gamboa R, Hugenholtz PG, Nadas AS. Accuracy of the phonocardiogram in assessing severity of aortic and pulmonic stenosis. Circulation 1964; 30:35–46.
   As pulmonic stenosis becomes more severe, S_2 becomes more widely split, the Q-ejection click interval narrows, and the harsh ejection murmur peaks later in systole.

8. Holt JH Jr, Eddleman EE Jr. The precordial movements in adults with pulmonic stenosis. Circulation 1967; 35:492–500.
   A correlative study between findings on the apexcardiogram and cardiac catheterization in 24 adult patients with valvular pulmonic stenosis.

9. Hultgren HN, Reeve R, Cohn K, McLeod R. The ejection click of valvular pulmonic stenosis. Circulation 1969; 40:631–40.
   A somewhat complicated analysis of why the ejection click in valvular pulmonic stenosis disappears during inspiration.

10. Leatham A, Weitzman D. Auscultatory and phonocardiographic signs of pulmonary stenosis. Br Heart J 1957; 19:303–17.
    An elegant phonocardiographic study of 70 patients with valvular pulmonic stenosis.

11. Roberts WC, Mason DT, Morrow AG, Braunwald E. Calcific pulmonic stenosis. Circulation 1968; 37:973–8.
    Survival into adulthood and severe valvular pulmonic stenosis are prerequisites for the development of calcification of the pulmonic valve.

12. Sharma S, Katdare AD, Munsi SC, Kinare SG. M-mode echographic detection of pulmonic valve infective endocarditis. Am Heart J 1981; 102:131–2.
    A case report that describes the features of pulmonic valve endocarditis on M-mode echocardiogram.

13. Vogelpoel L, Schrire V, Nellen M, Swanepoel A. The use of phenylephrine in the differentiation of Fallot's tetralogy from pulmonary stenosis with intact ventricular septum. Am Heart J 1960; 59:489–505.
    Phenylephrine causes a marked increase in pulmonary blood flow and intensity of the murmur in the patient with Fallot's tetralogy but minimal effect on these variables in the patient with pulmonic stenosis and an intact ventricular septum. Conversely, amyl nitrite causes a decrease in pulmonary blood flow and intensity of the murmur in the patient with Fallot's tetralogy but not in the patient with isolated pulmonic stenosis.

14. Vogelpoel L, Schrire V. The role of auscultation in the differentiation of Fallot's tetralogy from severe pulmonary stenosis with intact ventricular septum and right to left interatrial shunt. Circulation 1955; 11:714–32.
    An elegant discussion of the clinical features which help to distinguish between these two entities.

15. Weyman AE, Hurwitz RA, Girod DA, Dillon JC, Feigenbaum H, Green D. Cross-sectional echocardiographic visualization of the stenotic pulmonary valve. Circulation 1977; 56:769–74.

    With two-dimensional echocardiography, the stenotic pulmonic valve may be visualized frequently.

16. Yahini JH, Dulfano MJ, Toor M. Pulmonic stenosis, a clinical assessment of severity. Am J Cardiol 1960; 5:744–57.

    A presentation of clinical, phonocardiographic, electrocardiographic, vectorcardiographic, and roentgenographic findings in 34 patients with mild, moderate, and severe valvular pulmonic stenosis.

Prognosis and Therapy

17. Campbell M. Simple pulmonary stenosis: pulmonary valvular stenosis with a closed ventricular septum. Br Heart J 1954; 16:273–300.

    Pulmonary valvotomy is indicated in isolated valvular pulmonic stenosis for (1) a right ventricular systolic pressure over 100, (2) right ventricular strain on ECG, (3) severe symptoms, and (4) moderate or severe cardiomegaly.

18. Engle MA, Ito T, Goldberg HP. The fate of the patient with pulmonic stenosis. Circulation 1964; 30:554–61.

    Interestingly, 7 of 100 patients with valvular pulmonic stenosis in this series developed endocarditis.

19. Johnson LW, Grossman W, Dalen JE, Dexter L. Pulmonic stenosis in the adult: long-term follow-up results. N Engl J Med 1972; 287:1159–63.

    Long-term follow-up of adult patients with pulmonic stenosis shows that they do very well without surgery.

20. Kan JS, White RI Jr, Mitchell SE, Gardner TJ. Percutaneous balloon valvuloplasty: a new method for treating congenital pulmonary valve stenosis. N Engl J Med 1982; 307:540–2.

    A case report of pulmonic valve stenosis treated successfully by balloon dilatation.

21. Mirowski M, Shah KD. Neill CA, Taussig HB. Long-term (10 to 13 years) follow-up study after transventricular pulmonary valvotomy for pulmonary stenosis with intact ventricular septum. Circulation 1963; 28:906–14.

    This early study of 46 patients who survived pulmonary valvulotomy indicates that this procedure produces satisfactory results.

22. Roberts WC, Shemin RJ, Kent KM. Frequency and direction of interatrial shunting in valvular pulmonic stenosis with intact ventricular septum and without left ventricular inflow or outflow obstruction: an analysis of 127 patients treated by valvulotomy. Am Heart J 1980; 99:142–8.

    Of the 127 patients, 30 had shunting at the atrial level. The shunt was right-to-left in 19 (63%) and left-to-right in 8 (27%). The patients with an associated right-to-left shunt had severe pulmonic stenosis, whereas those with a left-to-right shunt had only mild pulmonic stenosis.

23. Snellen HA, Hartman H, Buis-Liem TN, Kole EH, Rohmer J. Pulmonic stenosis. Circulation 1968; 38(Suppl V):93–101.

    Patients with severe valvular pulmonic stenosis should be repaired surgically; if not operated on, they will eventually develop cyanosis and heart failure and die.

24. Tinker J, Howitt G, Markman P, Wade EG. The natural history of isolated pulmonary stenosis. Br Heart J 1965; 27:151–60.

    Patients with mild or moderate valvular pulmonic stenosis do well for many years and, therefore, do not require surgical intervention.

25. Eklund B, Freyschuss U. Congenital pulmonary stenosis at the age of 76. Acta Med Scand 1968; 183:455–6.

    A 76-year-old man with mild–moderate valvular pulmonic stenosis is reported.

PULMONIC REGURGITATION

Like most other valvular abnormalities, pulmonic regurgitation may be congenital or acquired. If it is acquired, it may be organic or functional. *Organic* pulmonic regurgitation is rare; it can be caused by pulmonic valve endocarditis, blunt or sharp chest trauma, or rheumatic scarring of the valve, or it can follow pulmonic valvotomy. *Functional* pulmonic regurgitation occurs more commonly and is seen in patients with severe pulmonary arterial hypertension (regardless of etiology) or idiopathic dilatation of the pulmonary artery.

The patient with functional pulmonic regurgitation usually complains of the symptoms induced by the underlying disease (e.g., dyspnea or fatigue in a patient with severe mitral stenosis). The patient with isolated organic pulmonic regurgitation may be asymptomatic for many years. When it is severe, however, right ventricular dilatation and failure eventually develop, leading to easy fatigability, dyspnea on exertion (due to a reduced cardiac output), peripheral edema, right upper quadrant abdominal discomfort (due to hepatic engorgement), and anorexia, nausea, and vomiting (due to venous congestion of the gastrointestinal tract).

If right ventricular failure has occurred, the patient may have jugular venous distention, hepatomegaly, peripheral edema, and even ascites. The cardiac examination reveals a palpable pulsation in the pulmonic area (second left intercostal space). On auscultation, the S_2 is widely split, and its pulmonic component is accentuated. There is a blowing, decrescendo diastolic murmur loudest in the second and third left intercostal spaces, which increases in intensity with inspiration. In addition, one often hears an associated systolic ejection murmur in the pulmonic area, due to increased flow across the pulmonic valve during systole. If right ventricular dilatation and failure have occurred, both a right-sided S_3 and a holosystolic murmur of tricuspid regurgitation may be audible at the left lower sternal border.

The chest x-ray demonstrates right ventricular enlargement and dilatation of the pulmonary artery. The hilar shadows may be prominent and may even be mistaken for a mediastinal tumor. On fluoroscopy, the pulmonary arteries pulsate vigorously. The ECG shows right axis deviation and right ventricular hypertrophy; there may be right bundle branch block. On M-mode echocardiography, one may see right ventricular dilatation and paradoxical motion of the interventricular septum during systole; occasionally, diastolic fluttering of the tricuspid valve leaflets is observed.

At the time of cardiac catheterization, the pulmonary arterial systolic pressure is usually normal, but the diastolic pressure is low. If pulmonic stenosis is not present, the right ventricular systolic and diastolic pressures are identical to those of the pulmonary artery. On pulmonary angiography, there is reflux of contrast material into the right ventricle.

If the pulmonic regurgitation is functional, the patient's prognosis is dependent on the severity of the underlying disease process (e.g., mitral stenosis, chronic obstructive lung disease). If it is organic, the course, for the most part, appears to be benign. However, when pulmonic regurgitation is due to an absent pulmonic valve (as occurs in a small percentage of patients with tetralogy of Fallot), the resulting marked dilatation of the proximal pulmonary arteries can cause respiratory embarrassment due to bronchial obstruction. If the regurgitation is only mild or moderate, it is likely that symptoms will never develop. In contrast, if the regurgitation is severe, the patient may eventually note symptoms of right ventricular failure, indicating that surgical intervention is warranted.

Even if the patient with pulmonic regurgitation is asymptomatic, he should receive antibiotic prophylaxis at the time of surgical procedures or dental manipulations. If symptoms appear, the patient should receive digitalis, and serious consideration should be given to valve replacement.

1. Collins NP, Braunwald E, Morrow AG. Isolated congenital pulmonic valvular regurgitation: diagnosis by cardiac catheterization and angiocardiography. Am J Med 1960; 28:159–64.
   An asymptomatic patient with isolated pulmonic regurgitation is described; at cardiac catheterization, pulmonary arterial and right ventricular pressures were identical.
2. Fish RG, Takaro T, Crymes T. Prognostic considerations in primary isolated insufficiency of the pulmonic valve. N Engl J Med 1959; 261:739–42.
   Mild or moderate isolated pulmonic regurgitation is well tolerated for many years.
3. Laneve SA, Uesu CT, Taguchi JT. Isolated pulmonic valvular regurgitation. Am J Med Sci 1962; 244:446–58.
   Most patients with isolated pulmonic regurgitation of mild or moderate degree tolerate it for many years without difficulty.
4. Levin HS, Runco V, Wooley CF, Ryan JM. Pulmonic regurgitation following staphylococcal endocarditis: an intracardiac phonocardiographic study. Circulation 1964; 30:411–6.
   A case report of a 30-year-old man with organic pulmonic regurgitation 5 years after an episode of successfully treated staphylococcal endocarditis.
5. Miller RA, Lev M, Paul MH. Congenital absence of the pulmonary valve: the clinical syndrome of tetralogy of Fallot with pulmonary regurgitation. Circulation 1962; 26:266–78.
   Six patients are described with tetralogy of Fallot and absence of the pulmonic valve.
6. Morton RF, Stern TN. Isolated pulmonic valvular regurgitation. Circulation 1956; 14:1069–72.
   Although isolated pulmonic stenosis is common, isolated pulmonic regurgitation is rare.
7. O'Toole JD, Wurtzbacher JJ, Wearner NE, Jain AC. Pulmonary valve injury and insufficiency during pulmonary artery catheterization. N Engl J Med 1979; 301:1167–8.
   A report of two cases of pulmonary valve insufficiency after a Swan-Ganz catheter had remained in the pulmonary artery for several days.
8. Price BO. Isolated incompetence of the pulmonic valve. Circulation 1961; 23:596–602.
   Two cases of isolated pulmonic regurgitation are presented; this is not a totally benign disorder, since it may lead to right ventricular failure.
9. Curtiss EI, Miller TR, Shapiro LS. Pulmonic regurgitation due to valvular tophi. Circulation 1983; 67:699–701.
   This article describes a 31-year-old man who had postmortem evidence of sterile gouty tophi on the pulmonic valve, causing valvular regurgitation.

TRICUSPID STENOSIS

Tricuspid stenosis is almost invariably due to rheumatic scarring of the valve, although occasionally functional tricuspid stenosis results from the protrusion of bacterial vegetations, thrombi, or tumors through the tricuspid orifice. Mild (and usually clinically inapparent) tricuspid stenosis occurs in 10 to 15 percent of patients with rheumatic heart disease, but hemodynamically significant tricuspid stenosis is uncommon, occurring in only 3 to 5 percent. Isolated rheumatic tricuspid stenosis (i.e., without concomitant mitral or aortic involvement) is extremely rare.

The patient with rheumatic tricuspid stenosis usually complains of symptoms caused by the predominant left-sided valvular lesion. Those that are attributable to tricuspid stenosis include easy fatigability (due to a reduced cardiac output), right upper quadrant abdominal discomfort (due to hepatomegaly), and peripheral edema. In addition, the patient may note anorexia, nausea, vomiting, and eructation, all due to passive venous congestion of the gastrointestinal tract. Less commonly, the patient with tricuspid stenosis may complain of syncope (or near-syncope), periodic cyanosis (due to right-to-left shunting through a patent foramen ovale), or vague retrosternal chest discomfort.

The physical examination of the patient with severe tricuspid stenosis reveals striking jugular venous distention with especially prominent A waves. Similar venous distention and pulsation may be visible in the more peripheral veins, such as the basilic veins or those in the dorsum of the hands. The peripheral venous pressure is elevated and increases with pressure over the right upper quadrant of the abdomen (hepatojugular reflux). The liver is enlarged and may be huge, and it may demonstrate a prominent presystolic pulsation. Ascites and peripheral edema are usually present. There may be evidence of unilateral or bilateral pleural effusions. Cyanosis or mild icterus may also be present.

On cardiac examination, the right heart border is usually displaced to the right; in fact, the dilated right atrium may even cause the right heart border to reach the right midclavicular line. On auscultation, there is usually concomitant mitral stenosis, aortic stenosis, or both. The S_1 is increased in intensity, as is the pulmonic component of the S_2 (due to pulmonary hypertension brought about by left-sided valvular disease). At the left lower sternal border, a rumbling mid-diastolic murmur that classically increases in intensity with inspiration is heard. Occasionally, this murmur is confused with that of mitral stenosis, but the latter usually is well localized to the apex. The murmur of tricuspid stenosis tends to be softer, higher pitched, and of shorter duration than the murmur of mitral stenosis. An opening snap may be audible before the diastolic murmur, following the P_2 by 0.06 to 0.08 seconds. The opening snap of tricuspid stenosis can be distinguished from that of mitral stenosis by its increasing intensity with inspiration as well as by the fact that it generally occurs after the mitral opening snap.

The chest x-ray in the patient with tricuspid stenosis shows right atrial enlargement, and the right lower cardiac contour is displaced to the right. The combination of left atrial enlargement (due to mitral stenosis) and right atrial enlargement (due to tricuspid stenosis) may produce double atrial concentric contours on the right side of the cardiac silhouette. Although patients with isolated tricuspid stenosis have clear lung fields, preexisting mitral stenosis can cause pulmonary venous congestion and Kerley B lines. The vascular shadow of the superior vena cava is widened and pulsates in presystole. The ECG demonstrates tall, peaked P waves in standard lead II, indicative of right atrial enlargement. The P–R interval is often slightly prolonged. Although atrial fibrillation may develop late in the course, regular sinus rhythm is frequent, even with coexisting mitral stenosis. On M-mode echocardiography, the tricuspid valve appears scarred and thickened, while on two-dimensional echocardiography both the stenosed tricuspid valve and the enlarged right atrium may be seen.

Ultimately, the diagnosis of tricuspid stenosis is determined by cardiac catheterization, although the jugular venous tracing, when considered in relation to other clinical findings, often permits an accurate noninvasive diagnosis. The diagnosis of tricuspid stenosis is particularly difficult when atrial fibrillation is present; since there are no prominent A waves in the jugular venous pulse, there is no characteristic presystolic murmur, and the auscultatory findings are often dominated by concomitant mitral stenosis. At cardiac catheterization, the patient with tricuspid stenosis demonstrates a diastolic pressure gradient across the tricuspid valve. Although a mean diastolic gradient of 3 mm Hg or more is suggestive of tricuspid stenosis, mean gradients as high as 5 mm Hg have been reported with predominant tricuspid regurgitation and a resultant increased flow across the tricuspid valve during diastole. Significant tricuspid stenosis may be missed at the time of cardiac catheterization unless right atrial and right ventricular pressures are recorded simultaneously, particularly in the patient with atrial fibrillation or a low cardiac output. The injection of radiographic contrast material into the right atrium may demonstrate delayed opacification of the right ventricle. In the right anterior oblique projection, one may visualize tricuspid valvular thickening and relative immobility.

The patient with isolated tricuspid stenosis may be totally asymptomatic for many years despite venous engorgement. Finally, however, symptoms of a low cardiac output appear, after which the patient begins a progressive downhill course. Tricuspid stenosis is almost always accompanied by mitral or aortic valvular disease, indicating a more severe and extensive rheumatic inflammation than in cases of mitral and aortic valve disease alone. As a result, the prognosis generally is poor in patients with combined tricuspid and left-sided valvular involvement. Without surgical correction, death eventually results from progressive right-sided failure, pulmonary embolism and infarction, or bronchopulmonary infection.

During the period before the appearance of symptoms, the patient with tricuspid stenosis should receive antibiotic prophylaxis against endocarditis. Once symptoms appear, the patient should be placed on salt restriction and diuretics. Digitalis is useful in the control of the ventricular rate if the patient is is in atrial fibrillation. Eventually, when the patient's activity becomes limited even on a good medical regimen, surgery should be performed. Valvuloplasty should be considered if the valve area is 2 cm² or less and the valve is mobile; tricuspid valve replacement should be recommended if the valve is unsuitable for valvuloplasty and the valve orifice area is 1.5 cm² or less. The risk of thrombosis on a tricuspid valvular prosthesis is greater than on a mitral prosthesis, since the papillary muscles and right ventricular free wall may impede the opening of a prosthesis in the tricuspid position. As a result, bioprostheses (e.g., the glutaraldehyde-preserved porcine prostheses) are the artificial valves of choice in the tricuspid position.

1. Bousvaros GA, Stubington D. Some auscultatory and phonocardiographic features of tricuspid stenosis. Circulation 1964; 29:26–33.
   An elegant phonocardiographic evaluation of 9 patients with tricuspid stenosis.
2. Gordon AJ, Genkins G, Grishman A, Nabatoff RA. Tricuspid stenosis. Report of a case, with hemodynamic studies at tricuspid commissurotomy. Am J Med 1957; 22:306–14.
   This article describes a rare case of isolated rheumatic tricuspid stenosis and provides a detailed hemodynamic assessment.
3. Hoffbrand AV, Lloyd-Thomas HG. Leiomyosarcoma of the inferior vena cava leading to obstruction of the tricuspid valve. Br Heart J 1964; 26:709–15.
   The clinical features of a patient with leiomyosarcoma of the inferior vena cava leading to its obstruction and to that of the tricuspid valve are described.
4. Joyner CR Jr, Hey EB Jr, Johnson J, Reid JM. Reflected ultrasound in the diagnosis of tricuspid stenosis. Am J Cardiol 1967; 19:66–73.
   An early description of the echocardiographic findings in tricuspid stenosis.

5. Killip T III, Lukas DS. Tricuspid stenosis: physiologic criteria for diagnosis and hemodynamic abnormalities. Circulation 1957; 16:3–13.
   At cardiac catheterization, 10 patients with tricuspid stenosis demonstrated abnormal mean diastolic pressure gradients across the tricuspid valve.

6. Killip T III, Lukas DS. Tricuspid stenosis: clinical features in twelve cases. Am J Med 1958; 24:836–52.
   A detailed review of 12 patients with this abnormality.

7. Kitchin A, Turner R. Diagnosis and treatment of tricuspid stenosis. Br Heart J 1964; 26:354–79.
   The diagnosis, circulatory effects, and surgical therapy of rheumatic tricuspid stenosis associated with mitral stenosis are discussed in 17 patients subjected to combined valvotomy.

8. Morgan JR, Forker AD, Coates JR, Myers WS. Isolated tricuspid stenosis. Circulation 1971; 44:729–32.
   A rare case of isolated rheumatic tricuspid stenosis is presented.

9. Patterson W, Baxley WA, Karp RB, Soto B, Bargeron LL. Tricuspid atresia in adults. Am J Cardiol 1982; 49:141–52.
   The findings at cardiac catheterization in 18 patients over the age of 15 years with tricuspid atresia are presented, and the surgical management of this condition is discussed.

10. Perloff JK, Harvey WP. Clinical recognition of tricuspid stenosis. Circulation 1960; 22:346–64.
    A phonocardiographic, electrocardiographic, and hemodynamic assessment of 13 patients with tricuspid stenosis.

11. Peterffy A. Surgical management of tricuspid valvular disease: ten years' experience of 141 consecutive patients. Scand J Thorac Cardiovasc Surg [Suppl] 1980; 26:1–65.
    An excellent review of one surgeon's experience with tricuspid valve replacement and annuloplasty in a large number of patients.

12. Peterffy A, Jonasson R, Henze A. Hemodynamic changes after tricuspid valve surgery: a recatheterization study in forty-five patients. Scand J Thorac Cardiovasc Surg 1981; 15:161–70.
    Both tricuspid valve replacement and tricuspid annuloplasty generally result in improved cardiac output, a decrease in pulmonary arterial and right atrial pressures, and an improvement in exercise capacity.

13. Reichek N, Shelburne JC, Perloff JK. Clinical aspects of rheumatic valvular disease. Prog Cardiovasc Dis 1973; 15:491–537.
    A good review of the clinical manifestations of mitral, aortic, and tricuspid stenosis and regurgitation. Includes 110 references.

14. Sanders CA, Harthorne JW, DeSanctis RW, Austen WG. Tricuspid stenosis: a difficult diagnosis in the presence of atrial fibrillation. Circulation 1966; 33:26–33.
    In 10 patients with tricuspid stenosis and atrial fibrillation, the diagnosis was made clincally in only 2 and by pullback recording from right ventricle to right atrium in only 3.

15. Vander Hauwaert LG, Corbeel L, Maldague P. Fibroma of the right ventricle producing severe tricuspid stenosis. Circulation 1965; 32:451–6.
    A report of a 16-month-old child with a right ventricular fibroma causing a hemodynamic picture of severe tricuspid stenosis.

16. Daniels SJ, Mintz GS, Kotler MN. Rheumatic tricuspid valve disease: two-dimensional echocardiographic, hemodynamic, and angiographic correlations. Am J Cardiol 1983; 51:492–6.
    Of 372 consecutive patients with rheumatic mitral valve disease, 23 (6%) had tricuspid valve involvement.

17. Thorburn CW, Morgan JJ, Shanahan MX, Chang VP. Long-term results of tricuspid valve replacement and the problem of prosthetic valve thrombosis. Am J Cardiol 1983; 51:1128–32.
    The tilting disc prosthetic valves have an unacceptably high rate of thrombosis in the tricuspid position, whereas the ball-in-cage and porcine prostheses appear to be satisfactory.

TRICUSPID REGURGITATION

Tricuspid regurgitation may be functional or due to intrinsic organic disease. Functional tricuspid regurgitation is more common than organic tricuspid regurgitation. *Functional* tricuspid regurgitation occurs when there is dilatation of the right ventricle, which is most often due to pulmonary hypertension (primary or secondary), pulmonic valvular or infundibular stenosis, or right ventricular infarction. With any of these conditions, tricuspid regurgitation is a reflection of right ventricular decompensation.

Organic tricuspid regurgitation can be due to (1) rheumatic heart disease, in which case it usually occurs in association with tricuspid valvular stenosis, (2) Ebstein's anomaly of the tricuspid valve, (3) right ventricular papillary muscle dysfunction, (4) myxomatous degeneration of the tricuspid valve, (5) the carcinoid syndrome, or (6) infective endocarditis. Tricuspid valve endocarditis is a common occurrence in intravenous drug abusers. Organic tricuspid regurgitation is frequently well tolerated in the absence of an elevated right ventricular systolic pressure. Indeed, the tricuspid valve can be resected in some patients with tricuspid valve endocarditis refractory to medical therapy without adverse hemodynamic effects. However, when right ventricular systolic pressures are elevated, peripheral edema, hepatic congestion and discomfort, as well as anorexia, nausea, vomiting, and eructation (due to chronic passive congestion of the gastrointestinal tract) may ensue. The patient may note mild icterus and easy fatigability (due to a reduced cardiac output). Occasionally, the patient may be cyanosed due to right-to-left shunting through a patent foramen ovale.

The physical examination of the patient with tricuspid regurgitation reveals distended jugular veins with an especially prominent regurgitant wave. The liver is enlarged, is often tender, and may pulsate prominently during systole. There may be massive peripheral edema and ascites. On cardiac examination, there may be characteristic seesaw movement of the anterior chest wall. The right heart border is displaced into the right chest. The S_1 is usually diminished. The S_2 may have an especially loud pulmonic component in the presence of pulmonary hypertension. A holosystolic murmur, loudest at the left lower sternal border, usually becomes distinctly louder during inspiration. However, when the regurgitation is massive or when the failing ventricle can no longer increase its stroke volume, this may not be appreciated. In addition, a right ventricular S_3 is usually audible. If the amount of regurgitation is large, a diastolic rumble (of "relative" tricuspid stenosis) may be audible.

Right atrial and right ventricular enlargement is present on the chest x-ray of the patient with tricuspid regurgitation. The superior vena cava may pulsate during systole. The ECG shows right axis deviation, right ventricular hypertrophy, and right atrial enlargement (peaked P waves in standard lead II). The rhythm may be atrial fibrillation, in which case P wave morphology is impossible to assess. Recently, two-dimensional echocardiography in conjunction with the peripheral venous injection of contrast material has been used to visualize directly the "to-and-fro" movement of contrast material across the tricuspid valve.

At the time of cardiac catheterization, right atrial and right ventricular diastolic pressures are elevated. When tricuspid regurgitation is severe, the right atrial pressure tracing may resemble the right ventricular pressure tracing. A right ventricular systolic pressure greater than 60 mm Hg generally implies that the tricuspid regurgitation is due to right ventricular decompensation rather than organic tricuspid valve disease; conversely, a systolic pressure less than 40 mm Hg suggests intrinsic valvular pathology. Right ventricular angiography shows regurgitation of dye into the right atrium and, in severe cases, into the superior or inferior vena cava. However, the quantitation of regurgitation by this technique is difficult.

Functional tricuspid regurgitation may improve markedly if the underlying disease process (e.g., mitral stenosis) is corrected. The need for an additional surgical procedure on the tricuspid valve in this setting is best assessed at the time of surgery. Definitive surgery for tricuspid regurgitation entails either tricuspid annuloplasty (with or without the use of a prosthetic ring) or replacement. Bioprostheses are preferred to mechanical prostheses in the tricuspid position because the low flow and local geometry favor stasis and the development of valvular thrombosis. If tricuspid regurgitation occurs as a result of end-stage right ventricular decompensation due to a process that is not surgically remediable, surgery is not indicated, and aggressive medical therapy should be pursued with digitalis and diuretics.

1. Aaron BL, Mills M, Lower RR. Congenital tricuspid insufficiency: definition and review. Chest 1976; 69:637–41.
   A review of 22 cases of congenital tricuspid regurgitation.
2. Arbulu A, Asfaw I. Tricuspid valvulectomy without prosthetic replacement: ten years of clinical experience. J Thorac Cardiovasc Surg 1981; 82:684–91.
   Tricuspid valvulectomy without prosthetic replacement is the treatment of choice in patients with intractable, right-sided infective endocarditis.
3. Breyer RH, McClenathan JH, Michaelis LL, McIntosh CL, Morrow AG. Tricuspid regurgitation: a comparison of nonoperative management, tricuspid annuloplasty, and tricuspid valve replacement. J Thorac Cardiovasc Surg 1976; 72:867–74.
   In this series, the surgical outcome for moderate or severe functional tricuspid regurgitation was better with prosthetic valve replacement than with annuloplasty.
4. Carpentier A, Deloche A, Hanania G, Forman J, Sellier P, Piwnica A, DuBost C. Surgical management of acquired tricuspid valve disease. J Thorac Cardiovasc Surg 1974; 67:53–65.
   In 150 patients, a Carpentier ring annuloplasty was successful in the treatment of tricuspid regurgitation in 135 (90%).
5. Chandraratna PAN, Littman BB, Wilson D. The association between atrial septal defect and prolapse of the tricuspid valve: an echocardiographic study. Chest 1978; 73:839–42.
   Of 52 patients with secundum ASDs, 6 had tricuspid valve prolapse by echocardiography. Repair of the ASD resulted in more severe tricuspid prolapse and marked tricuspid regurgitation in 1 patient.
6. Hansing CE, Rowe GG. Tricuspid insufficiency: a study of hemodynamics and pathogenesis. Circulation 1972; 45:793–9.
   This study assesses the utility of the indicator dilution technique to assess the presence and severity of tricuspid regurgitation in 90 patients at the time of cardiac catheterization.
7. Lieppe W, Behar VS, Scallion R, Kisslo JA. Detection of tricuspid regurgitation with two-dimensional echocardiography and peripheral vein injections. Circulation 1978; 57:128–32.
   This technique allows for the noninvasive visualization of tricuspid regurgitation.
8. McAllister RG Jr, Friesinger GC, Sinclair-Smith BC. Tricuspid regurgitation following inferior myocardial infarction. Arch Intern Med 1976; 136:95–9.
   A description of two patients without previous valvular disease in whom tricuspid regurgitation followed an inferior myocardial infarction, presumably due to right ventricular papillary muscle dysfunction.
9. Osborn JR, Jones RC, Jahnke EJ Jr. Traumatic tricuspid insufficiency. Hemodynamic data and surgical treatment. Circulation 1964; 30:217–22.
   A case report of a patient with isolated traumatic rupture of the anterior papillary muscle of the tricuspid valve, including clinical observations, hemodynamic data, and details of surgical treatment.

10. Pepine CJ, Nichols WW, Selby JH. Diagnostic tests for tricuspid insufficiency: how good? Cathet Cardiovasc Diagn 1979; 5:1–6.
    Tricuspid regurgitation is a difficult valvular lesion to evaluate precisely in the catheterization laboratory.
11. Reed GE, Boyd AD, Spencer FC, Engelman RM, Isom OW, Cunningham JN Jr. Operative management of tricuspid regurgitation. Circulation 1976; 54(Suppl III):96–101.
    In a large series of patients requiring surgical intervention for tricuspid regurgitation, tricuspid annuloplasty appeared superior to valve replacement.
12. Roberts WC, Sjoerdsma A. The cardiac disease associated with the carcinoid syndrome (carcinoid heart disease). Am J Med 1964; 36:5–34.
    The clinical and pathologic features of 17 patients with the carcinoid syndrome are reviewed; 9 had associated heart disease.
13. Salazar E, Levine HD. Rheumatic tricuspid regurgitation: the clinical spectrum. Am J Med 1962; 33:111–29.
    A complete description of 55 patients with rheumatic tricuspid regurgitation.
14. Sanfelippo PM, Giuliani ER, Danielson GK, Wallace RB, Pluth JR, McGoon DC. Tricuspid valve prosthetic replacement: early and late results with the Starr-Edwards prosthesis. J Thorac Cardiovasc Surg 1976; 71:441–5.
    A review of 154 patients at the Mayo Clinic who underwent tricuspid valve replacement with the Starr-Edwards valve, either alone or in combination with other valve replacements.
15. Silverman BD, Garabajal NR, Chorches MA, Taranto AI. Tricuspid regurgitation and acute myocardial infarction. Arch Intern Med 1982; 142:1394–5.
    A case report of a patient with tricuspid regurgitation following a right ventricular infarction who improved after tricuspid valve replacement.
16. Simon R, Oelert H, Brest HG, Lichtlen PR. Influence of mitral valve surgery on tricuspid incompetence concomitant with mitral valve disease. Circulation 1980; 62 (Suppl I):152–7.
    In 20 patients with tricuspid regurgitation who underwent isolated mitral valve surgery, tricuspid regurgitation decreased in 6, remained unchanged in 13, and was more severe in 1 postoperatively.
17. Ubago JL, Fugueroa A, Colman T, Ochoteco A, Rodriquez M, Duran CMG. Right ventriculography as a valid method for the diagnosis of tricuspid insufficiency. Cathet Cardiovasc Diagn 1981; 7:433–41.
    In 168 patients, right ventricular angiography using a balloon-tipped catheter was an effective technique for assessing tricuspid regurgitation.
18. Verel D, Sandler G, Mazurkie SJ. Tricuspid incompetence in cor pulmonale. Br Heart J 1962; 24:441–4.
    In patients with cor pulmonale and resultant tricuspid regurgitation, the characteristic holosystolic murmur radiates differently than in patients without lung disease.
19. Zone DD, Botti RE. Right ventricular infarction with tricuspid insufficiency and chronic right heart failure. Am J Cardiol 1976; 37:445–8.
    In some patients, right ventricular infarction can result in tricuspid regurgitation.

SUBACUTE BACTERIAL ENDOCARDITIS

Subacute bacterial endocarditis (SBE) usually occurs in patients with *previous valvular or congenital heart disease*. Since it can be caused by agents other than bacteria, the term *infective* endocarditis is preferred. Under normal conditions, the causative organisms are not very pathogenic, but in the patient with underlying endocardial disease, these organisms are capable of initiating and sustaining an infection. The most common causative organism is the streptococcus, among which the viridans group is most frequent, followed by microaerophilic streptococci, enterococci, anaerobic streptococci, and beta-hemolytic streptococci. Other organisms also can cause SBE. Although staphylococci usually cause acute bacterial endocarditis, they can occasionally cause a syndrome identical to SBE. The pneumococcus can cause subacute bacterial endocarditis, and a variety of gram-negative bacilli can cause it, including *Pseudomonas, Escherichia coli,* gonococci, and salmonellae. Fungal endocarditis often has the same clinical characteristics as SBE. Candidal endocarditis is especially frequent in intravenous drug abusers and in patients in whom endocarditis develops on a prosthetic valve.

The symptoms of SBE are nonspecific. They usually result from (1) the toxicity of the infection, (2) embolization by fragments of vegetations, and (3) destruction of the involved valves. The patient may complain of fever, but its magnitude and pattern may vary considerably. Chills, diaphoresis, fatigue, weakness, and anorexia with weight loss may be present. Low back pain is a common presenting complaint in about one-third of patients. Embolization of various organs is a cardinal feature of SBE. The patient may complain of left upper quadrant abdominal pain (due to splenic embolization with subsequent infarction), chest pain (due to coronary artery embolization), partial or total loss of vision (due to retinal artery embolization), hematuria (due to renal emboli), or a variety of neurologic symptoms, caused by central nervous system embolization (meningitis, hemiplegia, or a neuropsychiatric syndrome). Embolization of the large arteries of the extremities is uncommon with SBE but frequent with fungal endocarditis. Finally, if SBE is untreated, valvular destruction eventually causes congestive heart failure. In the modern era, treatment is usually administered early, and therefore, congestive failure is uncommon.

On initial physical examination, the patient may or may not have fever, but careful monitoring usually reveals a temperature spike sometime during the initial 24 to 48 hours of hospitalization. The fingernails may reveal splinter hemorrhages: the usual splinter is black, longitudinally oriented, and located in the distal third of the nail. Petechiae may appear on the conjunctivae, the mucous membranes inside the mouth, the soft or hard palate, or around the clavicles, lower neck, wrists, and legs. Osler's nodes (reddish-purple, tender cutaneous nodules of 1–10 mm in size) may appear in the pads of the distal fingers or toes as well as the palms, flanks, and sides of the fingers. Janeway lesions (numerous small hemorrhages with a slight nodular character in the palms of the hands and the soles of the feet) may appear late in the course of infective endocarditis. On funduscopic examination, Roth's spots (retinal hemorrhages, often with a pale or white center, located near the optic disc) may be single or multiple and may be oval, round, or fusiform in shape. The spleen may be palpable, and there may be clubbing of the fingers. The cardiac examination usually reveals the murmurs of the underlying valvular or congenital cardiac disease.

The patient with SBE usually has a mild or moderate anemia, a leukocytosis with a predominance of polymorphonuclear leukocytes, and an elevated erythrocyte sedimentation rate. If renal embolization has been extensive, the serum creatinine and blood urea nitrogen may be elevated. Autoimmune glomerulonephritis can occur in SBE. The serum globulin level may be elevated, and the rheumatoid factor may be transiently positive. The chest x-ray generally reflects the underlying valvular or congenital heart disease. If the endocarditis involves the right-sided cardiac valves, the lung fields may contain multiple foci of infection. The ECG also reflects the underlying cardiac disease. Echocardiography (both M-mode and two-dimensional) may allow one to visualize valvular vegetations if they are extensive and large (at least 2 mm in diameter) and may reveal the consequences of valvular regurgitation. In patients with aortic regurgitation, there may be fluttering of the anterior mitral leaflet and ventricular septum or even preclosure of the mitral valve; in the patient with mitral regurgitation, a flail leaflet or torn chordae may be seen.

The diagnosis of SBE is made (1) by having a high index of suspicion and (2) by growing the causative organism from the patient's blood. Thus, before treatment is initiated, blood samples should be obtained for culture. Three sets of blood cultures spaced over 24 hours will reveal the causative organism in 95 to 99 percent of cases. Even if the blood cultures are negative, one should treat the patient for SBE if one is sufficiently suspicious of its presence.

Before penicillin and other antibiotics, SBE was invariably fatal. Today, if effective antibiotic treatment is initiated, the vast majority of patients with SBE are cured. The effective therapy of SBE centers on the long-term (i.e., 4–6 weeks) administration of an antibiotic with proved efficacy against the causative organism. For viridans streptococci, high-dose intravenous penicillin is an extremely effective drug. It can be used either alone or in combination with streptomycin. For other types of streptococci, such as the enterococcus, a combination of antibiotics (e.g., penicillin and gentamicin) may be necessary. Staphylococcal endocarditis should be treated with high-dose intravenous nafcillin or oxacillin. Fungal endocarditis does not respond to medical therapy and should be treated surgically.

Although infective endocarditis may respond to antibiotic therapy, valve replacement may be necessary under several circumstances, including (1) severe congestive heart failure refractory to medical therapy, (2) failure of medical therapy to control the infection, (3) purulent pericarditis, (4) conduction disturbances due to a ventricular septal abscess, (5) systemic emboli, and (6) endocarditis due to certain organisms, particularly fungi and staphylococci. Congestive heart failure due to valvular destruction, particularly involving the aortic valve, is responsible for most deaths. The hemodynamic status of the patient rather than the duration or appropriateness of antibiotic therapy should determine the need for valve replacement, since the prognosis with medical therapy alone is dismal once heart failure occurs.

Clinical Characteristics

1. Andriole VT, Kravetz HM, Roberts WC, Utz JP. *Candida* endocarditis: clinical and pathologic studies. Am J Med 1962; 32:251–85.
   A review of the clinical manifestations of fungal endocarditis.
2. Bryan CS, Marney SR Jr, Alford RH, Bryant RE. Gram-negative bacillary endocarditis. Am J Med 1975; 58:209–15.
   A critical evaluation of the use of serum bactericidal testing to gauge the adequacy of antibiotic therapy in patients with infective endocarditis.
3. Cabane J, Godeau P, Herreman G, Acar J, Digeon M, Bach JF. Fate of circulating immune complexes in infective endocarditis. Am J Med 1979; 66:277–82.
   Circulating immune complexes are important in the pathogenesis of peripheral lesions in endocarditis.
4. Geraci JE, Wilson WR. Endocarditis due to gram-negative bacteria: report of 56 cases. Mayo Clin Proc 1982; 57:65–8.
   This study indicates an increasing incidence of gram-negative bacterial endocarditis (approximately 10% of endocarditis cases) and an improving cure rate (82%).
5. Hermans PE. The clinical manifestations of infective endocarditis. Mayo Clin Proc 1982; 57:13–9.
   Three sets of blood cultures obtained over several hours are sufficient for the diagnosis of SBE in approximately 95% of cases.
6. Jemsek JG, Greenberg SB, Gentry LO, Welton DE, Mattox KL. *Haemophilus para-influenzae* endocarditis: two cases and review of the literature in the past decade. Am J Med 1979; 66:51–7.
   A total of 25 cases of H. parainfluenzae *endocarditis are reviewed.*

7. Jones HR Jr, Siekert RG, Geraci JE. Neurologic manifestations of bacterial endocarditis. Ann Intern Med 1969; 71:21–8.
   Various neurologic manifestations are common in endocarditis, occurring in about 30% of patients.
8. Menda KB, Gorbach SL. Favorable experience with bacterial endocarditis in heroin addicts. Ann Intern Med 1973; 78:25–32.
   Twenty-three patients with bacterial endocarditis and heroin addiction are reported: because of early diagnosis and intensive management of complications all survived.
9. Pesanti EL, Smith IM. Infective endocarditis with negative blood cultures: an analysis of 52 cases. Am J Med 1979; 66:43–50.
   Of those patients who succumbed to their disease, death resulted primarily from major systemic emboli and from uncontrollable congestive heart failure.
10. Thell R, Martin FH, Edwards JE. Bacterial endocarditis in subjects 60 years of age and older. Circulation 1975; 51:174–82.
    Of 42 cases of endocarditis in elderly patients, the most common infecting organisms were staphylococci (14) and various types of streptococci (10).
11. Wilkowske CJ. Enterococci endocarditis. Mayo Clin Proc 1982; 57:51–5.
    Enterococci cause 10–20% of endocarditis. Combination therapy with penicillin G or ampicillin and an aminoglycoside is required for at least 4 weeks.
12. Wilson WR, Danielson GK, Giuliani ER, Geraci JE. Prosthetic valve endocarditis. Mayo Clin Proc 1982; 57:75–81.
    The frequency of prosthetic valve endocarditis is only 2%, but the mortality is over 50%. Staphylococci are most commonly associated with early onset infection and streptococci with late infection. Staphylococcal prosthetic valve endocarditis requires valve replacement.
13. Wilson WR, Jaumin PM, Danielson GK, Giuliani ER, Washington JA II, Geraci JE. Prosthetic valve endocarditis. Ann Intern Med 1975; 82:751–6.
    Forty-five patients with prosthetic valve endocarditis are reviewed; 25 (56%) patients died. Of the 20 survivors, medical therapy alone was curative in 12 (60%).

Diagnosis
14. Brandenburg RO, Giuliani ER, Wilson WR, Geraci JE. Infective endocarditis—a 25 year overview of diagnosis and therapy. JACC 1983; 1:280–91.
    An excellent overview of this subject by authorities in the field.
15. Dillon JC, Feigenbaum H, Konecke LL, Davis RH, Chang S. Echocardiographic manifestations of valvular vegetations. Am Heart J 1973; 86:698–704.
    M-mode echocardiography may be used to visualize vegetations at least 2 mm in diameter.
16. Martin RP, Meltzer RS, Chia BL, Stinson EB, Rakowski H, Popp RL. Clinical utility of two dimensional echocardiography in infective endocarditis. Am J Cardiol 1980; 46:379–85.
    In this study of 58 patients, two-dimensional echocardiography was superior to M-mode echocardiography in the recognition of vegetations.
17. Scanlan JG, Seward JB, Tajik AJ. Valve ring abscess in infective endocarditis: visualization with wide angle two-dimensional echocardiography. Am J Cardiol 1982; 49:1794–1800.
    Two dimensional echocardiography permitted visualization of a valve ring abscess complicating infective endocarditis in 4 patients.
18. Sheikh MU, Ali N, Covarrubias E, Fox LM, Morjaria M, Dejo J. Right-sided infective endocarditis: an echocardiographic study. Am J Med 1979; 66:283–7.
    Many patients with endocarditis of the tricuspid or pulmonic valves have echocardiographically visible vegetations.
19. Wann LS, Dillon JC, Weyman AE, Feigenbaum H. Echocardiography in bacterial endocarditis. N Engl J Med 1976; 295:135–9.
    The echocardiographic visualization of vegetations in patients with endocarditis is a bad prognostic sign, in that 20 of the 22 patients with visible vegetations died or underwent valve replacement for refractory congestive failure.
20. Washington JA II. The role of the microbiology laboratory in the diagnosis and antimicrobial treatment of infective endocarditis. Mayo Clin Proc 1982; 57:20–30.
    An excellent review of the isolation and identification of the infecting organism in SBE.

Therapy

21. Keys TF. Antimicrobial prophylaxis for patients with congenital or valvular heart disease. Mayo Clin Proc 1982; 57:91–5.
    Recommendations are given for selection of the most appropriate antibiotic for prophylaxis against endocarditis.
22. Richardson JV, Karp RB, Kirklin JW, Dismukes WE. Treatment of infective endocarditis: a 10-year comparative analysis. Circulation 1978; 58:589–97.
    Early surgical intervention is recommended in patients with endocarditis and concomitant moderate or severe heart failure.
23. Wilson WR, Danielson GK, Giuliani ER, Washington JA III, Jaumin PM, Geraci JE. Valve replacement in patients with active infective endocarditis. Circulation 1978; 58:585–8.
    The hemodynamic status of patients with infective endocarditis should be the determining factor in the timing of cardiac valve replacement.
24. Wilson WR, Giuliani ER, Geraci JE. Treatment of penicillin sensitive streptococcal infective endocarditis. Mayo Clin Proc 1982; 57:45–50.
    Patients with endocarditis due to penicillin-sensitive streptococci have an overall cure rate of 98%. Those unable to tolerate penicillin may be treated with vancomycin or a cephalosporin.
25. Brandenburg RO, Giuliani ER, Wilson WR, Geraci JE. Infective endocarditis—a 25-year overview of diagnosis and therapy. JACC 1983; 1:280–91.
    A good review of the clinical characteristics, diagnosis, and therapy of endocarditis in the 1980s.

ACUTE BACTERIAL ENDOCARDITIS

Acute bacterial endocarditis is a rapidly developing and usually fulminant disease, in which previously normal valves are affected by an especially virulent organism. In most instances, it is caused by *Staphylococcus aureus,* which gains access to the blood through an infection of the skin or by intravenous drug abuse. Less commonly, it may be caused by the pneumococcus or *Streptococcus pyogenes.*

The patient with acute bacterial endocarditis usually complains of high fever, shaking chills, and, in most instances, symptoms of congestive heart failure. The infecting organism invades and quickly damages the valvular and perivalvular tissues, resulting in regurgitation of the involved valves. If the aortic or mitral valve is involved, the clinical picture is that of acute aortic or mitral regurgitation, in which case the patient complains of symptoms of pulmonary vascular congestion (dyspnea, orthopnea, and paroxysmal nocturnal dyspnea). If the right-sided valves are involved, the patient may complain of dyspnea, cough, and pleuritic chest pain, and the chest x-ray often demonstrates multiple embolic abscesses. Pulmonary or systemic embolization of infected valvular tissue may produce additional symptoms, including dyspnea (due to recurrent pulmonary embolization), chest pain (due to embolization of the coronary arteries), various neurologic syndromes (due to cerebral embolization), or flank pain and hematuria (due to renal artery embolization). Cerebral embolization occurs in approximately 20 percent of patients with left-sided staphylococcal endocarditis.

On physical examination, the patient is usually febrile and may have rigors. The hands and feet often do not demonstrate the classic stigmata of subacute endocarditis (Osler's nodes, Janeway spots, and petechiae). The peripheral pulse is usually rapid. On cardiac examination, regurgitant murmurs of the involved valves are usually present but may be unimpressive. An S_3 and S_4 are usually audible. The overall heart size is normal or minimally enlarged. There is often evidence of pulmonary vascular congestion.

The patient with acute bacterial endocarditis usually has a normal hemoglobin and hematocrit, since the anemia characteristic of subacute endocarditis has not had time to develop. The white blood cell count is elevated, with a predominance of polymorphonuclear leukocytes, especially immature forms. The urinalysis may reveal hematuria. The appearance of the chest x-ray is dependent on which valves are involved: if the aortic or mitral valves are infected, the lung fields usually demonstrate pulmonary vascular redistribution. The left ventricle is not greatly enlarged, since the regurgitation has not been present long enough to cause left ventricular dilatation. Unilateral or bilateral pleural effusions may be present. The ECG usually does not show evidence of ventricular hypertrophy, since this has not had sufficient time to develop. Echocardiography may be very helpful in these patients, since it may demonstrate vegetations on the infected valves.

Untreated, acute bacterial endocarditis is a rapidly fatal disease, with the patient dying of overwhelming infection or cardiac failure. If proper antibiotics are initiated promptly, the chances of survival are improved, but they depend on which valve is involved. If the tricuspid valve is infected, medical therapy (with intravenous nafcillin or oxacillin for *S. aureus*) may be curative, but in some patients tricuspid valvulectomy (with or without a later valve replacement) may be required. In contrast, the patient with aortic valve involvement usually has severe hemodynamic decompensation; in addition, perivalvular abscess formation is common, and purulent pericarditis, conduction disturbances, and death are frequent if medical therapy alone is employed. Therefore, it is recommended that left-sided valve replacement be performed at the first sign of hemodynamic decompensation, since the major determinant of survival with acute bacterial endocarditis is the patient's hemodynamic status. If the patient's condition permits, cardiac catheterization may be particularly valuable before surgery to provide an assessment of (1) the presence and severity of valvular involvement, (2) the concomitant involvement of other valves, and (3) the presence of associated abnormalities, such as fistulae or aortic root abscesses.

Clinical Characteristics

1. Banks T, Fletcher R, Ali N. Infective endocarditis in heroin addicts. Am J Med 1973; 55:444–51.
   Valvular endocarditis, especially of the tricuspid valve, is a common occurrence in intravenous drug abusers.
2. Ramsey RG, Gunnar RM, Tobin JR Jr. Endocarditis in the drug addict. Am J Cardiol 1970; 25:608–18.
   Intravenous drug abusers are more likely to have right-sided endocarditis, usually due to Staphylococcus aureus.
3. Reyes MP, Palutke WA, Wylin RF, Lerner AM. *Pseudomonas* endocarditis in the Detroit Medical Center, 1969–1972. Medicine 1973; 52:173–94.
   A report of an unusually high incidence of right sided endocarditis due to Pseudomonas *in intravenous drug users.*
4. Sklaver AR, Hoffman TA, Greenman RL. Staphylococcal endocarditis in addicts. South Med J 1978; 71:638–43.
   In 50 drug addicts with staphylococcal endocarditis, the tricuspid valve was involved in all cases, whereas only 3 (5%) had left-sided involvement.
5. Thompson RL. Staphylococcal infective endocarditis. Mayo Clin Proc 1982; 57:56–64.

Staphylococcus aureus *causes an acute endocarditis, often involving previously normal valves. Despite prompt treatment and recognition of complications, the morbidity and mortality associated with this infection remain high.*

6. Dreyer NP, Fields BN. Heroin-associated infective endocarditis: a report of 28 cases. Am Intern Med 1973; 78:699–702.

Staphylococci were isolated in 68% of patients; Streptococcus, Candida, *and* Hemophilus *accounted for the remainder.*

Diagnosis

7. Andy JJ, Sheikh MU, Ali N, Barnes BO, Fox LM, Curry CL, Roberts WC. Echocardiographic observations in opiate addicts with active infective endocarditis: frequency of involvement of the various valves and comparison of echocardiographic features of right and left-sided cardiac valve endocarditis. Am J Cardiol 1977; 40:17–23.

In 25 opiate addicts, endocarditis involved only the tricuspid valve in 11, both right- and left-sided valves in 7, and only left-sided valves in 7. The infecting organism was Staphylococcus aureus *in 17 patients.*

8. Gintzon LE, Siegel RJ, Criley JM. Natural history of tricuspid valve endocarditis: a two-dimensional echocardiographic study. Am J Cardiol 1982; 49:1853–9.

With medical therapy, tricuspid valve vegetations usually decrease in size or disappear with time.

9. Davis RS, Strom JA, Frishman W, Becker R, Matsumoto M, LeJemtel TH, Sonnenblick EH, Frater RWM. The demonstration of vegetations by echocardiography in bacterial endocarditis: an indication for early surgical intervention. Am J Med 1980; 69:57–63.

The demonstration of vegetations by M-mode echocardiography identified a group of patients with severe disease in whom early operative intervention was required.

10. Stewart JA, Silimperi D, Harris P, Wise NK, Fraker TD Jr, Kisslo JA. Echocardiographic documentation of vegetative lesions in infective endocarditis: clinical implications. Circulation 1980; 61:374–80.

Although the detection of vegetations by echocardiography in patients with endocarditis identifies a group at risk of complications, decisions regarding clinical management made solely on the basis of the presence or absence of vegetations are hazardous. Management of such individuals should be based on the clinical condition of the patient.

Therapy

11. Arbulu A, Thomas NW, Wilson RF. Valvulectomy without prosthetic replacement. J Thorac Cardiovasc Surg 1972; 64:103–7.

Tricuspid valvulectomy without replacement is recommended for medically unresponsive tricuspid valve endocarditis.

12. Rapaport E. The changing role of surgery in the management of infective endocarditis. editorial. Circulation 1978; 58:598–9.

Patients with endocarditis and moderate or severe cardiac decompensation are best managed surgically.

13. Richardson JV, Karp RB, Kirklin JW, Dismukes WE. Treatment of infective endocarditis: a 10-year comparative analysis. Circulation 1978; 58:589–97.

Early valve replacement is recommended for the patient with moderate or severe heart failure. A particularly aggressive approach to acute staphylococcal endocarditis is recommended.

14. Wilson WR, Danielson GK, Giuliani ER, Washington JA II, Jaumin PM, Geraci JE. Valve replacement in patients with active infective endocarditis. Circulation 1978; 58:585–8.

The hemodynamic status of the patient with endocarditis, rather than the activity of the infection or the length of preoperative antimicrobial therapy, should be the determining factor in the timing of valve replacement.

15. Wilson WR, Giuliani ER, Danielson GK, Geraci JE. Management of complications of endocarditis. Mayo Clin Proc 1982; 57:82–90.

The complications of endocarditis may involve the heart and adjacent structures or may be extracardiac. Valve replacement is recommended if heart failure is unresponsive to medical therapy within 24–48 hours.

16. Sande MA, Scheld WM. Combination antibiotic therapy of bacterial endocarditis. Ann Intern Med 1980; 92:390–5.
   A succinct review of the preferred antibiotic therapy of endocarditis due to various organisms.

COMMON THERAPEUTIC APPROACHES
TO CARDIAC ABNORMALITIES

The digitalis glycosides have been used for over 3,000 years in the treatment of various edematous conditions, and presently they are among the most frequently prescribed medications in the United States. At the cellular level, these compounds inhibit sodium and potassium transport across the plasma membrane by impeding their transport enzyme, sodium-potassium–activated adenosine triphosphatase ([$Na^+ + K^+$]-ATPase). As a result, they cause a substantial efflux of potassium from the myocardium. The cardiac glycosides do not exert a direct effect on contractile proteins, intermediary metabolism, or substrate availability in cardiac muscle. Through their effect on ($Na^+ + K^+$)-ATPase, they increase the amount of calcium that is made available to the contractile element at the time of excitation-contraction coupling, and it is this increase in calcium availability that induces an increase in myocardial contractility.

The digitalis glycosides exert several discernible effects on the heart and vascular system. First, they have a direct positive inotropic effect on the ventricular myocardium, increasing the rate of development of intraventricular pressure at the onset of systole. This positive inotropic influence is demonstrable in the normal as well as the failing heart. In various experimental preparations, they induce a favorable shift in the ventricular function curve, so that at any given ventricular filling pressure, more stroke work is generated by the digitalized heart. Maximal tension development is augmented by the digitalis glycosides, and the time required to reach a given tension is reduced.

Second, the digitalis glycosides exert certain extracardiac hemodynamic effects. They induce arterial and venous constriction because of a local effect on vascular smooth muscle and an alpha-receptor–mediated stimulation of the central nervous system. They inhibit the tubular resorption of sodium when they are administered in large doses. In the experimental animal, the direct infusion of ouabain (a rapidly acting digitalis glycoside) into the renal artery inhibits renal ($Na^+ + K^+$)-ATPase and impairs concentrating and diluting abilities. However, it is unlikely that this direct effect on the kidney contributes importantly to the diuresis that occurs in the treatment of patients with congestive heart failure.

Third, the digitalis glycosides exert marked electrophysiologic effects and are used in the therapy of various tachyarrhythmias. Within the specialized conduction system, digitalis increases the refractory period and decreases conduction velocity, thus slowing the ventricular response in atrial fibrillation and flutter. In contrast, in the atrial and ventricular myocardium, the digitalis compounds shorten the refractory period and enhance automaticity.

Ouabain is the most rapidly acting of the digitalis glycosides that is available for clinical use. Following its intravenous administration, its onset of action is rapid (5–10 min), with a peak effect at 30 to 120 minutes. In normal subjects, its plasma half-life is about 21 hours. Since it is poorly absorbed from the gastrointestinal tract, it must be administered parenterally. Its mode of excretion is primarily renal, and the amount given must therefore be adjusted in patients with renal compromise.

Digoxin is the most widely prescribed digitalis glycoside. It can be given parenterally or orally, but in the latter case it is only 60- to 85-percent absorbed. Following its intravenous administration, it begins to act within 15 to 30 minutes, with its peak action coming 2 to 5 hours later. Its serum half-life is 36 hours. Like ouabain, it is excreted primarily by the kidney, and dosage adjustments must be made in patients with renal disease. *Digitoxin* is the most slowly excreted cardiac glycoside. Its gastrointestinal absorption is virtually complete, after which about 97 percent is bound to serum albumin. Following its administration, its peak effect comes in 4 to 12 hours. Its average serum half-life is 4 to 6 days, with excretion occurring primarily through the liver.

The clinical indications for the use of cardiac glycosides center on two broad areas. First, they are of potential value in patients with symptoms and signs of congestive heart failure due to ischemic, valvular, hypertensive, congenital, or primary myopathic heart disease. Through their direct positive inotropic effect, they increase cardiac output, promote a diuresis, and reduce filling pressures of the failing ventricles, thus relieving pulmonary and systemic venous congestion. They have no beneficial effect in patients with constrictive pericarditis or pericardial tamponade, and they may be deleterious in the patient with obstructive hypertrophic cardiomyopathy. Second, the digitalis glycosides are of potential use in the management of four types of supraventricular tachyarrhythmias. Paroxysmal supraventricular tachycardia usually responds to digitalization when simpler therapeutic measures are unsuccessful, and maintenance digitalis usually reduces the frequency of recurrent episodes. The digitalis glycosides slow the ventricular rate in patients with atrial fibrillation by increasing blockade at the AV junction. Similarly, they slow the ventricular rate in patients with atrial flutter. Lastly, some Wolff-Parkinson-White tachyarrhythmias may be terminated or prevented by digitalis. However, some patients with this syndrome have an extremely rapid ventricular response during atrial fibrillation, and digitalis may accelerate this response or contribute to the appearance of ventricular fibrillation.

Within the past 10 years, laboratory methods have become available for the accurate quantitation of the serum concentration of the commonly employed digitalis glycosides. Although several methods have been described, the radioimmunoassay is by far the most reliable and exact, allowing the measurement of amounts even smaller than a nanogram. Using this radioimmunoassay, it has been shown that digitalis intoxication is affected by many factors and that there is considerable overlap in the serum digitalis concentrations in patients with toxicity and those without. As a result, the serum digitalis concentration cannot be used as the only guide to digitalis dosage. At the same time, however, serum digitalis concentrations, when used in the overall clinical context in conjunction with other available information, can serve as a valuable aid to therapeutic decisions involving digitalis administration and dosage. The inotropic effects of digitalis appear to plateau at a serum level of approximately 1.1 ng per milliliter, whereas the toxic manifestations generally occur with a serum level above 2.0 ng per milliliter. However, in the presence of hypokalemia, digitalis toxicity can occur with serum levels as low as 1.1 ng per milliliter. Thus, the therapeutic-to-toxic margin is narrow.

Although digitalis is effective in the management of patients with congestive heart failure in sinus rhythm, the risk-benefit ratio of chronic therapy is of concern. Toxic manifestations of digitalis therapy comprise some of the most prevalent adverse drug reactions encountered in clinical practice. In the management of acute severe congestive heart failure (e.g., in the setting of acute myocardial infarction), dobutamine or dopamine are more powerful inotropic agents and more easily titrated than digitalis. Similarly, in patients with chronic congestive heart failure (particularly when due to ischemic heart disease or a congestive cardiomyopathy), the judicious use of diuretics with or without vasodilator therapy is generally adequate. In the patient on an adequate diuretic regimen, the addition or withdrawal of digitalis may not affect symptomatic status. In short, the use of digitalis in the patient with sinus rhythm and congestive heart failure should not be a reflex response but, rather, a carefully weighed decision.

1. Akera T, Larsen FS, Brody TM. Correlation of cardiac sodium- and potassium-activated adenosine triphosphatase activity with ouabain-induced inotropic stimulation. J Pharmacol Exp Ther 1970; 173:145–51.
   Cardiac (Na$^+$ + K$^+$)-ATPase activity is inhibited during inotropic stimulation by ouabain.
2. Arnold SB, Byrd RC, Meister W, Melmon K, Cheitlin MD, Bristow JD, Parmley WW, Chatterjee K. Long-term digitalis therapy improves left ventricular function in heart failure. N Engl J Med 1980; 303:1443–8.
   In this study, 9 patients with congestive heart failure showed an improvement in left ventricular function with acute and chronic digoxin therapy.
3. Beller GA, Smith TW, Abelmann WH, Haber E, Hood WB Jr. Digitalis intoxication: a prospective clinical study with serum level correlations. N Engl J Med 1971; 284:989–97.
   This study of patients in a large city hospital shows a high prevalence of digitalis intoxication (23% of those on digitalis), which is associated with a twofold increase in mortality.
4. Braunwald E, Bloodwell RD, Goldberg LI, Morrow AG. Studies on digitalis: IV. Observations in man on the effects of digitalis preparations on the contractility of the non-failing heart and on total vascular resistance. J Clin Invest 1961; 40:52–9.
   Digitalis augments the contractile force of the non-failing heart and constricts the systemic vascular bed.
5. Dreifus LS, Watanabe Y. Clinical correlates of the electrophysiologic action of digitalis on the heart. Semin Drug Treat 1972; 2:179–201.
   A detailed review of the electrophysiologic effects of digitalis. Includes 94 references.
6. Firth BG. Digoxin: help or hindrance in patients with ischemic heart disease? Int J Cardiol 1982; 2:233–5.
   Because of the inherent risks, the use of digitalis in patients with sinus rhythm and congestive heart failure should be a carefully weighed decision.
7. Firth BG, Dehmer GJ, Corbett JR, Lewis SE, Parkey RW, Willerson JT. Effect of chronic oral digoxin therapy on ventricular function at rest and peak exercise in patients with ischemic heart disease: assessment with equilibrium gated blood pool imaging. Am J Cardiol 1980; 46:481–90.
   In 14 patients with known ischemic heart disease on diuretics and/or nitrates, chronic oral digoxin therapy caused no change in ventricular function at rest and an improvement in ventricular function at peak exercise only in those with left ventricular ejection fractions greater than 0.50.
8. Fozzard HA. Excitation-contraction coupling and digitalis. Circulation 1973; 47:5–7.
   In all probability, digitalis exerts its positive inotropic effect by altering intracellular sodium concentration, which, in turn, affects calcium influx.
9. Gheorghiade M, Beller GA. Effects of discontinuing maintenance digoxin therapy in patients with ischemic heart disease and congestive heart failure in sinus rhythm. Am J Cardiol 1983; 51:1243–50.
   Digoxin withdrawal had no adverse clinical or hemodynamic effects in 24 patients with coronary artery disease and documented congestive heart failure who were on maintenance diuretic and/or vasodilator therapy.
10. Goldstein RA, Passamani ER, Roberts R. A comparison of digoxin and dobutamine in patients with acute infarction and cardiac failure. N Engl J Med 1980; 303:846–50.
    In this setting, dobutamine was a more powerful and effective inotropic agent than digoxin.
11. Green LH, Smith TW. The use of digitalis in patients with pulmonary disease. Ann Intern Med 1977; 87:459–65.

Patients with underlying pulmonary disease may be more susceptible to the toxic effects of cardiac glycosides.

12. Hyman AL, Jaques WE, Hyman ES. Observation on the direct effect of digoxin on renal excretion of sodium and water. Am Heart J 1956; 52:592–608.
    In dogs, a direct natriuretic and diuretic effect of digoxin can be demonstrated.

13. Karliner JS, Braunwald E. Present status of digitalis treatment of acute myocardial infarction. Circulation 1972; 45:891–902.
    Digitalis should not be given to patients with uncomplicated myocardial infarction who do not have cardiomegaly.

14. Langer GA. Effects of digitalis on myocardial ionic exchange. Circulation 1972; 46:180–7.
    By inhibiting $(Na^+ + K^+)$-ATPase, digitalis increases $Na^+ - Ca^{++}$ coupled transport, thereby increasing the influx of Ca^{++} to the myofilaments.

15. Lee DCS, Johnson RA, Bingham JB, Leahy M, Dinsmore RE, Goroll AH, Newell JB, Strauss HW, Haber E. Heart failure in outpatients: a randomized trial of digoxin versus placebo. N Engl J Med 1982; 306:699–705.
    Patients with the most severe heart failure showed the greatest response to digitalis. However, in patients who were given adequate amounts of diuretics, digitalis produced no further clinical improvement.

16. Lown B, Klein MD, Barr I, Hagemeijer F, Kosowsky BD, Garrison H. Sensitivity to digitalis drugs in acute myocardial infarction. Am J Cardiol 1972; 30:388–95.
    Most patients with acute myocardial infarction and heart failure can safely be treated with digitalis.

17. Lukas DS, DeMartino AG. Binding of digitoxin and some related cardenolides to human plasma proteins. J Clin Invest 1969; 48:1041–53.
    Digitoxin has a marked avidity for serum albumin, thus accounting for its lower rate of urinary excretion and its longer serum half-life.

18. Mason DT, Braunwald E. Studies on digitalis: X. Effects of ouabain on forearm vascular resistance and venous tone in normal subjects and in patients in heart failure. J Clin Invest 1964; 43:532–43.
    In normal subjects, ouabain increases forearm vascular resistance and venous tone.

19. Raabe DS Jr. Combined therapy with digoxin and nitroprusside in heart failure complicating acute myocardial infarction. Am J Cardiol 1979; 43:990–4.
    The addition of digoxin to nitroprusside in these patients caused an increase in cardiac output but no further decrease in pulmonary capillary wedge pressure.

20. Sellers TD Jr, Bashore TM, Gallagher JJ. Digitalis in the preexcitation syndrome: analysis during atrial fibrillation. Circulation 1977; 56:260–7.
    In some patients with the Wolff-Parkinson-White syndrome, digitalis induces ventricular fibrillation.

21. Shanbour LL, Jacobson ED. Digitalis and the mesenteric circulation. Am J Dig Dis 1972; 17:826–8.
    The cardiac glycosides clearly cause splanchnic vasoconstriction.

22. Shapiro W. Correlative studies of serum digitalis levels and the arrhythmias of digitalis intoxication. Am J Cardiol 1978; 41:852–9.
    Hypokalemic patients frequently manifest digitalis intoxication at serum digoxin levels well below 2 ng/mL.

23. Smith TW. Digitalis glycosides. N Engl J Med 1973; 288:719–22, 942–6.
    A brief discussion of the commonly prescribed digitalis preparations.

24. Smith TW, Haber E. Digitalis. N Engl J Med 1973; 289:945–52, 1010–5, 1063–72, 1125–9.
    A comprehensive review of digitalis, including a discussion of its clinical uses and mechanisms of action. Includes 336 references.

25. Sonnenblick EH, Williams JF Jr, Glick G, Mason DT, Braunwald E. Studies on digitalis: XV. Effects of cardiac glycosides on myocardial force-velocity relations in the nonfailing human heart. Circulation 1966; 34:532–9.
    In 6 patients who had undergone cardiac surgery, ouabain increased the velocity of shortening by 77% and intraventricular pressure rose by 23%.

26. Yankopoulos NA, Kawai C, Federici EE, Adler LN, Abelmann WH. The hemody-

namic effects of ouabain upon the diseased left ventricle. Am Heart J 1968; 76:466–80.
In 20 patients with left ventricular failure of various etiologies, ouabain consistently increased myocardial contractility.

INOTROPIC AGENTS

Those agents that increase myocardial contractility are important in the management of patients with acute and chronic severe left ventricular failure. Although several agents can be administered intravenously for the acute management of left ventricular failure, *digitalis* is the only inotropic agent approved for chronic oral use. *Isoproterenol,* the prototype beta-adrenergic receptor agonist, exerts a marked positive inotropic and chronotropic effect and has little effect on alpha-adrenergic receptors. Therefore, it causes an increase in the rate and force of ventricular contraction, a fall in left ventricular filling pressure, and either no change or a fall in systemic arterial pressure. In addition, it increases the rate of spontaneous depolarization of conducting tissue and may precipitate ventricular arrhythmias. In the setting of acute myocardial infarction, isoproterenol may increase myocardial oxygen consumption (due to the increase in heart rate and contractility), decrease myocardial oxygen supply (due to a reduction in coronary perfusion pressure), and potentiate arrhythmias. Thus, its use in this situation should be avoided. Even in patients without ischemic heart disease, isoproterenol's value is limited by its propensity to cause hypotension, tachycardia, and arrhythmias. In life-threatening situations where other positive inotropic agents are not available, isoproterenol may be administered at 0.5 to 5.0 µg per minute. Since its positive inotropic and chronotropic effects closely parallel one another, the dosage may be titrated against the change in heart rate in patients in a stable state.

In comparison to isoproterenol, *norepinephrine* is a more powerful alpha-adrenergic agonist and a much weaker beta-receptor agonist. It can be used in patients with cardiogenic shock to increase systolic and diastolic systemic arterial pressure and coronary perfusion, but it is not useful purely as a positive inotropic agent. The recommended intravenous dosage in the patient with cardiogenic shock is 0.5 to 5.0 µg per minute. Great care should be exercised to avoid extravasation of norepinephrine at the infusion site, since this can cause local tissue necrosis (due to its vasoconstrictive action). *Epinephrine* exerts effects that are intermediate between those of isoproterenol and norepinephrine. It is generally only used for the treatment of acute cardiac arrest and asystole, in which case it is administered as an intravenous bolus of 0.5 to 1.0 mg of a 1:10,000 solution.

Dopamine and *dobutamine* are catecholamine-like substances that presently are the preferred intravenous inotropic agents for the management of patients with severe acute or chronic left ventricular failure. In comparison to isoproterenol, epinephrine, and norepinephrine, they cause less tachycardia and are less arrhythmogenic. Dopamine releases norepinephrine from tissue stores and exerts a direct action on dopaminergic receptors. It increases myocardial contractility, systemic vascular resistance, and renal blood flow but exerts only a minimal effect on heart rate. It may also increase pulmonary capillary wedge pressure. The recommended dosage is 2 to 20 µg/kg/min. In contrast, dobutamine is a positive inotropic agent of similar potency but with *vasodilator* properties. As a result, it causes a fall in systemic arterial and pulmonary capillary wedge pressure. The recommended intravenous dosage is 2 to 30 μg/kg/min. Both of these agents are available only for intravenous administration and have short half-lives. Dopamine is generally used when severe hypotension persists, thus militating against the use of dobutamine. If systemic blood pressure is adequately maintained, a vasodilator (e.g., sodium nitroprusside) can be combined with dopamine, or dobutamine can be used. There is some evidence that dobutamine may have a deleterious effect on regional myocardial blood flow. Other studies have suggested that dopamine may lose some of its inotropic effect with prolonged administration (presumably because it depletes myocardial norepinephrine stores). Therefore, the preferred agent in the normotensive patient is presently a matter of physician preference. Indeed, there is some evidence that the combined use of dopamine and dobutamine (in approximately equal quantities) may be a rational and effective treatment of patients with severe left ventricular failure; with such combination therapy, myocardial contractility is improved, systemic blood pressure is maintained, renal blood flow is enhanced, and pulmonary capillary wedge pressure is reduced.

When dopamine or other alpha-adrenergic agonists are administered, care must be taken to insure that excessive blood flow to vital organs is not achieved at the expense of peripheral perfusion, which may cause vascular insufficiency or even gangrene. In general, the dosage of dopamine should not exceed 10 to 12 μg/kg/min. Beyond this range, its vasoconstrictive effects outweigh its positive inotropic effects, and the heart is compelled to work against an ever-increasing "afterload." For the same reason, the use of a pure alpha-adrenergic agonist, such as phenlyephrine or methoxamine, is contraindicated in the patient with severe left ventricular failure.

Amrinone is a new noncatecholamine, noncardiac glycoside agent with positive inotropic and vasodilator effects. It is available both as an intravenous and an oral preparation; however, only the intravenous preparation is approved for use in patients with severe left ventricular failure. The major adverse effect that limits the use of this agent is a dose-related thrombocytopenia. Other side effects include gastrointestinal disturbance, hepatotoxicity, and fever. The usual intravenous dosage is 3 to 20 μg/kg/min. A new cardiotonic agent with a chemical structure analogous to amrinone (at present designated WIN 47203) appears to be more potent than amrinone, effective both orally and intravenously, and devoid of clinical and laboratory manifestations of toxicity. At present it is available only for experimental use. Another experimental inotropic agent (MDL 17403) also appears to be a noncatecholamine, noncardiac glycoside in nature and to possess vasodilatory properties. It is effective intravenously and orally.

Dopamine and Dobutamine

1. Beregovich J, Bianchi C, Rubler S, Lomnitz E, Cagin N, Levitt B. Dose-related hemodynamic and renal effects of dopamine in congestive heart failure. Am Heart J 1974; 87:550–7.
   A detailed analysis of the effects of incremental dosages of dopamine in 9 patients with congestive heart failure. Tachycardia was significant at an infusion rate > 10 μg/kg/min.

2. Gillespie TA, Ambos HD, Sobel BE, Roberts R. Effects of dobutamine in patients with acute myocardial infarction. Am J Cardiol 1977; 39:588–94.
   This study concludes that dobutamine in doses sufficient to improve ventricular performance does not exacerbate myocardial injury or ventricular dysrhythmia.

3. Goldberg LI, Hsieh Y, Resnekov L. Newer catecholamines for treatment of heart failure and shock: an update on dopamine and a first look at dobutamine. Prog Cardiovasc Dis 1977; 19:327–40.
   A succinct review of both these agents. Includes 97 references.

4. Goldberg LI. Dopamine—clinical uses of an endogenous catecholamine. N Engl J Med 1974; 291:707–10.
   A detailed review of the mechanism of action and clinical uses of dopamine.
5. Hinds JE, Hawthorne EW. Comparative cardiac dynamic effects of dobutamine and isoproterenol in conscious instrumented dogs. Am J Cardiol 1975; 36:894–901.
   For the same inotropic effect, dobutamine produces a much smaller increase in heart rate than isoproterenol.
6. Leier CV, Heban PT, Huss P, Bush CA, Lewis RP. Comparative systemic and regional hemodynamic effects of dopamine and dobutamine in patients with cardiomyopathic heart failure. Circulation 1978; 58:466–75.
   This study in 13 patients with severe congestive heart failure concludes that dobutamine has many advantages over dopamine.
7. Loeb HS, Winslow EBJ, Rahimtoola SH, Rosen KM, Gunnar RM. Acute hemodynamic effects of dopamine in patients with shock. Circulation 1971; 44:163–73.
   The hemodynamic effects of dopamine in 62 patients with shock are described. The effects are compared to those of norepinephrine and isoproterenol.
8. Maekawa K, Liang CS, Hood WB Jr. Comparison of dobutamine and dopamine in acute myocardial infarction: effects on systemic hemodynamics, plasma catecholamines, blood flows and infarct size. Circulation 1983; 67:750–9.
   This study in chronically instrumented dogs suggests that dopamine loses its efficacy as an inotropic agent after 24 hours of administration.
9. Richard C, Ricome JL, Rimailho A, Bottineau G, Auzepy P. Combined hemodynamic effects of dopamine and dobutamine in cardiogenic shock. Circulation 1983; 67:620–6.
   In 8 patients with cardiogenic shock, the combination of dobutamine and dopamine, (7.5 µg/kg/min of each agent) was superior to 15 µg/kg/min of either agent alone.
10. Robie NW, Goldberg LI. Comparative systemic and regional hemodynamic effects of dopamine and dobutamine. Am Heart J 1975; 90:340–5.
    Although both dopamine and dobutamine are powerful positive inotropic agents, dopamine increases renal and mesenteric blood flow, whereas dobutamine does not.
11. Sonnenblick EH, Frishman WH, Le Jemtel TH. Dobutamine: a new synthetic cardioactive sympathetic amine. N Engl J Med 1979; 300:17–22.
    A succinct synopsis of the effects of dobutamine.
12. Stoner JD III, Bolen JL, Harrison DC. Comparison of dobutamine and dopamine in treatment of severe heart failure. Br Heart J 1977; 39:536–9.
    The effects of dobutamine in 12 patients with congestive heart failure were compared to the effects of dopamine in 10 clinically similar patients. Dopamine produced a considerably greater increase in heart rate for the same increase in cardiac output.
13. Tuttle RR, Mills J. Dobutamine: development of a new catecholamine to selectively increase cardiac contractility. Circ Res 1975; 36:185–96.
    The initial report of the effects of dobutamine and a description of its chemical structure and development.
14. Willerson JT, Hutton I, Watson JT, Platt MR, Templeton GH. Influence of dobutamine on regional myocardial blood flow and ventricular performance during acute and chronic myocardial ischemia in dogs. Circulation 1976; 53:828–33.
    This study in anesthetized dogs suggests that dobutamine in dosages sufficient to increase left ventricular dP/dt may increase myocardial ischemia.

Amrinone and Other New Inotropic Agents

15. Benotti JR, Grossman W, Braunwald E, Davolos DD, Alousi AA. Hemodynamic assessment of amrinone—a new inotropic agent. N Engl J Med 1978; 299:1373–7.
    One of the earliest reports of the beneficial effects of amrinone.
16. Le Jemtel TH, Keung E, Ribner HS, Davis R, Wexler J, Blaufox MD, Sonnenblick EH. Sustained beneficial effects of oral amrinone on cardiac and renal function in patients with severe congestive heart failure. Am J Cardiol 1980; 45:123–9.
    An early report of the efficacy of chronic oral amrinone therapy.

17. Maskin CS, Sinoway L, Chadwick B, Sonnenblick EH, LeJemtel TH. Sustained hemodynamic and clinical effects of a new cardiotonic agent, WIN 47203, in patients with severe congestive heart failure. Circulation 1983; 67:1065–70.
    A report of the acute and chronic efficacy of this experimental agent, a congener of amrinone, in 11 patients with severe congestive heart failure.
18. Uretsky BF, Generalovich T, Reddy PS, Spangenberg RB, Follansbee WP. The acute hemodynamic effects of a new agent, MDL 17,043, in the treatment of congestive heart failure. Circulation 1983; 67:823–8.
    The acute hemodynamic effects of this experimental agent, which is a non-catecholamine, non-cardiac glycoside, are described in 15 patients.
19. Weber KT, Andrews V, Janicki JS, Wilson JR, Fishman AP. Amrinone and exercise performance in patients with chronic heart failure. Am J Cardiol 1981; 48:164–9.
    This study suggests that amrinone improves cardiac function at rest and during exercise in patients with chronic heart failure refractory to digitalis, diuretics, and vasodilators.
20. Klein NA, Siskind SJ, Frishman WH, Sonnenblick EH, LeJemtel TH. Hemodynamic comparison of intravenous amrinone and dobutamine in patients with chronic congestive heart failure. Am J Cardiol 1981; 48:170–5.
    In patients with congestive failure, amrinone is comparable in effect to the optimal dose of dobutamine. With prolonged infusion (several hours), dobutamine's effects begin to lessen, whereas those of amrinone are sustained.
21. Siegel LA, Keung E, Siskind SJ, Forman R, Feinberg H, Strom J, Efstathakis D, Sonnenblick EH, LeJemtel TH. Beneficial effects of amrinone-hydralazine combination on resting hemodynamics and exercise capacity in patients with severe congestive heart failure. Circulation 1981; 63:838–44.
    In 9 patients with severe congestive heart failure, a combination of low-dose amrinone and hydralazine was markedly beneficial.

DIGOXIN-QUINIDINE INTERACTION

Digoxin and quinidine are frequently used in combination for the treatment of various cardiovascular disorders. Recent studies have demonstrated that the plasma digoxin concentration is increased approximately twofold when quinidine is administered concomitantly. In some individuals, this increase in the plasma concentration of digoxin induces digoxin toxicity.

Quinidine increases the plasma digoxin concentration by at least three mechanisms. First, quinidine displaces digoxin from its binding sites in the heart, skeletal muscle, and other tissues. Since digoxin is extensively bound to tissue, a relatively small change in tissue binding results in a pronounced rise in the plasma concentration of digoxin. Second, quinidine reduces the renal clearance of digoxin to about two-thirds of its value without quinidine. Since glomerular filtration is not altered when these drugs are administered concomitantly, the observed decrease in the renal clearance of digoxin during quinidine treatment probably results from a quinidine-induced inhibition of renal secretion of digoxin. Third, quinidine causes a decrease in the nonrenal clearance of digoxin, probably through a reduction in hepatic metabolism and biliary secretion.

Pharmacokinetic studies have demonstrated that the serum digoxin concentration begins to rise on the first day of concomitant quinidine administration and continues to rise until a new steady state is reached, usually in 4 to 5 days. The serum digoxin concentration then remains elevated as long as quinidine is continued. The alterations in the renal clearance of digoxin that are induced by quinidine occur even at subtherapeutic concentrations of the latter, although the overall magnitude of the reduction in renal digoxin clearance depends on the serum quinidine concentration.

Although quinidine clearly causes a rise in the plasma digoxin concentration, the overall clinical importance of this alteration is uncertain. In some individuals, the increased plasma digoxin concentration is associated with an increased incidence of the gastrointestinal symptoms of digoxin toxicity (nausea and vomiting), presumably due to the effect of a high plasma digoxin level on the area postrema of the medulla. Some studies also have suggested that the incidence of digoxin-toxic ventricular arrhythmias is increased by quinidine administration. Since digoxin binding to cardiac muscle is actually *reduced* by quinidine, however, the mechanism by which ventricular ectopy is induced is unknown. In light of this, it seems reasonable that the digoxin dosage should be reduced when quinidine therapy is initiated, and the serum digoxin concentration should be monitored carefully during the first several weeks of quinidine administration.

1. Hager WD, Fenster P, Mayersohn M, Perrier D, Graves P, Marcus FI, Goldman S. Digoxin-quinidine interaction: pharmacokinetic evaluation. N Engl J Med 1979; 300:1238–41.
   Quinidine reduces the renal clearance of digoxin and displaces digoxin from its tissue binding sites.
2. Leahey EB Jr, Reiffel JA, Drusin RE, Heissenbuttel RH, Lovejoy WP, Bigger JT Jr. Interaction between quinidine and digoxin. JAMA 1978; 240:533–4.
   In 27 patients on maintenance digoxin, quinidine increased the digoxin serum concentration from 1.4 to 3.2 ng/mL.
3. Doering W. Quinidine-digoxin interaction: pharmacokinetics, underlying mechanism and clinical implications. N Engl J Med 1979; 301:400–4.
   The addition of quinidine decreased renal digoxin clearance from 92 to 41 mL per minute. These authors suggest that when quinidine is given to a patient on digoxin, the digoxin dosage should be reduced by 30% to 50%.
4. Leahey EB Jr, Bigger JT Jr, Butler VP Jr, Reiffel JA, O'Connell GC, Scaffidi LE, Rottman JN. Quinidine-digoxin interaction: time course and pharmacokinetics. Am J Cardiol 1981; 48:1141–6.
   Changes in renal clearance of digoxin occur even at subtherapeutic concentrations of quinidine, and the magnitude of the decrease in renal digoxin clearance depends on the serum quinidine concentration.
5. Leahey EB Jr, Reiffel JA, Giardina EGV, Bigger JT Jr. The effect of quinidine and other oral antiarrhythmic drugs on serum digoxin. Ann Intern Med 1980; 92:605–8.
   In 22 patients already taking digoxin, quinidine raised the serum digoxin concentration from 1.2 to 2.4 nmol/L. Anorexia, nausea, and vomiting developed in 10 of the 22.
6. Ejvinsson G. Effect of quinidine on plasma concentrations of digoxin. Br Med J 1978; 1:279–80.
   One of the original articles describing an increase in the serum digoxin concentration during concomitant therapy with quinidine.
7. Hooymans PM, Merkus FWHM. Effect of quinidine on plasma concentration of digoxin. Br Med J 1978; 2:1022.
   These authors suggest that quinidine reduces the renal clearance of digoxin, thereby raising the serum digoxin concentration.
8. Fenster PE, Hager WD, Perrier D, Powell JR, Graves PE, Michael UF. Digoxin-quinidine interaction in patients with chronic renal failure. Circulation 1982; 66:1277–80.
   In patients who are essentially anephric, quinidine causes a decrease in digoxin clearance, which must be nonrenal in origin.
9. Goldman S, Hager WD, Olajos M, Perrier D, Mayersohn M. Effect of the ouabain-quinidine interaction on left ventricular and left atrial function in conscious dogs. Circulation 1983; 67:1054–8.
   This study demonstrates that the quinidine-induced increase in the serum digoxin concentration is accompanied by a decrease in the contractile response of the heart to digoxin.

10. Doherty JE, Straub KD, Murphy ML, deSoyza N, Bissett JK, Kane JJ. Digoxin-quinidine interaction: changes in canine tissue concentration from steady state with quinidine. Am J Cardiol 1980; 45:1196–1200.
    Quinidine causes the concentration of digoxin to increase in brain tissue; this increase in the brain digoxin concentration causes the clinical manifestations of digoxin toxicity.
11. Hirsh PD, Weiner HJ, North RL. Further insights into digoxin-quinidine interaction: lack of correlation between serum digoxin concentration and inotropic state of the heart. Am J Cardiol 1980; 46:863–8.
    Quinidine increases the serum digoxin concentration by displacing digoxin from cardiac binding sites. As a result, digoxin's positive inotropic effect is diminished.
12. Mungall DR, Robichaux RP, Perry W, Scott JW, Robinson A, Burelle T, Hurst D. Effects of quinidine on serum digoxin concentration: a prospective study. Ann Intern Med 1980; 93:689–93.
    Before quinidine therapy, 15 adults had a serum digoxin concentration of 0.75 ng/mL; after 4 days of quinidine, this rose to 1.41 ng/mL.
13. Ochs HR, Pabst J, Greenblatt DJ, Dengler HJ. Noninteraction of digitoxin and quinidine. N Engl J Med 1980; 303:672–4.
    In clinical terms, digitoxin can be coadministered with quinidine with no appreciable change in digitoxin kinetics.
14. Garty M, Sood P, Rollins DE. Digitoxin elimination reduced during quinidine therapy. Ann Intern Med 1981; 94:35–7.
    In this study of 5 healthy volunteers, quinidine substantially lengthened the digitoxin elimination half-life.
15. Fenster PE, Powell JR, Graves PE, Conrad KA, Hager WD, Goldman S, Marcus FI. Digitoxin-quinidine interaction: pharmacokinetic evaluation. Ann Intern Med 1980; 93:698–701.
    Quinidine prolonged digitoxin's elimination half-life and reduced its total body and renal clearance.

DIGITALIS INTOXICATION

Digitalis intoxication is a relatively common occurrence. In fact, recent studies of hospitalized patients have demonstrated that it occurs in 8 to 35 percent, with a mortality attributable to it ranging from 3 to 21 percent of those intoxicated. Although most of these studies have been performed retrospectively, a large prospective study of almost 1000 patients admitted to a general medical service showed that 23 percent of those taking a digitalis glycoside at the time of admission fulfilled the criteria for definite digitalis toxicity, and another 6 percent were judged to have possible toxicity. In short, digitalis intoxication occurs frequently, even in patients confined to the hospital and under close observation by experienced medical personnel.

The major manifestations of digitalis intoxication include disturbances of gastrointestinal and central nervous system function as well as cardiac rhythm abnormalities. Anorexia, nausea, and vomiting occur commonly and are probably caused by the direct effect of the digitalis glycosides on the area postrema of the medulla. Clinically, it is often difficult to attribute these symptoms to digitalis, since they may be caused by associated diseases or by mesenteric venous congestion due to right-sided congestive failure. The digitalis glycosides can cause a wide spectrum of neurologic disturbances, including headache, malaise, confusion, disorientation, delirium, and grand mal seizures. Visual symptoms, such as scotomas, halos, and changes in color perception, occur commonly. Skin rashes and gynecomastia occasionally appear as a manifestation of digitalis toxicity.

A variety of disturbances of cardiac rhythm can be induced by digitalis intoxication. The most frequent are ventricular premature beats (often with runs of bigeminy or trigeminy), junctional tachycardia, ventricular tachycardia, paroxysmal supraventricular tachycardia with AV block, sinus block, sinus arrest, and Mobitz type I (Wenckebach) second degree AV block. In short, almost any rhythm or conduction disturbance can be caused by digitalis intoxication. Rhythms that combine features of increased automaticity with impaired conduction (e.g., paroxysmal supraventricular tachycardia with AV block) are especially common in patients with digitalis intoxication.

In recent years it has become possible to measure the serum concentration of several cardiac glycoside preparations, including digoxin and digitoxin. From these measurements, it has become clear that patients intoxicated with digoxin usually have a serum concentration in excess of 2 ng per milliliter, whereas those intoxicated with digitoxin have a serum concentration greater than 30 ng per milliliter. Unfortunately, there is considerable overlap in measured values between individuals who are intoxicated and those in whom only a therapeutic serum concentration has been achieved. Thus, a digoxin level near 2 ng per milliliter or a digitoxin concentration of 25 ng per milliliter does not separate the toxic from the nontoxic patient. In addition, the propensity for digitalis intoxication is greatly accentuated by hypokalemia, so that an occasional patient with severe hypokalemia may manifest digitalis intoxication with a relatively low serum glycoside level. Even with the ready availability of serum glycoside levels, therefore, the diagnosis of digitalis intoxication remains largely a clinical one, though in many individuals the clinical diagnosis can be supported by the measurement of a serum concentration.

Massive overdoses of the digitalis glycosides occur occasionally and present special therapeutic problems. In the patient without underlying heart disease, massive digitalis ingestion usually induces severe sinus bradycardia and/or various degrees of AV block (first, second, or third degree). In these individuals, atropine is often successful in reversing these manifestations. Ventricular pacing can be employed if atropine does not work. Massive digitalis ingestion in the patient with underlying cardiac disease often leads to frequent ventricular premature beats, ventricular tachycardia, and ventricular fibrillation. Although phenytoin, lidocaine, or procainamide may be efficacious in some of these patients, the ventricular arrhythmias in this group are often fatal. At very high serum concentrations, the digitalis glycosides cause hyperkalemia that may be completely refractory to all therapeutic modalities. This elevation of serum potassium is probably due to an inhibition of sodium-potassium–activated adenosine triphosphatase throughout the body.

Digitalis intoxication should be treated by the prompt discontinuation of the offending medication. Bradyarrhythmias should be treated initially with atropine; if this is not successful, temporary transvenous ventricular pacing should be initiated. If drug therapy is needed, phenytoin and lidocaine are most efficacious in suppressing the ectopic impulses induced by digitalis. If rhythm disturbances occur in the setting of hypokalemia, potassium supplementation should be administered carefully. However, such supplements are contraindicated when conduction disturbances are present, since elevations of serum potassium may further impair AV conduction. Propranolol has been used occasionally to treat digitalis-induced arrhythmias, although it may cause bradycardia or sinus arrest. Quinidine and procainamide may depress sinoatrial nodal function and, in addition, may depress myocardial contractility. As a result, they should be used with great caution in the patient with digitalis intoxication. Direct current countershock is inadvisable in the presence of digitalis intoxication, since it may induce severe ventricular arrhythmias. However, it must sometimes be used as the only possible therapy for a life-threatening arrhythmia. The risk of DC shock is diminished when low energy levels are used.

Although still in their early stages of development, digoxin-specific antibodies, or Fab fragments thereof, may provide effective therapy for digitalis intoxication. After the Fab fragments are injected intravenously, they bind specifically to circulating digoxin molecules, rendering them inactive. The Fab-digoxin complexes are then excreted in the urine.

Incidence and Clinical Manifestations

1. Beller GA, Smith TW, Abelmann WH, Haber E, Hood WB Jr. Digitalis intoxication: a prospective clinical study with serum level correlations. N Engl J Med 1971; 284:989–97.

   Of 931 consecutive patients admitted to a general medical service, 140 (15%) were taking digitalis. Of these, 32 (23%) were definitely in a toxic condition, and another 8 (6%) were possibly toxic.

2. Bismuth C, Gaultier M, Conso F, Efthymiou ML. Hyperkalemia in acute digitalis poisoning: prognostic significance and therapeutic implications. Clin Toxicol 1973; 6:153–62.

   In 91 patients who had taken excessive doses of digitalis, there was a good relationship between the serum potassium concentration 3–18 hours after drug ingestion and mortality.

3. Lely AH, vanEnter CHJ. Non-cardiac symptoms of digitalis intoxication. Am Heart J 1972; 83:149–52.

   Of 179 individuals with digitalis intoxication, 170 (95%) had fatigue, 116 (65%) had psychological disturbances, and 143 (80%) had gastrointestinal complaints (nausea, vomiting, abdominal pain).

4. Evered DC, Chapman C. Plasma digoxin concentrations and digoxin toxicity in hospital patients. Br Heart J 1971; 33:540–5.

   Of 108 individuals on routine oral maintenance digoxin therapy, 22 were found to be in a toxic condition.

5. Lely AH, Van Enter CHJ. Large-scale digitoxin intoxication. Br Med J 1970; 3:737–40.

   Of a large number of digitalis-toxic patients, 95% had visual disturbances, including hazy vision, difficulty in reading, photophobia, and glitterings.

6. Shapiro W. Correlative studies of serum digitalis levels and the arrhythmias of digitalis intoxication. Am J Cardiol 1978; 41:852–9.

   This study of 73 patients with digitalis intoxication suggests that the serum glycoside concentration is limited as an independent indicator of toxicity. In the setting of hypokalemia, a digoxin serum level as low as 1.0 ng/mL may be associated with digitalis intoxication.

7. Schott A. Observations on digitalis intoxication—a plea. Postgrad Med J 1964; 40:628–43.

   Digitalis intoxication was present in 12% of hospitalized patients taking one of the digitalis preparations.

8. Smith TW, Willerson JT. Suicidal and accidental digoxin ingestion: report of 5 cases with serum digoxin level correlations. Circulation 1971; 44:29–36.

   A description of five patients with massive digoxin ingestion, including the arrhythmias they developed and their eventual outcome.

9. Kastor JA. Digitalis intoxication in patients with atrial fibrillation. Circulation 1973; 47:888–96.

   In the patient with atrial fibrillation, digitalis intoxication is signaled by a regularization of the ventricular response.

10. Sodeman WA. Diagnosis and treatment of digitalis toxicity. N Engl J Med 1965; 273:35–7, 93–5.

    A detailed discussion of the symptoms and electrocardiographic signs of digitalis intoxication.

11. Delman AJ, Stein E. Atrial flutter secondary to digitalis toxicity: report of three cases and review of the literature. Circulation 1964; 29:593–7.

    This paper emphasizes that atrial flutter is a very uncommon digitalis-toxic arrhythmia; only 16 cases can be collected from the medical literature.

12. Smith TW, Haber E. Digitalis. N Engl J Med 1973; 289:945–52, 1010–5, 1063–72, 1125–9.
    A very complete review of all aspects of digitalis usage, including intoxication.

Therapy
13. Bigger JT Jr, Strauss HC. Digitalis toxicity: drug interactions promoting toxicity and the management of toxicity. Semin Drug Treat 1972; 2:147–77.
    A very complete discussion of digitalis intoxication, including its electrocardiographic recognition and management. Includes 168 references.
14. Lown B, Kleiger R, Williams J. Cardioversion and digitalis drugs: changed threshold to electric shock in digitalized animals. Circ Res 1965; 17:519–31.
    In animals with digitalis intoxication, cardioversion is ineffective and even harmful, since it often provokes serious disturbances of rhythm.
15. Kleiger R, Lown B. Cardioversion and digitalis. II. Clinical studies. Circulation 1966; 33:878–87.
    In patients with atrial fibrillation in whom precardioversion ECGs suggested digitalis intoxication, DC shock was often accompanied by serious ventricular ectopy.
16. Smith TW, Haber E, Yeatman L, Butler VP Jr. Reversal of advanced digoxin intoxication with Fab fragments of digoxin-specific antibodies. N Engl J Med 1976; 294:797–800.
    Fab fragments were used successfully to treat this 39-year-old man after he had ingested 22.5 mg of digoxin.
17. Lloyd BL, Smith TW. Contrasting rates of reversal of digoxin toxicity by digoxin-specific IgG and Fab fragments. Circulation 1978; 58:280–3.
    Specific Fab fragments are better than intact IgG molecules for use in patients with life-threatening digoxin intoxication. The fragments have a more rapid distribution and elimination, and they accomplish a faster and more uniform reversal of advanced digoxin intoxication.
18. Smith TW, Butler VP Jr, Haber E, Fozzard H, Marcus FI, Bremner WF, Schulman IC, Phillips A. Treatment of life-threatening digitalis intoxication with digoxin-specific Fab antibody fragments: experience in 26 cases. N Engl J Med 1982; 307:1357–62.
    Of 26 individuals with life-threatening arrhythmias and (in some cases) hyperkalemia, 21 were treated effectively with purified Fab fragments of digoxin-specific antibodies.

DIURETICS

Diuretics increase the renal excretion of solute and water by inhibiting their tubular reabsorption. The *mercurials* exert their physiologic effect by inhibiting chloride reabsorption in the thick ascending limb of Henle. In addition, they inhibit the cation exchange pump in the distal tubule. Following their intramuscular administration, they begin to cause a diuresis in 30 to 60 minutes, with the peak diuresis occurring 2 to 3 hours later. Since the chloride pump is inhibited directly, the mercurials induce a disproportionate amount of chloride loss in the urine, leading to a hypochloremic alkalosis.

The mercurials usually cause a predictable diuresis without excessive potassium loss. Their disadvantages are (1) their relative lack of potency (compared to furosemide and ethacrynic acid), (2) the requirement that they be given intramuscularly, and (3) their ineffectiveness in patients with underlying metabolic alkalosis. In addition, they should not be administered to patients with renal compromise, since this may lead to mercurial toxicity. Finally, an occasional patient develops a hypersensitivity reaction, but these are relatively rare.

The *benzothiazides* exert their diuretic effect by inhibiting (1) the reabsorption of solute in the thick ascending limb of Henle and (2) the action of carbonic anhydrase in the proximal tubule. Clearly most of the diuretic potency of these compounds is attributable to their effect on the ascending limb of Henle. They are administered orally and exert a prolonged diuretic effect, resulting in a smoother diuresis than that obtained with the more potent short-acting diuretics. Their adverse effects include (1) a maculopapular skin rash, (2) occasional hyperglycemia, (3) hyperuricemia, (4) prerenal azotemia, and (5) mild hypercalcemia. Hypokalemic alkalosis is a common occurrence, resulting from an increased delivery of sodium to the distal tubule; the sodium, in turn, is exchanged for hydrogen and potassium by the cation exchange pump. The resultant hypokalemia increases the proximal reabsorption of bicarbonate, thus aggravating the already existing alkalosis.

The potent diuretics *furosemide* and *ethacrynic acid* exert their effect by inhibiting the reabsorption of solute in the medullary and cortical thick ascending limb of Henle. Following their intravenous administration, they act almost immediately, but their duration of action is shorter than that of the mercurials and thiazides. Both agents are effective irrespective of the patient's fluid-electrolyte or acid-base balance. Thus, they induce a diuresis in patients with hyponatremia, hypokalemia, or hypochloremia.

Both of these potent diuretics may predispose the patient to ototoxicity, but it appears that ethacrynic acid is associated with this complication more often than furosemide. Such ototoxicity is usually acute and transient, but permanent loss of hearing has been reported. Both drugs cause a reduction in glomerular filtration rate, leading to an elevation of the BUN, creatinine, and uric acid. Rarely, furosemide causes an increase in the urinary excretion of calcium, producing tetany. In a minority of patients, these diuretics cause hypokalemia. Although potassium supplementation need not be instituted when furosemide or ethacrynic acid is first prescribed, the serum potassium concentration should be checked 1 to 2 weeks after the initiation of diuretic therapy. If hypokalemia is present, potassium supplementation should be prescribed, or a potassium-sparing diuretic should be added to the patient's pharmacologic regimen.

The *carbonic anhydrase inhibitors,* such as *acetazolamide,* exert their effect by inhibiting carbonic anhydrase in the proximal tubule, causing an increased bicarbonate and potassium excretion as well as free water formation. Although they are used sparingly in clinical practice, they may be especially useful in the patient with metabolic alkalosis, since they promote bicarbonate excretion. They are not extremely powerful, and as a result, they exert only a limited effect in patients with massive edema. The carbonic anhydrase inhibitors are overwhelmingly safe and nontoxic, but occasionally they cause drowsiness or tingling of the fingers in patients receiving very large doses. The so-called *potassium-sparing diuretics, spironolactone* and *triamterene,* inhibit the cation exchange pump in the distal tubule. Spironolactone is a specific antagonist of aldosterone, whereas triamterene's effect is independent of aldosterone. Spironolactone is especially useful in the patient with secondary aldosteronism (e.g., one with cirrhosis and ascites). The disadvantage of these agents is their potential for causing hyperkalemia. This can be life-threatening, especially in the patient with renal compromise. Thus, potassium supplementation should not be administered with spironolactone or triamterene except under extremely rare and specific circumstances.

Finally, the *osmotic diuretics,* of which mannitol is the most commonly used, prevent the reabsorption of normal amounts of solute in the proximal tubule. As a result, a large amount of sodium and chloride is delivered distally, allowing for the increased generation of free water. These agents must be administered intravenously. They are most effective in restoring glomerular filtration during or after a transient episode of hypotension. If renal compromise is severe, the osmotic diuretics may lead to intravascular volume overload.

General
1. Frazier HS, Yager H. The clinical use of diuretics. N Engl J Med 1973; 288:246–9, 455–7.
   A succinct review of the mechanism of action and clinical uses of the various diuretics.

Mercurials
2. Cafruny EJ, Cho KC, Gussin RZ. The pharmacology of mercurial diuretics. Ann NY Acad Sci 1966; 139:362–74.
   A thorough discussion of the cellular mechanisms by which these compounds exert their effect.
3. Levitt MF, Goldstein MH, Lenz PR, Wedeen R. Mercurial diuretics. Ann NY Acad Sci 1966; 139:375–87.
   The data presented in this article suggest that the mercurial diuretics act within the distal tubule to block the reabsorption of salt (and, therefore, water).
4. Cafruny EJ. The site and mechanism of action of mercurial diuretics. Pharmacol Rev 1968; 20:89–116.
   An elegant and very thorough review of the manner in which these agents exert their effects. Includes 191 references.

Benzothiazides
5. Conway J, Palmero H. The vascular effect of the thiazide diuretics. Arch Int Med 1963; 111:203–7.
   Chlorothiazide produces about a 20% fall in peripheral vascular resistance; this effect is not dependent on the drug's diuretic effect.
6. Beyer KH. The mechanism of action of chlorothiazide. Ann NY Acad Sci 1958; 71:363–79.
   A thorough review of the mechanism of action and clinical uses of the thiazide diuretics.

Furosemide and Ethacrynic Acid
7. Kim KE, Onesti G, Moyer JH, Swartz C. Ethacrynic acid and furosemide: diuretic and hemodynamic effects and clinical uses. Am J Cardiol 1971; 27:407–15.
   A succinct review of the pharmacologic effects and clinical indications for these potent diuretics.
8. Meriwether WD, Mangi RJ, Serpick AA. Deafness following standard intravenous dose of ethacrynic acid. JAMA 1971; 216:795–8.
   Two nonuremic patients who developed transient deafness after receiving ethacrynic acid are described.
9. Schneider WJ, Becker EL. Acute transient hearing loss after ethacrynic acid therapy. Arch Int Med 1966; 117:715–7.
   This report describes 5 patients with compromised renal function in whom ethacrynic acid caused transient hearing loss.
10. Mukherjee SK, Katz MA, Michael UF, Ogden DA. Mechanisms of hemodynamic actions of furosemide: differentiation of vascular and renal effects on blood pressure in functionally anephric hypertensive patients. Am Heart J 1981; 101:313–8.
    It is concluded from these studies in 11 anephric patients that the early hypotensive effect of furosemide is mediated by its diuretic effects.
11. Schwartz GH, David DS, Riggio RR, Stenzel KH, Rubin AL. Ototoxicity induced by furosemide. N Engl J Med 1970; 282:1413–4.
    In 5 patients with compromised renal function, ototoxicity developed after they received large doses of furosemide.

12. Stason WB, Cannon PJ, Heinemann HO, Laragh JH. Furosemide: a clinical evaluation of its diuretic action. Circulation 1966; 34:910–20.
   The data presented in this article suggest that furosemide blocks sodium chloride reabsorption in the ascending limb of Henle's loop.

13. Wertheimer L, Almondhiry H, Khero B. Furosemide, a new diuretic in edematous states: clinical studies in patients with congestive heart failure and cirrhosis of the liver. Arch Int Med 1967; 119:189–94.
   Of 17 patients with severe fluid retention, oral or parenteral furosemide caused a good diuretic response in 15.

14. Maher JF, Schreiner GE. Studies on ethacrynic acid in patients with refractory edema. Ann Intern Med 1965; 62:15–29.
   In 38 patients with refractory edema, ethacrynic acid proved to be an effective diuretic despite adverse physiologic circumstances, such as hypoalbuminemia, hyponatremia, hypochloremia, hypokalemia, alkalosis, and a markedly diminished glomerular filtration rate.

15. Biddle TL, Yu PN. Effect of furosemide on hemodynamics and lung water in acute pulmonary edema secondary to myocardial infarction. Am J Cardiol 1979; 43:86–90.
   In 19 patients with left ventricular failure due to myocardial infarction, furosemide caused a fall in left- and right-sided filling pressures and a reduction in lung water. However, the latter reduction was delayed for several hours after the administration of furosemide.

16. Dikshit K, Vyden JK, Forrester JS, Chatterjee K, Prakash R, Swan HJC. Renal and extrarenal hemodynamic effects of furosemide in congestive heart failure after acute myocardial infarction. N Engl J Med 1973; 288:1087–90.
   The immediate effect of furosemide in patients with pulmonary congestion is not related to its diuretic properties but to its ability to increase venous capacitance.

Carbonic Anhydrase Inhibitors

17. Griggs RC, Engel WK, Resnick JS. Acetazolamide treatment of hypokalemic periodic paralysis. Prevention of attacks and improvement of persistent weakness. Ann Intern Med 1970; 73:39–48.
   In this study, 10 of 12 patients with hypokalemic periodic paralysis were markedly improved by acetazolamide therapy.

18. Berliner RW, Orloff J. Carbonic anhydrase inhibitors. Pharmacol Rev 1956; 8:137–74.
   A review of the effect of carbonic anhydrase inhibitors on the kidney, stomach, eye, pancreas, and salivary and sweat glands.

"Potassium-Sparing" Diuretics

19. Walker BR, Capuzzi DM, Alexander F, Familiar RG, Hoppe RC. Hyperkalemia after triamterene in diabetic patients. Clin Pharmacol Ther 1972; 13:643–51.
   Patients with moderate diabetes developed hyperkalemia during an intravenous glucose load while on triamterene therapy.

20. Liddle GW. Aldosterone antagonists and triamterene. Ann NY Acad Sci 1966; 139:466–70.
   Although triamterene and spironolactone cause similar changes in electrolyte excretion, they do so through totally different mechanisms.

21. Ginsberg DJ, Saad A, Gabuzda GJ. Metabolic studies with the diuretic triamterene in patients with cirrhosis and ascites. N Engl J Med 1964; 271:1229–35.
   Although the metabolic effects of triamterene resemble those that result from aldosterone antagonists, triamterene does not interfere directly with the action of mineralocorticoids.

Osmotic Diuretics

22. Morris CR, Alexander EA, Bruns FJ, Levinsky NG. Restoration and maintenance of glomerular filtration by mannitol during hypoperfusion of the kidney. J Clin Invest 1972; 51:1555–64.
   During severe renal hypoperfusion, mannitol can maintain or reestablish glomerular filtration, which otherwise could not be restored.

23. Barry KG, Malloy JP. Oliguric renal failure. Evaluation and therapy by the intra-venous infusion of mannitol. JAMA 1962; 179:510–3.
In 24 patients with impending renal failure, prompt mannitol therapy prevented it in 16.

ANTICOAGULANTS

Several groups of patients with cardiopulmonary disease may require acute or chronic anticoagulation. First, the patient with pulmonary embolic disease should receive anticoagulation provided, of course, that there is no strong contraindication. Second, the patient with mitral valve disease (stenosis, regurgitation, or mixed) and concomitant atrial fibrillation should be anticoagulated in an attempt to prevent systemic arterial embolism from the accumulation of left atrial thrombi. Third, the patient with a large and poorly functioning left ventricle (most often the result of extensive coronary artery disease or a congestive cardiomyopathy) should receive anticoagulation in an attempt to prevent the formation of left ventricular thrombi with subsequent systemic arterial embolism. Fourth, the patient in whom a metal or plastic prosthetic heart valve has been implanted should be anticoagulated, since thrombus commonly forms on such prostheses regardless of their anatomic position. In contrast, the patient with a homograft or heterograft prosthesis does not require anticoagulation. Fifth, the patient with cardiac disease who is hospitalized and whose activities are substantially curtailed should be considered for anticoagulant therapy, since these individuals are at increased risk of developing venous thromboses, with resultant embolic complications.

Heparin is the mainstay of parenteral anticoagulation. It is ineffective after oral administration, but it is well absorbed following intramuscular or subcutaneous injection. Its anticoagulant effect is achieved immediately after its intravenous administration. In the patient who requires full anticoagulation, heparin should be administered intravenously as a continuous infusion (of 1000–2000 units/hr) or by bolus injection (5000–7500 units every 4–6 hr). By either approach, the patient in whom full anticoagulation is desired should receive 25,000 to 40,000 units of heparin intravenously over 24 hours. The adequacy of heparin administration should be demonstrated by a prolongation of the Lee-White clotting time or the activated partial thromboplastin time to 2 to 2½ times control values.

Subcutaneous heparin, administered every 8 to 12 hours, effectively reduces the incidence of deep venous thrombosis and pulmonary embolism. In the patient who is immobilized in a surgical or medical setting, 10,000 to 15,000 units per day of subcutaneous heparin reduces the frequency of thromboembolic events without greatly increasing the incidence of serious hemorrhagic complications.

About half the heparin that is administered is eventually excreted unchanged in the urine. The other half is metabolized by the liver, after which it is also excreted in the urine. The commercially available heparin preparations are relatively nontoxic, and the incidence of adverse effects is low. Occasionally, heparin induces a reversible thrombocytopenia. Rarely, the patient may have a hypersensitivity or anaphylactic reaction, manifested clinically by severe asthma, giant urticaria, rhinitis, lacrimation, and fever. In some patients, transient alopecia appears several months after heparin administration. The major adverse effect of heparin is, of course, hemorrhage, most commonly hematuria, hemarthrosis, wound hematoma, and gastrointestinal bleeding. As a result, heparin is contraindicated in the patient with a bleeding diathesis as well as in those with threatened abortion, subacute bacterial endocarditis, suspected intracranial hemorrhage, peptic ulcer disease, or a history of heparin hypersensitivity.

The *coumarin* anticoagulants are used for chronic oral anticoagulation. They exert their effect by inhibiting the hepatic synthesis of clotting factors II, VII, IX, and X; in turn, this suppression is caused by the inhibition of vitamin K. After they are given orally, the coumarin drugs are absorbed erratically from the gastrointestinal tract, after which they are almost entirely bound to plasma protein. There is a 24- to 48-hour delay between the achievement of a peak plasma level and a substantial therapeutic response. The oral anticoagulants sometimes induce bleeding, most often hematuria, ecchymoses, epistaxis, bleeding gums, and hemoptysis. Extensive uterine bleeding has been observed occasionally. About 25 percent of all deaths from oral anticoagulant therapy are due to gastrointestinal bleeding, usually from unsuspected peptic ulcer disease. For this reason, oral anticoagulants are contraindicated in the patient with ulcerative lesions of the gastrointestinal tract, diverticulitis, colitis, subacute bacterial endocarditis, threatened abortion, or severe hepatic or renal disease. These drugs easily cross the placental barrier (whereas heparin does not), so that their use during pregnancy carries a sizable hemorrhagic risk for the fetus. The overall potency of a particular dose of oral anticoagulant is markedly affected by diet as well as concomitantly administered medications; therefore, the patient's prothrombin time should be checked often.

The treatment of hemorrhage due to oral anticoagulants should involve several maneuvers. First, the oral anticoagulants should be discontinued immediately. Second, vitamin K should be administered orally or parenterally. Third, if more rapid correction of the anticoagulation is required, fresh frozen plasma effectively reverses the drug-induced depression of factors II, VII, IX, and X.

Over the past few years, several agents that directly alter platelet function have been evaluated clinically, and their ability to reduce the frequency of postoperative thromboembolism in high-risk patients has been assessed. Aspirin reduces the incidence of deep venous thrombosis in men undergoing total hip replacement, and in some studies, its effect was equal to that of warfarin or low-molecular-weight dextran. A combination of dipyridamole and warfarin is more effective than warfarin alone in reducing the incidence of systemic arterial embolism in patients with prosthetic valves. However, dipyridamole given alone is not especially effective in patients with cerebrovascular disease or acute myocardial infarction. Sulfinpyrazone, a potent uricosuric agent used in the treatment of gout, reduces cardiovascular-related mortality in elderly male patients with a history of stroke or myocardial infarction. Although its mechanism of action is unclear, it appears to inhibit in vivo and in vitro platelet adhesion, aggregation, and the so-called release reaction induced by adenosine diphosphate, collagen, and antigen-antibody complexes. In addition, it is a potent inhibitor of platelet prostaglandin synthesis.

Heparin

1. Babcock RB, Dumper CW, Scharfman WB. Heparin-induced immune thrombocytopenia. N Engl J Med 1976; 295:237–41.
   Five patients with severe thrombocytopenia caused by heparin therapy are described.
2. Bell WR, Tomasulo PA, Alving BM, Duffy TP. Thrombocytopenia occurring during the administration of heparin: a prospective study in 52 patients. Ann Intern Med 1976; 85:155–60.

In a group of 52 patients receiving continuous intravenous heparin, 16 developed a platelet count below 100,000/mm³.

3. Gallus AS, Hirsh J, Tuttle RJ, Trebilcock R, O'Brien SE, Carroll JJ, Minden JH, Hudecki SM. Small subcutaneous doses of heparin in prevention of venous thrombosis. N Engl J Med 1973; 288:545–51.
   Subcutaneous heparin (5,000 units three times daily) was effective in reducing the frequency of venous thrombosis in a group of high-risk surgical and medical patients.

4. Genton E. Guidelines for heparin therapy. Ann Intern Med 1974; 80:77–82.
   A succinct review of the clinical uses of heparin.

5. Sherry S. Low-dose heparin prophylaxis for postoperative venous thromboembolism. N Engl J Med 1975; 293:300–2.
   The use of low-dose heparin should be encouraged, since it clearly reduces deep venous thrombosis and pulmonary embolism.

6. Hirsh J, van Aken WG, Gallus AS, Dollery CT, Cade JF, Yung WL. Heparin kinetics in venous thrombosis and pulmonary embolism. Circulation 1976; 53:691–5.
   Among 20 patients with venous thromboembolism treated with heparin, there were large individual variations in its anticoagulant effect.

Coumarin Anticoagulation

7. Koch-Weser J, Sellers EM. Drug interactions with coumarin anticoagulants. N Engl J Med 1971; 285:487–98, 547–58.
   A comprehensive review of the many drugs that interact with coumarin.

Platelet Inhibitors

8. Anturane Reinfarction Trial Research Group. Sulfinpyrazone in the prevention of cardiac death after myocardial infarction: The Anturane reinfarction trial. N Engl J Med 1978; 298:289–95.
   Sulfinpyrazone reduced cardiac deaths during the first year after myocardial infarction.

9. Harris WH, Salzman EW, Athanasoulis CA, Waltman AC, DeSanctis RW. Aspirin prophylaxis of venous thromboembolism after total hip replacement. N Engl J Med 1977; 297:1246–9.
   In men undergoing total hip replacement, aspirin reduced the risk of venous thromboembolism.

10. Genton E, Gent M, Hirsh J, Harker LA. Platelet-inhibiting drugs in the prevention of clinical thrombotic disease. N Engl J Med 1975; 293:1174–8, 1236–40, 1296–1300.
    A thorough review of the studies that have assessed the clinical efficacy of platelet-inhibiting agents.

11. Chesebro JH, Clements IP, Fuster V, Elveback LR, Smith HC, Bardsley WT, Frye RL, Holmes DR Jr, Vlietstra RE, Pluth JR, Wallace RB, Puga FJ, Orszulak TA, Piehler JM, Schaff HV, Danielson GK. A platelet-inhibitor drug trial in coronary artery bypass operations: benefit of perioperative dipyridamole and aspirin therapy on early postoperative vein-graft patency. N Engl J Med 1982; 307:73–8.
    Dipyridamole and aspirin in combination were effective in maintaining graft patency during the months after saphenous vein bypass grafting.

BETA-ADRENERGIC BLOCKING AGENTS

Numerous pharmacologic agents are available that provide an antagonistic effect to beta-adrenergic agonists and, therefore, are termed beta-adrenergic "blockers" or "antagonists" (Table 2). These compounds vary in overall potency, beta-adrenergic receptor selectivity, agonist activity, and membrane-stabilizing activity. Some (e.g., propranolol) are totally nonselective, in that they antagonize the effect of beta-adrenergic agonists on beta$_1$ (cardiac) and beta$_2$ (smooth muscle) receptors. Others (e.g., metoprolol and sotalol) are at least semiselective beta$_1$ antagonists, and they exert only minimal antagonistic effects on beta$_2$ receptors.

The beta-adrenergic antagonists have been used extensively in the treatment of patients with a variety of cardiovascular disorders. First, they have been used with great success in individuals with supraventricular and ventricular tachyarrhythmias. In the former instance, these agents are effective in (1) slowing the ventricular response in patients with atrial flutter or fibrillation and (2) converting the patient with paroxysmal supraventricular tachycardia to sinus rhythm. In the latter instance, some patients with frequent ventricular premature beats and ventricular tachycardia are effectively treated with a beta-adrenergic blocker. These agents are especially beneficial in patients with ventricular ectopic activity in association with the mitral valve prolapse syndrome. Finally, they often are effective in individuals with digitalis-induced arrhythmias.

Second, the beta-adrenergic blockers have been used widely in patients with exertional angina pectoris as well as in those hospitalized with unstable angina pectoris. In the setting of ischemic heart disease, these agents exert their beneficial effect by reducing the major determinants of myocardial oxygen consumption—heart rate, left ventricular contractility, and left ventricular wall tension. They exert no substantial effect on myocardial oxygen supply in patients with angina. Numerous trials have clearly shown that these agents reduce the frequency of angina and nitroglycerin consumption, and at the same time they increase exercise tolerance.

Third, the beta-adrenergic blockers reduce mortality in patients who have sustained a myocardial infarction when they are administered over the 6 to 12 months after infarction. The mechanism by which this beneficial effect is accomplished is unknown.

Fourth, the beta-adrenergic antagonists are effective antihypertensive agents, administered alone or—more often—in combination with a diuretic and a vasodilator. This antihypertensive effect is accomplished by (1) a direct renin-lowering influence and (2) an action on the central nervous system.

Fifth, the beta-adrenergic blockers are the therapy of choice for patients with hypertrophic cardiomyopathy. In these individuals, the negative inotropic effect of the beta blockers reduces the degree of left ventricular outflow tract obstruction and provides symptomatic improvement for most patients.

The beta-adrenergic blockers sometimes induce adverse effects. The most common complaints are generalized fatigue and lethargy. The patient may note depression, insomnia, and vivid dreams. An occasional male patient may complain of impotence. The nonselective beta blockers may induce bronchospasm in patients susceptible to it, and therefore, they should not be administered to a patient with a history of bronchospastic lung disease. Similarly, the use of beta-adrenergic blockers is contraindicated in patients with active congestive heart failure. Finally, since these agents prevent the clinical recognition of hypoglycemia, they should be administered to insulin-dependent diabetics only with considerable caution.

In an occasional patient with angina pectoris who is receiving a beta-adrenergic antagonist, the sudden discontinuation of this agent may lead to a distinct worsening of angina or even myocardial infarction—a phenomenon termed the "propranolol withdrawal syndrome." The mechanism by which this worsening of angina occurs is not fully understood, but it may result from the sudden unblocking of greatly increased numbers of cardiac beta receptors. If a patient with angina requires that his beta blocker be discontinued, its dosage should

Table 2. Beta-Adrenergic Antagonists

Name	Beta-Blockade Potency Ratio (Propranolol = 1.0)	Cardioselective*	Usual Therapeutic Dose Range (mg/day)	Elimination Half-life	Route of Excretion
Propranolol	1.0	0	80–480	3.5–6.0 hr	Urine
Timolol	6.0	0	5–40	4–5 hr	Urine
Oxprenolol	0.5–1.0	0	40–360	2 hr	Urine
Sotalol	0.3	0	80–480	5–13 hr	Urine
Metoprolol	1.0	+	100–800	3–4 hr	Urine
Pindolol	6.0	0	2.5–30.0	3–4 hr	Urine
Practolol	0.3	+	25–800	6–8 hr	Urine
Atenolol	1.0	+	100–400	6–9 hr	Approximately 40% of unchanged drug in urine
Alprenolol	0.3	0	200–800	2–3 hr	Urine
Acebutolol	0.3	+	400–800	8 hr	Uncertain

*Seen only at low dosage.

be tapered over a 3- to 4-day period. In addition, this gradual reduction of beta blocker dosage should probably be accomplished at a time when the patient's activities are somewhat restricted.

General

1. Shand DG. Propranolol. N Engl J Med 1975; 293:280–5.
   A succinct review of propranolol's therapeutic uses and adverse effects.
2. Frishman WH. β-adrenoceptor antagonists: new drugs and new indications. N Engl J Med 1981; 305:500–6.
   A solid discussion of the pharmacologic properties and uses of atenolol, metoprolol, nadolol, pindolol, propranolol, and timolol.
3. Koch-Weser J. Metoprolol. N Engl J Med 1979; 301:698–703.
   A discussion of metoprolol's clinical effectiveness, uses, and adverse effects. Includes 66 references.
4. Frishman WH. Nadolol: a new β-adrenoceptor antagonist. N Engl J Med 1981; 305:678–82.
   A concise review of the uses of nadolol, a nonselective beta-blocker.
5. Watanabe AM. Recent advances in knowledge about beta-adrenergic receptors: application to clinical cardiology. JACC 1983; 1:82–9.
   A good overview of beta-receptors and their pharmacologic blockade.

Treatment of Arrhythmias

6. Gibson D, Sowton E. The use of beta-adrenergic receptor blocking drugs in dysrhythmias. Prog Cardiovasc Dis 1969; 12:16–39.
   A complete review of beta-blockers in the therapy of various dysrhythmias. They were especially effective in reverting those arrhythmias precipitated by exercise or emotion, those associated with the Wolff-Parkinson-White syndrome, and those due to digitalis toxicity.
7. Coltart DJ, Gibson DG, Shand DG. Plasma propranolol levels associated with suppression of ventricular ectopic beats. Br Med J 1971; 1:490–1.
   Of 12 patients with frequent ventricular ectopy, a propranolol plasma level of 40–85 ng/mL suppressed the ectopy in 8.
8. Singh BN, Jewitt DE. β-adrenergic receptor blocking drugs in cardiac arrhythmias. Drugs 1974; 7:426–61.
   An extensive overview of beta-blockade for supraventricular and ventricular tachyarrhythmias.
9. Koppes GM, Beckmann CH, Jones FG. Propranolol therapy for ventricular arrhythmias 2 months after acute myocardial infarction. Am J Cardiol 1980; 46:322–8.
   In 32 patients 2 months after infarction, propranolol (average daily dose, 160 mg) effectively suppressed ventricular premature beats.
10. Nixon JV, Pennington W, Ritter W, Shapiro W. Efficacy of propranolol in the control of exercise-induced or augmented ventricular ectopic activity. Circulation 1978; 57:115–22.
    In 15 patients with exercise-induced or augmented VPBs, propranolol reduced their frequency in 10.

Treatment of Angina

11. Prichard BNC. Beta-adrenergic receptor blocking drugs in angina pectoris. Drugs 1974; 7:55–84.
    A thorough review of the use of all the beta-blockers in patients with angina.
12. Wolfson S, Heinle RA, Herman MV, Kemp HG, Sullivan JM, Gorlin R. Propranolol and angina pectoris. Am J Cardiol 1966; 18:345–53.
    Thirty-seven patients with severe angina were treated with propranolol, 160-280 mg/day, of which 30 (81%) reported marked improvement.
13. Thadani U, Parker JO. Propranolol in angina pectoris: comparison of therapy given two and four times daily. Am J Cardiol 1980; 46:117–23.

In patients with exertional angina, therapy with propranolol twice daily is as effective as therapy with this agent 4 times daily.

14. Olowoyeye JO, Thadani U, Parker JO. Slow release oxprenolol in angina pectoris: study comparing oxprenolol, once daily, with propranolol, four times daily. Am J Cardiol 1981; 47:1123–7.
    In this study, propranolol was better than oxprenolol in 23 patients with exertional angina.

15. Parker JO. Comparison of slow-release pindolol, standard pindolol, and propranolol in angina pectoris. Am J Cardiol 1983; 51:1062–6.
    These 3 agents were similarly effective in patients with exertional angina.

Treatment of Patients Following Myocardial Infarction

16. β-blocker heart attack study group: the β-blocker heart attack trial. JAMA 1981; 246:2073–4.
    In patients who had suffered myocardial infarction, propranolol reduced mortality by 26%.

17. Hjalmarson A, Herlitz J, Malek I, Ryden L, Vedin A, Waldenstrom A, Wedel H, Elmfeldt D, Holmberg S, Nyberg G, Swedberg K, Waagstein F, Waldenstrom J, Wilhelmsen L, Wilhelmsson C. Effect on mortality of metoprolol in acute myocardial infarction. Lancet 1981; 2:823–7.
    Metoprolol was 36% more effective than placebo in reducing mortality following myocardial infarction.

18. The Norwegian Multicenter Study Group: Timolol-induced reduction in mortality and reinfarction in patients surviving acute myocardial infarction. N Engl J Med 1981; 304:801–7.
    Long-term treatment with timolol (10 mg twice daily) in patients surviving acute myocardial infarction reduces mortality and the rate of reinfarction.

Treatment of Hypertension

19. Buhler FR, Laragh JH, Vaughan ED Jr, Brunner HR, Gavras H, Baer L. Antihypertensive action of propranolol: specific antirenin responses in high and normal renin forms of essential, renal, renovascular, and malignant hypertension. Am J Cardiol 1973; 32:511–22.
    In 74 patients with essential hypertension, propranolol was highly effective in those with normal or high serum renin concentrations, whereas it was ineffective in the 17 low-renin patients.

20. Zacharias FJ, Cowen KJ, Prestt J, Vickers J, Wall BG. Propranolol in hypertension: a study of long-term therapy, 1964–70. Am Heart J 1972; 83:755–61.
    Propranolol was given for the long-term therapy of hypertension in 311 patients. It was well tolerated and was very effective in lowering systemic arterial pressure.

21. Zacest R, Gilmore E, Koch-Weser J. Treatment of essential hypertension with combined vasodilation and beta-adrenergic blockade. N Engl J Med 1972; 286:617–22.
    A propranolol-hydralazine combination was very effective in 23 patients with moderate or severe essential hypertension.

Propranolol Withdrawal Syndrome

22. Alderman EL, Coltart J, Wettach GE, Harrison DC. Coronary artery syndromes after sudden propranolol withdrawal. Ann Intern Med 1974; 81:625–7.
    Six patients with stable exertional angina immediately developed unstable angina after cessation of propranolol therapy.

23. Goldstein RE, Corash LC, Tallman JF Jr, Lake CR, Hyde J, Smith CC, Capurro NL, Anderson JC. Shortened platelet survival time and enhanced heart rate responses after abrupt withdrawal of propranolol from normal subjects. Am J Cardiol 1981; 47:1115–22.
    This article offers an attractive hypothesis for the mechanism of the propranolol withdrawal syndrome.

CALCIUM ANTAGONISTS

The "calcium antagonists" or "slow channel calcium blockers" are useful in patients with a variety of cardiovascular disorders. By antagonizing the effect of calcium ions on the cardiac conducting system (particularly AV nodal tissue), the myocardium, and the smooth muscle of coronary and systemic arteries, these agents can be efficacious in the treatment of supraventricular tachyarrhythmias, systemic arterial hypertension, and a variety of ischemic heart disease syndromes. Although these drugs are classified as members of the same family, they differ substantially from one another in the magnitude of their influence on these tissues.

Verapamil prolongs AV conduction by depressing the portion of the conducting system immediately proximal to the bundle of His. As a result, it is an extremely effective agent—both acutely and chronically—for patients with (1) paroxysmal supraventricular tachycardia, (2) atrial flutter, or (3) atrial fibrillation. In the patient with recurrent episodes of paroxysmal supraventricular tachycardia, intravenous verapamil (5–10 mg by bolus injection) is often effective in converting the patient to sinus rhythm, and chronic oral verapamil (320–480 mg/day given in 3–4 divided doses) is usually successful in preventing recurrent episodes. For the patient with atrial flutter or fibrillation, verapamil (intravenous or oral) seldom induces a reversion to sinus rhythm, but it is an effective agent for controlling the ventricular response.

Verapamil exerts a modest influence as a systemic arterial dilator. Therefore, it is effective in patients with mild or moderate systemic arterial hypertension. It is a relatively powerful negative inotropic agent, and therefore, it has proved effective in many patients with hypertrophic cardiomyopathy. Finally, chronic oral verapamil (320–480 mg/day) is extremely efficacious in patients with Prinzmetal's variant angina, stable angina of effort, or unstable angina at rest. In patients with vasospastic (variant) angina, oral verapamil reduces the frequency of angina by about 70 percent. In those with angina of effort, its efficacy is similar to or even better than propranolol (in comparable doses). In patients with unstable angina at rest, oral verapamil alleviates angina and electrocardiographic evidence of recurrent myocardial ischemia.

Verapamil does not appear to be effective in the therapy of patients with (1) primary pulmonary hypertension (probably because of its negative inotropic influence on right ventricular function), (2) congestive heart failure (because of its powerful negative inotropic effect), (3) Raynaud's phenomenon, or (4) ventricular tachyarrhythmias. It can be administered concomitantly with propranolol in patients with especially severe angina of effort, but this must be done cautiously, since both agents exert a negative chronotropic and inotropic effect. The adverse effects seen most frequently during verapamil therapy include constipation and palpitations (due to an accelerated junctional rhythm caused by verapamil).

Nifedipine is an especially powerful arterial dilator with negligible negative chronotropic and inotropic effects. As a result, it is most effective in patients with (1) mild, moderate, or even severe systemic arterial hypertension, (2) primary pulmonary hypertension, (3) congestive heart failure of various causes (as an unloading agent), (4) Raynaud's phenomenon, or (5) variant angina, angina of effort, or unstable angina at rest. It is of only limited usefulness in patients with hypertrophic cardiomyopathy, and it exerts no effect in those with supraventricular tachyarrhythmias. Because it is such a powerful arterial dilator, most of its adverse effects center on excessive peripheral vasodilatation: pedal edema, headache, dizziness, orthostatic hypotension, and—on occasion—

syncope. Most of these side effects can be controlled effectively with a slight reduction in dosage. For all the above indications, nifedipine is administered orally 4 times daily in a total daily dosage of 60–120 mg.

Since nifedipine exerts no demonstrable effect on cardiac conduction or contractility, it appears to be an especially good agent in combination with a beta-adrenergic blocker, such as propranolol. Preliminary studies have shown that a propranolol-nifedipine combination is particularly efficacious in patients with angina of effort as well as in those with unstable angina at rest.

Diltiazem exerts a modest depressant effect on AV conduction and a modest vasodilating effect on peripheral arteries. It appears to be very effective in patients with variant angina, angina of effort, or unstable angina. It is administered 3 to 4 times daily in a total dosage of 120–360 mg per day. Its beneficial effect is unproved in patients with (1) systemic arterial hypertension, (2) primary pulmonary hypertension, (3) Raynaud's phenomenon, (4) hypertrophic cardiomyopathy, or (5) supraventricular tachyarrhythmias. The adverse effects most often associated with diltiazem are constipation and headache.

Verapamil

1. Rinkenberger RL, Prystowsky EN, Heger JJ, Troup PJ, Jackman WM, Zipes DP. Effects of intravenous and chronic oral verapamil administration in patients with supraventricular tachyarrhythmias. Circulation 1980; 62:996–1010.
   Intravenous verapamil is an effective antiarrhythmic drug for most patients with paroxysmal supraventricular tachycardia.

2. Mauritson DR, Winniford MD, Walker WS, Rude RE, Cary JR, Hillis LD. Oral verapamil for paroxysmal supraventricular tachycardia: a long-term double-blind, randomized trial. Ann Intern Med 1982; 96:409–12.
   In 11 patients with frequent paroxysmal supraventricular tachycardia, oral verapamil (240–480 mg/day) reduced the frequency and duration of tachycardic episodes.

3. Waxman HL, Myerburg RJ, Appel R, Sung RJ. Verapamil for control of ventricular rate in paroxysmal supraventricular tachycardia and atrial fibrillation or flutter: a double-blind randomized cross-over study. Ann Intern Med 1981; 94:1–6.
   Verapamil causes a significant slowing of the ventricular response in atrial fibrillation or flutter and is superior to placebo for converting paroxysmal supraventricular tachycardia to sinus rhythm.

4. Gould BA, Mann S, Kieso H, Subramanian VB, Raftery EB. The 24-hour ambulatory blood pressure profile with verapamil. Circulation 1982; 65:22–7.
   Oral verapamil (360–480 mg/day) produced a consistent reduction in systemic arterial pressure.

5. Rosing DR, Kent KM, Maron BJ, Epstein SE. Verapamil therapy: a new approach to the pharmacologic treatment of hypertrophic cardiomyopathy. II. Effects on exercise capacity and symptomatic status. Circulation 1979; 60:1208–13.
   In 19 patients with hypertrophic cardiomyopathy, verapamil improved exercise capacity and symptomatic status.

6. Johnson SM, Mauritson DR, Willerson JT, Hillis LD. A controlled trial of verapamil for Prinzmetal's variant angina. N Engl J Med 1981; 304:862–6.
   In comparison to placebo, oral verapamil was an effective agent in reducing the frequency of chest pain, nitroglycerin usage, and transient S–T segment deviations.

7. Johnson SM, Mauritson DR, Corbett JR, Woodward W, Willerson JT, Hillis LD. Double-blind, randomized, placebo-controlled comparison of propranolol and verapamil in the treatment of patients with stable angina pectoris. Am J Med 1981; 71:443–51.
   In 18 patients with angina of effort, verapamil was comparable to propranolol in relieving angina and improving exercise capability.

8. Pine MB, Citron PD, Bailly DJ, Butman S, Plasencia GO, Landa DW, Wong RK. Verapamil versus placebo in relieving stable angina pectoris. Circulation 1982; 65:17–22.

Verapamil (360–480 mg/day) was better than placebo in 18 patients with angina of effort.

9. Frishman WH, Klein NA, Strom JA, Willens H, LeJemtel TH, Jentzer J, Siegel L, Klein P, Kirschen N, Silverman R, Pollack S, Doyle R, Kirsten E, Sonnenblick EH. Superiority of verapamil to propranolol in stable angina pectoris: a double-blind, randomized cross-over trial. Circulation 1982; 65(Suppl I):51–9.
    Verapamil was better than placebo and propranolol in this group of 20 patients with angina of effort.

10. Winniford MD, Huxley RL, Hillis LD. Randomized, double-blind comparison of propranolol alone and a propranolol-verapamil combination in patients with severe angina of effort. JACC 1983; 1:492–8.
    In this study, propranolol and verapamil were administered together without problem; the combination exerted a more powerful antianginal effect than propranolol alone.

11. Mehta J, Pepine CJ, Day M, Guerrero JR, Conti CR. Short-term efficacy of oral verapamil in rest angina: a double-blind placebo controlled trial in CCU patients. Am J Med 1981; 71:977–82.
    Of 15 patients with unstable angina at rest, most responded markedly to oral verapamil, 320–480 mg/day.

Nifedipine

12. Guazzi MD, Fiorentini C, Olivari MT, Bartorelli A, Necchi G, Polese A. Short- and long-term efficacy of a calcium-antagonistic agent (nifedipine) combined with methyldopa in the treatment of severe hypertension. Circulation 1980; 61:913–9.
    In 23 patients with diastolic blood pressures > 120 mmHg, nifedipine and alpha-methyldopa reduced blood pressure substantially without worsening renal function.

13. Matsumoto S, Ito T, Sada T, Takahashi M, Su KM, Ueda A, Okabe F, Sato M, Sekine I, Ito Y. Hemodynamic effects of nifedipine in congestive heart failure. Am J Cardiol 1980; 46:476–80.
    In 8 patients with mild to moderate congestive heart failure, nifedipine (20 mg sublingually) increased cardiac index and decreased blood pressure and systemic vascular resistance.

14. Fioretti P, Benussi B, Scardi S, Klugmann S, Brower RW, Camerini F. Afterload reduction with nifedipine in aortic insufficiency. Am J Cardiol 1982; 49:1728–32.
    In 12 patients with severe aortic regurgitation, sublingual nifedipine reduced left ventricular end-diastolic pressure (from 19 to 9 mmHg) and increased forward cardiac index (from 3.8 to 4.4 L/min/m^2).

15. Winniford MD, Johnson SM, Mauritson DR, Rellas JS, Redish GA, Willerson JT, Hillis LD. Verapamil therapy for Prinzmetal's variant angina: comparison with placebo and nifedipine. Am J Cardiol 1982; 50:913–8.
    Nifedipine and verapamil were similarly effective in patients with vasospastic angina.

16. Hill JA, Feldman RL, Pepine CJ, Conti CR. Randomized double-blind comparison of nifedipine and isosorbide dinitrate in patients with coronary arterial spasm. Am J Cardiol 1982; 49:431–8.
    Both nifedipine and isosorbide dinitrate are effective in certain patients with coronary spasm; neither is clearly superior.

17. Moskowitz RM, Piccini PA, Nacarelli GV, Zelis R. Nifedipine therapy for stable angina pectoris: preliminary results of effects on angina frequency and treadmill exercise response. Am J Cardiol 1979; 44:811–6.
    In 10 patients with angina of effort, nifedipine reduced anginal frequency and prolonged exercise time.

18. Mueller HS, Chahine RA. Interim report of multicenter double-blind, placebo-controlled studies of nifedipine in chronic stable angina. Am J Med 1981; 71:645–57.
    In 66 patients with angina of effort, anginal frequency was reduced by 50% with nifedipine therapy.

19. Previtali M, Salerno JA, Tavazzi L, Ray M, Medici A, Chimienti M, Specchia G, Bobba P. Treatment of angina at rest with nifedipine: a short-term controlled study. Am J Cardiol 1980; 45:825–30.

In 14 patients with angina at rest, nifedipine was effective in relieving pain and preventing electrocardiographic evidence of ischemia.

20. Gerstenblith G, Ouyang P, Achuff SC, Bulkley BH, Becker LC, Mellits ED, Baughman KL, Weiss JL, Flaherty JT, Kallman CH, Llewellyn M, Weisfeldt ML. Nifedipine in unstable angina: a double-blind, randomized trial. N Engl J Med 1982; 306:885–9.

When added to a regimen of propranolol and nitrates, nifedipine (40–80 mg/day) was better than placebo in patients with rest angina. It was especially salutary in those whose chest pain was accompanied by transient S–T segment elevation.

21. Lynch P, Dargie H, Krikler S, Krikler D. Objective assessment of antianginal treatment: a double-blind comparison of propranolol, nifedipine, and their combination. Br Med J 1980; 281:184–7.

A combination of propranolol and nifedipine was superior to either agent alone in patients with angina of effort.

Diltiazem

22. Schroeder JS, Feldman RL, Giles TD, Friedman MJ, DeMaria AN, Kinney EL, Mallon SM, Pitt B, Meyer R, Basta LL, Curry RC Jr, Groves BM, MacAlpin RN. Multiclinic controlled trial of diltiazem for Prinzmetal's angina. Am J Med 1982; 72:227–32.

In 48 patients with variant angina, diltiazem (240 mg/day) reduced anginal frequency by 68%.

23. Pepine CJ, Feldman RL, Whittle J, Curry RC, Conti CR. Effect of diltiazem in patients with variant angina: a randomized double-blind trial. Am Heart J 1981; 101:719–25.

Diltiazem was markedly better than placebo in 12 patients with vasospastic angina.

24. Hossack KF, Bruce RA. Improved exercise performance in persons with stable angina pectoris receiving diltiazem. Am J Cardiol 1981; 47:95–101.

In 10 individuals with angina of effort, diltiazem increased the duration of exercise and the time to onset of angina.

25. Pool PE, Seagren SC, Bonanno JA, Salel AF, Dennish GW. The treatment of exercise-inducible chronic stable angina with diltiazem. Effect on treadmill exercise. Chest 1980; 78(Suppl):234–8.

Diltiazem (240 mg/day) increased exercise time from 8.0 to 9.8 minutes in 15 patients with angina of effort.

26. Wagniart P, Ferguson RJ, Chaitman BR, Achard F, Benacerraf A, Delanguenhagen B, Morin B, Pasternac A, Bourassa MG. Increased exercise tolerance and reduced electrocardiographic ischemia with diltiazem in patients with stable angina pectoris. Circulation 1982; 66:23–8.

Diltiazem decreases myocardial oxygen requirements during upright exercise and appears to increase myocardial oxygen delivery.

27. Subramanian VB, Khurmi NS, Bowles MJ, O'Hara M, Raftery EB. Objective evaluation of three dose levels of diltiazem in patients with chronic stable angina. JACC 1983; 1:1144–53.

In 21 patients with angina of effort, diltiazem given in substantial doses (270–360 mg/day) was effective in relieving angina.

LIDOCAINE

Intravenous lidocaine is frequently employed for the therapy of individuals with ventricular premature beats (VPBs) or ventricular tachycardia, especially in the setting of acute myocardial infarction. An initial intravenous bolus of 1.0 to 1.5 mg per kilogram of body weight is followed by a continuous intravenous infusion of 1 to 4 mg per minute. However, a lower maintenance dose should be used if heart failure or severe hepatic disease is present, since lidocaine is largely metabolized by the liver. In the setting of possible or definite myocardial infarction, intravenous lidocaine should be initiated in the patient with (1) frequent unifocal VPBs, (2) multifocal VPBs (even though infrequent), or (3) couplets or short runs of ventricular tachycardia. In some medical centers, lidocaine is administered routinely to all patients with suspected or obvious myocardial infarction for the first 24 to 48 hours after hospitalization. It is hoped that such "prophylactic" administration of intravenous lidocaine in the coronary care unit will prevent ventricular fibrillation. However, the benefits of prophylactic lidocaine administration must be balanced against the risk of lidocaine toxicity. In our coronary care unit, lidocaine is not given to all patients with suspected or definite infarction; rather, it is administered only to those with frequent (>5–8/min), multifocal, or coupled VPBs or with runs of ventricular tachycardia. Finally, *intravenously* administered lidocaine has been shown to prevent ventricular fibrillation, and such fibrillation is most likely to occur within minutes of infarction. Therefore, interest has arisen concerning the *intramuscular* administration of lidocaine "in the field," that is, before the patient's transfer to a hospital. Although some studies have suggested that intramuscular lidocaine is helpful in preventing early ventricular fibrillation, others have demonstrated no beneficial effect. At present, we do not recommend such prophylactic intramuscular lidocaine administration. Lidocaine is not used in patients with supraventricular tachyarrhythmias, although isolated anecdotal reports indicate that it is effective in some patients with paroxysmal supraventricular tachycardia. In addition, it may be efficacious in slowing the ventricular response in the patient with Wolff-Parkinson-White syndrome and rapidly conducted atrial fibrillation.

The patient with lidocaine toxicity often has slurred speech, mental confusion, lethargy, obtundation, and—on occasion—grand mal seizures. Toxicity is especially likely in (1) elderly individuals, (2) patients with primary hepatic dysfunction (due to hepatitis or cirrhosis), and (3) patients in whom hepatic blood flow is reduced (most often in the setting of right-sided congestive heart failure). For these individuals, the lidocaine dosage probably should not exceed 2 mg per minute, and it should be discontinued as early as possible. Lidocaine does not often produce adverse cardiovascular effects. On occasion, however, it has been shown to depress hemodynamic function in patients with severe left ventricular dysfunction and to induce AV block below the bundle of His in patients with bundle branch block. Finally, lidocaine may cause further slowing of the heart rate in the patient with sinus bradycardia, and it may induce sinus arrest in the individual with sick sinus syndrome. If signs of toxicity appear, the infusion should be discontinued immediately.

1. Dhingra RC, Deedwania PC, Cummings JM, Amat-y-Leon F, Wu D, Denes P, Rosen KM. Electrophysiologic effects of lidocaine on sinus node and atrium in patients with and without sinoatrial dysfunction. Circulation 1978; 57:448–54.
   In patients with sinus node dysfunction, lidocaine depressed the function of perinodal tissue. This may explain why sinus arrest occurs in some patients with conduction system disease during lidocaine administration.
2. Harrison DC. Should lidocaine be administered routinely to all patients after acute myocardial infarction? Circulation 1978; 58:581–4.
   In this editorial, the author recommends prophylactic lidocaine for all patients hospitalized with possible or definite infarction.
3. Josephson ME, Kastor JA, Kitchen JG III. Lidocaine in Wolff-Parkinson-White syndrome with atrial fibrillation. Ann Intern Med 1976; 84:44–5.

In an 18-year-old man with Wolff-Parkinson-White syndrome and atrial fibrillation, lidocaine immediately slowed the ventricular response by abolishing antegrade conduction over the accessory pathway.

4. LeLorier J, Grenon D, Latour Y, Caille G, Dumont G, Brosseau A, Solignac A. Pharmacokinetics of lidocaine after prolonged intravenous infusions in uncomplicated myocardial infarction. Ann Intern Med 1977; 87:700–2.
   In patients receiving intravenous lidocaine for more than 24 hours, the elimination half-life was 3.2 hours.

5. Ochs HR, Carstens G, Greenblatt DJ. Reduction in lidocaine clearance during continuous infusion and by coadministration of propranolol. N Engl J Med 1980; 303:373–7.
   The prolonged infusion of lidocaine and the simultaneous administration of propranolol reduce the clearance of lidocaine from the plasma.

6. Lie KI, Wellens HJ, vanCapélle FJ, Durrer D. Lidocaine in the prevention of primary ventricular fibrillation: a double-blind, randomized study of 212 consecutive patients. N Engl J Med 1974; 291:1324–6.
   Intravenous lidocaine was highly effective in preventing ventricular fibrillation in patients with acute myocardial infarction.

7. Valentine PA, Frew JL, Mashford ML, Sloman JG. Lidocaine in the prevention of sudden death in the pre-hospital phase of acute infarction: a double-blind study. N Engl J Med 1974; 291:1327–31.
   This study indicates that early intramuscular lidocaine administration may reduce mortality in the pre-hospital phase of acute myocardial infarction.

8. Lie KI, Liem KL, Louridtz WJ, Janse MJ, Willebrands AF, Durrer D. Efficacy of lidocaine in preventing primary ventricular fibrillation within 1 hour after a 300 mg intramuscular injection. A double-blind, randomized study of 300 hospitalized patients with acute myocardial infarction. Am J Cardiol 1978; 42:486–8.
   In this study, intramuscular lidocaine was ineffective in preventing ventricular fibrillation.

9. Thomson PD, Melmon KL, Richardson JA, Cohn K, Steinbrunn W, Cudihee R, Rowland M. Lidocaine pharmacokinetics in advanced heart failure, liver disease, and renal failure in humans. Ann Intern Med 1973; 78:499–508.
   Lidocaine clearance is greatly reduced in individuals with advanced heart failure or hepatic disease.

10. Zito RA, Reid PR. Lidocaine kinetics predicted by indocyanine green clearance. N Engl J Med 1978; 298:1160–3.
    In 26 patients with differing lidocaine clearance rates, indocyanine green clearance accurately reflected lidocaine clearance.

11. Collinsworth KA, Kalman SM, Harrison DC. The clinical pharmacology of lidocaine as an antiarrhythmic drug. Circulation 1974; 50:1217–30.
    A nice review of lidocaine's metabolism, electrophysiologic and hemodynamic effects, pharmacokinetics, and adverse effects.

12. Lichstein E, Chadda KD, Gupta PK. Atrioventricular block with lidocaine therapy. Am J Cardiol 1973; 31:277–81.
    A description of an 83-year-old man in whom 50 mg of lidocaine induced complete AV block. Prior to therapy, this patient had ECG evidence of trifascicular block.

13. Lippestad CT, Forfang K. Production of sinus arrest by lignocaine. Br Med J 1971; 1:537.
    A 77-year-old woman with the sick sinus syndrome developed sinus arrest with lidocaine administration.

14. Branch RA, Shand DG, Wilkinson GR, Nies AS. The reduction of lidocaine clearance by dl-propranolol: an example of hemodynamic drug interaction. J Pharmacol Exp Ther 1973; 184:515–9.
    In the dog, propranolol administration prolonged lidocaine's serum half-life.

15. Stargel WW, Shand DG, Routledge PA, Barchowsky A, Wagner GS. Clinical comparison of rapid infusion and multiple injection methods for lidocaine loading. Am Heart J 1981; 102:872–6.
    These authors loaded their patients with lidocaine by infusing 150 mg over 18 minutes following a 75 mg bolus. This was associated with minimal adverse effects.

QUINIDINE

Quinidine is frequently used in the therapy of patients with supraventricular and ventricular tachyarrhythmias. In the experimental animal, it exerts several effects on the electrical and mechanical functions of the heart. First, it increases the threshold to electrical stimulation, and in this way it depresses or abolishes ectopic impulse generation. Second, it prolongs the effective refractory period, exerting an especially prominent effect in the atria. Third, it increases the conduction interval in atrial and ventricular tissue, thus reducing the speed of depolarization. Fourth, it blocks vagal influences on the heart. As a result, despite its direct depressant effect on pacemaker tissue, quinidine increases the heart rate in unanesthetized animals and man. Finally, it reduces the developed tension in atrial and ventricular muscle. In therapeutic concentrations, this negative inotropic effect is modest, but in toxic concentrations, it can be substantial.

Clinically, quinidine is employed to suppress atrial and ventricular ectopic activity. First, quinidine often totally abolishes atrial premature beats. Second, it is an effective agent in converting atrial fibrillation or flutter to sinus rhythm, and once this is accomplished, continued quinidine administration helps to maintain the patient in sinus rhythm. In addition to quinidine maintenance, these individuals should receive long-term digitalis therapy. In such patients, a conversion from sinus rhythm to atrial fibrillation may be initiated by a short run of atrial flutter. Because of quinidine's vagolytic effect, the patient who is receiving quinidine alone (without concomitant digitalis) may develop 1:1 AV conduction (at a rate of 300/min), with resultant hypotension and poor peripheral perfusion. Thus, concomitant digitalis therapy is required to prevent such 1:1 AV conduction in the event the patient has an episode of atrial flutter or fibrillation. Third, quinidine is an effective agent for suppressing ventricular premature beats and ventricular tachycardia as well as for preventing their recurrence.

Quinidine is administered orally or intramuscularly; its intravenous administration may produce severe hypotension, and its absorption by the rectal route is poor and irregular. After its oral ingestion, it is completely absorbed from the gastrointestinal tract. Its maximal effects occur within 1 to 3 hours and persist for 6 to 8 hours. The usual oral dosage of quinidine sulfate is 300 to 500 mg 4 times daily. Most of it is excreted in the urine, with about half in the unchanged form.

As the quinidine plasma concentration rises above 2 μg per milliliter, the QRS and Q–T intervals widen progressively, and these alterations can be used to monitor therapy. Thus, a 25-percent increase in the QRS duration should be of concern, and a 50-percent increase should prompt a reduction in dosage. Similarly, the patient with the long Q–T syndrome, as well as the individual in whom therapeutic doses of quinidine induce a greatly prolonged Q–T interval, should not receive quinidine.

Quinidine has several potentially serious adverse effects. In the dosage generally used, the most common toxic manifestations are gastrointestinal: diarrhea is especially common in the patient with quinidine toxicity, and nausea and vomiting occasionally occur. Excess quinidine can induce a constellation of symptoms known as cinchonism, consisting of auditory and visual disturbances (tinnitus, nausea, blurring of vision, disturbed color perception, photophobia, diplopia, night blindness, scotomata, and mydriasis), gastrointestinal symptoms (nausea, vomiting, and diarrhea), cutaneous manifestations (warm and flushed skin; papular, scarlatiniform, or urticarial rash), and—when severe—

central nervous system symptoms (severe headache, fever, apprehension, excitement, confusion, delirium, and syncope). Death can even occur as the result of respiratory arrest and peripheral hypotension. Quinidine can cause substantial postural hypotension because of its alpha-adrenergic blocking action, especially when it is given intravenously.

An occasional patient may manifest an allergic reaction to quinidine, with resultant angioedema, vomiting, cramps, and diarrhea. Rarely, quinidine causes thrombocytopenic purpura. Finally, in an occasional patient receiving quinidine, sudden death occurs due to ventricular fibrillation. The underlying cause of this catastrophic event is unknown, but individuals with the prolonged Q–T syndrome or those who respond to quinidine with marked Q–T lengthening seem to be especially at risk.

In several clinical circumstances, quinidine should be used cautiously, if at all. In the patient with complete AV block, quinidine may suppress the AV nodal or idioventricular pacemaker, causing profound bradycardia or asystole. The patient in whom quinidine administration has previously induced thrombocytopenic purpura should not receive further quinidine. Quinidine should be given cautiously to the patient with digitalis intoxication, especially when the patient has AV conduction disturbances. Finally, because of its direct negative inotropic effect, quinidine should be used carefully in the patient with severe left ventricular dysfunction and resultant congestive heart failure.

1. Ochs HR, Greenblatt DJ, Woo E, Smith TW. Reduced quinidine clearance in elderly persons. Am J Cardiol 1978; 42:481–5.
   This study demonstrates that the hepatic biotransformation and renal excretion of quinidine decrease with age.
2. Kessler KM, Lowenthal DT, Warner H, Gibson T, Briggs W, Reidenberg MM. Quinidine elimination in patients with congestive heart failure or poor renal function. N Engl J Med 1974; 290:706–9.
   In this study, quinidine elimination was unimpaired in patients with poor renal function or congestive heart failure.
3. Conrad KA, Molk BL, Chidsey CA. Pharmacokinetic studies of quinidine in patients with arrhythmias. Circulation 1977; 55:1–7.
   This study suggests that quinidine's elimination or volume of distribution may be impaired or altered in patients with heart failure.
4. Markiewicz W, Winkle R, Binetti G, Kernoff R, Harrison DC. Normal myocardial contractile state in the presence of quinidine. Circulation 1976; 53:101–6.
   In experimental animals, quinidine (in therapeutic doses) does not depress left ventricular contractility.
5. Data JL, Wilkinson GR, Nies AS. Interaction of quinidine with anticonvulsant drugs. N Engl J Med 1976; 294:699–702.
   Phenobarbital and diphenylhydantoin each reduced the half-life of quinidine by about 50%.
6. Bloomfield SS, Romhilt DW, Chou TC, Fowler NO. Quinidine for prophylaxis of arrhythmias in acute myocardial infarction. N Engl J Med 1971; 285:979–86.
   Quinidine sulfate (300 mg 4 times daily) reduced the frequency of VPBs by 50% and of serious ventricular arrhythmias by 33% in patients with acute myocardial infarction.
7. Selzer A, Wray HW. Quinidine syncope: paroxysmal ventricular fibrillation occurring during treatment of chronic atrial arrhythmias. Circulation 1964; 30:17–26.
   In 8 patients receiving quinidine therapy, a total of 36 syncopal episodes occurred; most were due to ventricular fibrillation.
8. Winkle RA, Gradman AH, Fitzgerald JW. Antiarrhythmic drug effect assessed from ventricular arrhythmia reduction in the ambulatory electrocardiogram and treadmill test: comparison of propranolol, procainamide, and quinidine. Am J Cardiol 1978; 42:473–80.
   Of 13 patients treated with quinidine, VPB frequency was reduced in 11.

9. Ochs HR, Grube E, Greenblatt DJ, Woo E, Bodem G. Intravenous quinidine: pharmacokinetic properties and effects on left ventricular performance in humans. Am Heart J 1980; 99:468–75.

   In 10 healthy volunteers, 300 mg of quinidine (given intravenously) caused a mild increase in heart rate, Q–T interval, and left ventricular ejection fraction; blood pressure was unaltered.

10. DiMarco JP, Garan H, Ruskin JN. Quinidine for ventricular arrhythmias: value of electrophysiologic testing. Am J Cardiol 1983; 51:90–5.

    When selected on the basis of invasive electrophysiologic testing, quinidine provides effective long-term prophylaxis against recurrent ventricular arrhythmias.

11. Baker BJ, Gammill J, Massengill J, Schubert E, Karin A, Doherty JE. Concurrent use of quinidine and disopyramide: evaluation of serum concentrations and electrocardiographic effects. Am Heart J 1983; 105:12–5.

    In 16 normal, healthy adults, this drug combination produced no substantial problems. Both drugs produced prolongation of the Q–T interval.

12. Koenig W, Schinz AM. Spontaneous ventricular flutter and fibrillation during quinidine medication. Am Heart J 1983; 105:863–5.

    Patients showing marked Q–T prolongation during quinidine medication may be at high risk for developing ventricular tachyarrhythmias.

PROCAINAMIDE

Like quinidine, procainamide is effective in the treatment of individuals with atrial and ventricular tachyarrhythmias, and its electrophysiologic and hemodynamic actions are similar to those of quinidine. Specifically, procainamide (1) depresses the excitability of the atria and the ventricles to electrical stimulation, (2) slows conduction through the atria and ventricles, (3) prolongs the refractory period of the atria and, to a lesser extent, the ventricles, (4) has certain anticholinergic properties and, as a result, sometimes accelerates the heart rate, and (5) elevates the threshold of the atria and ventricles to electrically induced fibrillation. Aside from these electrophysiologic influences, procainamide exerts a modest negative inotropic effect, but this depression of contractility is of a lesser magnitude than that induced by quinidine.

Orally administered procainamide is rapidly and almost completely absorbed from the gastrointestinal tract, achieving a peak plasma concentration in about 60 minutes. Alternatively, it can be administered intramuscularly or intravenously. Most of the drug is bound to diffusible constituents of plasma, and as a result, its concentration in most tissues (except the brain) exceeds that in plasma. Of each dose of procainamide, about half is excreted unchanged in the urine, whereas the other half is acetylated by the liver to N-acetylprocainamide (NAPA), which is also excreted in the urine. When renal function declines, the plasma procainamide concentration rises substantially, and a larger fraction of it is converted to NAPA. Similarly, some individuals acetylate procainamide very rapidly and, as a result, have especially high concentrations of NAPA in the blood. Recent studies have demonstrated that NAPA is an effective antiarrhythmic agent in some patients and, furthermore, that NAPA administration is not accompanied by the lupus erythematosus–like adverse effects that often occur with long-term procainamide therapy.

Procainamide is efficacious in the therapy of individuals with atrial or ventricular premature beats as well as supraventricular or ventricular tachyarrhythmias. It may abolish atrial and ventricular premature beats completely. It is often effective in converting the individual with atrial fibrillation or flutter to sinus rhythm, and it is a good agent for maintaining these patients in sinus rhythm once it is achieved. Finally, it may prevent recurrences of ventricular tachycardia.

When possible, procainamide should be administered orally, in which case an initial loading dose of 1 to 2 gm over 4 to 6 hours is followed by a maintenance dose of 0.5 to 1.0 gm every 3 to 6 hours. Its intravenous administration is reserved for patients with severe, life-threatening arrhythmias. A total dose of 0.5 to 1.0 gm is infused slowly (at a rate of 25–50 mg/min), during which the systemic arterial pressure is observed closely. Subsequently, the procainamide infusion is maintained at 1 to 4 mg per minute. As a therapeutic plasma concentration is achieved, the QRS complex widens slightly, the P–R and Q–T intervals become prolonged, and minor T wave abnormalities appear. The desired therapeutic plasma concentration is 3 to 10 mg per liter. Recent studies have demonstrated that large doses of procainamide (i.e., 750–1500 mg every 4 hours with a resultant plasma concentration of 10–25 mg/L) may be effective in treating some individuals with recurrent ventricular tachycardia.

Procainamide therapy may be associated with several adverse effects. First, if it is given alone to the patient with atrial flutter, it may induce 1:1 AV conduction at a rate of 280 to 320 per minute, leading to diminished peripheral perfusion and pulmonary venous congestion. Therefore, in the patient who receives procainamide to prevent recurrent atrial fibrillation or flutter, digitalis should be administered concomitantly to prevent 1:1 AV conduction should atrial flutter occur. Second, procainamide commonly causes anorexia, nausea, and vomiting. Third, agranulocytosis has been reported with procainamide, and therefore, the white blood cell count should be monitored in the patient on procainamide therapy. Fourth, an occasional patient receiving procainamide develops a clinical and serologic syndrome of systemic lupus erythematosus, with skin rash, arthralgias, pulmonary fibrosis, and pericarditis but without cerebral and renal involvement. Leukopenia, anemia, thrombocytopenia, and hyperglobulinemia are distinctly uncommon. The entire syndrome regresses when procainamide is discontinued.

Procainamide

1. Greenspan AM, Horowitz LN, Spielman SR, Josephson ME. Large dose procainamide therapy for ventricular tachyarrhythmia. Am J Cardiol 1980; 46:453–62.
   Large dose procainamide therapy (500–1,500 mg every 4 hours) is quite effective in the treatment of recurrent inducible ventricular tachyarrhythmia; furthermore, the improved efficacy of large-dose over small-dose therapy may be achieved without a greatly increased incidence of toxic adverse effects.

2. Engle TR, Meister SG, Luck JC. Modification of ventricular tachycardia by procainamide in patients with coronary artery disease. Am J Cardiol 1980; 46:1033–8.
   In 15 patients with ventricular tachycardia and underlying coronary artery disease, procainamide slowed but did not prevent induced ventricular tachycardia.

3. Giardina EGV, Fenster PE, Bigger JT Jr, Mayersohn M, Perrier D, Marcus FI. Efficacy, plasma concentrations, and adverse effects of a new sustained release procainamide preparation. Am J Cardiol 1980; 46:855–62.
   In this study, a new sustained release form of procainamide (given every 8 hours) was effective in abolishing ventricular ectopy. Adverse effects were generally minor.

4. Strasberg B, Sclarovsky S, Erdberg A, Duffy CE, Lam W, Swiryn S, Agmon J, Rosen KM. Procainamide-induced polymorphous ventricular tachycardia. Am J Cardiol 1981; 47:1309–14.
   In 7 cases, oral or intravenous procainamide induced a polymorphous ventricular tachycardia.

5. Burton JR, Mathew MT, Armstrong PW. Comparative effects of lidocaine and procainamide on acutely impaired hemodynamics. Am J Med 1976; 61:215–20.
   In 15 patients with moderately impaired hemodynamics (pulmonary capillary

wedge pressure > 15 mmHg and/or cardiac index < 2.5 L/min/m²), intravenous procainamide (500–600 mg over about 25 minutes) caused no change in these variables.

6. Ghose MK. Pericardial tamponade: a presenting manifestation of procainamide-induced lupus erythematosus. Am J Med 1975; 58:581–5.

    A 75-year-old woman who had procainamide-induced lupus pericarditis with tamponade is described. This occurrence is extremely uncommon.

7. Giardina EGV, Heissenbuttel RH, Bigger JT Jr. Intermittent intravenous procaine amide to treat ventricular arrhythmias: correlation of plasma concentration with effect on arrhythmia, electrocardiogram, and blood pressure. Ann Intern Med 1973; 78:183–93.

    In 20 patients with ventricular arrhythmias, intravenous procainamide abolished the arrhythmia in 17 and partially suppressed it in 2.

8. Waxman HL, Buxton AE, Sadowski LM, Josephson ME. The response to procainamide during electrophysiologic study for sustained ventricular tachyarrhythmias predicts the response to other medications. Circulation 1983; 67:30–7.

    In 126 patients with inducible sustained ventricular tachyarrhythmias, the response to procainamide accurately predicted the response to other conventional antiarrhythmic agents during invasive electrophysiologic study.

N-Acetylprocainamide (NAPA)

9. Roden DM, Reele SB, Higgins SB, Wilkinson GR, Smith RF, Oates JA, Woosley RL. Antiarrhythmic efficacy, pharmacokinetics, and safety of N-acetylprocainamide in human subjects: comparison with procainamide. Am J Cardiol 1980; 46:463–8.

    NAPA appears to be effective in some patients with ventricular arrhythmias, yet it is much less likely than procainamide to induce the lupus syndrome.

10. Kluger J, Drayer D, Reidenberg M, Ellis G, Lloyd V, Tyberg T, Hayes J. The clinical pharmacology and antiarrhythmic efficacy of acetylprocainamide in patients with arrhythmias. Am J Cardiol 1980; 45:1250–7.

    In 16 patients, NAPA reduced the frequency of arrhythmias by more than 75% in 9.

11. Winkle RA, Jaillon P, Kates RE, Peters F. Clinical pharmacology and antiarrhythmic efficacy of N-acetylprocainamide. Am J Cardiol 1981; 47:123–30.

    In 11 patients with chronic ventricular arrhythmias, NAPA induced a 90% reduction in arrhythmia frequency in only 2.

12. Kluger J, Leech S, Reidenberg MM, Lloyd V, Drayer DE. Long-term antiarrhythmic therapy with acetylprocainamide. Am J Cardiol 1981; 48:1124–32.

    In 19 patients treated long-term with NAPA, 8 died or withdrew because of arrhythmia recurrence; 7 required a reduction in dosage or drug discontinuation; and the remainder continued to show a beneficial effect for 3 years.

13. Kluger J, Drayer DE, Reidenberg MM, Lahita R. Acetylprocainamide therapy in patients with previous procainamide-induced lupus syndrome. Ann Intern Med 1981; 95:18–23.

    In 11 patients with previous procainamide-induced lupus syndrome, NAPA did not cause a recurrence of this adverse effect.

14. Sung RJ, Juma Z, Saksena S. Electrophysiologic properties and antiarrhythmic mechanisms of intravenous N-acetylprocainamide in patients with ventricular dysrhythmias. Am Heart J 1983; 105: 811–9.

    In patients with inducible ventricular arrhythmias, NAPA was effective in suppressing these arrhythmias in only about half.

DIPHENYLHYDANTOIN

Diphenylhydantoin (phenytoin) has been used extensively in patients with various kinds of seizures. In addition, it has been utilized in patients with atrial and ventricular arrhythmias due to digitalis excess. As such, it is used most often in patients with digitalis-induced paroxysmal supraventricular tachycardia with block, ventricular premature beats, and ventricular tachycardia. Its effects on digitalis-induced sinus arrest or sinoatrial block are unknown. It is relatively ineffective in individuals with atrial or ventricular tachyarrhythmias not related to digitalis intoxication.

Phenytoin should be administered intravenously or orally, since it is erratically and unpredictably absorbed following its intramuscular injection. By the intravenous route, an initial loading dose of 700 to 1000 mg is administered at a rate of 100 mg every 5 minutes. Subsequently, a maintenance dosage of 300 mg per day is infused, usually 100 mg every 8 hours. Since the vehicle that is provided to solubilize this agent has a pH of 11.0, it may cause a severe phlebitis if it is infused into a small peripheral vein. To avoid this, phenytoin should be infused into a large vein, and after each dose the vein should be flushed thoroughly with normal saline or a dilute glucose solution. By the oral route, an initial loading dose of 1000 mg is given on the first day and 500 to 600 mg on the second and third days. Then, maintenance therapy (300–400 mg/day in divided doses) is prescribed.

Phenytoin is a relatively safe agent. The patient with mild intoxication may have unsteadiness of gait, dizziness, nystagmus, and difficulty with rapid alternating movements. In addition to these, the individual with moderate intoxication usually has some behavioral abnormalities, such as inappropriate laughter or weeping. The patient with severe phenytoin intoxication has a so-called restless coma, marked by periods of excitation alternating with periods of depression. The patient may also have decerebrate posturing and even respiratory paralysis. During long-term oral therapy, the patient may develop hyperglycemia, hypocalcemia with osteomalacia, skin rash, a megaloblastic anemia, and even a syndrome of lymphadenopathy and gingival hyperplasia that resembles malignant lymphoma.

1. Damato AN. Diphenylhydantoin: pharmacological and clinical use. Prog Cardiovasc Dis 1969; 12:1–15.
   Phenytoin appears to have special utility in the treatment of ventricular arrhythmias, especially those which are digitalis-induced.
2. Stone N, Klein MD, Lown B. Diphenylhydantoin in the prevention of recurring ventricular tachycardia. Circulation 1971; 43:420–7.
   In 10 patients with recurrent ventricular tachycardia, phenytoin was uniformly ineffective in preventing recurrences.
3. Garson A Jr, Kugler JD, Gilette PC, Simonelli A, McNamara DG. Control of late postoperative ventricular arrhythmias with phenytoin in young patients. Am J Cardiol 1980; 46:290–4.
   In 6 patients following surgical correction of congenital heart abnormalities, phenytoin was effective in suppressing ventricular ectopy.
4. Mercer EN, Osborne JA. The current status of diphenylhydantoin in heart disease. Ann Intern Med 1967; 67:1084–1107.
   Phenytoin is especially effective in patients with digitalis-induced arrhythmias.

DISOPYRAMIDE

Disopyramide appears to be an effective antiarrhythmic agent, especially for the management of patients with ventricular tachyarrhythmias. In addition, preliminary studies from abroad have demonstrated that this agent is sometimes helpful in converting supraventricular tachyarrhythmias to sinus rhythm as well as in maintaining sinus rhythm after cardioversion. Following its oral administration, disopyramide is almost completely absorbed from the gastrointestinal tract. Maximal plasma concentrations are usually achieved 1 to 3 hours after ingestion, and the drug's plasma half-life is about 6 hours. The usual therapeutic plasma concentration is 2 to 4 mg per milliliter, a level usually attained with an oral dosage of 100 to 150 mg 4 times daily. About 50 percent of disopyramide is excreted unchanged in the urine, and an additional 20 percent is eliminated in the urine in the form of the mono-N-dealkylated metabolite. The remainder is excreted through the biliary tract into the feces.

Electrophysiologic studies have demonstrated that disopyramide shortens the spontaneous cycle length; prolongs the relative refractory period of the atria, His-Purkinje system, and ventricles; and increases both P wave and QRS duration. Apart from these depressant effects on conduction, disopyramide exerts a direct anticholinergic influence. In patients with normal left ventricular function, the drug produces no measurable hemodynamic effect, but it may cause myocardial depression in the patient with already abnormal left ventricular function.

Disopyramide occasionally causes adverse effects, the most serious of which are related to its anticholinergic properties: dryness of the mouth and tongue, urinary retention, constipation, abdominal discomfort, blurred vision, dizziness, and headache. Especially prone to the development of urinary retention are male patients with benign prostatic hypertrophy. Less commonly, mental depression and impotence occur. Hypoglycemia has been reported in an occasional individual. In the patient with marginal left ventricular function, disopyramide may induce congestive heart failure. Interestingly, this negative inotropic effect is accentuated by hyperkalemia and (at least partially) alleviated by hypokalemia. Because of these potential problems, disopyramide is contraindicated in the patient with acute pulmonary edema, uncontrolled congestive heart failure, cardiogenic shock, glaucoma, and urinary retention. In addition, the drug may be harmful in patients with sinus node dysfunction, sinus pauses, or sinoatrial exit block.

1. Jensen G, Sigurd B, Uhrenholt A. Hemodynamic effects of intravenous disopyramide in heart failure. Eur J Clin Pharmacol 1975; 8:167–73.
   In 11 patients with borderline cardiac function, intravenous disopyramide reduced cardiac index by 28% and raised intracardiac filling pressures.
2. Hartel G, Louhija A, Konttinen A. Disopyramide in the prevention of recurrence of atrial fibrillation after electroconversion. Clin Pharmacol Ther 1974; 15:551–5.
   In patients undergoing electroversion for atrial fibrillation, disopyramide maintained 72% in sinus rhythm over the subsequent 3 months, whereas placebo maintained only 30% in sinus rhythm.
3. Luoma PV, Kujala PA, Juustila HJ, Takkunen JT. Efficacy of intravenous disopyramide in the termination of supraventricular arrhythmias. J Clin Pharmacol 1978; 18:293–301.
   Intravenous disopyramide was given to 57 patients with supraventricular tachyarrhythmias; it induced a reversion to sinus rhythm in 24 (42%).
4. Mathur PP. Cardiovascular effects of a newer antiarrhythmic agent, disopyramide phosphate. Am Heart J 1972; 84:764–70.
   In comparison to equipotent doses of quinidine, disopyramide exerted a marked cardiodepressant effect.
5. Danilo P Jr, Rosen MR. Cardiac effects of disopyramide. Am Heart J 1976; 92:532–6.
   Electrophysiologically, the effects of disopyramide closely resemble those of quinidine.
6. Kotter V, Linderer T, Schroder R. Effects of disopyramide on systemic and coronary hemodynamics and myocardial metabolism in patients with coronary artery disease: comparison with lidocaine. Am J Cardiol 1980; 46:469–75.

In patients with severe coronary artery disease, disopyramide induced coronary arterial vasoconstriction.

7. Podrid PJ, Schoeneberger A, Lown B. Congestive heart failure caused by oral disopyramide. N Engl J Med 1980; 302:614–7.
   Of 100 patients receiving oral disopyramide, 16 had congestive heart failure. Disopyramide exerts a profound negative myocardial inotropic effect that is unique among the antiarrhythmic agents in current use.

8. Swiryn S, Bauernfeind RA, Wyndham CRC, Dhingra RC, Palileo E, Strasberg B, Rosen KM. Effects of oral disopyramide phosphate on induction of paroxysmal supraventricular tachycardia. Circulation 1981; 64:169–75.
   In 16 patients with inducible paroxysmal supraventricular tachycardia, disopyramide prevented or limited its induction in 10 (63%).

9. Goldberg IJ, Brown LK, Rayfield EJ. Disopyramide (Norpace)-induced hypoglycemia. Am J Med 1980; 69:463–6.
   The case report of an 88-year-old woman in whom disopyramide caused severe hypoglycemia.

10. Leach AJ, Brown JE, Armstrong PW. Cardiac depression by intravenous disopyramide in patients with left ventricular dysfunction. Am J Med 1980; 68:839–44.
    In 9 patients with left ventricular dysfunction, intravenous disopyramide caused a fall in systemic arterial pressure and cardiac index as well as a rise in intracardiac filling pressures.

11. LaBarre A, Strauss HC, Scheinman MM, Evans GT, Bashore T, Tiedeman JS, Wallace AG. Electrophysiologic effects of disopyramide phosphate on sinus node function in patients with sinus node dysfunction. Circulation 1979; 59:226–35.
    This drug should be administered cautiously to patients with sinus node dysfunction, particularly those with sinus pauses, sinoatrial exit block, or secondary pauses.

12. Yu PN. Disopyramide phosphate (Norpace): a new antiarrhythmic drug. Circulation 1979; 59:236–7.
    A brief but thorough review of disopyramide's uses and contraindications.

13. Lerman BB, Waxman HL, Buxton AE, Josephson ME. Disopyramide: evaluation of electrophysiologic effects and clinical efficacy in patients with sustained ventricular tachycardia or ventricular fibrillation. Am J Cardiol 1983; 51:759–64.
    Of 50 patients studied, disopyramide prevented induction of sustained ventricular tachyarrhythmias in 17 (34%).

14. Riccioni N, Castiglioni M, Bartolomei C. Disopyramide-induced QT prolongation and ventricular tachyarrhythmias. Am Heart J 1983; 105:870–1.
    A report of a 66-year-old woman who developed torsade de pointes during relatively low-dose disopyramide therapy.

15. Kowey PR, Friedman PL, Podrid PJ, Zielonka J, Lown B, Wynne J, Holman BL. Use of radionuclide ventriculography for assessment of changes in myocardial performance induced by disopyramide phosphate. Am Heart J 1982; 104:769–74.
    Patients with left ventricular dysfunction are particularly susceptible to the cardiodepressant effects of disopyramide.

BRETYLIUM TOSYLATE

Bretylium tosylate has been used outside the United States as an antihypertensive and antiarrhythmic agent. In the experimental setting, it increases the electrical threshold for ventricular fibrillation, and in some animals it even causes a conversion of ventricular fibrillation to sinus rhythm. In man, bretylium reduces the frequency and severity of ventricular ectopic activity. It is especially effective in suppressing life-threatening ventricular tachyarrhythmias unresponsive to other agents. Even ventricular fibrillation that fails to respond to repeated DC countershock may respond to the combination of bretylium and countershock. It is ineffective in patients with supraventricular tachyarrhythmias.

At present, bretylium is available in the United States only in the parenteral form (to be given intramuscularly or intravenously). In the therapy of ventricular fibrillation, it must be given as an intravenous bolus. Following bolus injection, its onset of action is immediate. The usual dosage is 5 to 10 mg per kilogram of body weight. For maintenance therapy, the same dosage is administered every 6 to 8 hours as an infusion of 1 to 2 mg per minute.

Bretylium is generally well tolerated. It often causes a transient and modest increase in systemic arterial pressure, after which it commonly induces mild hypotension. In an occasional individual, it induces a severe fall in blood pressure. This has prevented its use in patients with ventricular tachyarrhythmias in association with myocardial infarction. In contrast to most antiarrhythmic agents, bretylium exerts a positive inotropic action. Nausea and vomiting occur rarely. During chronic oral therapy, many patients have parotid pain and swelling, but these have not occurred during bretylium's short-term parenteral administration.

1. Allen JD, Zaidi SA, Shanks RG, Pantridge JF. The effects of bretylium on experimental cardiac dysrhythmias. Am J Cardiol 1972; 29:641–9.
   In the dog with ventricular dysrhythmias, bretylium was less effective than propranolol.
2. Heissenbuttel RH, Bigger JT Jr. Bretylium tosylate: a newly available antiarrhythmic drug for ventricular arrhythmias. Ann Intern Med 1979; 91:229–38.
   An excellent review of this agent's pharmacokinetics and clinical uses. Includes 68 references.
3. Greene HL, Werner JA, Gross BW, Sears GK. Failure of bretylium to suppress inducible ventricular tachycardia. Am Heart J 1983; 105:717–21.
   In 5 patients with inducible ventricular tachycardia, intravenous bretylium did not suppress inducibility in any patient.
4. Dhurandhar RW, Teasdale SJ, Mahon WA. Bretylium tosylate in the management of refractory ventricular fibrillation. Can Med Assoc J 1971; 105:161–5.
   In 18 patients with recurrent episodes of ventricular fibrillation, intramuscular bretylium lowered or abolished its occurrence.
5. Bernstein JG, Koch-Weser J. Effectiveness of bretylium tosylate against refractory ventricular arrhythmias. Circulation 1972; 45:1024–34.
   In 30 patients with ventricular tachycardia/fibrillation unresponsive to conventional therapy, bretylium suppressed the tachyarrhythmia completely in 18 and partially in 5. It was ineffective in the remaining 7 individuals.
6. Luomanmaki K, Heikkila J, Hartel G. Bretylium tosylate: adverse effects in acute myocardial infarction. Arch Intern Med 1975; 135: 515–8.
   Of 16 patients with acute myocardial infarction given bretylium, marked hypotension developed in 7.
7. Holder DA, Sniderman AD, Fraser G, Fallen EL. Experience with bretylium tosylate by a hospital cardiac arrest team. Circulation 1977; 55:541–4.
   In 27 consecutive patients with resistant ventricular fibrillation, intravenous bretylium was useful in restoring sinus rhythm in 20, 12 of whom eventually were discharged from the hospital.
8. Patterson E, Gibson JK, Lucchesi BR. Prevention of chronic canine ventricular tachyarrhythmias with bretylium tosylate. Circulation 1981; 64:1045–50.
   Bretylium was effective in preventing reentrant ventricular rhythms in dogs 3–6 days after myocardial infarction.
9. Haynes RE, Chinn TL, Copass MK, Cobb LA. Comparison of bretylium tosylate and lidocaine in management of out of hospital ventricular fibrillation: a randomized clinical trial. Am J Cardiol 1981; 48:353–6.
   In 146 victims of out of hospital ventricular fibrillation, bretylium and lidocaine afforded similar advantages and disadvantages.

10. Bauernfeind RA, Hoff JV, Swiryn S, Palileo E, Strasberg B, Scagliotti D, Rosen KM. Electrophysiologic testing of bretylium tosylate in sustained ventricular tachycardia. Am Heart J 1983; 105:973–80.
In 10 patients with inducible sustained ventricular tachycardia, bretylium prevented its induction in only 1.

AMIODARONE

Amiodarone has been evaluated extensively in experimental animals and in man outside the United States and has been shown to be effective in the control of supraventricular and ventricular tachyarrhythmias. Specifically, it is an extremely good agent for suppressing episodes of recurrent paroxysmal atrial flutter and fibrillation and supraventricular tachycardia, including those that occur in patients with the Wolff-Parkinson-White syndrome. It is effective in the suppression of ventricular tachycardia in many patients in whom other antiarrhythmic agents have been unsuccessful. Its efficacy in patients with ventricular ectopy appears to be good regardless of the underlying cardiac disease. Thus, amiodarone has successfully controlled ventricular tachycardia in patients with congestive cardiomyopathy or ischemic heart disease.

Oral amiodarone is administered in a dosage of 500 to 2000 mg per day for 4 to 8 days, after which the dosage is reduced to 200 to 1200 mg per day. Its onset of action may require 7 to 14 days, and its elimination may require even a longer period of time. In fact, 30 days after its discontinuation, its concentration has diminished by only 16 to 34 percent. In contrast to the established antiarrhythmic agents, the results of invasive electrophysiologic testing during amiodarone therapy often do not reflect its long-term efficacy. Thus, in the electrophysiology laboratory, amiodarone may not prevent the induction of supraventricular or ventricular tachycardia, yet it is a clinically efficacious agent in these same patients.

Constipation and skin rash occur in about 10 percent of patients receiving amiodarone, but they seldom mandate its discontinuation. Since each molecule of amiodarone contains two iodine atoms, its administration may uncover a subclinical form of hypothyroidism or hyperthyroidism. Similar to other iodine-containing compounds, amiodarone is excreted by the lacrimal glands and is deposited in the superficial layers of the cornea. As a result, corneal microdeposits develop in nearly all patients on long-term amiodarone therapy and occasionally cause blurring of vision. These microdeposits gradually disappear when amiodarone is discontinued, although this may take several months. Their appearance can be minimized by the use of eyedrops containing methylcellulose. Like quinidine and procainamide, amiodarone should not be administered to the patient with intraventricular or atrioventricular block. Finally, an occasional patient receiving amiodarone develops pulmonary fibrosis.

1. Rosenbaum MB, Chiale PA, Halpern MS, Nau GJ, Przybylski J, Levi RJ, Lazzari JO, Elizari MV. Clinical efficacy of amiodarone as an antiarrhythmic agent. Am J Cardiol 1976; 38:934–44.
With amiodarone, total suppression and control was provided in 92.4% of those with supraventricular arrhythmias and in 82% of those with ventricular arrhythmias.
2. Wellens HJJ, Lie KI, Bar FW, Wesdorp JC, Dohmen HJ, Duren DR, Durrer D. Effect of amiodarone in the Wolff-Parkinson-White syndrome. Am J Cardiol 1976; 38:189–94.

The effect of amiodarone in prolonging the refractory period of the accessory pathway makes it especially useful in patients with the Wolff-Parkinson-White syndrome and atrial fibrillation.

3. Ward DE, Camm AJ, Spurrell RAJ. Clinical antiarrhythmic effects of amiodarone in patients with resistant paroxysmal tachycardias. Br Heart J 1980; 44:91–5.
   In 72 patients, 54 with supraventricular tachyarrhythmias and 18 with ventricular tachyarrhythmias, amiodarone completely or partially abolished tachyarrhythmias in 57 (79%).

4. Podrid PJ, Lown B. Amiodarone therapy in symptomatic, sustained refractory atrial and ventricular tachyarrhythmias. Am Heart J 1981; 101:374–9.
   In 70 patients with sustained refractory tachyarrhythmias, amiodarone was highly effective in controlling their recurrence.

5. Nademanee K, Hendrickson JA, Cannom DS, Goldreyer BN, Singh BN. Control of refractory life-threatening ventricular tachyarrhythmias by amiodarone. Am Heart J 1981; 101:759–68.
   In 22 patients with recurrent symptomatic ventricular tachyarrhythmias refractory to 2 or more conventional antiarrhythmic agents, amiodarone (600–1,200 mg/day) was an extremely potent and safe agent.

6. Kaski JC, Girotti LA, Messuti H, Rutitzky B, Rosenbaum MB. Long-term management of sustained, recurrent, symptomatic ventricular tachycardia with amiodarone. Circulation 1981; 64:273–9.
   Of 23 patients with sustained, recurrent, symptomatic ventricular tachycardia, amiodarone was highly effective in 20 (87%). In these individuals, it took an average of 9½ days to reach antiarrythmic efficacy.

7. Heger JJ, Prystowsky EN, Jackman WM, Naccarelli GV, Warfel KA, Rinkenberger RL, Zipes DP. Amiodarone: clinical efficacy and electrophysiology during long-term therapy for recurrent ventricular tachycardia or ventricular fibrillation. N Engl J Med 1981; 305:539–45.
   Of 45 patients with these tachyarrhythmias, amiodarone successfully controlled 9 of the 16 who had recurrent ventricular fibrillation and 21 of the 29 who had recurrent ventricular tachycardia. In these individuals, the induction of arrhythmia during therapy often did not predict long-term therapeutic efficacy.

8. Morady F, Scheinman MM, Shen E, Shapiro W, Sung RJ, DiCarlo L. Intravenous amiodarone in the acute treatment of recurrent symptomatic ventricular tachycardia. Am J Cardiol 1983; 51:156–9.
   Of 15 patients with recurrent ventricular tachycardia treated with intravenous amiodarone, 12 were successfully controlled.

9. Leak D, Eydt JN. Control of refractory cardiac arrhythmias with amiodarone. Arch Intern Med 1979; 139:425–8.
   Amiodarone suppressed tachyarrhythmias in 17 of 19 patients previously unresponsive to conventional antiarrhythmic therapy.

10. Hamer AW, Finerman WB Jr, Peter T, Mandell WJ. Disparity between the clinical and electrophysiologic effects of amiodarone in the treatment of recurrent ventricular tachyarrythmias. Am Heart J 1981; 102:992–1000.
    The clinical efficacy of amiodarone in patients with ventricular arrythmias may not be reliably predicted by electrophysiologic studies.

11. Harris L, McKenna WJ, Rowland E, Holt DW, Storey GCA, Krikler DM. Side effects of long-term amiodarone therapy. Circulation 1983; 67:45–51.
    A complete review of all the adverse effects seen in 140 patients on chronic amiodarone therapy.

12. Marcus FI, Fontaine GH, Frank R, Grosgogeat Y. Clinical pharmacology and therapeutic applications of the antiarrythmic agent, amiodarone. Am Heart J 1981; 101:480–93.
    A thorough review of amiodarone's efficacy and adverse effects. Includes 68 references.

NEW ANTIARRHYTHMIC AGENTS

Over the past few years, a number of agents have been tested extensively in patients with supraventricular and ventricular ectopic activity, and it is likely that at least some of them will become available for general use in the near future.

Tocainide hydrochloride is an oral analog of lidocaine that has been shown to suppress ventricular ectopic activity and ventricular tachycardia. Similar to lidocaine, it is not effective in suppressing or reverting supraventricular tachyarrhythmias. In most individuals, there is a good relationship between the antiarrhythmic efficacy of intravenous lidocaine and oral tocainide. It is administered 2 or 3 times daily, with the total daily dose ranging from 1.0 to 2.5 gm. Its serum half-life in patients with ventricular ectopy is 14 to 16 hours. The minimal plasma concentration that affords antiarrhythmic efficacy is 3.5 to 7.0 μg per milliliter, whereas central nervous system toxicity occurs at a plasma concentration of 10 to 15 μg per milliliter. As a result, there is a relatively narrow difference between therapeutic and toxic plasma concentrations. To minimize tocainide toxicity, it is recommended that it be administered every 8 hours rather than every 12 hours.

Adverse effects due to tocainide are relatively common, occurring in 25 to 70 percent of patients. Gastrointestinal complaints, most often nausea and vomiting, are very common, followed by central nervous system symptoms, including vertigo, dizziness, diplopia, blurred vision, unsteadiness of gait, and tremor. No abnormalities of renal, hepatic, or hematologic function have been observed. In addition, tocainide does not markedly depress myocardial function.

Aprindine appears to be effective in controlling both supraventricular and ventricular tachyarrhythmias. In the setting of acute myocardial infarction, its efficacy in patients with ventricular ectopy is similar to that of lidocaine. It is beneficial following intravenous or oral administration, and it may be given only every 12 hours. Its total daily dose is usually 200 mg, with which a plasma concentration of 1 to 2 μg per milliliter is achieved. During its administration, blood pressure and heart rate are not altered, but it exerts a modest negative inotropic influence, and the P–R, QRS, and Q–T intervals are prolonged slightly.

The most frequent untoward effects of aprindine are dizziness and tremor. With very high doses, convulsions may occur. If these adverse effects appear, the dosage of aprindine should be decreased, or the drug should be discontinued. It does not appear to exert a deleterious influence on the renal or hepatic systems, but it has been reported to cause agranulocytosis on occasion. A derivative of aprindine, moxaprindine, appears to be a promising antiarrhythmic agent that is not associated with many of these adverse effects.

Flecainide acetate is a membrane-stabilizing antiarrhythmic agent that appears to be extremely effective in a variety of supraventricular and ventricular tachyarrhythmias. Electrophysiologic studies have demonstrated that it prolongs all cardiac conduction intervals, exerting a particularly marked effect on His-Purkinje and ventricular myocardial conduction. Although it has little effect on the refractoriness of normal cardiac tissue, it substantially prolongs the refractoriness of accessory pathways. Because of these electrophysiologic effects, flecainide has been shown to be an effective agent in patients with reentrant tachycardias utilizing an AV accessory pathway and in patients with complex ventricular ectopy.

Flecainide acetate may be administered intravenously in a dosage of 2 mg per kilogram of body weight over a 5-minute period. For long-term oral therapy, it is given every 12 hours, beginning with a dose of 100 mg and increasing gradually to a maximal dose of 250 to 300 mg every 12 hours. Its average elimination half-life is about 20 hours. Its peak plasma concentration 3 hours after an oral dose ranges widely from one patient to another, so that it is difficult to establish accurately the relation between therapeutic and toxic plasma concentrations. In most studies, flecainide prolonged the P–R, QRS, and Q–T intervals in parallel with the reduction in arrhythmia frequency. Adverse effects are relatively infrequent when flecainide is administered in the dosages mentioned. The most frequent side effects are blurring of vision, dizziness, lightheadedness, abnormal taste sensation, flushing, tinnitus, sleepiness, paresthesias, headache, and a mild elevation of the serum alkaline phosphatase. Flecainide does not exert a depressant effect on left ventricular performance.

Encainide is a benzanilide derivative that appears promising in patients with refractory, life-threatening recurrent ventricular tachycardia and fibrillation as well as in those with frequent ventricular premature beats. In many ways, its chemical structure resembles that of procainamide; however, unlike procainamide and other conventional antiarrhythmic agents, it is extraordinarily active in nanogram concentrations and has only minimal adverse effects. In most individuals, it is administered orally in a total daily dose of 150 to 250 mg, usually 3 or 4 times daily. Following its ingestion, there is large interpatient variability in its bioavailability and clearance, so that the relationship between its plasma concentration and its therapeutic effect is poor. However, since encainide induces a predictable widening of the QRS complex, this variable can be used as a reliable indicator of the drug's effect on the cardiac conducting system. In general, the dosage of encainide is adjusted to provide a 30- to 50-percent widening of the QRS complex.

Encainide is generally well tolerated, although an occasional patient complains of dizziness, mild ataxia, tremor, and difficulty with visual accommodation. Gastrointestinal disturbances occasionally occur, especially nausea and constipation. Finally, some patients receiving chronic encainide therapy may note headache.

Mexiletine is an antiarrhythmic agent structurally similar to lidocaine. Preliminary studies have demonstrated that it suppresses ventricular arrhythmias associated with acute and chronic ischemic heart disease as well as those that appear in patients with apparently normal hearts. It appears to be capable of suppressing ventricular ectopy that is unresponsive to conventional antiarrhythmic agents. Furthermore, mexiletine has been combined with quinidine in the treatment of individuals with ectopy that is especially difficult to control with either agent alone, with apparently good results.

Mexiletine is generally administered orally in an initial daily dose of 600 mg, usually given in 3 equal doses. Subsequently, the dosage is titrated upward until dose-related toxicity occurs or a maximal dose of 1200 mg per day is achieved. At present, plasma concentrations of mexiletine are not available. Adverse effects related to the drug are fairly frequent and are severe enough to require its discontinuation in 10 to 15 percent of patients. Most commonly, mexiletine causes gastrointestinal symptoms, including nausea and vomiting, and neurologic complaints, such as light-headedness, tremor, ataxia, confusion, and blurred vision.

Ethmozin, a phenothiazine derivative, has been evaluated extensively in the Soviet Union in patients with complex ventricular ectopy and recurrent supraventricular tachyarrhythmias, and preliminary studies in this country have provided support for the enthusiasm voiced by Russian investigators. At this point, its optimal therapeutic dose is not known, since it has been administered in short-term studies in daily doses ranging from 225 to 600 mg. Following the initiation of therapy with this agent, antiarrhythmic activity does not appear for 24 hours; the reason for this prolonged latency in onset of antiarrhythmic effect has not been determined. In early studies, the adverse effects associated with ethmozin appear to be minimal.

Lorcainide is a new antiarrhythmic agent that appears to be especially effective in suppressing ventricular tachyarrhythmias. It can be administered either intravenously or orally. Its serum half-life ranges from 6 to 23 hours. Most patients are able to tolerate an oral dosage of 100 mg twice daily. On this regimen, adverse effects are minimal.

Tocainide Hydrochloride

1. LeWinter MM, Engler RL, Karliner JS. Tocainide therapy for treatment of ventricular arrhythmias: assessment with ambulatory electrocardiographic monitoring and treadmill exercise. Am J Cardiol 1980; 45:1045–52.
   In 10 patients not receiving quinidine, procainamide, or disopyramide, tocainide (1,200 mg/day in 3 equal doses) was effective in suppressing ventricular arrhythmias.

2. Winkle RA, Meffin PJ, Fitzgerald JW, Harrison DC. Clinical efficacy and pharmacokinetics of a new orally effective antiarrhythmic, tocainide. Circulation 1976; 54:884–9.
   Premature ventricular contractions were suppressed by more than 70% in 11 of 15 patients with tocainide therapy.

3. Woosley RL, McDevitt DG, Nies AS, Smith RF, Wilkinson GR, Oates JA. Suppression of ventricular ectopic depolarizations by tocainide. Circulation 1977; 56:980–4.
   In 8 of 12 individuals with frequent VPBs, tocainide effectively suppressed ectopic activity.

4. Winkle RA, Meffin PJ, Harrison DC. Long-term tocainide therapy for ventricular arrhythmias. Circulation 1978; 57:1008–16.
   In 17 patients with complex ventricular ectopy, chronic tocainide therapy (300–700 mg every 8 hours) was unsuccesesful in 8 but effective in the other 9.

5. Ryan W, Engler R, LeWinter M, Karliner JS. Efficacy of a new oral agent (tocainide) in the acute treatment of refractory ventricular arrhythmias. Am J Cardiol 1979; 43:285–91.
   Of 30 patients with ventricular ectopy who received tocainide, a satisfactory response occurred in 18 (60%).

6. Engler R, Ryan W, LeWinter M, Bluestein H, Karliner JS. Assessment of long-term antiarrhythmic therapy: studies on the long-term efficacy and toxicity of tocainide. Am J Cardiol 1979; 43:612–8.
   In 21 individuals tocainide was successful in acutely suppressing VPBs and ventricular tachycardia. Four patients had adverse reactions requiring tocainide withdrawal.

Aprindine

7. Strasberg B, Palileo E, Prechel D, Bauernfeind R, Swiryn S, Wyndham CR, Dhingra RC, Kehoe R, Rosen KM. Ventricular tachycardia: prediction of response to oral aprindine with intravenous aprindine. Am J Cardiol 1981; 47:676–82.
   The administration of intravenous aprindine to patients with ventricular tachycardia is helpful in predicting the subsequent response to oral aprindine.

8. Zipes DP, Gaum WE, Foster PR, Rosen KM, Wu D, Amat-y-Leon F, Noble RJ. Aprindine for treatment of supraventricular tachycardias—with particular application to Wolff-Parkinson-White syndrome. Am J Cardiol 1977; 40:586–96.
   Aprindine was given to 10 patients with recurrent or continuous supraventricular tachycardia, 9 of whom had the Wolff-Parkinson-White syndrome; it was generally effective in 8.

9. Fasola AF, Noble RJ, Zipes DP. Treatment of recurrent ventricular tachycardia and fibrillation with aprindine. Am J Cardiol 1977; 39:903–9.

In 23 patients with recurrent ventricular tachycardia and fibrillation, aprindine was effective in 21.

10. Troup PJ, Zipes DP. Aprindine treatment of recurrent ventricular tachycardia in patients with mitral valve prolapse. Am Heart J 1979; 97:322–8.
   In 7 patients with mitral valve prolapse and life-threatening ventricular arrhythmias, aprindine caused a 91% reduction in the number of VPBs.

11. Greene HL, Reid PR, Schaeffer AH. Prolongation of cardiac conduction times by intravenous aprindine in man. Am J Cardiol 1978; 42:1002–6.
   In 48 patients receiving aprindine during electrophysiologic study, this agent prolonged conduction transiently in the atria, the AV node, the His-Purkinje system, and the ventricles.

12. van Leeuwen R, Meyboom RHB. Agranulocytosis and aprindine. letter. Lancet 1976; 2:1137.
   A letter describing 8 patients who developed agranulocytosis during aprindine therapy.

13. Waleffe A, Mary-Rabine L, Kulbertus HE. Study of moxaprindine with programmed electrical stimulation of the heart in patients with reentrant tachyarrhythmias. Am J Cardiol 1980; 45:640–7.
   Moxaprindine, a derivative of aprindine but with less toxicity, exerted a potent antiarrhythmic effect in 19 individuals with recurrent episodes of reentrant tachyarrhythmias.

Flecainide Acetate

14. Duff HJ, Roden DM, Maffucci RJ, Vesper BS, Conard GJ, Higgins SB, Oates JA, Smith RF, Woosley RL. Suppression of resistant ventricular arrhythmias by twice daily dosing with flecainide. Am J Cardiol 1981; 48:1133–40.
   During oral flecainide therapy, 11 patients had almost complete abolition of ventricular ectopic activity.

15. Somani P. Antiarrhythmic effects of flecainide. Clin Pharmacol Ther 1980; 27:464–70.
   Intravenous flecainide suppressed ventricular ectopy in 7 of 10 individuals without causing changes in QRS, P–R, or Q–T intervals.

16. Hellestrand KJ, Nathan AW, Bexton RS, Spurrell RAJ, Camm AJ. Cardiac electrophysiologic effects of flecainide acetate for paroxysmal reentrant junctional tachycardias. Am J Cardiol 1983; 51:770–6.
   Flecainide exerted a depressant effect on conduction through the accessory atrioventricular pathway.

17. Anderson JL, Stewart JR, Perry BA, Van Hamersveld DD, Johnson TA, Conard GJ, Chang SF, Kvam DC, Pitt B. Oral flecainide acetate for the treatment of ventricular arrhythmias. N Engl J Med 1981; 305:473–7.
   In 13 patients with chronic ventricular ectopy, flecainide was effective and well-tolerated.

18. Flecainide-Quinidine Research Group. Flecainide versus quinidine for treatment of chronic ventricular arrhythmias: a multicenter clinical trial. Circulation 1983; 67:1117–23.
   In a multicenter study involving 280 patients with ventricular ectopy, flecainide was more effective than quinidine in suppressing ventricular arrhythmias.

Encainide

19. Winkle RA, Peters F, Kates RE, Tucker C, Harrison DC. Clinical pharmacology and antiarrhythmic efficacy of encainide in patients with chronic ventricular arrhythmias. Circulation 1981; 64:290–6.
   An initial assessment of this antiarrhythmic agent in 9 patients with frequent and complex VPBs. In 8 of the 9, encainide produced a greater than 90% suppression of ventricular ectopy.

20. Sami M, Mason JW, Peters F, Harrison DC. Clinical electrophysiologic effects of encainide, a newly developed antiarrhythmic agent. Am J Cardiol 1979; 44:526–32.
   In 10 patients with coronary artery disease, intravenous encainide prolonged the H–V and QRS intervals by 31% and 18%, respectively; at the same time, it exerted no effect on heart rate, A–H interval, or corrected sinus node recovery time.

21. Mason JW, Peters FA. Antiarrhythmic efficacy of encainide in patients with re-fractory recurrent ventricular tachycardia. Circulation 1981; 63:670–5.

   Encainide, 150–250 mg/day in 4–6 equal doses, is a safe, well-tolerated antiar-rhythmic agent that is often effective against previously drug-refractory ventricu-lar tachycardia.

22. Roden DM, Reele SB, Higgins SB, Mayol RF, Gammans RE, Oates JA, Woosley RL. Total suppression of ventricular arrhythmias by encainide: pharmacokinetic and electrocardiographic characteristics. N Engl J Med 1980; 302:877–82.

   In 10 of 11 patients with high-frequency ventricular arrhythmias, encainide to-tally suppressed all ectopic activity.

Mexiletine

23. Waspe LE, Waxman HL, Buxton AE, Josephson ME. Mexiletine for control of drug-resistant ventricular tachycardia: clinical and electrophysiologic results in 44 patients. Am J Cardiol 1983; 51:1175–81.

   When used alone, mexiletine has limited efficacy as an antiarrhythmic agent; ad-verse effects are relatively common.

24. Duff HJ, Roden D, Primm RK, Oates JA, Woosley RL. Mexiletine in the treatment of resistant ventricular arrhythmias: enhancement of efficacy and reduction of dose-related side effects by combination with quinidine. Circulation 1983; 67:1124–8.

   In 17 patients, quinidine and mexiletine were given in combination, with generally good results.

25. Mehta J, Conti CR. Mexiletine, a new antiarrhythmic agent, for treatment of pre-mature ventricular complexes. Am J Cardiol 1982; 49:455–60.

   Mexiletine appears to be an effective antiarrhythmic agent in the long-term man-agement of VPBs.

26. Podrid PJ, Lown B. Mexiletine for ventricular arrhythmias. Am J Cardiol 1981; 47:895–902.

   Both acutely and chronically, oral mexiletine is effective and generally well toler-ated in patients with ventricular arrhythmias resistant to standard antiar-rhythmic drugs.

27. DiMarco JP, Garan H, Ruskin JN. Mexiletine for refractory ventricular arrhyth-mias: results using serial electrophysiologic testing. Am J Cardiol 1981; 47:131–8.

   By invasive electrophysiologic testing, mexiletine was effective in most patients with recurrent ventricular arrhythmias.

Ethmozin

28. Podrid PJ, Lyakishev A, Lown B, Mazur N. Ethmozin, a new antiarrhythmic drug for suppressing ventricular premature complexes. Circulation 1980; 61:450–7.

   In patients given 600 mg/day of ethmozin, ventricular ectopy was controlled in 54%.

Lorcainide

29. Somani P. Pharmacokinetics of lorcainide, a new antiarrhythmic drug, in patients with cardiac rhythm disorders. Am J Cardiol 1981; 48:157–63.

   In 10 patients with ventricular tachyarrhythmias, lorcainide was an effective an-tiarrhythmic agent.

HYPOLIPIDEMIC AGENTS

Epidemiologic studies over the past 10 to 15 years have demonstrated that in-dividuals with an abnormally elevated serum cholesterol concentration have an increased risk of coronary artery disease. Similarly, elevated serum triglyc-eride values have been shown to bear a relationship with coronary disease, particularly in patients less than 60 years of age. Although a serum cholesterol concentration of 220 mg/100 ml is considered abnormal, treatment usually is not initiated unless this level exceeds 250 mg/100 ml. Likewise, therapy for hypertriglyceridemia is not recommended unless the serum triglyceride concentration exceeds 150 mg/100 ml.

Dietary treatment of hyperlipidemia can substantially influence serum lipoprotein concentrations. Specifically, a diet that is restricted in fats and low in cholesterol can reduce serum cholesterol and triglyceride levels. This diet should contain approximately 20-percent protein, 40-percent carbohydrates, and 40-percent fat, with 300 mg of total cholesterol and a polyunsaturated-saturated fat ratio of 1.5:2.0. Such dietary therapy is modestly effective in lowering serum lipids: the serum cholesterol concentration declines an average of 12 percent and the serum triglyceride value an average of 17 percent. This reduction in serum triglycerides is most marked in patients who lose weight during dietary treatment.

Several pharmacologic agents are available for the treatment of individuals with hyperlipidemia. *Nicotinic acid* (niacin) reduces the serum concentrations of very low density lipoprotein (VLDL) and low density lipoprotein (LDL). It is administered orally in a dosage of 1 to 3 gm 3 times daily. During therapy with this agent, serum cholesterol concentrations fall by 17 to 39 percent, whereas serum triglyceride levels decline by as much as 90 percent. In general, the most striking results are seen in patients with the highest lipid levels before the institution of therapy. Hepatic function should be monitored during nicotinic acid therapy, since hepatotoxicity has been reported. Other side effects include pruritus, hyperuricemia, diminished glucose tolerance, nausea, vomiting, and diarrhea. As a result of these potential adverse effects, this agent should be used with caution—if at all—in patients with liver disease, gout, or diabetes mellitus.

Cholestyramine and *colestipol*, quaternary ammonium anion exchange resins with a molecular weight of about 1 million, bind bile salts in the intestine and, therefore, promote their loss from the gastrointestinal tract. These agents usually lower the serum cholesterol concentration by about 20 percent. At the same time, they do nothing to reduce the serum triglyceride level, and in fact, this concentration may even rise slightly. Cholestyramine is given in a dosage of 4 to 8 gm orally 4 times daily, administered 30 to 60 minutes before meals, whereas colestipol is administered in a total daily dose of 15 to 20 gm. Their associated adverse effects include constipation, bloating, and nausea; some patients require laxatives to combat the constipating effect of these drugs. Cholestyramine and colestipol interfere with several other medications that some patients with coronary artery disease may take. First, anticoagulation with warfarin is sufficiently difficult during their administration that another pharmacologic agent should be substituted for cholestyramine or colestipol if anticoagulation is mandatory. Second, in the patient being treated for hypothyroidism who requires cholestyramine or colestipol, periodic monitoring of thyroid function is necessary, since thyroxine binds to these agents and, therefore, may not be absorbed. Third, digitalis absorption may be impeded by cholestyramine or colestipol.

D-Thyroxine is effective in reducing the serum cholesterol concentration; it is often administered concomitantly with propranolol to control its calorigenic and cardiac effects. Recent data have suggested that patients with underlying coronary artery disease have an increased risk of sudden death during D-thyroxine therapy, so that this agent is contraindicated in patients with any form of organic heart disease, hypertension, or advanced liver or kidney disease. The maintenance dosage is 4 to 8 mg per day.

Clofibrate (Atromid-S) is the most widely used hypolipidemic agent, having been administered for long periods with good patient tolerance and few side effects. It causes only a minimal reduction in serum cholesterol, but it is very effective in lowering the serum triglyceride concentration. Clofibrate exerts a beneficial effect on morbidity in patients with coronary heart disease, but interestingly, this effect is not related to the drug's hypolipidemic action. Instead, it may be caused by clofibrate's inhibition of platelet aggregation. Although this agent has an antidiuretic hormone–like action, substantial water retention and weight gain as a result of its use have rarely occurred. An occasional patient receiving clofibrate develops alopecia or hepatic dysfunction, and a rare patient may have agranulocytosis. The usual maintenance dosage is 1 gm orally twice daily.

Probucol is a relatively new hypercholesterolemic agent with a chemical structure different from that of any of the other drugs that lower serum lipids. In most studies, it has been shown to lower serum cholesterol by 10 to 15 percent, whereas it exerts little, if any, effect on the serum triglyceride concentration. Its most frequent adverse effects are diarrhea and flatulence. The usual dosage is 500 mg twice daily.

Combination drug treatment may be beneficial in individuals with hyperlipidemia, since some of these agents may act by alternate mechanisms. Clofibrate and cholestyramine as well as nicotinic acid and cholestyramine have been shown to exert a synergistic influence. Such drug combinations are usually reserved for patients with resistant hyperlipidemia.

Finally, *ileal bypass surgery* promotes an increased fecal loss of bile acids and can cause both malabsorption and diarrhea. *Portacaval shunt surgery* has been reported to be beneficial in some individuals with homozygous hypercholesterolemia, and monthly *plasma exchange* has also been used with some success in these patients.

General

1. Levy RI, Morganroth J, Rifkind BM. Treatment of hyperlipidemia. N Engl J Med 1974; 290:1295–1301.
   A succinct review of all the hypolipidemic agents.
2. Samuel P. Drug treatment of hyperlipidemia. Am Heart J 1980; 100:573–7.
   A concise review of the major hypolipidemic agents, including an estimate of their cost (in dollars/month) to the patient.

Dietary Therapy

3. Levy RI, Frederickson DS, Shulman R, Bilheimer DW, Breslow JL, Stone NJ, Lux SE, Sloan HR, Krauss RM, Herbert PN. Dietary and drug treatment of primary hyperlipoproteinemia. Ann Intern Med 1972; 77:267–94.
   For all kinds of hyperlipidemia, dietary restriction is the cornerstone of successful therapy. Includes 138 references.
4. Levy RI, Bonnell M, Ernst ND. Dietary management of hyperlipoproteinemia. J Am Diet Assoc 1971; 58:406–16.
   A general review of the types of hyperlipidemia and the dietary approach to each.
5. Keys A, Anderson JT, Grande F. Serum cholesterol response to changes in diet. II. The effect of cholesterol in the diet. Metabolism 1965; 14:759–65.
   This article emphasizes that changes in dietary cholesterol do not greatly affect the serum concentration.
6. Hall Y, Stamler J, Cohen DB, Mojonnier L, Epstein MB, Berkson DM, Whipple IT, Catchings S. Effectiveness of a low saturated fat, low cholesterol, weight-reducing diet for the control of hypertriglyceridemia. Atherosclerosis 1972; 16:389–403.
   Most adults with hyperlipidemia, including hypertriglyceridemia, can be managed successfully with a diet low in carbohydrate and saturated fat.
7. Turpeinen O. Effect of cholesterol-lowering diet on mortality from coronary heart disease and other causes. Circulation 1979; 59:1–7.

A replacement of dairy fats by vegetable oils was followed by a substantial reduction in mortality from coronary heart disease.

8. Spritz N. Diet in the treatment of hyperlipidemia. Am Heart J 1980; 100:924–7.
This brief article offers general guidelines for dietary modifications for patients with hyperlipidemia.

Nicotinic Acid

9. Carlson LA, Oro L. Effect of treatment with nicotinic acid for one month on serum lipids in patients with different types of hyperlipidemia. Atherosclerosis 1973; 18:1–9.
In 188 patients with various kinds of hyperlipidemia, nicotinic acid (3 grams daily) lowered serum cholesterol and triglyceride concentrations.

Cholestyramine and Colestipol

10. Nazir DJ, Horlick L, Kudchodkar BJ, Sodhi HS. Mechanisms of action of cholestyramine in treatment of hypercholesterolemia. Ciriculation 1972; 46:95–102.
In 4 subjects with hypercholesterolemia, cholestyramine (12 grams/day) caused a 24–28% fall in serum cholesterol.

11. Levy RI, Fredrickson DS, Stone NJ, Bilheimer DW, Brown WV, Glueck CJ, Gotto AM, Herbert PN, Kwiterovich PO, Langer T, LaRosa J, Lux SE, Rider AK, Shulman RS, Sloan HR. Cholestyramine in type II hyperlipoproteinemia: a double-blind trial. Ann Intern Med 1973; 79:51–8.
In 47 patients with hyperlipidemia, cholestyramine (16 grams/day) lowered plasma cholesterol from 333 to 264 mg/100 mL.

12. Miller NE, Clifton-Bligh P, Nestel PJ. Effects of colestipol, a new bile-acid-sequestering resin, on cholesterol metabolism in man. J Lab Clin Med 1973; 82:876–90.
In 8 hypercholesterolemic patients, colestipol reduced the serum cholesterol concentration by an average of 54 mg/100 mL.

D-Thyroxine

13. Krikler DM, Lefevre D, Lewis B. Dextrothyroxine with propranolol in treatment of hypercholesterolemia. Lancet 1971; 1:934–6.
Of 26 patients with hypercholesterolemia treated with these agents, serum cholesterol concentrations fell to normal in 16 and were substantially reduced in 4 others.

Clofibrate

14. Hunninghake DB, Tucker DR, Azarnoff DL. Long-term effects of clofibrate (Atromid-S) on serum lipids in man. Circulation 1969; 39:675–83.
In 45 patients treated with clofibrate, serum triglyceride levels fell by at least 25%, but serum cholesterol fell less impressively.

15. Krasno LR, Kidera GJ. Clofibrate in coronary heart disease: effect on morbidity and mortality. JAMA 1972; 219:845–51.
Those treated with clofibrate had a substantial fall in the incidence of nonfatal myocardial infarction.

Probucol

16. LeLorier J, DuBreuil-Quidoz S, Lussier-Cacan S, Huang YS, Davignon J. Diet and probucol in lowering cholesterol concentrations. Arch Intern Med 1977; 137:1429–34.
A combination of diet and probucol lowered serum cholesterol concentrations by 25–30%.

17. Salel AF, Zelis R, Sodhi HS, Price J, Mason DT. Probucol: a new cholesterol-lowering drug effective in patients with type II hyperlipoproteinemia. Clin Pharmacol Ther 1976; 20:690–4.
In 11 patients with hyperbetalipoproteinemia, probucol lowered serum cholesterol from 353 to 291 mg/100 mL. There were no untoward effects.

Combination Drug Treatment

18. Moutafis CD, Myant NB, Mancini M, Oriente P. Cholestyramine and nicotinic acid in the treatment of familial hyperbetalipoproteinemia in the homozygous form. Atherosclerosis 1971; 14:247–58.

In a handful of these patients, this drug combination appeared to be effective in lowering the cholesterol concentration.

19. Coronary Drug Project Research Group. Clofibrate and niacin in coronary heart disease. JAMA 1975; 231:360–81.
    This study provides no evidence that either clofibrate or nicotinic acid are beneficial to patients with hyperlipidemia and coronary artery disease.

20. Kane JP, Malloy MJ, Tun P, Phillips NR, Freedman DD, Williams ML, Rowe JS, Havel RJ. Normalization of low-density lipoprotein levels in heterozygous familial hypercholesterolemia with a combined drug regimen. N Engl J Med 1981; 304:251–8.
    A combined regimen of colestipol and nicotinic acid reduced serum cholesterol by 55% in patients with heterozygous familial hypercholesterolemia.

21. Stein EA, Heimann KW. Colestipol, clofibrate, cholestyramine, and combination therapy in the treatment of familial hyperbetalipoproteinemia. S Afr Med J 1975; 49:1252–6.
    During therapy with a clofibrate-colestipol or a clofibrate-cholestyramine combination, serum cholesterol fell 32% and triglyceride fell 20%.

22. Mabuchi H, Sakai T, Sakai Y, Yoshimura A, Watanabe A, Wakasugi T, Koizumi J, Takeda R. Reduction of serum cholesterol in heterozygous patients with familial hypercholesterolemia: additive effects of compactin and cholestyramine. N Engl J Med 1983; 308:609–13.
    A combination of these two hypolipidemic agents reduced serum cholesterol from 356 to 217 mg/100 mL.

Surgical Treatment

23. Thompson GR, Gotto AM Jr. Ileal bypass in the treatment of hyperlipoproteinemia. Lancet 1973; 2:35–6.
    Although ileal bypass is effective in lowering serum cholesterol, so too is diet and cholestyramine.

24. Starzl TE, Putnam CW, Koep LJ. Portacaval shunt and hyperlipidemia. Arch Surg 1978; 113:71–4.
    In the 3 cases described here, a portacaval shunt procedure reduced the serum cholesterol concentration by 40–60%.

Plasma Exchange Therapy

25. Thompson GR, Lowenthal R, Myant NB. Plasma exchange in the management of homozygous familial hypercholesterolemia. Lancet 1975; 1:1208–11.
    Three young women with homozygous familial hypercholesterolemia underwent plasma exchange every 3 weeks, with a dramatic lowering of serum cholesterol levels.

26. King MEE, Breslow JL, Lees RS. Plasma-exchange therapy of homozygous familial hypercholesterolemia. N Engl J Med 1980; 302:1457–9.
    In 2 children with this metabolic disorder, plasma exchange therapy (performed every 2 weeks) lowered the serum cholesterol level, and xanthomas regressed.

UNLOADING AGENTS

Cardiac performance can be influenced by alterations in the inotropic state of the heart and by changes in loading conditions. Vasodilator (or "unloading") agents generally exert no intrinsic effect on the heart but act by reducing *preload* (the degree of filling or stretching of the left ventricle), *afterload* (the opposition to left ventricular emptying), or both. These agents can be particularly useful in the patient with severe congestive heart failure, and they may be life-saving in the patient with an acute ventricular septal defect or mitral regurgitation complicated by congestive failure. In general, a reduction in preload diminishes pulmonary congestion but does not increase cardiac output;

conversely, a reduction in afterload increases cardiac output but may not reduce pulmonary congestion. Depending on clinical circumstances, a reduction in preload, afterload, or both may be desirable.

Unloading agents can be classified according to their predominant site of action as *arteriolar dilators* (afterload reducing agents), *venodilators* (preload reducing agents), or *balanced* arteriolar and venodilators. *Hydralazine* is the prototype arteriolar dilator that exerts little or no effect on the venous capacitance vessels. It increases cardiac output when given intravenously or orally. Although intravenous hydralazine can be used acutely to reduce afterload, its duration of action makes it unsuitable for easy dosage titration or prolonged intravenous use. Chronic oral hydralazine therapy (25–100 mg 4 times daily) may lead to fluid retention, peripheral neuropathy, or drug-induced lupus erythematosus. It generally causes a slight increase in heart rate and decrease in blood pressure. Since a reflex increase in contractility may occur due to enhanced sympathetic nervous system activity, hydralazine should be used with caution in patients with ischemic heart disease for fear of provoking angina pectoris. Its efficacy may be enhanced by the concomitant administration of nitrates. *Minoxidil* exerts an effect similar to that of hydralazine, but fluid retention is often severe and may limit its usefulness in patients with congestive heart failure. *Nifedipine* is a calcium antagonist that exerts major effects on afterload. Similar to the other afterload reducing agents, it increases cardiac output but may cause hypotension, tachycardia, and fluid retention. It is not suitable for intravenous administration, but a rapid effect (within 10–15 min) can be achieved with sublingual administration if the capsule is punctured and the gelatinous contents are allowed to escape. The usual oral dosage is 10 to 20 mg 3 times daily.

Nitroglycerin and its analogs (administered orally, sublingually, topically, or intravenously) are venodilators at low dosages but have arteriolar dilating properties at higher dosages. The acute administration of intravenous nitroglycerin may reduce blood pressure and increase cardiac output; however, with chronic usage, the nitrates are mainly venodilators that can be used alone or in combination with arteriolar dilators. Headache is the major adverse effect associated with nitrates. Some patients cannot tolerate sublingual nitroglycerin or isosorbide dinitrate but may be more tolerant of topical nitrate preparations, since the latter have a more sustained action. Nitrates are particularly useful in patients with congestive heart failure and ischemic heart disease and may reduce the need for concomitant diuretic therapy.

Sodium nitroprusside is a powerful intravenous agent that has a balanced effect on the arterial and venous vascular beds. It is widely used, alone or in conjunction with positive inotropic agents, in patients with severe congestive heart failure or a low output state in an intensive care unit setting. It acts rapidly, has a short half-life, causes minimal change in heart rate, and can be readily titrated to obtain the desired hemodynamic effect. Although intravenous therapy may be continued for several days with nitroprusside, thiocyanate toxicity may occur after 4 to 5 days of therapy. The usual intravenous dosage ranges from 0.25 to 4.0 μg/kg/min. An oral preparation is not available. *Phentolamine* is a nonselective alpha-adrenergic receptor antagonist, available both as an intravenous and an oral preparation. It produces a balanced effect on the arterial and venous systems. It is not used widely because it is expensive, intravenous dosage titration is difficult, and it produces a brisk tachycardia. *Prazosin hydrochloride* is a selective, postsynaptic (α_2) alpha-adrenergic receptor antagonist that produces balanced effects on preload and afterload. Because of its selective effects on postsynaptic alpha-adrenergic receptors, tachycardia is less of a problem than with phentolamine. The usual oral dosage is 2 to 7 mg 4 times daily. Prazosin's major adverse effect is marked postural hypotension. Its chronic efficacy in patients with congestive heart failure is uncertain, since tolerance to its effects are common and may occur as early as the fifth dose. Fluid retention is seldom a substantial problem.

Captopril is a balanced arteriolar and venous dilator that acts by blocking the conversion of angiotensin I to angiotensin II. The usual oral dosage is 25 to 100 mg 3 times daily. It is an effective unloading agent and has well-documented, beneficial long-term effects. It offers the distinct advantage of allowing the dosage of concomitantly administered diuretics to be reduced. However, when administered acutely, captopril may cause marked hypotension and even acute renal failure. Therefore, it should be used with great caution and under carefully controlled conditions in patients who are marginally hypotensive before the commencement of therapy. Its other adverse effects include proteinuria (due to a glomerulonephritis), fever, skin rash, and taste alterations. Despite these, it appears to be the most consistently effective unloading agent for the chronic management of congestive heart failure; it has been shown to cause hemodynamic as well as objective and subjective clinical improvement in patients with chronic congestive failure.

The efficacy of a particular unloading agent can be assessed by determining its acute or chronic effects on invasively determined hemodynamic variables or by assessing its effects on objectively determined measurements of exercise capacity. Noninvasive techniques, including echocardiography and radionuclide ventriculography, are frequently not sufficiently sensitive to assess changes produced by these agents, and purely subjective clinical assessments may be misleading. Finally, the injudicious use of these agents may cause an excessive reduction in preload (with a resultant decrease in cardiac output), an excessive reduction in afterload (with resultant postural hypotension, reflex tachycardia, and diminished perfusion of the coronary, renal, and other essential circulations), or both. Thus, although it is not imperative to assess the efficacy of a particular agent using invasive techniques in every patient, such invasive monitoring is essential in the patient with a tenuous hemodynamic state.

General

1. Chatterjee K, Parmley WW. The role of vasodilator therapy in heart failure. Prog Cardiovasc Dis 1977; 19:301–25.
   A thorough review of the pathophysiology of heart failure and the mechanisms by which vasodilator therapy is effective. Includes 133 references.
2. Cohn JN. Vasodilator therapy for heart failure: the influence of impedance on left ventricular performance. Circulation 1973; 48:5–8.
   A review of the role of vasodilator therapy in the treatment of congestive heart failure.
3. Firth BG, Dehmer GJ, Markham RV Jr, Willerson JT, Hillis LD. Assessment of vasodilator therapy in patients with severe congestive heart failure: limitations of measurements of left ventricular ejection fraction and volumes. Am J Cardiol 1982; 50:954–9.
   Vasodilator therapy may produce a marked change in cardiac output and pulmonary capillary wedge pressure without detectable changes in radionuclide-determined left ventricular ejection fraction or volumes.
4. Haq A, Rakowski H, Baigrie R, McLaughlin P, Burns R, Tihal H, Hilton D, Feiglin D. Vasodilator therapy in refractory congestive heart failure: a comparative analysis of hemodynamic and non-invasive studies. Am J Cardiol 1982; 49:439–44.
   The changes produced by vasodilators may be detectable by invasive techniques but not by noninvasive techniques, such as echocardiography and radionuclide ventriculography.
5. Miller RR, Vismara LA, Williams DO, Amsterdam EA, Mason DT. Pharmacological mechanisms for left ventricular unloading in clinical congestive heart failure:

differential effects of nitroprusside, phentolamine, and nitroglycerin on cardiac function and peripheral circulation. Circ Res 1976; 39:127–33.
The hemodynamic effects of each of these agents in the treatment of congestive heart failure are characterized.

6. Shah PK. Ventricular unloading in the management of heart disease: role of vasodilators (parts I and II). Am Heart J 1977; 93:256–60, 403–6.
A thorough review of the indications for unloading therapy in the management of various types of heart disease.

7. Sonnenblick EH, Downing SE. Afterload as a primary determinant of ventricular performance. Am J Physiol 1963; 204:604–10.
A careful experimental analysis of the importance of afterload as a determinant of cardiac performance.

8. Cohn JN. Physiologic basis of vasodilator therapy for heart failure. Am J Med 1981; 71:135–9.
A succinct discussion of the principles of vasodilator therapy.

Hydralazine

9. Franciosa JA, Weber KT, Levine TB, Kinasewitz GT, Janicki JS, West J, Henis MMJ, Cohn JN. Hydralazine in the long-term treatment of chronic heart failure: lack of difference from placebo. Am Heart J 1982; 104:587–94.
Therapy with hydralazine for 6 months was not superior to placebo.

10. Leier CV, Magorien RD, Desch CE, Thompson MJ, Unverferth DV. Hydralazine and isosorbide dinitrate: comparative central and regional hemodynamic effects when administered alone or in combination. Circulation 1981; 63:102–9.
A detailed account of the effects of these two agents, alone and in combination. Hydralazine, alone or in combination with isosorbide, increases renal and limb blood flow in congestive heart failure in proportion to the augmentation of cardiac output. In contrast, isosorbide dinitrate alone does not alter blood flow to these regions.

11. Packer M, Meller J, Medina N, Gorlin R, Herman MV. Importance of left ventricular chamber size in determining the response to hydralazine in severe chronic heart failure. N Engl J Med 1980; 303:250–5.
Patients with moderate or severe cardiomegaly had a good response to long-term hydralazine therapy; those without cardiomegaly did not respond well to this agent.

12. Packer M, Meller J, Medina N, Yushak M, Gorlin R. Provocation of myocardial ischemic events during initiation of vasodilator therapy for severe chronic heart failure: clinical and hemodynamic evaluation of 52 consecutive patients with ischemic cardiomyopathy. Am J Cardiol 1981; 48:939–46.
Of these 52 individuals given hydralazine, 12 (23%) had ischemic events.

Minoxidil

13. McKay CR, Chatterjee K, Ports TA, Holly AN, Parmley WW. Minoxidil therapy in chronic congestive heart failure: acute plus long-term hemodynamic and clinical study. Am Heart J 1982; 104:575–80.
Minoxidil is effective in the chronic management of congestive heart failure, but fluid retention is a major problem.

14. Packer M, Meller J, Medina N, Yushak M. Sustained effectiveness of minoxidil in heart failure after development of tolerance to other vasodilator drugs. Am J Cardiol 1981; 48:375–9.
In a 78-year-old man who developed tolerance to hydralazine and captopril, minoxidil exerted a sustained beneficial effect.

Nifedipine

15. Matsumoto S, Ito T, Sada T, Takahashi M, Su KM, Ueda A, Okabe F, Sato M, Sekine I, Ito Y. Hemodynamic effects of nifedipine in congestive heart failure. Am J Cardiol 1980; 46:476–80.
In 8 patients with congestive failure, nifedipine increased cardiac index and reduced systemic arterial pressure.

16. Polese A, Fiorentini C, Olivari MT, Guazzi MD. Clinical use of a calcium antago-

nistic agent (nifedipine) in acute pulmonary edema. Am J Med 1979; 66:825–30.
In patients with acute pulmonary edema of various etiologies, nifedipine reduced systemic pressure and increased cardiac output.

Nitroglycerin
17. Chiariello M, Gold HK, Leinbach RC, Davis MA, Maroko PR. Comparison between the effects of nitroprusside and nitroglycerin on ischemic injury during acute myocardial infarction. Circulation 1976; 54:766–73.
Nitroglycerin may be preferable to nitroprusside for reducing preload and afterload in patients with acute myocardial infarction.
18. Leier CV, Huss P, Magorien RD, Unverferth DV. Improved exercise capacity and differing arterial and venous tolerance during chronic isosorbide dinitrate therapy for congestive heart failure. Circulation 1983; 67:817–22.
In patients with congestive heart failure, 12 weeks of oral isosorbide dinitrate therapy improved resting and exercise hemodynamics, exercise capacity, and clinical status.
19. Mantle JA, Russell RO Jr, Moraski RE, Rackley CE. Isosorbide dinitrate for the relief of severe heart failure after myocardial infarction. Am J Cardiol 1976; 37:263–8.
Seven patients with anterior infarction and severe heart failure were given isosorbide dinitrate; symptomatic pulmonary venous hypertension was effectively relieved without compromising left ventricular function.
20. Williams DO, Bommer WJ, Miller RR, Amsterdam EA, Mason DT. Hemodynamic assessment of oral peripheral vasodilator therapy in chronic congestive heart failure: prolonged effectiveness of isosorbide dinitrate. Am J Cardiol 1977; 39:84–90.
Isosorbide dinitrate may produce a sustained reduction in left ventricular filling pressure without a pronounced effect on cardiac output.

Sodium Nitroprusside
21. Chatterjee K, Swan HJC, Kaushik VS, Jobin G, Magnusson P, Forrester JS. Effects of vasodilator therapy for severe pump failure in acute myocardial infarction on short-term and late prognosis. Circulation 1976; 53:797–802.
In 43 patients with severe pump failure complicating myocardial infarction, nitroprusside improved short-term prognosis but did not affect long-term survival.
22. Guiha NH, Cohn JN, Mikulic E, Franciosa JA, Limas CJ. Treatment of refractory heart failure with infusion of nitroprusside. N Engl J Med 1974; 291:587–92.
Sodium nitroprusside was given to 18 patients with intractable heart failure and produced a prompt reduction of left ventricular filling pressure and a rise in cardiac output.
23. Harshaw CW, Grossman W, Munro AB, McLaurin LP. Reduced systemic vascular resistance as therapy for severe mitral regurgitation of valvular origin. Ann Intern Med 1975; 83:312–6.
Seven patients who had severe mitral regurgitation were given nitroprusside with substantial improvement in hemodynamics.
24. Miller RR, Vismara LA, DeMaria AN, Saler AF, Mason DT. Afterload reduction therapy with nitroprusside in severe aortic regurgitation: improved cardiac performance and reduced regurgitant volume. Am J Cardiol 1976; 38:564–7.
Twelve patients with aortic regurgitation were studied before and after nitroprusside. Afterload reduction in patients with aortic regurgitation may improve cardiac performance, decrease left ventricular preload, and reduce aortic regurgitant volume.
25. Hockings BEF, Cope GD, Clarke GM, Taylor RR. Randomized controlled trial of vasodilator therapy after myocardial infarction. Am J Cardiol 1981; 48:345–52.
Fifty patients with infarction and a pulmonary capillary wedge pressure > 20 mmHg were given nitroprusside or furosemide. There was no difference in morbidity or mortality.

Prazosin Hydrochloride
26. Colucci WS, Wynne J, Holman BL, Braunwald E. Long-term therapy of heart failure with prazosin: a randomized double-blind trial. Am J Cardiol 1980; 45:337–44.

Prazosin produced a subjective and objective improvement in 22 patients with congestive heart failure.

27. Harper RW, Claxton H, Middlebrook K, Anderson S, Pitt A. The acute and chronic hemodynamic effects of prazosin in severe congestive cardiac failure. Med J Aust 1980; 2(Suppl):36–8.
    In 16 patients with severe heart failure, the acute beneficial effects of prazosin were markedly attenuated with chronic usage.
28. Markham RV Jr, Corbett JR, Gilmore A, Pettinger WA, Firth BG. Efficacy of prazosin in the management of chronic congestive heart failure: a 6-month, randomized, double-blind, placebo-controlled study. Am J Cardiol 1983; 51:1346–52.
    Long-term prazosin therapy produced no demonstrable subjective or objective improvement when compared to placebo in this group of patients on stable digitalis and diuretic therapy.
29. Packer M, Meller J, Gorlin R, Herman MV. Hemodynamic and clinical tachyphylaxis to prazosin-mediated afterload reduction in severe chronic congestive heart failure. Circulation 1979; 59:531–9.
    The first of several reports to document the development of tolerance to prazosin in congestive heart failure.

Captopril
30. Kramer BL, Massie BM, Topic N. Controlled trial of captopril in chronic heart failure: a rest and exercise hemodynamic study. Circulation 1983; 67:807–16.
    Captopril produced a sustained improvement in hemodynamics and exercise capacity during 3 months of therapy.
31. Massie B, Kramer BL, Topic N, Henderson SG. Hemodynamic and radionuclide effects of acute captopril therapy for heart failure: changes in left and right ventricular volumes and function at rest and during exercise. Circulation 1982; 65:1374–81.
    A detailed account of the acute hemodynamic effects of captopril in 14 patients with congestive heart failure.

ANTIHYPERTENSIVE AGENTS

Numerous pharmacologic agents are available for the long-term therapy of patients with essential hypertension. In addition to them, the patient with this disorder should be encouraged (1) to restrict salt intake, (2) to restrict caloric intake (if the patient is obese), and (3) to participate in some form of regular exercise, as permitted by the individual's cardiovascular status. In most individuals with essential hypertension, a *diuretic* is the cornerstone of long-term medical therapy. These agents reduce systemic arterial pressure primarily by causing a sodium diuresis, with resultant intravascular volume depletion. The thiazide diuretics inhibit the reabsorption of sodium chloride in the cortical thick ascending limb of Henle. As a result, an increased amount of sodium is delivered to the distal nephron, where sodium-potassium exchange occurs, leading to kaliuresis. The thiazide diuretics are usually administered once or twice daily. Following their oral administration, they exert a steady and sustained diuresis, lasting 8 to 15 hours. They are associated with several potential adverse effects, most frequently hypokalemia, hyperuricemia, hyperglycemia, hypercalcemia, skin rash, thrombocytopenia, and granulocytopenia. Many patients to whom the thiazides are administered require potassium supplementation to prevent hypokalemia.

Furosemide and ethacrynic acid are extremely potent but relatively short-acting diuretics. They act by inhibiting the reabsorption of sodium chloride in the medullary and cortical thick ascending limb of Henle. They are highly effective regardless of the patient's underlying fluid-electrolyte or acid-base balance. Similar to the thiazide diuretics, these agents may cause hypokalemia, so that some patients receiving them may require potassium supplementation. They are occasionally associated with transient hearing loss when they are given in very high doses. Although furosemide and ethacrynic acid are more powerful diuretics than the thiazides, their brief duration of action (5–6 hr) makes their long-term outpatient administration difficult. Therefore, for the patient with essential hypertension for whom a diuretic is indicated, a thiazide is preferable to these more potent agents.

Two *sympatholytic agents,* methyldopa and clonidine, are available for the treatment of essential hypertension. These agents act on the sympathetic nervous system centers in the brain to reduce vasomotor tone, thus causing peripheral vasodilatation. Methyldopa is administered in a total daily dose of 500 to 3000 mg, given in 2 to 4 equal doses. Its most common adverse effects include fatigue, lethargy (especially at doses above 2000 mg daily), and impotence; less frequently, it may be associated with bradycardia, psychological depression, hepatitis, leukopenia, thrombocytopenia, and a Coombs-positive hemolytic anemia. Clonidine is administered in a total daily dose of 0.2 to 2.4 mg, usually in 2 equal doses, although in an occasional patient a single dose at bedtime is sufficient to achieve adequate blood pressure control. It exerts no effect on glucose homeostasis and, therefore, can be administered safely to individuals with diabetes mellitus. Its most frequent adverse effects are lethargy and drowsiness, dry mouth, constipation, and impotence. It should not be administered in combination with methyldopa, beta-adrenergic blockers, sedatives, or tricyclic antidepressants. If clonidine withdrawal is desired, it should be done slowly, since an occasional patient develops severe hypertension following abrupt clonidine discontinuation.

The *beta-adrenergic blocking agents* are used widely in patients with essential hypertension, yet even today their precise mechanism of action is not understood completely. Although these agents exert a negative inotropic and chronotropic influence on the heart, the blood pressure control that is achieved with their chronic administration does not result from these effects. Similarly, although the beta-adrenergic blockers inhibit the secretion of renin by the juxtaglomerular apparatus of the kidney, their antihypertensive effect is not dependent on enhanced renin activity. Finally, some of the beta-adrenergic blockers cross the blood-brain barrier and may, therefore, exert their effect by a central nervous system mechanism. However, other beta blockers that do not penetrate the central nervous system nevertheless are effective antihypertensive agents. In short, the manner in which the beta-adrenergic blocking agents exert their effect on systemic arterial pressure is not understood.

The beta-adrenergic blocker propranolol has been used extensively in patients with essential hypertension. It is given in a total daily dose of 80 to 480 mg, usually in 2 or 3 equal doses. Its most frequent adverse effects are psychological depression, fatigue, and impotence. The beta-adrenergic blockers should not be administered to the patient with congestive heart failure, diabetes mellitus, bronchospastic pulmonary disease, or severe peripheral vascular disease with resultant claudication. They may be administered concomitantly with diuretics and vasodilators.

The *alpha-adrenergic blocking agent* prazosin induces a fall in systemic arterial pressure without a concomitant increase in heart rate. It is administered in a total daily dose of 6 to 20 mg, given 3 times daily. It can be added to any antihypertensive regimen if further blood pressure reduction is desired. Its most frequent adverse effects include drowsiness, weakness, postural dizziness, palpitations, and depression. Therapy with this agent must be initiated with care, since a small percentage of patients develop weakness, lassitude, and transient faintness when they are first given it, even in doses as small as 1 mg. The alpha blocking agents phentolamine and phenoxybenzamine are not used for the chronic therapy of patients with essential hypertension, since their administration is frequently accompanied by severe postural hypotension, impotence, and nasal stuffiness.

The *postganglionic blocking agents* reserpine and guanethidine are used less extensively now than they were 10 to 20 years ago. Reserpine prevents the binding of norepinephrine in the granular pool, which leads to cytoplasmic degradation of the neurotransmitter by mitochondrial monoamine oxidase. It is administered as a single daily dose of 0.1 to 0.25 mg. Its most frequent adverse effects are lassitude, lethargy, dry mouth, and impotence. In an occasional patient, it may cause bradycardia. Guanethidine exerts its antihypertensive action by interfering with neurotransmitters at the adrenergic postganglionic nerve terminals, thus diminishing arteriolar vasoconstriction. It is administered in a single daily dose of 10 to 150 mg. Its use is frequently associated with weakness, impotence, and postural dizziness, and for these reasons, it is not frequently prescribed today.

The *direct vasodilators* hydralazine and minoxidil have been used extensively in patients with essential hypertension, especially those with severely elevated arterial pressure. They are most effective when given concomitantly with a beta-adrenergic blocker, since the latter prevents the reflex tachycardia induced by peripheral vasodilatation. Hydralazine is given in a total daily dose of 50 to 400 mg; it is usually administered 3 or 4 times daily. Its most frequent adverse effects are headache, palpitations, postural hypotension, and dizziness. An occasional patient who is receiving large doses of hydralazine develops a lupus-like syndrome. Minoxidil is given in a total daily dose of 10 to 40 mg, usually in 4 equal doses. It is especially efficacious for patients with severe hypertension that is unresponsive to other medications. Its most troublesome adverse effects are headache, hypertrichosis, peripheral edema, and reflex tachycardia, which may induce angina in the patient with severe coronary artery disease.

Finally, the *calcium antagonists* verapamil, nifedipine, and diltiazem appear to exert an effective antihypertensive effect in patients with mild or moderate essential hypertension, administered either alone or in combination with a beta-adrenergic blocker or methyldopa. Of these agents, nifedipine appears to be the best antihypertensive, since it is the most powerful systemic arterial dilator. (See the Calcium Antagonists, p. 288, for the details concerning their use.)

Diuretics

1. Conway J, Lauwers P. Hemodynamic and hypotensive effects of long-term therapy with chlorothiazide. Circulation 1960; 21:21–7.
   In 83 unselected ambulatory patients with hypertension, chlorothiazide was effective in 55 (66%).

2. Leth A. Changes in plasma and extracellular fluid volumes in patients with essential hypertension during long-term treatment with hydrochlorothiazide. Circulation 1970; 42:479–85.
   Thiazides have a volume-depleting effect that is maintained during long-term treatment of patients with essential hypertension.

3. Anderson J, Godfrey BE, Hill DM, Munro-Faure AD, Sheldon J. A comparison of the effects of hydrochlorothiazide and of furosemide in the treatment of hypertensive patients. Q J Med 1971; 40:541–60.
   In comparison to 40 mg twice daily of furosemide, hydrochlorothiazide (50 mg twice daily) produced a more salutary effect on blood pressure.

Sympatholytic Drugs

4. Gillespie L Jr, Oates JA, Crout JR, Sjoerdsma A. Clinical and chemical studies with alpha-methyldopa in patients with hypertension. Circulation 1962; 25:281–91.

   An early study in 52 patients with essential hypertension, showing that methyldopa is an effective antihypertensive agent.

5. Leonard JW, Gifford RW Jr, Humphrey DC. Treatment of hypertension with methyldopa alone or combined with diuretics and/or guanethidine. Am Heart J 1965; 69:610–8.

   In 63 patients treated for up to 2 years, methyldopa was safe and effective, especially when combined with a diuretic and/or guanethidine.

6. Mroczek WJ, Leibel BA, Finnerty FA Jr. Comparison of clonidine and methyldopa in hypertensive patients receiving a diuretic: a double-blind crossover study. Am J Cardiol 1972; 29:712–7.

   In 41 outpatients, clonidine and methyldopa were similarly effective in the control of blood pressure.

7. Hoobler SW, Kashima T. Central nervous system actions of clonidine in hypertension. Mayo Clin Proc 1977; 52:395–8.

   The patient who is taking more than 1.2 mg daily of clonidine is especially likely to have rebound hypertension if the drug is withdrawn abruptly.

8. Horwitz D, Pettinger WA, Orvis H, Thomas RE, Sjoerdsma A. Effects of methyldopa in fifty hypertensive patients. Clin Pharmacol Ther 1967; 8:224–34.

   Methyldopa was highly effective in two-thirds of these patients.

9. Whitsett TL, Chrysant SG, Dillard BL, Anton AH. Abrupt cessation of clonidine administration: a prospective study. Am J Cardiol 1978; 41:1285–90.

   In 20 patients, clonidine was abruptly discontinued without rebound hypertension.

10. Rodman JS, Deutsch DJ, Gutman SI. Methyldopa hepatitis: a report of six cases and review of the literature. Am J Med 1976; 60:941–8.

    This article describes 6 cases of methyldopa-induced hepatitis, 2 of which resulted in death.

11. Pettinger WA. Clonidine, a new antihypertensive drug. N Engl J Med 1975; 293:1179–80.

    A brief review of the pharmacology and toxicity of clonidine, as well as a discussion of its interactions with other drugs.

12. Hoobler SW, Sagastume E. Clonidine hydrochloride in the treatment of hypertension. Am J Cardiol 1971; 28:67–73.

    Over a treatment period of 6 months to 2 years, clonidine (combined with a diuretic) was an effective antihypertensive agent in 57 patients.

Beta-Adrenergic Blockers

13. Zacharias FJ, Cowen KJ, Presst J, Vickers J, Wall BG. Propranolol in hypertension: a study of long-term therapy, 1964–70. Am Heart J 1972; 83:755–61.

    Propranolol was an effective and well-tolerated antihypertensive agent in 311 patients.

14. Bravo EL, Tarazi RC, Dustan HP. β-adrenergic blockade in diuretic-treated patients with essential hypertension. N Engl J Med 1975; 292:66–70.

    In 17 of 20 patients with essential hypertension already on diuretic therapy, propranolol (160 mg per day) lowered mean arterial pressure by more than 10 mmHg.

15. Brogden RN, Heel RC, Speight TM, Avery GS. Metoprolol: a review of its pharmacological properties and therapeutic efficacy in hypertension and angina pectoris. Drugs 1977; 14:321–48.

    An elegant review of the use of this beta-blocker in patients with hypertension and angina.

16. Hansson BG, Dymling JF, Hedeland H, Hulthen UL. Long-term treatment of moderate hypertension with the beta$_1$-receptor blocking agent, metoprolol. I. Effect on maximal working capacity, plasma catecholamines and renin, urinary aldosterone, blood pressure, and pulse rate under basal conditions. Eur J Clin Pharmacol 1977; 11:239–45.

In 9 men with moderate hypertension, metoprolol reduced blood pressure in the supine and upright positions.

17. Holland OB, Kaplan NM. Propranolol in the treatment of hypertension. N Engl J Med 1976; 294:930–6.
   A thorough review of propranolol's uses and side effects in patients with hypertension. Includes 89 references.

Alpha-Adrenergic Blockers

18. Brogden RN, Heel RC, Speight TM, Avery GS. Prazosin: a review of its pharmacological properties and therapeutic efficacy in hypertension. Drugs 1977; 14:163–97.
   A very thorough review of this agent's pharmacology and therapeutic uses.

19. Graham RM, Pettinger WA. Prazosin. N Engl J Med 1979; 300:232–6.
   A succinct review of this agent and its clinical uses.

Postganglionic Blocking Agents

20. Dollery CT, Emslie-Smith D, Milne MD. Clinical and pharmacological studies with guanethidine in the treatment of hypertension. Lancet 1960; 2:381–7.
   Of 80 patients treated with guanethidine over a period of 9 months, good or fair control of blood pressure was attained in 68 (85%).

21. Woosley RL, Nies AS. Guanethidine. N Engl J Med 1976; 295:1053–7.
   A good review of this drug's uses and adverse effects.

Direct Vasodilators

22. Chidsey CA III, Gottlieb TB. The pharmacologic basis of antihypertensive therapy: the role of vasodilator drugs. Prog Cardiovasc Dis 1974; 17:99–113.
   A good review of the pharmacokinetics, metabolism, and clinical utility of hydralazine and the other vasodilators.

23. Koch-Weser J. Hydralazine. N Engl J Med 1976; 295:320–3.
   A succinct review of this drug's uses, metabolism, and adverse effects.

24. Pettinger WA, Mitchell HC. Minoxidil—an alternative to nephrectomy for refractory hypertension. N Engl J Med 1973; 289:167–71.
   In 11 patients with malignant or accelerated hypertension, minoxidil reduced blood pressure dramatically.

25. Koch-Weser J. Diazoxide. N Engl J Med 1976; 294:1271–4.
   Diazoxide is a highly useful drug for the emergency treatment of elevated arterial pressure, as in patients with hypertensive encephalopathy.

26. Zacest R, Gilmore E, Koch-Weser J. Treatment of essential hypertension with combined vasodilation and beta-adrenergic blockade. N Engl J Med 1972; 286:617–22.
   A hydralazine-propranolol-diuretic combination was shown to be very effective in 21 of 23 patients with moderate or severe essential hypertension.

Calcium Antagonists

27. Gould BA, Mann S, Kieso H, Subramanian VB, Raftery EB. The 24-hour ambulatory blood pressure profile with verapamil. Circulation 1982; 65:22–7.
   Verapamil exerted a substantial and consistent antihypertensive effect in 16 patients with mild or moderate hypertension.

28. Olivari MT, Bartorelli C, Polese A, Fiorentini C, Moruzzi P, Guazzi MD. Treatment of hypertension with nifedipine, a calcium antagonistic agent. Circulation 1979; 59:1056–62.
   Nifedipine was an effective antihypertensive agent in 27 patients with essential hypertension.

INTRA-AORTIC BALLOON COUNTERPULSATION

Over the past 15 years, intra-aortic balloon counterpulsation has been used extensively in the treatment of several cardiac abnormalities. In the *medical* setting, it has been employed in some centers for the treatment of patients with cardiogenic shock due to acute myocardial infarction. It is believed to be somewhat beneficial in reducing mortality in these individuals. Counterpulsation has been used to stabilize the patient with a ventricular septal defect or severe mitral regurgitation in the setting of acute infarction. In patients with continuing chest pain at rest, it has been utilized to alleviate symptoms and electrocardiographic evidence of ongoing ischemia. In an occasional individual, counterpulsation has been employed to control malignant ventricular ectopy due to recurrent ischemia. In the experimental animal, it has been shown to exert a salutary effect on the extent of myocardial ischemic injury, and its beneficial effect in this setting is especially marked when it is initiated in combination with other beneficial agents.

In the *surgical* setting, intra-aortic balloon counterpulsation has enjoyed even wider application. In patients with severe coronary artery disease in whom transient episodes of systemic arterial hypotension may be particularly deleterious, balloon counterpulsation is often instituted preoperatively to insure that the induction of anesthesia is accomplished without a profound decline in blood pressure. In the immediate postoperative period, it is often helpful in the patient with transient left ventricular dysfunction of any cause.

The intra-aortic balloon can be inserted by direct vision (i.e., by femoral arterial cutdown) or by the percutaneous technique. From the femoral artery, it is passed retrograde to the descending thoracic aorta (just distal to the left subclavian artery). It usually measures 4 to 5 inches in length and has a capacity of 30 to 40 cc. A large polyethylene catheter connects the balloon to a mechanical apparatus that remains at the patient's bedside. During each cardiac cycle, the balloon is inflated during left ventricular diastole (immediately after the T wave) and deflated just before systole (at the beginning of the QRS complex). Properly timed intra-aortic balloon counterpulsation augments aortic diastolic pressure and reduces the impedance to left ventricular systolic emptying. As a result, several hemodynamic alterations occur during counterpulsation: (1) left ventricular and systolic aortic pressures fall modestly; (2) left ventricular end-diastolic pressure falls slightly in the absence of severe hypotension and precipitously in the setting of severe hypotension; (3) left ventricular stroke work diminishes, since left ventricular systolic and end-diastolic pressures are reduced; and (4) aortic diastolic pressure increases. In the normotensive individual, balloon counterpulsation transiently augments coronary blood flow, but coronary autoregulation quickly causes such blood flow to return to baseline levels. However, in the patient with severe hypotension, intra-aortic balloon counterpulsation causes a sustained increase in coronary blood flow, since it reduces left ventricular afterload and augments coronary arterial perfusion pressure.

The initiation and maintenance of intra-aortic balloon counterpulsation may be associated with certain complications. In almost all patients in whom the balloon is used, moderate thrombocytopenia occurs, due to the mechanical destruction of platelets by the balloon. Red blood cell destruction may also occur, but a substantial fall in hemoglobin and hematocrit is unusual. Insertion of the balloon may be accompanied by aortic dissection or perforation. Finally, the device may cause arterial embolization or insufficiency of the bowel or leg.

The use of intra-aortic balloon counterpulsation is contraindicated in the patient with severe peripheral vascular disease, since its initiation is difficult and its maintenance often accompanied by peripheral arterial insufficiency. It is contraindicated in the patient with aortic regurgitation, since diastolic augmentation of aortic pressure in such a patient may cause more severe regurgitation. Once the balloon is inserted, a heparin infusion is generally used to prevent arterial thrombosis. In the patient in whom such anticoagulation is contraindicated, balloon counterpulsation is associated with an increased risk and, therefore, is inadvisable.

Clinical Uses

1. Braunwald E, Maroko PR. Intraaortic balloon counterpulsation: an assessment. Ann Intern Med 1972; 76:659–61.
   A brief review of the various uses of balloon counterpulsation.
2. Dunkman WB, Leinbach RC, Buckley MJ, Mundth ED, Kantrowitz AR, Austen WG, Sanders CA. Clinical and hemodynamic results of intraaortic balloon pumping and surgery for cardiogenic shock. Circulation 1972; 46:465–77.
   In patients with cardiogenic shock as a result of myocardial infarction, balloon counterpulsation is an effective means of supporting the circulation during angiography and surgery.
3. Gold HK, Leinbach RC, Sanders CA, Buckley MJ, Mundth ED, Austen WG. Intraaortic balloon pumping for ventricular septal defect or mitral regurgitation complicating acute myocardial infarction. Circulation 1973; 47:1191–6.
   Balloon counterpulsation reduces the amount of mitral regurgitation and diminishes the left-to-right shunt in patients with acute VSD.
4. Gold HK, Leinbach RC, Sanders CA, Buckley MJ, Mundth ED, Austen WG. Intraaortic balloon pumping for control of recurrent myocardial ischemia. Circulation 1973; 47:1197–1203.
   Balloon counterpulsation is often effective in controlling ischemic pain that is resistant to maximal medical therapy.
5. Leinbach RC, Gold HK, Harper RW, Buckley MJ, Austen WG. Early intraaortic balloon pumping for anterior myocardial infarction without shock. Circulation 1978; 58:204–10.
   In patients with recent anterior infarction, balloon counterpulsation was successful in diminishing the extent of ischemic injury only in patients who had residual patency of the involved left anterior descending coronary artery.
6. Levine FH, Gold HK, Leinbach RC, Daggett WM, Austen WG, Buckley MJ. Management of acute myocardial ischemia with intraaortic balloon pumping and coronary bypass surgery. Circulation 1978; 58(Suppl I):69–72.
   When balloon counterpulsation is used to control recurrent ischemia, patients with refractory angina can be safely revascularized and have a favorable long-term prognosis.
7. McEnany MT, Kay HR, Buckley MJ, Daggett WM, Erdmann AJ, Mundth ED, Rao RS, deToeuf J, Austen WG. Clinical experience with intraaortic balloon pump support in 728 patients. Circulation 1978; 58(Suppl I):124–32.
   Earlier and more liberal use of balloon counterpulsation has led to increased survival in a large number of patients with various complications of acute myocardial ischemia.
8. Scheidt S, Wilner G, Mueller H, Summers D, Lesch M, Wolff G, Krakauer J, Rubenfire M, Fleming P, Noon G, Oldham N, Killip T, Kantrowitz A. Intraaortic balloon counterpulsation in cardiogenic shock: report of a cooperative clinical trial. N Engl J Med 1973; 288:979–84.
   Of 87 patients with cardiogenic shock treated with balloon support, 35 survived, 15 of whom left the hospital.
9. Sturm JT, McGee MG, Fuhrman TM, Davis GL, Turner SA, Edelman SK, Norman JC. Treatment of postoperative low output syndrome with intraaortic balloon pumping: experience with 419 patients. Am J Cardiol 1980; 45:1033–6.
   Of 419 patients with low output postoperatively treated with balloon support, 226

(54%) were successfully weaned from pumping support, and 188 (45%) were subsequently discharged from the hospital.

10. Bregman D, Nichols AB, Weiss MB, Powers ER, Martin EC, Casarella WJ. Percutaneous intraaortic balloon insertion. Am J Cardiol 1980; 46:261–4.
    Percutaneous balloon insertion permits the rapid institution of circulatory support and broadens the applications of balloon pumping.

11. Vignola PA, Swaye PS, Gosselin AJ. Guidelines for effective and safe percutaneous intraaortic balloon pump insertion and removal. Am J Cardiol 1981; 48:660–4.
    This article emphasizes that meticulous attention to percutaneous insertion and removal technique and adequate anticoagulation must be employed to assure effective and safe balloon pumping.

12. DeWood MA, Notske RN, Hensley GR, Shields JP, O'Grady WP, Spores J, Goldman M, Ganji JH. Intraaortic balloon counterpulsation with and without reperfusion for myocardial infarction shock. Circulation 1980; 61:1105–12.
    When performed early after infarction, counterpulsation and surgical reperfusion are beneficial. When initiated late after infarction (i.e., more than 18 hours after the onset of symptoms), counterpulsation alone is most efficacious.

13. Scanlon PJ, O'Connell J, Johnson SA, Moran JM, Gunnar R, Pifarre R. Balloon counterpulsation following surgery for ischemic heart disease. Circulation 1976; 54(Suppl III):90–3.
    Of 40 patients placed on balloon support postoperatively, 28 were successfully weaned from such support, and 22 of these were discharged from the hospital.

14. Willerson JT, Curry GC, Watson JT, Leshin SJ, Ecker RR, Mullins CB, Platt MR, Sugg ML. Intraaortic balloon counterpulsation in patients in cardiogenic shock, medically refractory left ventricular failure, and/or recurrent ventricular tachycardia. Am J Med 1975; 58:183–91.
    Most patients who require balloon support have such extensive disease that they cannot be weaned from the balloon and cannot tolerate corrective surgery.

15. Williams DO, Korr KS, Gewirtz H, Most AS. The effect of intraaortic balloon counterpulsation on regional myocardial blood flow and oxygen consumption in the presence of coronary artery stenosis in patients with unstable angina. Circulation 1982; 66:593–7.
    Reduction of myocardial oxygen consumption is the most likely mechanism by which counterpulsation relieves ischemia in patients with unstable angina.

Problems and Complications

16. Alpert J, Bhaktan EK, Gielchinsky I, Gilbert L, Brener BJ, Brief DK, Parsonnet V. Vascular complications of intraaortic balloon pumping. Arch Surg 1976; 111:1190–5.
    Of 79 patients undergoing balloon counterpulsation, 36 lived long enough to have the balloon removed. Of these, 13 (36%) had vascular complications.

17. Pace PD, Tilney NL, Lesch M, Couch NP. Peripheral arterial complications of intraaortic balloon counterpulsation. Surgery 1977; 82:685–8.
    Of 104 patients in whom the intra-aortic balloon was inserted, 64 complications occurred in 32 patients (31%). Of these, 21 patients (20%) sustained one or more life-threatening or limb-threatening complications.

18. Isner JM, Cohen SR, Virmani R, Lawrinson W, Roberts WC. Complications of the intraaortic balloon counterpulsation device: clinical and morphologic observations in 45 necropsy patients. Am J Cardiol 1980; 45:260–8.
    Of 45 patients who died after insertion of the intra-aortic balloon, 16 (36%) had one or more complications, including aortic dissection (9), arterial perforation (3), arterial thrombosis (3), arterial emboli (3), limb ischemia (1), and local infection (1).

MISCELLANEOUS CONDITIONS AND ISSUES

Idiopathic or primary pulmonary hypertension is a disease entity character-ized by an abnormally elevated pulmonary arterial pressure and resistance. Its etiology is unknown. On pathologic examination, the pulmonary arterioles demonstrate intimal and medial thickening, necrotizing arteritic changes, and—if the disease is far advanced—so-called plexiform lesions (dilated and thin-walled branches of the pulmonary arterioles).

The patient with primary pulmonary hypertension is usually young and fe-male. In fact, the female-male ratio is roughly 5:1. The disease most often oc-curs between the ages of 15 and 40 years. The patient may complain of dizzi-ness or syncope on physical exertion, emotional excitement, or exposure to cold. She may have chest pain that closely resembles angina pectoris in its character, location, and frequency. The pain is usually provoked by physical exertion and is often accompanied by dyspnea. The patient may note dyspnea, weakness, and extreme fatigue, all made worse by physical exertion. Eventually, the pa-tient with primary pulmonary hypertension begins to have symptoms of right ventricular dilatation and failure: abdominal discomfort (due to hepatomegaly and ascites) and peripheral edema. On occasion, the patient may note hoarse-ness (due to compression of the recurrent laryngeal nerve by a dilated pulmo-nary arterial trunk), hemoptysis (due to the rupture of plexiform lesions), or prominent jugular venous pulsations.

On physical examination, the patient may be slightly cyanotic, due to a re-duced cardiac output and a greatly increased peripheral extraction of oxygen. The cyanosis is usually peripheral and not central. The systemic arterial pulse pressure is narrow. The jugular veins are usually prominent, with unusually distinctive A waves. There may be ascites and peripheral edema, and the en-larged liver may pulsate with each systole, indicating tricuspid regurgitation.

On cardiac examination, there is a right ventricular lift along the lower left sternal border. At the pulmonic area (second left intercostal space), one may palpate the systolic impulse of a dilated and hypertensive pulmonary trunk, the pulmonic component of the S_2, and a pulmonic ejection sound. On auscul-tation, the S_1 is normal; the S_2 is widely split, and its pulmonic component is loud and "popping." A pulmonic ejection sound is heard best at the pulmonic area; it usually diminishes in intensity during inspiration. Immediately follow-ing the ejection sound, a crescendo-decrescendo murmur is audible, resulting from the ejection of blood into a dilated pulmonary trunk.

At the lower left sternal border, a holosystolic murmur of tricuspid regurgi-tation may be audible if right ventricular failure has developed. This murmur usually becomes louder with inspiration. A decrescendo diastolic murmur of pulmonic regurgitation may be audible at the upper left sternal border. An S_3 is often audible along the left sternal border; it may increase in intensity with inspiration, indicating its right ventricular origin.

The chest x-ray of the patient with primary pulmonary hypertension dem-onstrates enlargement of the pulmonary trunk and its main branches, but the distal branches are diminished and the peripheral lung fields clear (so-called pruned appearance). The aorta appears small compared with the dilated pul-monary trunk. Right ventricular and right atrial enlargement may be severe. The ECG shows right axis deviation and right ventricular hypertrophy. The P waves in standard lead II and in lead VI may be peaked, reflecting right atrial enlargement. M-mode echocardiography reveals right ventricular enlargement with paradoxical systolic motion of the interventricular septum.

Cardiac catheterization identifies the presence and severity of the pulmonary hypertension in these patients. If there are no discernible causes of the hypertension (enumerated under Secondary Pulmonary Hypertension, p. 332), the assumption is made that it is primary. A lung biopsy reveals hypertrophy of the media of the pulmonary arterioles, as well as intimal proliferation and fibrosis, thrombosis, and atherosclerosis.

The patient with symptomatic primary pulmonary hypertension usually follows a rapidly downhill course. Some die suddenly, whereas others succumb because of severe right ventricular failure and diminished cardiac output. Once symptoms appear, most patients are dead within 1 to 2 years. Longevity is directly related to the severity of pulmonary hypertension.

For the patient with primary pulmonary hypertension, an anticoagulant has been administered commonly in the hope of preventing venous thrombosis. Its beneficial effects, however, have not been demonstrated clearly. Once right ventricular dilatation and failure develop, digitalis and diuretics may be of some help in controlling the peripheral edema. At present, there are no surgical procedures that are of benefit to the patient with primary pulmonary hypertension.

Over the past few years, several vasodilators have proved to be beneficial in some patients with primary pulmonary hypertension. These agents, such as hydralazine, captopril, and nifedipine, reduce pulmonary arteriolar resistance both acutely and chronically (i.e., for at least 6 months). It is presumed that even the most severely diseased pulmonary vascular bed maintains some reversible arterial tone, so that a powerful vasodilating agent can exert an effect.

Clinical Characteristics, Diagnosis, and Prognosis

1. Chapman DW, Abbott JP, Latson J. Primary pulmonary hypertension: review of literature and results of cardiac catheterization in 10 patients. Circulation 1957; 15:35–46.
   Ten patients with primary pulmonary hypertension are reported, and their poor prognosis is emphasized.
2. Hood WB, Spencer H, Lass RW, Daley R. Primary pulmonary hypertension: familial occurrence. Br Heart J 1968; 30:336–43.
   Three cases of primary pulmonary hypertension occurring in 2 women and a girl in one generation of one family are described.
3. Melmon KL, Braunwald E. Familial pulmonary hypertension. N Engl J Med 1963; 269:770–5.
   Two proved cases and 3 presumptive cases of primary pulmonary hypertension occurring in 3 generations of one family are described.
4. Perloff JK. Auscultatory and phonocardiographic manifestations of pulmonary hypertension. Prog Cardiovasc Dis 1967; 9:303–40.
   A complete description of physical findings in patients with pulmonary hypertension.
5. Sleeper JC, Orgain ES, McIntosh HD. Primary pulmonary hypertension: review of clinical features and pathologic physiology with a report of pulmonary hemodynamics derived from repeated catheterization. Circulation 1962; 26:1358–69.
   Sixteen patients with this disorder are described in detail. In these patients, the clinical course was highly variable and unaffected by any mode of therapy.
6. Wagenvoort CA, Wagenvoort N. Primary pulmonary hypertension: a pathologic study of the lung vessels in 156 clinically diagnosed cases. Circulation 1970; 42:1163–84.
   Of 156 autopsies of patients given a clinical diagnosis of primary pulmonary hypertension, 110 showed morphologic evidence of arteriolar lesions initiated by vasoconstriction.
7. Suarez LD, Sciandro EE, Llera JJ, Perosio AM. Long-term follow-up in primary pulmonary hypertension. Br Heart J 1979; 41:702–8.

Two patients with severe primary pulmonary hypertension who lived for many years after the initial diagnosis are described. They were physically active with only minimal limitation.

8. Kanemoto N, Furuya H, Etoh T, Sasamoto H, Matsuyama S. Chest roentgenograms in primary pulmonary hypertension. Chest 1979; 76:45–9.
   A review of chest x-ray findings in 59 patients with this disorder. In most of these patients, the main pulmonary arteries were remarkably dilated.

9. Goodman DJ, Harrison DC, Popp RL. Echocardiographic features of primary pulmonary hypertension. Am J Cardiol 1974; 33:438–43.
   In 9 patients with primary pulmonary hypertension, M-mode echocardiography revealed a reduced diastolic slope of the anterior mitral valve leaflet, probably related to a reduced rate of left ventricular filling.

Therapy

10. Guadagni DN, Ikram H, Maslowski AH. Hemodynamic effects of prostacyclin (PGI_2) in pulmonary hypertension. Br Heart J 1981; 45:385–8.
    In 4 patients with primary pulmonary hypertension, PGI_2 caused a decline in both pulmonary and systemic vascular resistances.

11. Ruskin JN, Hutter AM Jr. Primary pulmonary hypertension treated with oral phentolamine. Ann Intern Med 1979; 90:772–4.
    The case report of a 29-year-old man with primary pulmonary hypertension who obtained marked short- and long-term benefit from phentolamine.

12. Cohen ML, Kronzon I. Adverse hemodynamic effects of phentolamine in primary pulmonary hypertension. Ann Intern Med 1981; 95:591–2.
    The case report of a 38-year-old woman with this disease in whom phentolamine caused a substantial increase in pulmonary arterial pressure (66 to 86 mmHg, mean pressure).

13. Rubin LJ, Peter RH. Oral hydralazine therapy for primary pulmonary hypertension. N Engl J Med 1980; 302:69–73.
    In 4 patients with this disorder, oral hydralazine caused considerable hemodynamic and symptomatic improvement.

14. Klinke P, Gilbert JAL. Diazoxide in primary pulmonary hypertension. N Engl J Med 1980; 302:91–2.
    The report of a 19-year-old woman who obtained marked benefit from short- and long-term diazoxide therapy.

15. Buch J, Wennevold A. Hazards of diazoxide in pulmonary hypertension. Br Heart J 1981; 46:401–3.
    A description of 3 patients with pulmonary hypertension who responded poorly to diazoxide, including one who sustained a cardiac arrest.

16. Young TE, Lundquist LJ, Chesler E, Weir EK. Comparative effects of nifedipine, verapamil, and diltiazem on experimental pulmonary hypertension. Am J Cardiol 1983; 51:195–200.
    In dogs with experimentally induced pulmonary hypertension, nifedipine reduced pulmonary vascular resistance, whereas diltiazem exerted no effect and verapamil was deleterious.

17. Leier CV, Bambach D, Nelson S, Hermiller JB, Huss P, Magorien RD, Unverferth DV. Captopril in primary pulmonary hypertension. Circulation 1983; 67:155–61.
    In 7 women with this disease, captopril reduced systemic vascular resistance but did not alter pulmonary hemodynamics.

18. DeFeyter PJ, Kerkkamp HJJ, deJong JP. Sustained beneficial effect of nifedipine in primary pulmonary hypertension. Am Heart J 1983; 105:333–4.
    The case report of a young woman (age 27) with primary pulmonary hypertension who derived substantial benefit from nifedipine over a 6-month period of observation.

SECONDARY PULMONARY HYPERTENSION

Secondary pulmonary hypertension occurs when the pulmonary arterial pressure is abnormally high because of an identifiable underlying disease process. Several pathologic entities can cause pulmonary hypertension. First, any disorder that causes an elevation of the pulmonary capillary or left atrial pressure can lead to an abnormally high pulmonary arterial pressure, including left ventricular dilatation and failure, mitral stenosis, left atrial myxoma or thrombus causing mitral valve obstruction, cor triatriatum, and congenital or acquired stenosis of the pulmonary veins. Second, pulmonary arterial hypertension can result from a reduction in the cross-sectional area of the pulmonary vascular bed, caused by pulmonary embolic disease or any disorder that causes progressive fibrosis and obliteration of the pulmonary vasculature. Third, a marked increase in pulmonary blood flow (due to a left-to-right intracardiac shunt) can lead to an elevation of pulmonary arterial pressure. Finally, marked alveolar hypoventilation associated with pulmonary parenchymal disease (e.g., chronic bronchitis or emphysema) can lead to hypoxic pulmonary arterial vasoconstriction. If pulmonary hypertension is initiated by any of these disease processes, subsequent morphologic changes within the remaining pulmonary arterioles lead to a further elevation of pulmonary vascular resistance.

By the time substantial secondary pulmonary arterial hypertension develops, the patient usually has symptoms similar to those of the patient with primary pulmonary hypertension: dizziness or syncope on exertion, chest discomfort that closely resembles angina pectoris, dyspnea, weakness, and easy fatigability. If right ventricular dilatation and failure occur, the patient may note abdominal discomfort (due to hepatomegaly) and peripheral edema. On physical examination, jugular venous distention, hepatomegaly, and peripheral edema may be present. On precordial palpation, a right ventricular lift and an impulse at the pulmonic area (second left intercostal space) are often felt. On auscultation, a loud pulmonic component of the S_2, a pulmonic ejection click, a right ventricular S_3, and a systolic murmur of tricuspid regurgitation may be heard. Finally, if the pulmonary hypertension is severe and prolonged, a murmur of pulmonic regurgitation may be audible. The physical examination may also reveal evidence of the underlying disease process that has caused pulmonary hypertension. For instance, the patient with pulmonary hypertension due to mitral stenosis has physical signs of this valvular abnormality.

The chest x-ray of the patient with secondary pulmonary hypertension demonstrates enlargement of the pulmonary trunk and its main branches. The right ventricle and atrium are usually enlarged. The cardiac contour may suggest underlying valvular or congenital cardiac disease (i.e., mitral stenosis, atrial septal defect, or ventricular septal defect). The ECG usually reflects right ventricular hypertrophy and right atrial enlargement. If the pulmonary hypertension is due to left ventricular disease, it may demonstrate biventricular hypertrophy. By M-mode echocardiography, one sees an enlarged right ventricular chamber. At cardiac catheterization, the pulmonary arterial pressure and resistance are elevated. Catheterization may also demonstrate the underlying cause of pulmonary hypertension (i.e., mitral valve disease, atrial tumor, multiple pulmonary emboli, or the presence of an intracardiac shunt). A lung biopsy reveals varying severity of intimal and medial thickening and fibrosis of the pulmonary arterioles.

The prognosis and therapy of the patient with secondary pulmonary hypertension depend on its underlying cause. For instance, if pulmonary hypertension results from mitral stenosis, the surgical correction of the stenosis will alleviate the elevation of pulmonary arterial pressure. In contrast, severe pulmonary hypertension due to intracardiac shunting (Eisenmenger syndrome), with a resultant right-to-left shunt, does not regress after surgical closure of the shunt, leading to severe right ventricular failure. In the patient with pulmonary hypertension, therefore, it is important both prognostically and therapeutically to attempt to identify and correct a remediable cause of the pulmonary hypertension.

1. Arnett EN, Battle WE, Russo JV, Roberts WC. Intravenous injection of talc-containing drugs intended for oral use: a cause of pulmonary granulomatosis and pulmonary hypertension. Am J Med 1976; 60:711–8.
   Intravenous drug abusers may develop secondary pulmonary hypertension because of repeated embolization of the pulmonary arterioles with talc particles.
2. Robertson CH Jr, Reynolds RC, Wilson JE III. Pulmonary hypertension and foreign body granulomas in intravenous drug abusers: documentation by cardiac catheterization and lung biopsy. Am J Med 1976; 61:657–64.
   Pulmonary hypertension was shown by cardiac catheterization in 4 intravenous drug abusers with biopsy-proven foreign body granulomas in the pulmonary vasculature.
3. Young RH, Mark GJ. Pulmonary vascular changes in scleroderma. Am J Med 1978; 64:998–1004.
   Of 30 patients with scleroderma examined at postmortem, 14 had moderate or marked abnormalities of the pulmonary arterial tree.
4. Eisenberg H, Dubois EL, Sherwin RP, Balchum OJ. Diffuse interstitial lung disease in systemic lupus erythematosus. Ann Intern Med 1973; 79:37–45.
   The incidence of diffuse interstitial pulmonary disease in patients with systemic lupus is small, probably somewhere between 1–3%.
5. Jones MB, Osterholm RK, Wilson RB, Martin FH, Commers JR, Bachmayer JD. Fatal pulmonary hypertension and resolving immune-complex glomerulonephritis in mixed connective tissue disease: a case report and review of the literature. Am J Med 1978; 65:855–63.
   Pulmonary hypertension due to mixed connective tissue disease is very uncommon.
6. Salerni R, Rodnan GP, Leon DF, Shaver JA. Pulmonary hypertension in the CREST syndrome variant of progressive systemic sclerosis (scleroderma). Ann Intern Med 1977; 86:394–9.
   Ten patients are described with severe pulmonary hypertension in association with the CREST syndrome (calcinosis, Raynaud's phenomenon, esophageal dysfunction, sclerodactyly, and telangiectasia).
7. Kleiger RE, Boxer M, Ingham RE, Harrison DC. Pulmonary hypertension in patients using oral contraceptives: a report of 6 cases. Chest 1976; 69:143–7.
   Six women are described who had severe pulmonary hypertension after long-term ingestion of oral contraceptives. It is hypothesized that oral contraceptives can produce vascular intimal proliferation within the pulmonary arterial branches.
8. Dalen JE, Matloff JM, Evans GL, Hoppin FG Jr, Bhardwaj P, Harken DE, Dexter L. Early reduction of pulmonary vascular resistance after mitral valve replacement. N Engl J Med 1967; 277:387–94.
   Within 8–10 days of mitral valve replacement, mean pulmonary arterial pressure fell from 71 to 35 mmHg, and pulmonary arteriolar resistance declined from 2067 to 463 dynes/s/cm^{-5}.
9. Zener JC, Hancock EW, Shumway NE, Harrison DC. Regression of extreme pulmonary hypertension after mitral valve surgery. Am J Cardiol 1972; 30:820–6.
   Even extreme degrees of pulmonary hypertension and increased pulmonary vascular resistance due to mitral valve disease regress markedly if surgery adequately decompresses the left atrium.
10. Harvey RM, Ferrer MI, Richards DW, Cournand A. Influence of chronic pulmonary disease on the heart and circulation. Am J Med 1951; 10:719–38.
    In patients with underlying pulmonary disease, both anatomic destruction of the pulmonary vasculature and hypoxia contribute to the development and maintenance of pulmonary hypertension.

11. Kane RD, Hawkins HK, Miller JA, Noce PS. Microscopic pulmonary tumor emboli associated with dyspnea. Cancer 1975; 36:1473–82.
Eight patients are reported who complained of dyspnea; at postmortem, they had widespread microscopic tumor emboli throughout their lungs.

PRIMARY CARDIAC TUMORS

Primary tumors of the heart are extremely rare. Morphologically, about 75 percent are termed benign; the remaining 25 percent are malignant. Of those that are classified as benign, myxoma is by far the most common, followed by lipoma, papillary fibroelastoma, and rhabdomyoma. Of the malignant primary cardiac tumors, angiosarcoma and rhabdomyosarcoma comprise about two-thirds.

Myxomas are the most common type of primary cardiac tumor, comprising 30 to 50 percent of all primary tumors (benign and malignant). They have been reported in patients as young as 3 years and as old as 83 years, but most occur between the ages of 30 and 60. On occasion, they have been noted in successive generations, in which case they appear to be transmitted as an autosomal dominant trait. Over 90 percent occur in the atria, with three to four times as many occurring in the left atrium as the right. They rarely occur in the other cardiac chambers. A very rare individual may have myxomas in more than one cardiac chamber. On gross examination, they are usually pedunculated and average 4 to 8 cm in diameter. Atrial myxomas are typically attached to the interatrial septum in the area of the fossa ovalis.

The patient with an atrial myxoma may present with one of several symptom complexes. First, he may be totally asymptomatic. Second, he may complain of symptoms identical to those of mitral stenosis or regurgitation: dyspnea, orthopnea, and possibly pedal edema and fatigue, all due to impingement of the myxoma on normal mitral valve function. At times, these symptoms may be sudden in onset, intermittent, and related to the patient's body position. In fact, the occurrence of paroxysmal symptoms that occur only in a particular body position and are out of proportion to the findings on physical examination should raise the possibility of a left atrial myxoma.

Third, the patient with a left atrial myxoma may come to medical attention after an episode of systemic arterial embolism. Thus, the patient may present with the sudden onset of a neurologic deficit, chest pain, and evidence of acute myocardial infarction, visceral organ infarction, or vascular insufficiency of an arm or leg. Lastly, the patient with a myxoma may complain of nonspecific constitutional symptoms similar in many respects to those of subacute bacterial endocarditis: malaise, low-grade fever, weight loss, and arthralgias.

The patient with a right atrial myxoma may have similar constitutional symptoms to those described for left atrial myxoma. Systemic embolization, of course, is uncommon. These patients may have marked peripheral venous congestion (due to interference of the myxoma with normal tricuspid valve function) or recurrent pulmonary emboli.

On physical examination, the patient with a left or right atrial myxoma may have an elevated jugular venous pressure. The peripheral pulse is regular, since the patient usually remains in sinus rhythm, unlike many patients with mitral stenosis. On cardiac examination, many of the findings in the patient with a left atrial myxoma simulate those of the patient with rheumatic mitral stenosis: a loud S_1, a loud pulmonary component of the S_2, and a diastolic rumble. In addition, a loud but low-pitched sound occurs 0.1 to 0.16 seconds after the aortic component of the S_2 and may be mistaken for an opening snap or an S_3; in actuality, it is a "tumor plop." It may be distinguished from an opening snap by its lower frequency and by the unusually long A_2–plop interval (the A_2–plop interval is usually 0.1–0.16 sec, whereas the A_2–OS interval is considerably shorter, usually 0.05–0.1 sec). The differentiation of the tumor plop from an S_3 may be difficult, since each occurs at about the same time after the S_2. Classically, the tumor plop has a higher frequency than an S_3. The diastolic murmur, tumor plop, and symptoms may vary with the patient's position. They may be most marked in the erect position and diminish when the patient is supine.

The laboratory examination may reveal anemia, leukocytosis, an increased erythrocyte sedimentation rate, and hypergammaglobulinemia—all hematologic signs that may suggest subacute bacterial endocarditis. The chest x-ray may appear identical to that of the patient with rheumatic mitral stenosis, including an enlarged left atrium, pulmonary vascular redistribution, and an enlarged right ventricle. However, the left atrial appendage is usually not prominent. Occasionally, the tumor may be calcified, and the ECG may show atrial fibrillation or evidence of right ventricular enlargement.

Several clinical clues may help to distinguish a left atrial myxoma from rheumatic mitral stenosis. In comparison to the patient with rheumatic mitral valve disease, the patient with a left atrial myxoma generally provides no history of acute rheumatic fever and has a relatively rapid onset and progression of symptoms. There may be a poor correlation among the physical findings, radiologic abnormalities, and severity of symptoms. The patient with a left atrial myxoma often has marked positional variation in symptoms, blood pressure, and auscultatory findings. Finally, an occasional patient with an atrial myxoma may have intracardiac calcification, whereas the patient with rheumatic mitral valve disease has calcification within the valve leaflets.

The diagnosis of a left atrial myxoma is best made by echocardiography. The anterior leaflet of the mitral valve moves normally, but dense echoes from the atrial tumor are seen posterior to it. With a right atrial myxoma, there are dense echoes behind the tricuspid valve. Since myxomas may occur biatrially, it is vital to visualize both atria by echocardiography. These tumors may also be visualized by gated blood pool scintigraphy. In the cardiac catheterization laboratory, a left atrial myxoma is best demonstrated by filming the levophase of a pulmonary arteriogram. When the left atrium fills with contrast material, a filling defect is visible. A right atrial myxoma is easily visualized with the injection of contrast material into the superior or inferior vena cava. Since these tumors are somewhat friable, it is recommended that one not traumatize them with a catheter, thus minimizing the risk of catheter-induced embolization.

The therapy of a myxoma, regardless of its location, is surgical excision. Since tumor recurrence may occur, many surgeons prefer to remove a rim of normal interatrial septal tissue in addition to the tumor. Dislodging tumor fragments constitutes a major risk of operation and may result in peripheral or pulmonary emboli or seeding of small metastases. To minimize this risk, manipulation of the heart prior to cardiopulmonary bypass should be avoided, if possible.

Rhabdomyomas, the most common primary cardiac tumors of childhood, frequently occur as part of tuberous sclerosis. They most frequently appear in the ventricles. Although many children with rhabdomyomas are asymptomatic, some complain of syncope or congestive heart failure, and an occasional child may die suddenly. As with myxomas, the optimal therapy is surgical removal.

Of the primary cardiac tumors that are malignant, sarcomas are by far the most common. They are most likely to involve the right or left atria. The patient may complain of symptoms of rapidly progressive congestive heart failure or precordial pain; in addition, he may have evidence on physical examination and noninvasive evaluation of pericardial effusion, arrhythmias and conduction disturbances, or obstruction to right-sided venous inflow. Finally, the patient may have sudden death as the initial manifestation of a sarcoma. The patient with a primary cardiac sarcoma has a very poor prognosis, and death often occurs within a few weeks of diagnosis. When it occurs, death is attributable to widespread infiltration of the myocardium, obstruction of flow within the heart, or distant metastases.

Finally, other primary cardiac tumors are extremely rare. Certain benign tumors of the pericardium, including teratomas and dermoid cysts, usually originate near the origin of the great vessels and extend into the pericardium as pedunculated masses. Although most cause no symptoms, some may be responsible for electrocardiographic abnormalities, obstruction to ventricular outflow, arrhythmias and conduction defects, syncope, and even sudden death.

Myxoma

1. Carter JB, Cramer R Jr, Edwards JE. Mitral and tricuspid lesions associated with polypoid atrial tumors, including myxoma. Am J Cardiol 1974; 33:914–9.
   Atrial myxomas may cause traumatic damage of the atrioventricular valves.

2. Croxson RS, Jewitt D, Bentall HH, Cleland WP, Kristinsson A, Goodwin JF. Long-term follow-up of atrial myxoma. Br Heart J 1972; 34:1018–23.
   The authors advise careful removal of all the tumor (including resecting part of the atrial septum) in order to minimize the chance of recurrence.

3. Ghahramani AR, Arnold JR, Hildner FJ, Sommer LS, Samet P. Left atrial myxoma: hemodynamic and phonocardiographic features. Am J Med 1972; 52:525–32.
   Two cases of left atrial myxoma are presented, and helpful clinical clues are given to distinguish this entity from intrinsic mitral valve disease.

4. Liebler GA, Magovern GJ, Park SB, Cushing WJ, Begg FR, Joyner CR. Familial myxomas in 4 siblings. J Thorac Cardiovasc Surg 1976; 71:605–8.
   Of these 4 siblings with myxomas, 3 had 2 or more myxomas.

5. Nasser WK, Davis RH, Dillon JC, Tavel ME, Helman CH, Feigenbaum H, Fisch C. Atrial myxoma: II. Phonocardiographic, echocardiographic, hemodynamic, and angiographic features in 9 cases. Am Heart J 1972; 83:810–24.
   Of these 9 cases, 7 were left atrial and 2 right atrial in location.

6. Penny JL, Gregory JJ, Ayres SM, Giannelli S, Rossi P. Calcified left atrial myxoma simulating mitral insufficiency. Circulation 1967; 36:417–21.
   A diagnosis of mitral regurgitation was mimicked by a calcified left atrial myxoma in a 48-year-old woman.

7. Siltanen P, Tuuteri L, Norio R, Tala P, Ahrenberg P, Halonen PI. Atrial myxoma in a family. Am J Cardiol 1976; 38:252–6.
   A family is described in which the mother and 3 of the 7 children had atrial myxomas. The authors emphasize that first-degree relatives of patients with myxoma should be evaluated medically.

8. Sung RJ, Ghahramani AR, Mallon SM, Richter SE, Sommer LS, Gottlieb S, Myerburg RJ. Hemodynamic features of prolapsing and nonprolapsing left atrial myxoma. Circulation 1975; 51:342–9.
   Some left atrial myxomas prolapse from the left atrium into the left ventricle during each cardiac cycle, whereas others do not. This paper emphasizes the hemodynamic findings of each type.

9. Gonzalez A, Altieri PI, Marquez E, Cox RA, Castillo M. Massive pulmonary embolism associated with a right ventricular myxoma. Am J Med 1980; 69:795–8.

A case report of a 12-year-old boy with a huge pulmonary embolism due to a myxoma of the right ventricle.

10. Zager J, Smith JO, Goldstein S, Franch RH. Tricuspid and pulmonary valve obstruction relieved by removal of a myxoma of the right ventricle. Am J Cardiol 1973; 32:101–4.
    A 30-year-old woman is described who had tricuspid and pulmonic valvular pressure gradients due to a right ventricular myxoma. When the tumor was excised, the gradients disappeared.

11. Bulkley BH, Hutchins GM. Atrial myxomas: a fifty year review. Am Heart J 1979; 97:639–43.
    Of these 24 patients with atrial myxomas, 17 (70%) were women, and the average age at diagnosis was 50 years.

12. Pohost GM, Pastore JO, McKusick KA, Chiotellis PN, Kapellakis GZ, Myers GS, Dinsmore RE, Block PC. Detection of left atrial myxoma by gated radionuclide cardiac imaging. Circulation 1977; 55:88–92.
    In 7 patients with left atrial myxoma, gated blood pool scintigraphy allowed tumor visualization in all.

13. Perry LS, King JF, Zeft HJ, Manley JC, Gross CM, Wann LS. Two-dimensional echocardiography in the diagnosis of left atrial myxoma. Br Heart J 1981; 45:667–71.
    Of 11 patients with left atrial myxoma, M-mode echocardiography identified 9. Of the 7 patients in this group who underwent 2-dimensional echocardiography, all were correctly identified, including one not visualized by M-mode.

14. Massumi R. Bedside diagnosis of right heart myxomas through detection of palpable tumor shocks and audible plops. Am Heart J 1983; 105:303–10.
    Four cases of right-sided myxomas were diagnosed on physical examination through the detection of a palpable tumor shock and audible tumor plop.

Rhabdomyoma

15. Fenoglio JJ Jr, McAllister HA Jr, Ferrans VJ. Cardiac rhabdomyoma: a clinicopathologic and electron microscopic study. Am J Cardiol 1976; 38:241–51.
    Rhabdomyoma is almost exclusively a tumor of infancy and early childhood. In this autopsy series of 36 patients, 25 (70%) died during the first year of life.

16. Mair DD, Titus JL, Davis GD, Ritter DG. Cardiac rhabdomyoma simulating mitral atresia. Chest 1977; 71:102–5.
    In this infant, a left atrial rhabdomyoma completely obstructed the mitral valvular orifice, leading to an initial clinical diagnosis of mitral atresia and the hypoplastic left heart syndrome.

17. Shaher RM, Mintzer J, Farina M, Alley R, Bishop M. Clinical presentation of rhabdomyoma of the heart in infancy and childhood. Am J Cardiol 1972; 30:95–103.
    Of 4 infants described with rhabdomyoma, 2 were siblings. All 4 had tuberous sclerosis.

Sarcoma

18. Whorton CM. Primary malignant tumor of the heart. Cancer 1949; 2:245–60.
    Of the initial 100 patients reported with primary malignant cardiac tumors, the diagnosis was made antemortem in only 4.

19. Glancy DL, Morales JB, Roberts WC. Angiosarcoma of the heart. Am J Cardiol 1968; 21:413–9.
    Of the 41 patients described in this report, 32 had clinical evidence of obstruction to filling of the right-sided cardiac chambers.

20. Rossi NP, Kioschos JM, Aschenbrener CA, Ehrenhaft JL. Primary angiosarcoma of the heart. Cancer 1976; 37:891–4.
    The patient described herein—a 17-year-old student—is the youngest yet reported with a cardiac angiosarcoma.

21. Panella JS, Paige ML, Victor TA, Semerdjian RA, Hueter DC. Angiosarcoma of the heart: diagnosis by echocardiography. Chest 1979; 76:221–3.
    In this 40-year-old man, a right-sided angiosarcoma was visualized by M-mode echocardiography.

SECONDARY CARDIAC TUMORS

Cardiac involvement by tumor metastases occurs 20 to 40 times more frequently than primary cardiac tumors. Such metastatic involvement of the heart has been reported to occur in 0.1 to 6.4 percent of unselected autopsies and in 1.5 to 20.6 percent of patients dying of malignant neoplasms. The incidence of cardiac involvement by tumor metastases has increased over the past 5 to 10 years, probably due to improved patient survival because of more effective therapeutic modalities.

Pericardial metastases are more common than those that involve the myocardium or endocardium. They are especially frequent in patients with intrathoracic neoplasms, in which case they occur by direct invasion of malignant tissue or by lymphatic spread. Direct tumor invasion is particularly common with mediastinal lymphoma, whereas lymphatic spread to the pericardium occurs frequently in patients with carcinoma of the bronchus or breast. In contrast, myocardial and endocardial metastases usually result from hematogenous dissemination of neoplastic cells; therefore, they occur in direct proportion to coronary blood flow. As a result, endocardial and valvular metastases are unusual, since these areas are relatively avascular.

Although cardiac involvement by tumor metastases occurs with all kinds of tumors (including carcinomas, leukemias, lymphomas, and sarcomas), malignant melanomas are especially likely to involve the heart. Microscopic or gross evidence of myocardial infiltration by melanoma has been shown to occur in half the patients with this malignancy. Myocardial infiltration is also very frequent in patients with leukemia or lymphoma, especially reticulum cell sarcoma.

The symptoms and signs produced by cardiac metastases depend on the location and extent of tissue infiltration. Thus, pericardial involvement may cause (1) an acute pericarditis, with chest pain, fever, and an audible pericardial friction rub; (2) a painless and silent pericardial effusion; or (3) pericardial tamponade due to the rapid accumulation of an effusion, with resultant dyspnea and peripheral venous congestion. Myocardial infiltration of tumor tissue may cause (1) progressive biventricular congestive heart failure, with dyspnea, orthopnea, and peripheral edema; (2) bradyarrhythmias, tachyarrhythmias, or AV block, all due to involvement of the cardiac conduction system; (3) angina pectoris or acute myocardial infarction, both due to tumor tissue impinging on the coronary blood flow; or (4) rarely, myocardial rupture, with resultant pericardial tamponade and sudden death. Endocardial involvement rarely occurs but can lead to valvular stenoses or regurgitation.

Electrocardiographically, nonspecific abnormalities are common in the patient with cardiac involvement by tumor metastases. ST–T wave abnormalities occur frequently. Various degrees of AV block or bundle branch block may be present. If pericardial involvement leads to an effusion, the QRS voltage may be diminished. Supraventricular tachyarrhythmias, many of which respond poorly to antiarrhythmic medications, are frequent. M-mode and two-dimensional echocardiography can be used to visualize neoplastic tissue that protrudes into the cardiac chambers or pericardial space. On occasion, neoplastic tissue can be identified after the injection of a radioactive tracer material, such as gallium citrate or technetium pertechnetate. Cineangiography remains the best method for delineating the presence, location, and size of metastatic tumor foci.

If tumor infiltration has produced a pericardial effusion, pericardiocentesis will permit a direct cytologic diagnosis and will relieve tamponade. Surgical therapy for metastatic involvement of the heart usually does not allow a total resection of tumor tissue and, therefore, is not curative. Palliative irradiation or systemic chemotherapy usually reduces the size of the tumor mass, thus affording relief of obstructive or infiltrative symptoms. However, such therapy eventually may lead to pericarditis or pericardial constriction. If pericardial effusion with tamponade is a recurrent problem, a pericardiectomy may be necessary.

1. Berge T, Sievers J. Myocardial metastases: a pathological and electrocardiographic study. Br Heart J 1968; 30:383–90.
   Of 122 cases of myocardial metastases, the highest frequency was found among melanomas. Electrocardiography was generally of no help in establishing the diagnosis.
2. Biran S, Hochman A, Levij IS, Stern S. Clinical diagnosis of secondary tumors of the heart and pericardium. Chest 1969; 55:202–8.
   Of 26 patients with postmortem evidence of cardiac metastases, only 6 were suspected during life.
3. Glancy DL, Roberts WC. The heart in malignant melanoma: a study of 70 autopsy cases. Am J Cardiol 1968; 21:555–71.
   Cardiac metastases were present at postmortem in 45 of 70 patients dying of malignant melanoma. Of the 45, 11 had clinical evidence of cardiac dysfunction.
4. Roberts WC, Glancy DL, DeVita VT Jr. Heart in malignant lymphoma (Hodgkin's disease, lymphosarcoma, reticulum cell sarcoma, and mycosis fungoides): a study of 196 autopsy cases. Am J Cardiol 1968; 22:85–107.
   Of 196 patients with malignant lymphoma, 48 (24%) had cardiac involvement on postmortem examination.
5. Terry LN Jr, Kligerman MM. Pericardial and myocardial involvement by lymphomas and leukemias: the role of radiotherapy. Cancer 1970; 25:1003–8.
   Radiotherapy is often efficacious in patients with cardiac involvement by lymphomas and leukemias.
6. Goldman BS, Pearson FG. Malignant pericardial effusion: review of hospital experience and report of a case successfully treated by talc poudrage. Can J Surg 1965; 8:157–61.
   A proportion of patients with clinically important malignant pericardial effusion may benefit from the pericardial instillation of a sclerosing agent.
7. Hanfling SM. Metastatic cancer to the heart: review of the literature and report of 127 cases. Circulation 1960; 22:474–83.
   Of 694 consecutive deaths from cancer, cardiac metastases were observed at postmortem examination in 127 (18%).
8. Hanburg WJ. Secondary tumors of the heart. Br J Cancer 1960; 14:23–7.
   The most common tumors involving the heart by metastatic spread were malignant melanoma and carcinoma of the bronchus.
9. Harris TR, Copeland GD, Brody DA. Progressive injury current with metastatic tumor of the heart: case report and review of the literature. Am Heart J 1965; 69:392–400.
   A report of a patient with electrocardiographic alterations of an acute myocardial infarction due to cardiac involvement by tumor metastases.
10. Onuigbo WIB. The spread of lung cancer to the heart, pericardium, and great vessels. Jpn Heart J 1974; 15:234–8.
    Of 100 consecutive autopsies on patients with lung cancer, there was spread to the pericardium in 27.
11. Roberts WC, Bodey GP, Wertlake PT. The heart in acute leukemia: a study of 420 autopsy cases. Am J Cardiol 1968; 21:388–412.
    Of 420 consecutive autopsies on leukemic patients, 156 (37%) had leukemic infiltrates in the heart, and cardiac hemorrhages were observed in 228 (54%).
12. Biran S, Brufman G, Klein E, Hochman A. The management of pericardial effusion in cancer patients. Chest 1977; 71:182–6.
    The authors advocate an aggressive approach to malignant pericardial effusions, including pericardiectomy, if necessary.
13. Flannery EP, Gregoratos G, Corder MP. Pericardial effusions in patients with malignant diseases. Arch Int Med 1975; 135:976–7.

In 6 patients with malignant pericardial effusions, catheter drainage allowed adequate drainage.

14. Smith FE, Lane M, Hudgins PT. Conservative management of malignant pericardial effusion. Cancer 1974; 33:47–57.

The 5 patients described herein had malignant pericardial effusions and were treated with local instillation of a chemotherapeutic agent with or without radiotherapy. Four had good responses to this therapeutic approach.

SYPHILITIC INVOLVEMENT OF THE HEART AND GREAT VESSELS

The causative organism of syphilis is *Treponema pallidum*. Although the primary infection with this organism is acquired by sexual contact with an infected person, its cardiovascular manifestations usually do not become manifest until at least 10 to 20 years later. Pathologically, the patient with cardiovascular syphilis develops a destructive aortitis, which usually involves the ascending or transverse thoracic aorta. Initially, the infecting organism invades the aortic wall through its vasa vasorum, resulting in an inflammatory reaction of the adventitia and media. As this inflammation resolves, the aortic wall becomes thickened and stretched, with a characteristic "tree bark" appearance. Such aortic involvement, in turn, may lead to dysfunction of the aortic valve or coronary ostia.

The patient with cardiovascular syphilis is most often an elderly man, usually of a lower socioeconomic group. Over the past 3 to 4 decades, the average age of the patient with luetic aortitis has gradually risen: in the preantibiotic era, this disease entity usually became clinically apparent in patients between the ages of 35 and 55, whereas today it becomes manifest in patients in their sixties or seventies.

Most patients with cardiovascular syphilis have mild aortitis and, therefore, are asymptomatic. In a small percentage, luetic aortitis causes major cardiovascular problems. If dilatation of the ascending aorta is severe, coaptation of the aortic valvular cusps cannot occur during diastole, resulting in aortic regurgitation. The aortic cusps themselves are not involved by the luetic process, but secondary changes (characterized by thickened, everted edges) may develop in the cusps. Such valvular aortic regurgitation is the most common complication of syphilitic aortitis. Like other causes of aortic regurgitation, luetic valvular regurgitation can lead to symptoms and signs of left ventricular failure.

In 33 percent of patients with syphilitic aortitis, there is at least some narrowing of one or both coronary ostia, and severe narrowing is present in 20 to 26 percent. Most patients with ostial narrowing have concomitant aortic regurgitation. Luetic aortitis usually involves only the coronary ostia. A more diffuse syphilitic coronary arteritis, involving the proximal 3 to 4 cm of both coronary arteries, is extremely rare. In most patients, the development of coronary ostial stenoses is very slow, thus allowing for the appearance of extensive collaterals in the coronary circulation. Therefore, patients with syphilitic aortitis and coronary ostial involvement may have angina pectoris but rarely myocardial infarction.

Syphilitic aortitis may eventually lead to a large saccular aneurysm. Although such aneurysms appear in only 5 to 10 percent of patients with luetic aortitis, this disease entity nonetheless is the second most common cause of aortic aneurysms, being responsible for about 20 percent. The resultant symptoms depend on the location of the aneurysm and the structures adjacent to it.

For example, if an ascending aortic aneurysm expands anteriorly and laterally, it may cause no symptoms except for a pulsatile mass in the first and second right intercostal spaces. Alternatively, enlarging aneurysms of the transverse aorta are more likely to produce early symptoms, such as dysphagia, cough, hoarseness, or chest pain. Dissecting aortic aneurysms due to syphilitic aortitis are very rare.

Apart from luetic aortitis, a very rare patient with cardiovascular syphilis has gummatous myocarditis. Although this disorder usually causes no symptoms, AV block or an interventricular conduction defect occurs occasionally if a gumma impinges on the conducting system. On occasion, gummas at the base of the heart impinge on the cardiac valves and cause pseudostenosis. Finally, a gumma may produce an electrocardiographic picture similar to that of myocardial infarction.

On physical examination, the patient with luetic aortic regurgitation usually has the peripheral and central manifestations of this abnormality: a widened pulse pressure, water-hammer pulses, Quincke's pulses, and Hill's sign, as well as a decrescendo diastolic murmur, an S_3, and an Austin Flint murmur. Classically, the decrescendo diastolic murmur in these patients is loudest at the right sternal border, since the ascending aorta is severely dilated.

In the patient with cardiovascular syphilis, the FTA-ABS test is positive. The VDRL is usually positive but may be nonreactive. On the chest x-ray, there is a dilated and somewhat tortuous ascending aorta, which may contain calcium in its walls. If aortic regurgitation is present, the left ventricle may be dilated. The ECG may reveal left ventricular hypertrophy. The M-mode echocardiogram demonstrates a dilated aortic root, an enlarged left ventricular chamber, and diastolic fluttering of the anterior leaflet of the mitral valve. The diagnosis of cardiovascular syphilis is usually made by serologic confirmation of luetic infection in the patient with clear-cut aortitis with or without aortic valvular regurgitation.

Following the primary infection with *T. pallidum,* the patient remains asymptomatic for 10 to 25 years, after which he begins to complain of (1) symptoms of left ventricular failure (dyspnea, orthopnea, and paroxysmal nocturnal dyspnea), (2) angina pectoris, or (3) symptoms of organ compression in the mediastinum by a saccular aortic aneurysm. Once symptoms of congestive heart failure appear, life expectancy ranges from 2 to 14 years, with an average of about 6 years. The 10-year survival rate once symptoms appear is only 30 to 40 percent. In the absence of congestive failure, the 15-year survival rate is approximately 56 percent.

The patient with cardiovascular syphilis should receive sufficient antibiotics to eliminate the infecting organism: (1) benzathine penicillin G, 2.4 million units intramuscularly weekly for 3 weeks, (2) aqueous procaine penicillin G, 600,000 units intramuscularly daily for 10 days, or (3) tetracycline or erythromycin, 500 mg orally 4 times daily for at least 30 days. There is no evidence that antibiotic treatment of patients with the fully established cardiovascular complications of syphilis alters the natural history of the disease. If aortic regurgitation is severe, the patient should have an aortic valve replacement. Finally, if angina pectoris due to ostial disease is incapacitating, coronary artery bypass grafting should be performed.

Clinical Characteristics, Diagnosis, and Prognosis
1. Heggtveit HA. Syphilitic aortitis: autopsy experience at the Ottawa General Hospital since 1950. Can Med Assoc J 1965; 92:880–1.
   Of 26 cases of syphilitic aortitis identified at autopsy, 10 had aneurysms, 9 had coronary ostial stenoses, and 5 had aortic regurgitation.

2. Heggtveit HA. Syphilitic aortitis: a clinicopathologic autopsy study of 100 cases, 1950 to 1960. Circulation 1964; 29:346–55.
   Of these 100 cases, 29 had aortic insufficiency, and 26 had coronary ostial narrowing.
3. Kalz F, Scott AI. Follow-up studies in cardiovascular syphilis. Can Med Assoc J 1955; 72:274–9.
   Those patients with mild luetic aortitis have a normal life expectancy.
4. Leonard JC, Smith WG. Syphilitic aortic incompetence with special reference to prognosis and effect of treatment. Lancet 1957; 1:234–40.
   Of those patients with syphilitic aortic regurgitation, the presence of concomitant heart failure carried a bad prognosis—only 15% survived 5 years.
5. Prewitt TA. Syphilitic aortic insufficiency: its increased incidence in the elderly. JAMA 1970; 211:637–9.
   Of 56 patients with syphilitic aortic insufficiency, the VDRL was nonreactive in 17 (30%), whereas the FTA-ABS was negative in only 1 (1.9%).
6. McCann JS, Porter DC. Calcification of the aorta as an aid to the diagnosis of syphilis. Br Med J 1956; 1:826–7.
   Calcification of the ascending aorta is a reliable sign of syphilitic involvement.
7. Smith WG, Leonard JC. The radiological features of syphilitic aortic incompetence. Br Heart J 1959; 21:162–6.
   Although linear calcification of the ascending aorta is a specific radiographic sign of syphilitic aortitis, it is found in only about 40% of patients with this disorder.
8. Phillips PL, Amberson JB, Libby DM. Syphilitic aortic aneurysm presenting with the superior vena cava syndrome. Am J Med 1981; 71:171–3.
   A case report of a 65-year-old man with superior vena cava obstruction due to a luetic aneurysm.

Therapy

9. Connolly JE, Eldridge FL, Calvin JW, Stemmer EA. Proximal coronary artery obstruction: its etiology and treatment by transaortic endarterectomy. N Engl J Med 1964; 271:213–9.
   An early report of coronary endarterectomy for a severe luetic ostial stenosis.
10. Kampmeier RH, Morgan HJ. The specific treatment of syphilitic aortitis. Circulation 1952; 5:771–8.
    Even penicillin therapy probably is not effective in altering the patient's prognosis once cardiovascular syphilis is present.

DISSECTING AORTIC ANEURYSM

A dissection of the aorta is said to exist when a tear in the aortic intima is followed by an accumulation of blood in the media. It occurs most commonly in individuals whose aortic media lacks strength and durability. Specifically, patients with systemic arterial hypertension or cystic medial necrosis most often have dissection. In addition, aortic dissection occurs with increased frequency during the last trimester of pregnancy as well as in those with extensive aortic atherosclerotic involvement, bicuspid aortic valves, or coarctation of the aorta. Finally, blunt chest trauma can lead to an aortic dissection.

Aortic dissections are classified anatomically into three types. A type I dissection begins in the ascending aorta and extends at least into the aortic arch and possibly even the descending thoracic aorta and abdominal aorta. A type II dissection begins in the ascending aorta but ends before the innominate artery, whereas a type III dissection begins at or distal to the left subclavian artery and, therefore, involves only the descending aorta.

The patient with an aortic dissection almost always complains of severe chest or back pain. Although it is sometimes described as "tearing," "lacerating," or "as if something has torn loose," it may closely simulate angina pectoris or acute myocardial infarction. Many other symptoms and signs may appear if the aortic dissection compromises blood flow to specific organs. For example, the patient may complain of hemiplegia or transient blindness; he may have evidence of dissection-induced aortic regurgitation; he may note epigastric pain, vomiting, melena, and hematemesis (due to involvement of the mesenteric arteries); he may have oliguria or hematuria (due to renal arterial involvement); or he may complain of hoarseness (due to stretching of the recurrent laryngeal nerve) or Horner's syndrome (due to involvement of the stellate ganglion).

On physical examination, the pulses in the extremities are usually equal, but 30 to 40 percent of patients with an aortic dissection have a unilateral reduction in blood pressure and pulse in an upper extremity. If the dissection involves the pericardium, the patient may have evidence of pericardial effusion or tamponade, including jugular venous distention, a pulsus paradoxus, a quiet precordium with muffled heart sounds, and occasionally, a pericardial friction rub. If the dissection involves the aortic valve, a murmur of aortic regurgitation is usually present. Dullness to percussion and auscultation at the base of one lung, due to a bloody pleural effusion, may be present. Finally, a variety of neurologic abnormalities may appear if the cerebral or spinal cord vessels are involved.

The chest x-ray of the patient with ascending aortic dissection usually demonstrates a widening of the superior mediastinum, but such widening may not be present when the dissection is distal. The trachea may be deviated to the right, and a unilateral pleural effusion may be present. The ECG often shows left ventricular hypertrophy. Although it usually does not demonstrate the changes of an acute myocardial infarction, these alterations may be present if the dissection involves a coronary artery. An echocardiogram may demonstrate a true and false aortic lumen, but the absence of two lumens does not exclude the diagnosis of aortic dissection. The definitive diagnosis of aortic dissection is best made by aortography. In some patients, one may visualize the true and false aortic lumens, whereas in others the angiographic evidence of dissection is more subtle, including compression of the true aortic lumen, thickening of the aortic wall, or an abnormal catheter position within the aorta.

The patient with an aortic dissection of any type should be placed in an intensive care unit and given sufficient trimethaphan to reduce systemic arterial pressure to the lowest level compatible with adequate cerebral, cardiac, and renal perfusion; in most individuals, this is a systolic arterial pressure of 100 to 110 mm Hg. Since tachyphylaxis to trimethaphan develops within 24 to 36 hours, additional antihypertensive agents should be initiated, such as alphamethyldopa and beta-adrenergic blocking agents. Such intensive pharmacologic therapy is successful in 80 to 90 percent of patients. Once blood pressure is controlled, aortography is performed to localize the intimal tear and to determine if major vessels are involved. Immediate surgical therapy is warranted for any of the following: (1) severe aortic regurgitation, (2) pericardial tamponade, (3) leakage of the aneurysm, (4) occlusion of a major systemic artery, (5) a dissection originating in the ascending aorta, or (6) progressive enlargement of the aneurysm. In addition, some authors have suggested that a persistent communication between the true and false aortic lumens carries a poor outlook with medical therapy and, therefore, should be corrected surgically. In general, type III aortic dissections are well treated medically. Indeed, the risk of neurologic sequelae with operative intervention for a type III dissection makes surgical therapy unattractive.

Without aggressive therapy, aortic dissection is a rapidly fatal disease in most individuals. Although most patients reach the hospital alive, 50 percent die within 48 hours. Even in those treated surgically, subsequent medical therapy with agents to control blood pressure and to reduce left ventricular contractility is required. Finally, the prophylactic use of beta-adrenergic blocking agents in patients with connective tissue abnormalities (e.g., Marfan's syndrome) is recommended to prevent aortic dissection.

1. Brown OR, Popp RL, Kloster FE. Echocardiographic criteria for aortic root dissection. Am J Cardiol 1975; 36:17–20.
   Some patients without clinical aortic dissection demonstrate many of its echocardiographic features.
2. Debakey ME, Henly WS, Cooley DA, Morris GC Jr, Crawford ES, Beall AC Jr. Surgical management of dissecting aneurysms of the aorta. J Thorac Cardiovasc Surg 1965; 49:130–49.
   A description of the 3 anatomic types of dissection as well as their surgical treatment.
3. Hirst AE Jr, Johns VJ Jr, Kime SW Jr. Dissecting aneurysm of the aorta: a review of 505 cases. Medicine 1958; 37:217–79.
   An exhaustive review of the etiology, pathogenesis, clinical manifestations, therapy, and prognosis of this entity. Includes 346 references.
4. Lindsay J Jr, Hurst JW. Clinical features and prognosis in dissecting aneurysm of the aorta: a re-appraisal. Circulation 1967; 35:880–8.
   A review of 62 patients with dissection. In many ways, dissection of the ascending aorta behaves differently from that of the descending aorta.
5. McFarland J, Willerson JT, Dinsmore RE, Austen WG, Buckley MJ, Sanders CA, DeSanctis RW. The medical treatment of dissecting aortic aneurysms. N Engl J Med 1972; 286:115–9.
   Of 33 patients with aortic dissection treated medically, 17 (52%) survived, with an average follow-up of 3½ years.
6. Moothart RW, Spangler RD, Blount SG Jr. Echocardiography in aortic root dissection and dilatation. Am J Cardiol 1975; 36:11–16.
   Of 6 patients with aortic dissection, echo was diagnostic in 5 and suggestive in the other.
7. Murdoch JL, Walker BA, Halpern BL, Kuzma JW, McKusick VA. Life expectancy and causes of death in the Marfan syndrome. N Engl J Med 1972; 286:804–8.
   Many patients with Marfan syndrome die at a young age of cardiac problems, including aortic dilatation and dissection.
8. Nanda NC, Gramiak R, Shah PM. Diagnosis of aortic root dissection by echocardiography. Circulation 1973; 48:506–13.
   Demonstration of enlargement of the aortic root with marked parallel widening of anterior or posterior walls appears to be specific for aortic root involvement in dissecting aneurysm of the aorta.
9. Palmer RF, Wheat MW Jr. Treatment of dissecting aneurysm of the aorta. Ann Thorac Surg 1967; 4:38–52.
   With medical treatment of aortic dissection, the overall success rate approaches 90%.
10. Shuford WH, Sybers RG, Weens HS. Problems in the aortographic diagnosis of dissecting aneurysm of the aorta. N Engl J Med 1969; 280:225–31.
    The aortographic diagnosis of dissection can be extremely difficult.
11. Slater EE, DeSanctis RW. The clinical recognition of dissecting aortic aneurysm. Am J Med 1976; 60:625–33.
    Almost all the 125 patients with aortic dissection had chest or back pain and an abnormal chest x-ray.
12. Wheat MW Jr, Palmer RF. Dissecting aneurysms of the aorta: present status of drug versus surgical therapy. Prog Cardiovasc Dis 1968; 11:198–210.
    Surgical intervention is necessary only if aortic regurgitation, aneurysmal leakage, or occlusion of a major branch of the aorta develops.
13. Roberts WC. Aortic dissection: anatomy, consequences, and causes. Am Heart J 1981; 101:195–214.
    An extensive review of the anatomic features, causes, and consequences of aortic dissection.

14. Moncada R, Churchill R, Reynes C, Gunnar RM, Salinas M, Love L, Demos T, Pifarre R. Diagnosis of dissecting aortic aneurysm by computed tomography. Lancet 1981; 1:238–41.

The results of computed tomography with contrast injection in 16 patients suspected of having aortic dissection are presented. All 11 with aortic dissection were recognized correctly by CT.

15. Victor MF, Mintz GS, Kotler MN, Wilson AR, Segal BL. Two dimensional echocardiographic diagnosis of aortic dissection. Am J Cardiol 1981; 48:1155–9.

Two-dimensional echocardiography detected the intimal flap in 12 of 15 patients with dissection, whereas it missed the other 3; in addition, it suggested one false positive.

16. Cooley DA, Ott DA, Frazier OH, Walker WE. Surgical treatment of aneurysms of the transverse aortic arch: experience with 25 patients using hypothermic techniques. Ann Thorac Surg 1981; 32:260–72.

Surgical methods of correcting this difficult kind of aortic dissection are discussed.

17. Crawford ES, Walker HSJ III, Saleh SA, Normann NA. Graft replacement of aneurysm in descending thoracic aorta: results without bypass or shunting. Surgery 1981; 89:73–85.

The surgical results in 148 patients with aneurysms confined to the thoracic aorta between the left subclavian artery and the diaphragm are described.

18. Arciniegas JG, Soto B, Little WC, Papapietro SE. Cineangiography in the diagnosis of aortic dissection. Am J Cardiol 1981; 47:890–4.

In this series of 20 patients with acute dissection, cineangiography was helpful in diagnosing and localizing the dissection.

19. Wheat MW Jr. Acute dissecting aneurysms of the aorta: diagnosis and treatment—1979. Am Heart J 1980; 99:373–87.

A concise review of the pathogenesis, clinical and radiographic findings, and therapy of aortic dissection.

ACUTE RHEUMATIC FEVER

Acute rheumatic fever develops because of an unusual host reaction to pharyngitis caused by group A streptococci. Although it occurs randomly in about 0.3 percent of patients with pharyngitis in whom beta-hemolytic group A streptococci are cultured, its incidence may be as high as 3 percent during epidemics caused by more virulent streptococcal group A strains. Acute rheumatic fever occurs most commonly in patients between 3 and 15 years of age; it is rare before age 2 and after age 25. It occurs most frequently in children living in crowded conditions and is especially common during cold weather. Among industrialized nations, Mexico, Greece, and Israel have the highest attack rates, and the large cities of the northern United States have a tenfold higher incidence than cities in the south. Improved economic conditions with resultant less crowding have caused a decline in the incidence of rheumatic fever. In addition, the use of effective antibiotics has greatly reduced its frequency.

Approximately 65 to 70 percent of patients with rheumatic fever have noted a recent pharyngitis or upper respiratory infection, whereas the remaining 30 to 35 percent cannot remember such an infection. Nevertheless, by serologic testing, these individuals have an elevation of serum antibodies to streptococcal antigens consistent with a recent silent pharyngitis. The patient who develops acute rheumatic fever manifests an immune response to streptococcal antigen that differs from the patient who does not develop rheumatic fever. The individual who develops rheumatic fever produces an abundance of antibodies to streptococcal polysaccharide A, but these antibodies have a lower binding affinity for the antigen than those that are produced by patients without rheumatic fever. In the patient with rheumatic fever, a high antibody titer to streptococcal polysaccharide A may persist for years despite penicillin prophylaxis and no further streptococcal infection. In contrast, those in whom rheumatic fever does not develop have a rapid decline in antibody titer after the acute streptococcal infection resolves. Since streptococcal polysaccharide A closely resembles a glycoprotein in mammalian heart valves, this chronic persistence of antibody may predispose the patient to continuing valvular damage.

Following a streptococcal infection, the time of onset of the symptoms and signs of acute rheumatic fever varies substantially from one patient to the next. The acute pharyngitis usually resolves in 5 to 7 days, after which there is a latent period of 7 to 10 days. Subsequently, a number of symptoms and signs may appear. A *relapsing fever* is often the first symptom of acute rheumatic fever. A migratory *polyarthritis* usually appears early in the course of the disease, and it may be severe and disabling. It usually involves the large joints of the lower extremities. The synovial membrane of the involved joints is covered with fibrin and polymorphonuclear leukocytes, and the joint fluid usually has a diminished viscosity and numerous polymorphonuclear cells (2,000–10,000/ mm^3). Permanent bony destruction and soft tissue damage are rare. Acute rheumatic *carditis* may appear concomitant with the polyarthritis or up to several weeks afterward. The patient may complain of dyspnea and fatigue, and on examination he may have cardiomegaly, a persistent tachycardia, a left-sided valvular regurgitant murmur (most often mitral), or a ventricular gallop. In addition, a mitral mid-diastolic rumble (the so-called Carey-Coombs murmur) may be audible. In children with acute rheumatic fever, *erythema marginatum* and *subcutaneous nodules* may appear in conjunction with the polyarthritis. *Sydenham's chorea* may occur on occasion. In general, it appears much later (often as long as 2 months) after the other manifestations of rheumatic fever.

The patient with acute rheumatic carditis may have several alterations on the chest x-ray, most commonly generalized cardiomegaly with straightening of the left heart border. Additional x-ray findings depend on the valves that are involved, the hemodynamic importance of the valvular lesions, the presence or absence of a pericardial effusion, and the chronicity of the alterations. Electrocardiographically, 30 to 35 percent of patients with acute carditis have a prolonged P–R interval, but this also occurs in some patients with streptococcal infection without carditis. Nonspecific S–T and T wave abnormalities are noted in the majority, and second or third degree heart block and premature atrial or ventricular beats are seen in some. The laboratory findings in the patient with acute rheumatic fever include an elevated erythrocyte sedimentation rate (ESR) and C-reactive protein during the active phase of inflammation. Since the C-reactive protein may fall 1 to 2 weeks before the ESR, it may be used to determine the optimal timing for ambulation or hospital discharge. The antistreptolysin (ASO) titer, antistreptococcal hyaluronidase, and antistreptococcal DNAase can be used to demonstrate a recent streptococcal infection in more than 95 percent of patients.

A variety of infectious or inflammatory conditions should be considered in the patient with the symptoms and signs described above. Subacute bacterial endocarditis may appear clinically similar to acute rheumatic fever, and therefore, the patient should be examined for splinter hemorrhages, Osler's nodes, and splenomegaly, and several blood samples should be obtained for culture. Several other viral and bacterial infections may mimic acute rheumatic fever, including hepatitis B, brucellosis, miliary tuberculosis, cat-scratch fever, staphylococcal osteomyelitis, gonnococcal arthritis, and meningococcal arthritis. Similarly, several acute inflammatory conditions may be confused with it, such as rheumatoid arthritis, systemic lupus erythematosus, and serum sickness.

To prevent the development of acute rheumatic fever, streptococcal pharyngitis should be treated early in its course (i.e., before the eighth or ninth day after its onset). The child should receive 600,000 to 900,000 units of benzathine penicillin G and the adult 1.2 million units. Alternatively, the child or adult may be given 250,000 units of oral penicillin G 4 times daily for 10 days. If the patient is allergic to penicillin, he should receive erythromycin in divided doses for 10 days. Once the diagnosis of acute rheumatic fever is made, the patient with polyarthritis or carditis should be treated with bed rest and high doses of aspirin (i.e., 650 mg orally every 4 hr). After the polyarthritis has been controlled successfully for 2 weeks, the aspirin dosage should be tapered down to 650 mg 3 to 4 times daily for an additional 6 weeks. The patient should be allowed to ambulate and return home when the ESR and C-reactive protein have returned to normal. If active congestive heart failure occurs with acute rheumatic carditis, steroid therapy should be initiated. Specifically, prednisone, 40 to 60 mg daily, should be administered for 2 to 3 weeks, after which the dosage is tapered slowly over 3 weeks. A clinical or laboratory "rebound" of rheumatic activity may occur when aspirin or steroid therapy is abruptly discontinued. Finally, the patient with rheumatic carditis should be placed at bed rest for a minimum of 6 weeks.

The most effective rheumatic fever prophylaxis is the monthly intramuscular administration of 1.2 million units of benzathine penicillin G. Alternatively, oral penicillin may be administered on a daily basis. Those patients who require prophylaxis include those with a previous episode of rheumatic fever who are under the age of 30, and those patients, even though they may be older than 30, who are regularly exposed to young children.

1. Bisno AL, Pearce IA, Wall HP, Moody MD, Stollerman GH. Contrasting epidemiology of acute rheumatic fever and acute glomerulonephritis: nature of the antecedent streptococcal infection. N Engl J Med 1970; 283:561–5.
   The strains of streptococci that cause pyoderma do not lead to acute rheumatic fever.
2. Spagnuolo M, Pasternack B, Taranta A. Risk of rheumatic fever recurrences after streptococcal infections: prospective study of clinical and social factors. N Engl J Med 1971; 285:641–7.
   Those individuals with a high risk of recurrent episodes of rheumatic fever included (1) those with symptomatic pharyngitis, (2) those of young age, and (3) those who had recently sustained an episode of rheumatic fever.
3. McDanald EC, Weisman MH. Articular manifestations of rheumatic fever in adults. Ann Intern Med 1978; 89:917–20.
   Six adult patients are described who had a lower-extremity, large joint polyarthritis following a streptococcal infection. The authors suggest that this syndrome be called poststreptococcal arthritis rather than acute rheumatic fever.
4. Gibney R, Reinick HJ, Bannayan GA, Stein JH. Renal lesions in acute rheumatic fever. Ann Intern Med 1981; 94:322–6.
   Transient abnormalities of the urinary sediment may occur with acute rheumatic fever. This article describes 4 patients with such findings, including the results of renal biopsies.
5. Feinstein AR, Spagnuolo M. The clinical patterns of acute rheumatic fever: a reappraisal. Medicine 1962; 41:279–305.
   An elegant and thorough review of this disease entity, including 115 references.
6. Czoniczer G, Amezcua F, Pelargonio S, Massell BF. Therapy of severe rheumatic

carditis: comparison of adrenocortical steroids and aspirin. Circulation 1964; 29:813–9.
In 145 patients with rheumatic carditis, steroids were more effective than aspirin in preventing death and hastening recovery.

7. Stollerman GH. Factors determining the attack rate of rheumatic fever. JAMA 1961; 177:823–8.
The frequency with which rheumatic fever follows a streptococcal infection is related to the intensity of the antigenic stimulus, which, in turn, is related to strain virulence.

8. Stollerman GH. Nephritogenic and rheumatogenic group A streptococci. J Infect Dis 1969; 120:258–63.
A succinct review of the 2 broad categories of group A streptococci—those producing rheumatic fever following pharyngitis but apparently incapable of producing glomerulonephritis at the same time, and those producing glomerulonephritis following skin or throat infections but seemingly incapable of producing rheumatic fever.

9. Wannamaker LW. Differences between streptococcal infections of the throat and of the skin. N Engl J Med 1970; 282:23–31, 78–85.
A thorough review of the clinical and laboratory features of the 2 most common streptococcal infections—pharyngitis and impetigo/pyoderma.

10. Johnson EE, Stollerman GH, Grossman BJ. Rheumatic recurrences in patients not receiving continuous prophylaxis. JAMA 1964; 190:407–13.
In patients with prior rheumatic fever not receiving antibiotic prophylaxis, recurrences of rheumatic fever were common in adolescents and much less common in adults.

11. Goldstein I, Halpern B, Robert L. Immunological relationship between streptococcus A polysaccharide and the structural glycoproteins of heart valve. Nature 1967; 213:44–7.
In the experimental animal, antibodies to human valvular tissue also react with those from group A streptococci.

12. Pader E, Elster SK. Studies of acute rheumatic fever in the adult: I. Clinical and laboratory manifestations in 30 patients. Am J Med 1959; 26:424–41.
Rheumatic fever in the adult differs from childhood rheumatic fever in the higher incidence of arthritis as compared to carditis, as well as the extremely low incidence of subcutaneous nodules, chorea, and erythema marginatum.

13. Massell BF, Fyler DC, Roy SB. The clinical picture of rheumatic fever: diagnosis, immediate prognosis, course, and therapeutic implications. Am J Cardiol 1958; 1:436–49.
Of 490 children and adolescents with rheumatic fever, 113(23%) had chorea; 260(53%) had heart murmurs; 39(8%) developed congestive heart failure; 59(12%) had subcutaneous nodules; and 54(11%) had erythema marginatum.

14. Rosenthal A, Czoniczer G, Massell BF. Rheumatic fever under 3 years of age: a report of 10 cases. Pediatrics 1968; 41:612–9.
Rheumatic fever in the first few years of life is rare but not nonexistent. It comprised 0.5% of all cases in children under age 16.

15. Stollerman GH. Prognosis and treatment of acute rheumatic fever: the possible effect of treatment on subsequent cardiac disease. Prog Cardiovasc Dis 1960; 3:193–203.
Corticosteroids and aspirin are both helpful in the management of patients with severe rheumatic carditis.

16. Tierney RC, Kaplan S. Treatment of Sydenham's chorea. Am J Dis Child 1965; 109:408–11.
In 28 patients with chorea, chlorpromazine was effective in decreasing the motor manifestations and shortening the course of the disease.

17. DiSciascio G, Taranta A. Rheumatic fever in children. Am Heart J 1980; 99:635–58.
A thorough review of the epidemiology, clinical manifestations, laboratory findings, treatment, and prevention of rheumatic fever in children, including 149 references.

18. Escudero J, Stanislawsky E, Escudero X. Fulminant acute rheumatic fever with multisystem involvement. Am Heart J 1983; 105:161–2.
This case report describes a 14-year-old boy with fatal acute rheumatic carditis.

CONNECTIVE TISSUE DISEASES AND THE HEART

Systemic lupus erythematosus (SLE) can involve the endocardium, myocardium, or pericardium. Libman-Sachs verrucous endocarditis is one of the most common cardiac manifestations of SLE, occurring in about 50 percent of patients. The Libman-Sachs valvular lesions are wart-like, pink, and somewhat granular in consistency. They vary from 0.5 to 4.0 mm in diameter. Although they may form anywhere on the endocardial surface, they most frequently appear in the angles of the mitral and tricuspid valves as well as on the underside of the mitral valve. Aortic valve involvement has been described in an occasional patient. Only rarely do these lesions become large enough to interfere with valvular function.

Since the small-vessel vasculitis of SLE often involves the arterioles that supply the myocardium, a diffuse myocarditis with poor systolic and diastolic ventricular function may occur. Subclinical myocarditis is common in patients with SLE, whereas more obvious myocardial involvement occurs uncommonly. The cardiac conducting system may be involved by the inflammatory process, leading to atrial and ventricular arrhythmias. Rarely, the arteritis of SLE occurs in the larger coronary arteries, causing angina pectoris or myocardial infarction. Independent of the vasculitis that sometimes involves the myocardium in patients with SLE, many of these individuals have renal involvement, with resultant systemic arterial hypertension and hypertensive heart disease.

Pericarditis is extremely common in patients with SLE, occurring in 60 to 70 percent in most series gathered at postmortem. Of these, about half have symptomatic pericarditis. The acute pericardial inflammation is often accompanied by a pericardial effusion, which ranges from clear to sanguinous in consistency. The effusion may be voluminous in amount. On occasion, a rapidly accumulating effusion may cause tamponade, but only rarely does the pericarditis and effusion of SLE lead to chronic constriction. In most patients, episodes of pericarditis occur randomly and independently of the systemic disease.

Electrocardiographically, the patient with SLE usually has nonspecific ST–T wave abnormalities. If a pericardial effusion is present, the QRS amplitude may be diminished. Left bundle branch block or episodes of high-degree AV block may occur. Atrial arrhythmias, most commonly atrial fibrillation and flutter, occur in 5 to 10 percent of patients with SLE. Left ventricular hypertrophy secondary to systemic arterial hypertension is a common finding.

If congestive heart failure occurs in the patient with SLE, digitalis, diuretics, and salt restriction should be prescribed. Occasionally, corticosteroids may be required to suppress the acute inflammatory process. Strict control of systemic arterial pressure is mandatory. If pericardial tamponade occurs, pericardiocentesis and even pericardiectomy may be required.

Periarteritis nodosa is a necrotizing vasculitis that usually involves medium- and large-sized muscular arteries. The coronary arteries are occasionally involved, resulting in angina pectoris or myocardial infarction. The renal arteries are usually extensively involved, and as a result, systemic arterial hypertension, often severe, occurs frequently, leading eventually to hypertensive heart disease. Although pericarditis (with or without effusion) occurs occasionally in the patient with periarteritis nodosa, endocardial and valvular involvement does not occur.

Clinically, periarteritis nodosa commonly leads to left ventricular failure due to severe, long-standing hypertension. Angina pectoris and myocardial infarction occur infrequently, as do cardiac arrhythmias. On the ECG, nonspecific ST–T wave abnormalities are often present, believed secondary to patchy myocardial fibrosis, and left ventricular hypertrophy is common. Right or left bundle branch block, AV block, and supraventricular tachycardia occur infrequently. The routine chest x-ray may demonstrate left ventricular dilatation and pulmonary vascular redistribution. Peripheral arteriography may show multiple small aneurysms of the medium and large arteries.

If periarteritis nodosa involves the heart, glucocorticosteroids should be administered in large doses. In some patients with severe, refractory congestive heart failure, steroid therapy may induce a dramatic response. In addition, the usual pharmacologic agents for the treatment of heart failure (digitalis and diuretics) should be administered. Systemic arterial hypertension should be controlled with whatever medications are necessary.

Scleroderma most often involves the myocardium, causing the gradual replacement of left ventricular myocytes with nonvascular connective tissue. Although this process may involve all cardiac chambers, it most commonly involves the left ventricle, including the papillary muscles. Pericarditis with or without effusion occurs frequently in patients with scleroderma, and in one report it was shown to be present in two-thirds of scleroderma patients at the time of postmortem examination. However, pericardial tamponade and constriction are distinctly rare. Since patients with scleroderma commonly have pulmonary and/or systemic arterial hypertension, right and left ventricular hypertrophy, dilatation, and failure may eventually appear.

The cardiac manifestations of scleroderma usually are not prominent until late in the course of the disease, at which time the patient has symptoms of left- and right-sided congestive heart failure: dyspnea on exertion, orthopnea, paroxysmal nocturnal dyspnea, ankle edema, abdominal swelling due to ascites, and easy fatigability. Pericardial involvement may cause the clinical picture of acute pericarditis. The ECG demonstrates various degrees of AV block or bundle branch block, and right or left ventricular hypertrophy may be present. Diffuse myocardial fibrosis often is reflected by nonspecific ST–T wave abnormalities. If pericardial involvement is present, S–T segment elevation and diminished QRS amplitude may be present. The chest radiograph usually demonstrates generalized cardiomegaly.

There is no specific therapy for sclerodermal cardiac disease. Digitalis, diuretics, and salt restriction may induce some improvement. Pericarditis with or without effusion may respond to nonsteroidal anti-inflammatory agents or corticosteroids.

Although cardiac involvement is frequent in patients with *dermatomyositis,* it is usually not of great clinical importance. In many patients, microscopic infiltration of the myocardial interstitium with fibrous tissue is observed pathologically, but symptoms of left ventricular dysfunction are uncommon. Alternatively, pulmonary hypertension due to primary lung involvement may cause right ventricular hypertrophy, dilatation, and failure. Pericarditis is rare in the patient with dermatomyositis. Electrocardiographically, one usually sees nonspecific ST–T wave abnormalities, but on occasion, the patient with dermatomyositis may have atrial arrhythmias, AV block, or bundle branch block. If cardiac involvement with dermatomyositis is clinically apparent, the patient should receive corticosteroids, and the usual therapeutic measures (digitalis, diuretics, and salt restriction) should be initiated.

Although the heart is frequently involved by the inflammatory process of *rheumatoid arthritis,* its overall function is rarely affected. First, many individuals (as many as 50%) with rheumatoid arthritis have a subclinical form of fibrinous pericarditis, but only a small number of these (about 1–2%) develop symptomatic and clinically apparent pericardial involvement. Of patients whose arthritis is severe enough to require hospitalization, symptomatic pericarditis occurs in about 10 percent. The pericarditis of rheumatoid arthritis may appear without relation to the duration of the arthritis, and on occasion it may even precede the onset of more active arthritis. Second, most patients whose rheumatoid arthritis is accompanied by subcutaneous rheumatoid nodules have pathologic evidence of nodular granulomas within the myocardium and endocardium. Only rarely do these granulomas compromise myocardial or valvular function, but on occasion they may achieve large enough proportions to produce severe valvular regurgitation. Third, some patients with severe rheumatoid arthritis have microscopic evidence of a diffuse myocarditis, which may cause biventricular congestive heart failure. Fourth, about 20 percent of patients with rheumatoid arthritis have evidence on postmortem examination of coronary arteritis, but only rarely does this inflammatory process cause angina pectoris or myocardial infarction.

Some patients with *ankylosing spondylitis* have valvular, myocardial, or pericardial involvement. Aortic regurgitation results from a thickening and shortening of the valve cusps as well as aortic root dilatation due to the destruction of aortic elastic tissue. Less commonly, patients with spondylitis have a diffuse infiltration of the myocardium with fibrous tissue and mucinous ground substance, leading to the clinical picture of a congestive cardiomyopathy. Pericarditis may be observed at postmortem examination but is seldom apparent clinically.

The acute stage of *Reiter's disease* may be accompanied by clinical and electrocardiographic evidence of pericarditis and myocarditis. Similar to patients with ankylosing spondylitis, these individuals occasionally have aortic regurgitation.

Systemic Lupus Erythematosus

1. Borenstein DG, Fye WB, Arnett FC, Stevens MB. The myocarditis of systemic lupus erythematosus: association with myositis. Ann Intern Med 1978; 89:619–24.
   Most patients with myocarditis due to SLE have clinically evident myositis, suggesting a generalized inflammatory process directed against striated muscle.
2. Brigden W, Bywaters E, Lessof M, Ross IP. The heart in systemic lupus erythematosus. Br Heart J 1960; 22:1–16.
   At postmortem examination, most patients with SLE have pericarditis.
3. Bulkley BH, Roberts WC. The heart in systemic lupus erythematosus and the changes induced in it by corticosteroid therapy: a study of 36 necropsy patients. Am J Med 1975; 58:243–64.
   Although often vital in the management of SLE, corticosteroids have a deleterious effect on the heart: systemic hypertension and left ventricular hypertrophy appear or, when present, worsen; congestive cardiac failure increases; epicardial and myocardial fat increases; and coronary atherosclerosis is accelerated.
4. Hejtmancik MR, Wright JC, Quint R, Jennings FL. The cardiovascular manifestations of systemic lupus erythematosus. Am Heart J 1964; 68:119–30.
   Of 142 patients with SLE, 24(17%) had clinical evidence of pericarditis, 30(21%) of myocarditis, and 9(6%) of endocarditis. Congestive heart failure occurred in 10(7%) and was usually due to myocarditis.
5. Paget SA, Bulkley BH, Grauer LE, Seningen R. Mitral valve disease of systemic lupus erythematosus: a cause of severe congestive heart failure reversed by valve replacement. Am J Med 1975; 59:134–9.

Although Libman-Sachs endocarditis occurs in about half the patients with SLE, it does not always cause an audible murmur, it is rarely associated with clinically severe valvular dysfunction, and, therefore, it is not usually recognized during life. This article describes an 18-year-old woman whose Libman-Sachs endocarditis was severe enough to require mitral valve replacement.

6. Strauer BE, Brune I, Schenk H, Knoll D, Perings E. Lupus cardiomyopathy: cardiac mechanics, hemodynamics, and coronary blood flow in uncomplicated systemic lupus erythematosus. Am Heart J 1976; 92:715–22.
   Invasive studies in 5 women with SLE demonstrated impaired pump function, reduced contractility, increased myocardial stiffness, and decreased coronary vascular reserve.
7. Bidani AK, Roberts JL, Schwartz MM, Lewis EJ. Immunopathology of cardiac lesions in fatal systemic lupus erythematosus. Am J Med 1980; 69:849–58.
   Immune reactants can be demonstrated in the cardiac tissues of most patients with severe active and fatal SLE, indicating a major pathogenetic role for immune complexes in the mediation of cardiac injury in SLE.
8. Pritzker MR, Ernst JD, Caudill C, Wilson CS, Weaver WF, Edwards JE. Acquired aortic stenosis in systemic lupus erythematosus. Ann Intern Med 1980; 93:434–6.
   Two patients are described with SLE and valvular aortic stenosis resulting from massive thrombotic deposits on the valve.

Periarteritis Nodosa
9. Holsinger DR, Osmundson PJ, Edwards JE. The heart in periarteritis nodosa. Circulation 1962; 25:610–8.
   Of 66 patients with periarteritis, 41 had evidence at postmortem of a necrotizing arteritis of the coronary arteries.
10. Griffith GC, Vural IL. Polyarteritis nodosa: correlation of clinical and postmortem findings in 17 cases. Circulation 1951; 3:481–91.
    Of 17 cases of periarteritis examined at postmortem, 13 had cardiac abnormalities.

Scleroderma
11. Gladman DD, Gordon DA, Urowitz MB, Levy HL. Pericardial fluid analysis in scleroderma (systemic sclerosis). Am J Med 1976; 60:1064–8.
    Pericardial involvement is the most common form of cardiac involvement in scleroderma.
12. McWhorter JE, LeRoy EC. Pericardial disease in scleroderma (systemic sclerosis). Am J Med 1974; 57:566–75.
    In postmortem studies, pericardial involvement is present in 60–65% of patients with scleroderma.
13. Ridolfi RL, Bulkley BH, Hutchins GM. The cardiac conduction system in progressive systemic sclerosis: clinical and pathologic features of 35 patients. Am J Med 1976; 61:361–6.
    The conduction system is uncommonly involved by the myocardial fibrotic changes of scleroderma. The high incidence of conduction disturbances is a result of damage to working myocardium.
14. Sackner MA, Heinz ER, Steinberg AJ. The heart in scleroderma. Am J Cardiol 1966; 17:542–59.
    The most frequent site of cardiac involvement in patients with scleroderma is the pericardium; also common is right ventricular hypertrophy due to pulmonary hypertension.
15. Smith JW, Clements PJ, Levisman J, Furst D, Ross M. Echocardiographic features of progressive systemic sclerosis (PSS): correlation with hemodynamic and postmortem studies. Am J Med 1979; 66:28–33.
    In a large group of patients with scleroderma, pericardial effusion was demonstrable by echocardiography in 22 (41%), although it was suspected clinically in only 7 patients.
16. Pisko E, Gallup K, Turner R, Parker M, Nomeir AM, Box J, Davis J, Box P, Rothberger H. Cardiopulmonary manifestations of progressive systemic sclerosis: associations with circulating immune complexes and fluorescent antinuclear antibodies. Arthritis Rheum 1979; 22:518–23.

Sixteen patients with scleroderma were evaluated, and 4 (25%) had echocardiographic abnormalities.

17. Clements PJ, Furst DE, Cabeen W, Tashkin D, Paulus HE, Roberts N. The relationship of arrhythmias and conduction disturbances to other manifestations of cardiopulmonary disease in progressive systemic sclerosis (PSS). Am J Med 1981; 71:38–46.

    Of 46 ambulatory patients with scleroderma, conduction disturbances (sinus node dysfunction, first degree AV block, pre-excitation), supraventricular and ventricular arrhythmias were observed by Holter monitoring in 26 (57%).

18. Roberts NK, Cabeen WR Jr, Moss J, Clements PJ, Furst DE. The prevalence of conduction defects and cardiac arrhythmias in progressive systemic sclerosis. Ann Intern Med 1981; 94:38–40.

    In 50 patients with scleroderma, 31(62%) had serious electrical abnormalities, including supraventricular tachyarrhythmias, conduction disturbances, coupled ventricular extrasystoles, and ventricular tachycardia.

19. Duska F, Bradna P, Novak J, Kubicek J, Vizda J, Kafka P, Mazurova Y, Blaha V. Pyrophosphate heart scan in patients with progressive systemic sclerosis. Br Heart J 1982; 47:90–3.

    Of 17 patients with scleroderma, 7 had evidence by pyrophosphate scanning of myocardial damage.

20. Botstein GR, LeRoy EC. Primary heart disease in systemic sclerosis (scleroderma): advances in clinical and pathologic features, pathogenesis, and new therapeutic approaches. Am Heart J 1981; 102:913–9.

    A good overall review of the various ways in which scleroderma may affect the heart.

Dermatomyositis

21. Schaumburg HH, Nielsen SL, Yurchak PM. Heart block in polymyositis. N Engl J Med 1971; 284:480–1.

    Polymyositis in a 26-year-old man involved the cardiac conduction system, with the initial appearance of AV block and eventually persistent ventricular asystole.

22. Oka M, Raasakka T. Cardiac involvement in polymyositis. Scand J Rheumatol 1978; 7:203–8.

    Sixteen cases of polymyositis are described, 11 of whom (69%) had cardiac involvement.

23. Reid JM, Murdoch R. Polymyositis and complete heart block. Br Heart J 1979; 41:628–9.

    A 37-year-old man is described with polymyositis who developed complete heart block.

24. Kehoe RF, Bauernfeind R, Tommaso C, Wyndham C, Rosen KM. Cardiac conduction defects in polymyositis: electrophysiologic studies in 4 patients. Ann Intern Med 1981; 94:41–3.

    This study provides electrophysiologic data localizing the site of spontaneously occurring AV block to the infra-AV nodal region.

Rheumatoid Arthritis

25. Khan AH, Spodick DH. Rheumatoid heart disease. Semin Arthritis Rheum 1972; 1:327–37.

    A concise yet thorough discussion of cardiac abnormalities in patients with rheumatoid arthritis.

26. Kirk J, Cosh J. The pericarditis of rheumatoid arthritis. Q J Med 1969; 38:397–423.

    An extremely detailed discussion of this disease entity.

27. Bacon PA, Gibson DG. Cardiac involvement in rheumatoid arthritis: an echocardiographic study. Ann Rheum Dis 1974; 33:20–4.

    Of 44 patients with rheumatoid arthritis, 15 (34%) had a pericardial effusion by echocardiography; of the subgroup, with subcutaneous nodules, 50% had an effusion.

28. Lebowitz WB. The heart in rheumatoid arthritis (rheumatoid disease): a clinical and pathological study of 62 cases. Ann Intern Med 1963; 58:102–23.

An excellent overview of the many kinds of cardiac involvement that may appear in patients with rheumatoid arthritis.

Ankylosing Spondylitis

29. Kinsella TD, Johnson LG, Sutherland RI. Cardiovascular manifestations of ankylosing spondylitis. Can Med Assoc J 1974; 111:1309–11.
    Of 97 patients with ankylosing spondylitis, 8 had isolated aortic regurgitation, 3 had isolated heart block, 2 had combined aortic regurgitation and heart block, and 1 had mitral regurgitation.
30. Malette WG, Eiseman B, Danielson GK, Mozzoleni A, Rams JJ. Rheumatoid spondylitis and aortic insufficiency: an operable combination. J Thorac Cardiovasc Surg 1969; 57:471–4.
    The cases of 3 successful aortic valve replacements in patients with spondylitis are presented and discussed.
31. Demoulin JC, Lespagnard J, Bertholet M, Soumagne D. Acute fulminant aortic regurgitation in ankylosing spondylitis. Am Heart J 1983; 105:859–61.
    A case report of a 19-year-old male with ankylosing spondylitis and severe aortic regurgitation requiring valve replacement.

Reiter's Disease

32. Paulus HE, Pearson CM, Pitts W Jr. Aortic insufficiency in 5 patients with Reiter's syndrome: a detailed clinical and pathological study. Am J Med 1972; 53:464–72.
    In patients with Reiter's syndrome in whom aortic regurgitation develops, the arthritic syndrome tends to be very severe.
33. Neu LT Jr, Reider RA, Mack RE. Cardiac involvement in Reiter's disease: report of a case with review of the literature. Ann Intern Med 1960; 53:215–20.
    The incidence of cardiac involvement in this syndrome is approximately 12%.

PREGNANCY AND CARDIOVASCULAR ABNORMALITIES

The most prominent cardiovascular alteration induced by pregnancy is a 30- to 40-percent increase in cardiac output during the first 6 months, reaching its highest value at 20 to 24 weeks of gestation. Subsequently, cardiac output plateaus and then declines during the last 8 weeks of pregnancy. This fall in cardiac output during the later stages of pregnancy is caused by an obstruction of the inferior vena cava and the aortoiliac arteries by the enlarging uterus. Since heart rate increases by about 10 beats per minute during pregnancy, the increase in cardiac output is accomplished primarily by an increase in stroke volume.

Total blood volume increases substantially during pregnancy, beginning around the sixth week and gradually rising throughout the remainder of pregnancy. In fact, it may be augmented by as much as 45 to 50 percent in comparison to the nonpregnant state. This expansion of blood volume is caused by a major increase in plasma volume and a smaller increase in red cell volume. The augmentation of blood volume enlarges the vascular beds of the expanding uteroplacental circulation and the developing mammary glands; it helps to dissipate increased heat caused by an accelerated metabolic rate; and it protects against the deleterious effects of impaired venous return, with resultant sequestration of blood in the lower extremities.

These physiologic alterations that occur during pregnancy may make the recognition of heart disease difficult. Alternatively, they may induce major physiologic changes in patients with underlying cardiac disease, resulting in increased morbidity or even mortality. The enlarging uterus elevates the diaphragm and, therefore, may induce a change in the electrocardiographic QRS axis as well as in overall heart size. It also compresses the vena cava, which may cause ankle edema. The augmented cardiac output and stroke volume often cause an S_3, a systolic ejection murmur, and radiographic evidence of pulmonary vascular redistribution. Increased flow through the mammary vessels may cause a systolic or even a continuous murmur. Finally, a decrease in systemic vascular resistance may result in a diminution of the murmurs of aortic and mitral regurgitation.

Because of the increased demands that pregnancy places on the heart, the woman with valvular, congenital, or myocardial disease may not tolerate it. Pulmonary and peripheral venous congestion become especially prominent during the last 3 months of pregnancy, when total blood volume is maximal. Thus, the woman with valvular stenosis or regurgitation who is compensated hemodynamically before pregnancy may require additional medical therapy during pregnancy to maintain such compensation. The woman with severe pulmonary hypertension (primary or secondary) or cyanotic congenital heart disease often tolerates pregnancy poorly. As a result, these patients should avoid pregnancy or undergo therapeutic abortion if it occurs. Any woman with valvular disease should receive antibiotic prophylaxis during delivery, since transient bacteremia frequently occurs during the puerperium. Finally, women with prosthetic cardiac valves usually tolerate pregnancy without difficulty from a hemodynamic standpoint, but their continued anticoagulation throughout pregnancy and delivery requires a great deal of physician input.

1. Conradsson TB, Werko L. Management of heart disease in pregnancy. Prog Cardiovasc Dis 1974; 16:407–19.
   A review of the physical findings induced by pregnancy as well as its effects in women with underlying heart disease. Includes 87 references.
2. Burch GE. Heart disease and pregnancy. Am Heart J 1977; 93:104–16.
   A complete review of the management of pregnant patients with organic heart disease, including valvular, congenital, and hypertensive.
3. Lees MM, Taylor SH, Scott DB, Kerr MG. A study of cardiac output at rest throughout pregnancy. J Obstet Gynecol Br Comm 1967; 74:319–28.
   During pregnancy, cardiac output increases by 30–40%. Most of this increase is established by the end of the first trimester.
4. Lund CJ, Donovan JC. Blood volume during pregnancy: significance of plasma and red cell volumes. Am J Obstet Gynecol 1967; 98:393–403.
   In pregnancy, plasma volume begins to increase at about 6 weeks of gestation, rises rapidly to about 24 weeks, then rises more slowly until term is reached.
5. Cutforth R, MacDonald CB. Heart sounds and murmurs in pregnancy. Am Heart J 1966; 71:741–7.
   Of 50 pregnant women, 42 (84%) developed an S_3, and 46 (92%) developed a systolic ejection murmur. These sounds appeared 12–20 weeks into pregnancy and disappeared within a week of delivery.
6. Selzer A. Risks of pregnancy in women with cardiac disease. JAMA 1977; 238:892–3.
   This article attempts to provide guidelines for prepregnancy counseling based on the severity of underlying cardiac disease.
7. Marcus FI, Ewy GA, O'Rourke RA, Walsh B, Bleich AC. The effect of pregnancy on the murmurs of mitral and aortic regurgitation. Circulation 1970; 41:795–805.
   In most women with aortic or mitral regurgitation, pregnancy induces a diminution in the murmur.
8. Turner AF. The chest radiograph in pregnancy. Clin Obstet Gynecol 1975; 18:65–74.
   A concise but thorough review of the radiographic changes in the heart and lungs induced by pregnancy.

9. Cannell DE, Vernon CP. Congenital heart disease and pregnancy. Am J Obstet Gynecol 1963; 85:744–53.
   In this series of 47 patients with ASD, PDA, coarctation of the aorta, VSD, and other assorted congenital lesions, pregnancy was, for the most part, tolerated without great difficulty.
10. Pitts JA, Crosby WM, Basta LL. Eisenmenger's syndrome in pregnancy: does heparin prophylaxis improve the maternal mortality rate? Am Heart J 1977; 93:321–6.
    The very high mortality of Eisenmenger's syndrome during pregnancy (5 of 7 in this series) is not modified by prophylactic heparin.
11. Deal K, Wooley CF. Coarctation of the aorta and pregnancy. Ann Intern Med 1973, 78:706–10.
    Although early reports indicated that pregnancy was prohibitively dangerous in women with coarctation, this study suggests that the risk is not as great as once thought.
12. Kolibash AJ, Ruiz DE, Lewis RP. Idiopathic hypertrophic subaortic stenosis in pregnancy. Ann Intern Med 1975; 82:791–4.
    Despite increasing symptoms, most women with obstructive hypertrophic cardiomyopathy can tolerate pregnancy and a vaginal delivery.
13. Limet R, Grondin CM. Cardiac valve prostheses, anticoagulation, and pregnancy. Ann Thorac Surg 1977; 23:337–41.
    The pregnant woman with a prosthetic valve can safely receive oral anticoagulants.
14. Ibarra-Perez C, Arevalo-Toledo N, Alvarez-de la Cadena O, Noriega-Guerra L. The course of pregnancy in patients with artificial heart valves. Am J Med 1976; 61:504–12.
    In this report of 28 pregnancies in 25 women with prosthetic heart valves, it is concluded that such women can have children if their management is closely supervised and if extreme care is exercised with the use of oral anticoagulants.
15. Carruth JE, Mirvis SB, Brogan DR, Wenger NK. The electrocardiogram in normal pregnancy. Am Heart J 1981; 102:1075–8.
    A detailed description of the ECG alterations in 157 pregnant women without clinical evidence of heart disease.
16. Blake S, O'Neill H, MacDonald D. Haemodynamic effects of pregnancy in patients with heart failure. Br Heart J 1982; 47:495–6.
    In 4 patients with congestive failure during pregnancy, all demonstrated improvement during the third trimester because of obstruction of the inferior vena cava.
17. Rotmensch HH, Elkayam U, Frishman W. Antiarrhythmic drug therapy during pregnancy. Ann Intern Med 1983; 98:487–97.
    A thorough review of which antiarrhythmic agents are preferable in pregnant women. Includes 169 references.

OBESITY AND THE HEART

Extreme obesity may affect the cardiovascular system in several ways. Although epidemiologic studies have demonstrated that obesity is not a major risk factor for the development of arteriosclerotic coronary artery disease, it often occurs in conjunction with well-established risk factors (e.g., hypertension and diabetes mellitus), and as a result, obesity is frequently linked to coronary artery disease. In fact, the combination of obesity, glucose intolerance, and a low high-density lipoprotein concentration is associated with an especially high risk of coronary artery disease, particularly in women.

Morbid obesity may induce certain physiologic alterations in cardiovascular function. In response to it, cardiac output and stroke volume increase, so that cardiac work is elevated in proportion to the severity of obesity. In addition, many severely obese patients have concomitant systemic arterial hypertension. As a result, *left ventricular hypertrophy* develops, eventually causing an elevation in left ventricular filling pressure. Some individuals with severe obesity develop alveolar hypoventilation, cyanosis, intermittent somnolence, and secondary polycythemia, a combination of findings called the Pickwickian syndrome. This may eventually lead to pulmonary hypertension, which, in turn, may induce *right ventricular hypertrophy* and an elevation in right ventricular filling pressure. In its early stages, therefore, the cardiac dysfunction caused by obesity is primarily an abnormality of ventricular compliance, so that left and right ventricular filling pressures are elevated. Eventually, ventricular systolic function deteriorates as well, leading to a worsening of heart failure.

The patient with an abnormally elevated left or right ventricular filling pressure due to extreme obesity most often complains of dyspnea, but orthopnea and paroxysmal nocturnal dyspnea are relatively uncommon. Other symptoms may include somnolence, fatigue, peripheral edema, and abdominal distention due to ascites. On physical examination, the patient may have pitting edema of the legs, abdominal enlargement (due to hepatomegaly or ascites), and jugular venous distention. On cardiac examination, one may detect a holosystolic murmur along the lower left sternal border of tricuspid regurgitation, and a right ventricular S_3 may be audible. The ECG usually reveals right atrial enlargement, right axis deviation, and right ventricular hypertrophy. Because of a greatly thickened chest wall, the amplitude of the precordial QRS complexes may be diminished. The chest x-ray confirms the presence of massive obesity, and the cardiothoracic ratio is usually increased. On M-mode and two-dimensional echocardiography, the right ventricular chamber is dilated, and both the left and right ventricular walls may be hypertrophied.

The massively obese patient with resultant cardiac dysfunction can be treated effectively only by weight reduction. In most patients a substantial reduction of body weight eliminates (or at least attenuates) systemic arterial hypertension, glucose intolerance, and abnormalities of serum high-density lipoprotein. Left ventricular stroke work returns toward normal, hypoventilation and somnolence resolve, and pulmonary arterial, left, and right ventricular pressures return to normal. Ventricular failure due to obesity can be treated with digitalis, diuretics, and salt restriction. If these conventional measures are unsuccessful in controlling heart failure, afterload reducing agents, such as hydralazine or captopril, may be cautiously administered.

1. Alexander JK. Obesity and cardiac performance. Am J Cardiol 1964; 14:860–5.
   Obesity requires that cardiac workload be increased considerably. Of 50 extremely obese individuals, cardiac enlargement and increased heart weight increased in proportion to the amount of excess body weight.
2. Epstein FH, Ostrander LD Jr, Johnson BC, Payne MW, Hayner NS, Keller JB, Francis T Jr. Epidemiological studies of cardiovascular disease in a total community—Tecumseh, Michigan. Ann Intern Med 1965; 62:1170–87.
   Among men, obesity was independently associated with coronary artery disease.
3. Gordon T, Castelli WP, Hjortland MC, Kannel WB, Dawber TR. Diabetes, blood lipids, and the role of obesity in coronary heart disease risk for women: the Framingham study. Ann Intern Med 1977; 87:393–7.
   In women, the triad of obesity, glucose intolerance, and a low concentration of high-density lipoprotein cholesterol carries an especially high risk of coronary artery disease.
4. Kannel WB, Brand N, Skinner JJ Jr, Dawber TR, McNamara PM. The relation of adiposity to blood pressure and development of hypertension: the Framingham study. Ann Intern Med 1967; 67:48–59.

Obesity predisposes and contributes to the development of hypertension in men and women over age 30.

5. Kannel WB, Lebauer EJ, Dawber TR, McNamara PM. Relation of body weight to development of coronary heart disease: the Framingham study. Circulation 1967; 35:734–44.

   An excess risk of angina pectoris and sudden death was present in obese men, probably because obesity imposed an increased workload on the heart.

6. Stamler J, Lindberg HA, Berkson DM, Shaffer A, Miller W, Poindexter A. Prevalence and incidence of coronary heart disease in strata of the labor force of a Chicago industrial corporation. J Chronic Dis 1960; 11:405–20.

   In a study of 784 men, obesity, hypertension, and diabetes melliltus were associated with an increased incidence of coronary artery disease.

7. Amad KH, Brennan JC, Alexander JK. The cardiac pathology of chronic exogenous obesity. Circulation 1965; 32:740–5.

   In 12 obese patients examined at postmortem, all had an increased heart weight, and 9 had left ventricular hypertrophy.

8. Alexander JK, Peterson KL. Cardiovascular effects of weight reduction. Circulation 1972; 45:310–8.

   In 9 markedly obese subjects, cardiac function was assessed before and after the loss of 39–84 kg. With weight loss, heart size decreased, but left ventricular filling pressure did not change.

9. Kaltman AJ, Goldring RM. Role of circulatory congestion in the cardiorespiratory failure of obesity. Am J Med 1976; 60:645–53.

   In patients who are massively obese, a high cardiac output is maintained despite marked circulatory congestion, which may result in generalized anasarca and increased ventricular filling pressures.

10. de Divitiis O, Fazio S, Petitto M, Maddalena G, Contaldo F, Mancini M. Obesity and cardiac function. Circulation 1981; 64:477–82.

    In 10 obese subjects without associated abnormalities, left ventricular diastolic function was distinctly abnormal. The degree of impairment of cardiac function paralleled the degree of obesity.

11. Alexander JK, Pettigrove JR. Obesity and congestive heart failure. Geriatrics 1967; 22:101–8.

    Of 9 patients weighing more than 300 pounds, autopsy revealed increased heart weight and left ventricular hypertrophy in all.

12. Hubert HB, Feinleib M, McNamara PM, Castelli WP. Obesity as an independent risk factor for cardiovascular disease: a 26-year follow-up of participants in the Framingham heart study. Circulation 1983; 67:968–77.

    Weight gain after the young adult years conveys an increased risk of cardiovascular disease in both sexes, particularly women.

ACCELERATED ATHEROGENESIS IN PATIENTS WITH CHRONIC RENAL FAILURE

Over the past 10 to 15 years, many patients have been maintained on long-term hemodialysis for chronic renal failure, and it has become clear that these individuals have a greatly increased morbidity and mortality from atherosclerotic vascular disease, specifically myocardial infarction and cerebrovascular accident. Patients with chronic renal failure requiring maintenance hemodialysis have a mortality from vascular events that is 3 to 4 times higher than that of persons of similar age without renal failure.

Pathologically, patients who are on maintenance hemodialysis have accelerated atherogenesis, the pathogenesis of which is complex and multifactorial. First, many of these patients are hypertensive, and in some the hypertension is severe and responds poorly to medical therapy. Wide fluctuations in intravascular volume contribute to this problem. Second, almost all these patients retain phosphate and, as a result, develop secondary hyperparathyroidism, which leads to an increased calcium-phosphorus product and the extraosseous deposition of calcium. These calcium complexes often accumulate in atherosclerotic plaques. In addition, they are occasionally deposited in the myocardium, leading to AV block or congestive heart failure. Third, almost all patients with chronic renal failure on maintenance hemodialysis have some evidence of glucose intolerance. Although their fasting blood glucose may be normal, its rate of decline during the several hours after ingestion is slowed. This defective handling of glucose is only partially corrected by hemodialysis. Fourth, 40 to 70 percent of patients with chronic renal failure on maintenance hemodialysis have hypertriglyceridemia; in addition, many of them have elevated very low density lipoprotein (VLDL) and depressed levels of high-density lipoprotein (HDL). The hypertriglyceridemia is caused by (1) a diminished clearance of triglycerides from the plasma, due to a deficiency in lipoprotein lipase, and (2) an increased hepatic synthesis of triglycerides, presumably due to insulin resistance and possibly high serum levels of growth hormone. In addition, some of these patients are given androgens in an attempt to stimulate erythropoiesis; such androgen therapy accentuates hypertriglyceridemia.

For the patient with hypertriglyceridemia without concomitant renal failure, weight reduction, a limitation of ethanol intake, and a reduction in carbohydrate consumption are usually successful in lowering the serum triglyceride concentration. However, the patient with hypertriglyceridemia and renal failure is often not obese and does not consume ethanol. In addition, a reduction in carbohydrate intake may be difficult to achieve because of the limitations imposed on the patient's diet by virtue of a reduced protein intake. For these individuals, a diet high in polyunsaturated fats appears to be effective in lowering the serum triglyceride concentration. If dietary alterations are ineffective, clofibrate may be administered. However, it must be given cautiously, since it is metabolized by the kidney. If the patient receives an excessive amount of clofibrate, myositis may occur.

1. Bagdade JD, Albers JJ. Plasma high-density lipoprotein concentrations in chronic hemodialysis and renal transplant patients. N Engl J Med 1977; 296:1436–9.
   In patients on hemodialysis and in those who have received transplants, HDL concentrations are lower than normal, and the VLDL/HDL ratio is higher than normal.
2. Lindner A, Charra B, Sherrard DJ, Scribner BH. Accelerated atherosclerosis in prolonged maintenance hemodialysis. N Engl J Med 1974; 290:697–701.
   This study clearly demonstrates that accelerated atherosclerosis is a major risk in patients on long-term maintenance hemodialysis.
3. Cattran DC, Fenton SSA, Wilson DR, Steiner G. Defective triglyceride removal in lipemia associated with peritoneal dialysis and hemodialysis. Ann Intern Med 1976; 85:29–33.
   In this study, 60% of the patients requiring dialysis had hypertriglyceridemia due to impaired triglyceride removal from the plasma.
4. Bagdade JD, Porte D Jr, Bierman EL. Hypertriglyceridemia: a metabolic consequence of chronic renal failure. N Eng J Med 1968; 279:181–5.
   One of the original articles emphasizing that hypertriglyceridemia is a frequent finding in patients with chronic renal failure.
5. Curry RC Jr, Roberts WC. Status of the coronary arteries in the nephrotic syndrome: analysis of 20 necropsy patients aged 15 to 35 years to determine if coronary atherosclerosis is accelerated. Am J Med 1977; 63:183–92.
   These patients with the nephrotic syndrome had much more postmortem evidence of coronary atherosclerosis than a group of age-matched controls.

6. Horton ES, Johnson C, Lebovitz HE. Carbohydrate metabolism in uremia. Ann Intern Med 1968; 68:63–74.
   In a group of uremic patients challenged with intravenous glucose, insulin resistance was demonstrated, the etiology of which is not understood.
7. Reaven GM, Weisinger JR, Swenson RS. Insulin and glucose metabolism in renal insufficiency. Kidney Int 1974; 6:S63–9.
   Most patients with azotemia have glucose intolerance which results from insulin resistance. The cause of this insulin resistance is not clear.
8. Wochos DN, Anderson CF, Mitchell JC III. Serum lipids in chronic renal failure. Mayo Clin Proc 1976; 51:660–4.
   Of 100 consecutive patients with chronic renal failure, 43 had hypertriglyceridemia. The lipoprotein abnormality bore no relation to the degree of renal impairment, the type of renal disease, or the patient's age, sex, weight, or diet.
9. Francis GS, Sharma B, Collins AJ, Helseth HK, Comty CM. Coronary artery surgery in patients with end-stage renal disease. Ann Intern Med 1980; 92:499–503.
   The authors report that coronary artery bypass grafting can be performed with an acceptable risk in patients on maintenance hemodialysis.
10. Sanfelippo ML, Swensen RS, Reaven GM. Reduction of plasma triglycerides by diet in subjects with chronic renal failure. Kidney Int 1977; 11:54–61.
    Hypertriglyceridemia occurs frequently in patients with moderate or severe chronic renal failure. A reduction in carbohydrate intake and an increase in polyunsaturated fat ingestion promptly reduces serum triglyceride concentrations in these patients.
11. Murase T, Cattran DC, Rubenstein B, Steiner G. Inhibition of lipoprotein lipase by uremic plasma, a possible cause of hypertriglyceridemia. Metabolism 1975; 24:1279–86.
    Uremic plasma appears to contain an inhibitor of lipoprotein lipase.
12. Mordasini R, Frey F, Flury W, Klose G, Greten H. Selective deficiency of hepatic triglyceride lipase in uremic patients. N Engl J Med 1977; 297:1362–6.
    Hypertriglyceridemia in patients with renal disease may be a consequence of low hepatic lipoprotein lipase activity.
13. Goldberg AP, Harter HR, Patsch W, Schechtman KB, Province M, Weerts C, Kuisk I, McCrate MM, Schonfeld G. Racial differences in plasma high-density lipoproteins in patients receiving hemodialysis: a possible mechanism for accelerated atherosclerosis in white men. N Engl J Med 1983; 308:1245–52.
    In this study of a large group of patients on maintenance hemodialysis, the white men had high serum levels of triglycerides, low serum levels of high density lipoproteins, and a greatly increased cardiovascular mortality.

NONCARDIAC SURGERY IN PATIENTS WITH CORONARY ARTERY DISEASE

As life expectancy has improved, a group of patients in whom underlying cardiac disease is frequent has appeared. In these elderly individuals, coronary artery disease is common, as is systemic arterial hypertension, with resultant hypertensive heart disease. These patients, many of whom have cardiac disease, may require a noncardiac surgical procedure. Because of their underlying heart disease, they enter the perioperative period at an increased risk when compared to patients of similar age without such disease.

During and immediately following a noncardiac surgical procedure, the metabolic requirements of the tissues affected by the operation increase. In response, cardiac output rises, and myocardial oxygen demands increase. If the patient has coronary artery disease, this increase in oxygen demand may lead to myocardial ischemia or infarction. Conversely, if cardiac disease prevents cardiac output from increasing sufficiently, congestive heart failure may result. During the perioperative period, several complications may appear, any of which is particularly dangerous to the patient with cardiac disease. Hemorrhage with resultant hypotension may lead to inadequate coronary perfusion, causing myocardial ischemia or infarction. Impaired ventilation (especially likely to occur in patients undergoing intrathoracic or high intra-abdominal surgical procedures) may lead to hypoxemia, which, in turn, may cause myocardial injury. Thromboembolic complications are likely to occur in patients with cardiac disease, and such events are tolerated poorly by these patients. Finally, infections in the immediate postoperative period may increase myocardial oxygen requirements, leading to an imbalance between oxygen supply and demand in patients with coronary artery disease.

The administration of an anesthetic can have a profound effect on the cardiovascular system. At concentrations that produce light surgical anesthesia, all general anesthetics depress the mechanical performance of the isolated heart and reduce cardiac ouput. In addition, some general anesthetics depress systemic arterial pressure, and in the patient with coronary artery disease, this fall in perfusion pressure may lead to ischemia. Spinal or epidural anesthesia blocks sympathetic constrictor outflow to arterioles and veins, making hypotension a common occurrence. In short, both general and local anesthesia can depress cardiac function and reduce coronary arterial perfusion pressure.

Patients with coronary artery disease—especially those with myocardial infarction in the preceding 6 months—who require noncardiac surgery have an increased risk of morbidity and mortality when compared to patients of a similar age without coronary artery disease. Several uncontrolled studies have suggested that coronary artery bypass surgery lowers the perioperative risk in patients undergoing subsequent noncardiac surgical procedures. Therefore, it may be advisable to perform coronary artery bypass grafting before or at the same time as other operations when severe and symptomatic coronary artery disease coexists with diseases that require surgery.

Some physicians routinely administer digitalis to the patient with underlying cardiac disease who is scheduled to have a noncardiac procedure. It is hoped that digitalis will abolish the myocardial depressant effect of anesthesia, help the heart to meet increased demands in the immediate postoperative period, help to maintain the patient in normal sinus rhythm, and help to control the ventricular response if an atrial tachyarrhythmia appears. Despite anecdotal reports, a controlled and randomized trial of digitalis during the perioperative period in patients with cardiac disease has not been reported. Since recent studies have emphasized the high incidence of digitalis intoxication, we recommend that digitalis be administered prophylactically only to patients having noncardiac surgery if congestive heart failure or atrial tachyarrhythmias are present. Similarly, although temporary transvenous pacing has been used in patients with cardiac disease during noncardiac operative procedures, no controlled study has been reported that determines which patients actually require pacing. We recommend that patients with second or third degree AV block and those with a history of Stokes-Adams attacks be temporarily paced during the perioperative period. In contrast, patients with unifascicular or chronic bifascicular block probably do not require a temporary pacemaker.

Finally, many patients with coronary artery disease who undergo noncardiac surgical procedures are taking propranolol or a calcium antagonist for their angina pectoris. Because of its negative inotropic and chronotropic effects, propranolol may cause hemodynamic instability in the perioperative period. As a result, some physicians recommend that it be gradually discontinued prior to surgery. However, we prefer to continue propranolol and the calcium antagonists until the day of surgery. In the postoperative period, they can be reinstituted when the patient can receive oral medications.

1. Hillis LD, Cohn PF. Noncardiac surgery in patients with coronary artery disease: risks, precautions, and perioperative management. Arch Intern Med 1978; 138:972–5.
   A brief review of perioperative management of patients with coronary artery disease.
2. Goldman L, Caldera DL, Nussbaum SR, Southwick FS, Krogstad D, Murray B, Burke DS, O'Malley TA, Goroll AH, Caplan CH, Nolan J, Carabello B, Slater EE. Multifactorial index of cardiac risk in noncardiac surgical procedures. N Engl J Med 1977; 297:845–50.
   In a study of over 1,000 patients, the authors identified 9 correlates of life-threatening or fatal cardiac complications in patients having noncardiac procedures: S_3; infarction in the preceding 6 months; frequent VPBs; any rhythm other than sinus; age > 70 years; intraperitoneal, intrathoracic, or aortic operation; emergency operation; valvular aortic stenosis; and poor general medical condition.
3. Goldman L. Noncardiac surgery in patients receiving propranolol: case reports and a recommended approach. Arch Intern Med 1981; 141:193–6.
   In patients on maintenance propranolol, its continuation up to the time of surgery appears safe from an anesthetic standpoint and may also help to minimize the risk of the propranolol withdrawal syndrome.
4. Kopriva CJ, Brown MB, Pappas G. Hemodynamics during general anesthesia in patients receiving propranolol. Anesthesiology 1978; 48:28–33.
   The continued administration of propranolol until time of operation is not associated with adverse hemodynamic events.
5. Goldman L, Caldera DL, Southwick FS, Nussbaum SR, Murray B, O'Malley TA, Goroll AH, Caplan CH, Nolan J, Burke DS, Krogstad D, Carabello B, Slater EE. Cardiac risk factors and complications in noncardiac surgery. Medicine 1978; 57:357–70.
   A review of the clinical, electrocardiographic, and radiographic features that determine operative risk in patients with heart disease.
6. McCollum CH, Garcia-Rinaldi R, Graham JM, DeBakey ME. Myocardial revascularization prior to subsequent major surgery in patients with coronary artery disease. Surgery 1977; 81:302–4.
   An uncontrolled report suggesting that myocardial revascularization should be performed prior to other major operative procedures in patients with coronary artery disease.
7. Mauney FM Jr, Ebert PA, Sabiston DC Jr. Postoperative myocardial infarction: a study of predisposing factors, diagnosis, and mortality in a high risk group of surgical patients. Ann Surg 1970; 172:497–503.
   Of 365 patients with coronary artery disease undergoing noncardiac surgical procedures, there was a direct correlation between the incidence of postoperative myocardial infarction and both the length of the operative procedure and the occurrence of intraoperative hypotension.
8. Bernhard VM, Johnson WD, Peterson JJ. Carotid artery stenosis: association with surgery for coronary artery disease. Arch Surg 1972; 105:837–40.
   In patients who require both carotid and coronary artery surgery, a simultaneous approach is better than performing the carotid endarterectomy before the coronary bypass procedure.
9. Deutsch S, Dalen JE. Indications for prophylactic digitalization. Anesthesiology 1969; 30:648–56.
   The authors recommend prophylactic digitalization preoperatively in all patients with clinical, electrocardiographic, or radiologic evidence of organic heart disease.
10. Shields TW, Ujiki GT. Digitalization for prevention of arrhythmias following pulmonary surgery. Surg Gynecol Obstet 1968; 126:743–6.
    In elderly patients undergoing noncardiac intrathoracic surgery, prophylactic digitalization may be beneficial.
11. Perlroth MG, Hultgren HN. The cardiac patient and general surgery, JAMA 1975; 232:1279–80.

A general review of the care of the cardiac patient during and after a noncardiac surgical procedure.

12. Skinner JF, Pearce ML. Surgical risk in the cardiac patient. J Chron Dis 1964; 17:57–72.

    Perioperative mortality in patients with cardiac disease is directly related to the magnitude of the surgical procedure and the patient's preoperative functional class.

13. Wells PH, Kaplan JA. Optimal management of patients with ischemic heart disease for noncardiac surgery by complementary anesthesiologist and cardiologist interaction. Am Heart J 1981; 102:1029–37.

    This article describes an integrated approach of the anesthesiologist and cardiologist in minimizing the risk of noncardiac surgery in patients with coronary artery disease.

14. Goldman L. Cardiac risks and complications of noncardiac surgery. Ann Intern Med 1983; 98:504–13.

    In patients undergoing noncardiac surgery, perioperative risk can be estimated from the severity of underlying heart failure, the occurrence of a recent myocardial infarction, the presence of aortic stenosis, the patient's age, the type of planned surgery, and the patient's general medical condition.

THYROTOXICOSIS AND THE HEART

Thyroid hormone exerts a profound effect on a number of metabolic processes in almost all tissues, with the heart being especially sensitive to its effects. Many of the cardiovascular effects of hyperthyroidism are caused by increased activity of the sympathetic nervous system, due at least in part to a thyroxine-induced increase in the concentration of beta-adrenergic receptors in the myocardium. Independent of augmented sympathetic nervous system activity, thyroid hormone appears to alter cardiac function directly. Thus, the increased heart rate and myocardial contractility observed in experimental hyperthyroidism are not totally reversed by sympathetic or parasympathetic blockade. Furthermore, thyroxine enhances the rate of contraction of cardiac muscle even in the presence of adrenergic blockade. This direct effect of thyroid hormone on the heart appears to be mediated by an increase in protein synthesis, so that the activity of a number of vital intracellular enzymes is augmented.

The younger patient with thyrotoxicosis often complains of palpitations, dyspnea, weight loss, diarrhea, and heat intolerance. Nervousness and excitability are also frequent complaints. On physical examination, the heart rate is usually rapid ($>$ 90 beats/min), and there is often systolic hypertension, with a resultant widened pulse pressure. The skin is often warm and moist. The patient may demonstrate a fine tremor, lid lag, exophthalmos, a widened palpebral fissure with a resultant "stare," and hyperactive deep tendon reflexes. The precordium is unusually active, with an easily palpable point of maximal impulse. The S_1 is usually loud, as is the pulmonic component of the S_2. An S_3 may be audible. A systolic ejection murmur is frequently heard at the aortic area and along the left sternal border; in addition, a systolic scratch—the so-called Means-Lerman scratch—is occasionally heard in the second left intercostal space during expiration. This sound is presumably caused by the rubbing together of normal pleural and pericardial surfaces by the hyperdynamic heart.

In contrast to the younger patient, the elderly individual with hyperthyroidism may not manifest many of the aforementioned symptoms or signs of a hyperdynamic circulation. Instead, these patients may complain only of dyspnea, orthopnea, and paroxysmal nocturnal dyspnea—the symptoms of pulmonary vascular congestion. Alternatively, they may note angina pectoris with exertion or even at rest. On physical examination, the pulse is often irregularly irregular, reflecting the presence of atrial fibrillation. There is usually mild or moderate cardiomegaly as well as evidence of pulmonary congestion (rales at both bases). The patient may even have peripheral edema.

The ECG usually demonstrates either sinus tachycardia or atrial fibrillation. Intra-atrial conduction disturbances, manifested by prolongation or notching of the P wave and prolongation of the P–R interval, may occur in some individuals. About 15 percent have an intraventricular conduction delay, most commonly right bundle branch block. The Q–T interval may be shortened, and diffuse, nonspecific ST–T wave abnormalities are frequent. The chest x-ray usually demonstrates mild or moderate cardiomegaly, and there may be evidence of pulmonary venous hypertension. M-mode or two-dimensional echocardiography usually reveals a mildly dilated but vigorously contracting left ventricle. At cardiac catheterization, the patient is noted to have (1) systolic hypertension, with a widened pulse pressure; (2) an augmented cardiac output, sometimes as high as 5 to 7 L/min/m^2; (3) normal systolic left ventricular function; and (4) a diminished systemic vascular resistance. Intracardiac filling pressures are usually normal.

The therapy of the patient with thyrotoxic heart disease centers on (1) correction of the hypermetabolic manifestations of the disease and (2) definitive correction of the hyperthyroid state. The hypermetabolic manifestations of the disease are treated effectively with propranolol, a beta-adrenergic blocking agent. For the patient with the usual cardiovascular manifestations of hyperthyroidism, propranolol (80–240 mg/day orally in 3–4 divided doses) slows heart rate, diminishes systolic arterial and pulse pressure, reduces cardiac output, and increases systemic vascular resistance. Since propranolol is a myocardial depressant, it must be used cautiously in patients with congestive heart failure. For these individuals, a cardiac glycoside, such as digitalis, should be administered instead of (or in combination with) a beta-adrenergic blocker. In this setting, it must be kept in mind that the serum concentration of digitalis is diminished because of a thyroid-induced increase in this drug's volume of distribution.

Although beta-adrenergic blockade and/or digitalis induces an improvement in the cardiovascular status of patients with hyperthyroidism, the correction of the underlying metabolic defect requires specific therapy directed at reducing the production of thyroid hormone. Thus, propylthiouracil, radioactive iodine, or surgical subtotal thyroidectomy have each been used successfully to render the thyrotoxic patient euthyroid. The choice of therapy depends on the patient's age, sex, and preference for medical versus surgical therapy.

1. Williams LT, Lefkowitz RJ, Watanabe AM, Hathaway DR, Besch HR Jr. Thyroid hormone regulation of beta-adrenergic receptor number. J Biol Chem 1977; 252:2787–9.
   Exogenous thyroid hormone causes an increased number of cardiac beta-adrenergic receptors. This may be responsible, at least in part, for the enhanced catecholamine sensitivity in hyperthyroid individuals.
2. Davis PJ, Davis FB. Hyperthyroidism in patients over the age of 60 years: clinical features in 85 patients. Medicine 1974; 53:161–81.
   In these elderly patients, atrial fibrillation was present in 33 (39%) but was often associated with a ventricular response below 100/min.
3. DeGroot WJ, Leonard JJ. Hyperthyroidism as a high cardiac output state. Am Heart J 1970; 79:265–75.

A succinct review of the hemodynamic alterations and clinical characteristics of hyperthyroidism.

4. Hoffman I, Lowrey RD. The electrocardiogram in thyrotoxicosis. Am J Cardiol 1960; 6:893–904.
   Of 123 patients with hyperthyroidism, 46 had sinus tachycardia; 11 had PR prolongation; 28 had ST–T wave abnormalities; and 21 had a shortened Q–T interval.

5. Levey GS. The heart and hyperthyroidism. Med Clin North Am 1975; 59:1193–1201.
   A concise review of the use of propranolol in patients with thyrotoxicosis and cardiovascular symptoms and signs.

6. Grossman W, Robin NI, Johnson LW, Brooks HL, Selenkow HA, Dexter L. The enhanced myocardial contractility of thyrotoxicosis: role of the beta adrenergic receptor. Ann Intern Med 1971; 74:869–74.
   This study of 10 hyperthyroid individuals demonstrates that the tachycardia, shortened circulation time, and widened pulse pressure of thyrotoxicosis are apparently mediated by beta-adrenergic influences, whereas the heightened ventricular function associated with thyrotoxicosis seems to be independent of beta-adrenergic influences and, therefore, probably represents a primary effect of thyroxine on the heart.

7. Grossman W, Robin NI, Johnson LW, Brooks H, Selenkow HA, Dexter L. Effects of beta blockade on the peripheral manifestations of thyrotoxicosis. Ann Intern Med 1971; 74:875–9.
   The tremor, stare, hyperreflexia, lid-lag, and globe-lag of thyrotoxicosis are mediated by the beta-adrenergic nervous system.

8. Nixon JV, Anderson RJ, Cohen ML. Alterations in left ventricular mass and performance in patients treated effectively for thyrotoxicosis: a comparative echocardiographic study. Am J Med 1979; 67:268–76.
   In 15 thyrotoxic patients, antithyroid therapy caused a substantial reduction in left ventricular mass and the velocity of circumferential fiber shortening.

9. Abrahamsen AM, Haarstad J, Ovlie C. Hemodynamic studies in thyrotoxicosis before and after treatment. Acta Med Scand 1963; 174:463–7.
   In 29 patients with thyrotoxicosis, therapy caused a substantial fall in cardiac index and heart rate.

10. Cohen MV, Schulman IC, Spenillo A, Surks MI. Effects of thyroid hormone on left ventricular function in patients treated for thyrotoxicosis. Am J Cardiol 1981; 48:33–8.
    In 9 patients with hyperthyroidism studied repetitively before and after therapy, corrected left ventricular ejection time increased, and the velocity of circumferential fiber shortening decreased.

11. Feely J, Stevenson IH, Crooks J. Increased clearance of propranolol in thyrotoxicosis. Ann Intern Med 1981; 94:472–4.
    In 6 patients with thyrotoxicosis treated with propranolol, the pharmacokinetics of propranolol were altered in the thyrotoxic state in comparison to the euthyroid state.

12. Channick BJ, Adlin EV, Marks AD, Denenberg BS, McDonough MT, Chakko CS, Spann JF. Hyperthyroidism and mitral valve prolapse. N Engl J Med 1981; 305:497–500.
    Of 40 patients with hyperthyroidism, 17 (43%) had mitral valve prolapse, compared to 18% in a control group.

13. Merillon JP, Passa P, Chastre J, Wolf A, Gourgon R. Left ventricular function and hyperthyroidism. Br Heart J 1981; 46:137–43.
    With the induction of euthyroidism, cardiac output, dP/dt, ejection fraction, and mean velocity of fiber shortening decreased. In addition, left ventricular mass was reduced by therapy.

14. Iskandrian AS, Rose L, Hakki AH, Segal BL, Kane SA. Cardiac performance in thyrotoxicosis: analysis of 10 untreated patients. Am J Cardiol 1983; 51:349–52.
    Using radionuclide ventriculography, these authors demonstrated that left ventricular performance in patients with thyrotoxicosis is normal at rest, but during exercise abnormalities occur in some individuals.

HYPOTHYROIDISM AND THE HEART

Hypothyroidism results from a reduced secretion of both triiodothyronine and thyroxine. In most patients, this occurs as a consequence of destruction of the thyroid gland, usually by an inflammatory process. Less commonly, hypothyroidism is the result of a diminished secretion of thyrotropin, due to pituitary or hypothalamic disease. In either event, the resultant deficiency of circulating thyroid hormone reduces myocardial oxygen consumption and the sensitivity of the myocardium to catecholamines.

The cardiac disease that accompanies hypothyroidism may manifest itself in three ways. First, many individuals with long-standing thyroid hormone deficiency have pericardial effusions. It is estimated that such effusions are demonstrable in 35 to 40 percent of patients with hypothyroidism. In most individuals, they accumulate slowly, so that pericardial tamponade is distinctly uncommon but has been reported to occur in a rare patient.

Second, patients with hypothyroidism are at increased risk of developing atherosclerosis because of the frequent occurrence of hypercholesterolemia, hypertriglyceridemia, and an impairment of free fatty acid mobilization. Studies in both animals and man have demonstrated clearly that hypothyroidism causes an acceleration of the atherosclerotic process. As a result, the patient with long-standing hypothyrodism may complain of angina pectoris or may sustain a myocardial infarction. These are especially likely to occur when thyroid replacement therapy is administered to the patient with a long history of hypothyroidism.

Third, the contractile state of the myocardium is reduced in the hypothyroid patient, and there is a diminished sensitivity of cardiac muscle to circulating catecholamines. As a result, cardiac output is often reduced in these patients. Although left ventricular contractility is clearly depressed in these individuals, intracardiac filling pressures are usually normal, and therefore, venous congestion (pulmonary or peripheral) is unusual.

In the adult patient, the symptoms of hypothyroidism begin insidiously. The patient (or patient's family) may note the gradual appearance of weakness, malaise, fatigue, and lethargy. He may complain of a worsening memory, cold intolerance, a modest gain in weight, a deepening voice, constipation, or dry and unusually coarse skin. Cardiac symptoms are uncommon early in the development of hypothyroidism. Eventually, however, the patient may complain of angina pectoris, exertional dyspnea, orthopnea, and peripheral edema, the last due to increased capillary permeability rather than an increased peripheral venous pressure.

On physical examination, the patient usually has a sinus bradycardia and a narrowed pulse pressure. The skin is dry and cool, and the tongue may be large and somewhat reddened. There may be alopecia of the eyebrows. The deep tendon reflexes are slowed. On cardiac examination, the point of maximal impulse may not be palpable, but if it is, it is often displaced laterally. On auscultation, the S_1 and S_2 may be muffled. Murmurs, rubs, or extra sounds are usually not present.

The ECG often reveals (1) sinus bradycardia, (2) a prolonged Q–T interval, (3) diffusely diminished QRS voltage, and (4) nonspecific ST–T wave flattening. Intraventricular conduction disturbances occur commonly. On the chest x-ray, the cardiac silhouette is enlarged, sometimes massively, but the lung fields do not show evidence of vascular congestion. An occasional patient may have unilateral or bilateral pleural effusions. Echocardiography often shows a pericardial effusion. At cardiac catheterization, the cardiac output is reduced, intra-cardiac filling pressures are normal, left ventricular ejection fraction is usually in the normal range, and the coronary arteries may be narrowed by the ather-osclerotic process.

Many of the cardiovascular symptoms of hypothyroidism do not respond to conventional therapy unless thyroid replacement is instituted. In the patient with underlying atherosclerotic coronary artery disease, however, such thyroid replacement must be initiated slowly and very carefully, else it may precipitate worsening angina or even a myocardial infarction. Thus, thyroxine is begun at an extremely small dose (i.e., 0.0125 mg/day), then gradually increased every 10 to 14 days until a daily dose of 0.1 to 0.125 mg is reached. If angina worsens during thyroid replacement therapy and is unresponsive to medical therapy, coronary artery bypass grafting should be performed, after which thyroid re-placement can proceed.

1. Kerber RE, Sherman B. Echocardiographic evaluation of pericardial effusion in myxedema: incidence and biochemical and clinical correlations. Circulation 1975; 52:823–7.
   By echocardiography, 10 of 33 patients (30%) with hypothyroidism had pericardial effusions.
2. Alsever RN, Stjernholm MR. Cardiac tamponade in myxedema. Am J Med Sci 1975; 269:117–21.
   A 43-year-old woman with a myxedematous pericardial effusion which caused tamponade is reported.
3. Smolar EN, Rubin JE, Avramides A, Carter AC. Cardiac tamponade in primary myxedema and review of the literature. Am J Med Sci 1976; 272:345–52.
   Despite the common occurrence of pericardial effusion in myxedema, cardiac tamponade is extremely rare.
4. Aber CP, Thompson GS. The heart in hypothyroidism. Am Heart J 1964; 68:428–30.
   Cardiac failure in uncomplicated hypothyroidism is exceedingly uncommon.
5. Steinberg AD. Myxedema and coronary artery disease—a comparative autopsy study. Ann Intern Med 1968; 68:338–44.
   In comparison to age-, sex-, and race-matched controls, patients with hypothyroidism have an increased incidence of coronary atherosclerosis.
6. Paine TD, Rogers WJ, Baxley WA, Russell RO Jr. Coronary arterial surgery in patients with incapacitating angina pectoris and myxedema. Am J Cardiol 1977; 40:226–31.
   Both coronary arteriography and bypass surgery can be performed safely in patients with severe hypothyroidism.
7. Crowley WF Jr, Ridgway EC, Bough EW, Francis GS, Daniels GH, Kourides IA, Myers GS, Maloof F. Noninvasive evaluation of cardiac function in hypothyroidism: response to gradual thyroxine replacement. N Engl J Med 1977; 296:1–6.
   In 15 patients with severe hypothyroidism, thyroid replacement caused an improvement in noninvasively-determined markers of left ventricular performance.
8. Hamolsky MW, Kurland GS, Freedberg AS. The heart in hypothyroidism. J Chronic Dis 1961; 14:558–69.
   Left ventricular failure only rarely, if ever, results from hypothyroidism.
9. Levine HD. Compromise therapy in the patient with angina pectoris and hypothyroidism: a clinical assessment. Am J Med 1980; 69: 411–8.
   Of 51 patients with hypothyroidism and coronary artery disease, angina control during thyroid replacement therapy was unsatisfactory in one-third.
10. Hay ID, Duick DS, Vlietstra RE, Maloney JD, Pluth JR. Thyroxine therapy in hypothyroid patients undergoing coronary revascularization: a retrospective analysis. Ann Intern Med 1981; 95:456–7.
    In a review of 18 patients from the Mayo Clinic, coronary artery surgery in hypothyroid patients was not accompanied by perioperative or postoperative mortality.

PARADOXICAL EMBOLISM

Paradoxical embolization occurs when a thrombus arising in the venous system or right side of the heart passes through an intracardiac communication to become a systemic arterial embolus. In almost all reported cases, the source of the emboli has been venous thrombosis in the lower extremities, and the intracardiac communication has been a patent foramen ovale. Rarely, such paradoxical embolization occurs through a ventricular septal defect (VSD) or a patent ductus arteriosus (PDA). Although paradoxical embolization is occasionally discovered premortem, it is usually an unexpected postmortem finding; less than 10 percent of all reported cases have been discovered during life.

The patient with paradoxical embolization presents with obvious evidence of arterial occlusion: a cerebrovascular accident, a myocardial infarction, or the sudden development of arterial insufficiency to a visceral organ or an extremity. When such an event occurs without evidence of a source of emboli in the left side of the heart (e.g., mitral valve disease with atrial fibrillation or a left ventricular aneurysm), paradoxical embolism should be considered, and the patient should be questioned and examined to determine if venous thrombosis and pulmonary embolism have occurred. *When arterial embolization occurs in association with thrombophlebitis or pulmonary embolism, it should alert the physician to the possibility that the arterial embolism is of venous origin.*

To confirm the presence of paradoxical embolism, a right-to-left intracardiac shunt must be demonstrated. Such shunting can occur in one of three clinical settings. First, the patient with *cyanotic congenital heart disease* has right-to-left shunting through an atrial septal defect (ASD, VSD, or PDA); the presence of cyanosis and clubbing should focus attention to this possibility.

Second, the patient with *acyanotic congenital heart disease* with a resultant left-to-right intracardiac shunt (most frequently an uncomplicated secundum ASD) may have an associated small right-to-left shunt, due to the streaming of venous blood from the inferior vena cava toward the region of the fossa ovalis and across the ASD. If venous thromboembolism occurs in such a patient, there is a small but finite risk of paradoxical embolism.

Third, the patient with a *patent foramen ovale* (without intracardiac shunting) may develop a small right-to-left interatrial shunt if right atrial pressure exceeds that in the left atrium, as in the patient with recurrent pulmonary embolism and a resultant increase in pulmonary arterial pressure. Thus, if pulmonary embolism occurs and is sufficiently large to induce right ventricular failure, it may cause a right-to-left intracardiac shunt through a patent foramen ovale. If further venous thromboembolism occurs in this setting, the thrombi may pass across the patent foramen, leading to a systemic arterial embolism. On physical examination, individuals with this condition usually have evidence of pulmonary hypertension (a palpable pulmonary arterial impulse in the left second intercostal space and a right ventricular lift along the lower left sternal border) and right ventricular dilatation and failure (a holosystolic murmur of tricuspid regurgitation at the lower left sternal border, which increases in intensity with inspiration, as well as a right ventricular S_3). The patent foramen ovale itself produces no abnormality on physical examination.

The chest x-ray of the patient with paradoxical embolization across a patent foramen ovale may demonstrate prominent pulmonary arteries and an enlarged right ventricle, and the ECG may show right axis deviation and right ventricular overload. By M-mode or two-dimensional echocardiography, one may see a dilated right atrium and ventricle. The left atrium and ventricle are normal in size and do not demonstrate an intracavitary filling defect suggestive of a thrombus.

At cardiac catheterization, the patient who has previously sustained a paradoxical embolism may have residual pulmonary hypertension. By the indicator dilution technique, one can demonstrate a right-to-left intracardiac shunt, which is usually of small size. In some patients, shunting may be demonstrable only during maneuvers that disproportionately increase right atrial pressure, such as the Valsalva maneuver.

If the patient is shown to have paradoxical embolization, treatment should be directed at preventing a recurrence of venous thromboembolism: chronic anticoagulation or venous interruption. If the intracardiac shunt is occurring through a patent foramen ovale, it does not require surgical closure. In fact, the indications to close the intracardiac defect should be based on the usual indications for surgical correction rather than on the occurrence of paradoxical embolism alone.

1. Meister SG, Grossman W, Dexter L, Dalen JE. Paradoxical embolism. Am J Med 1972; 53:292–8.
   Five patients with paradoxical embolism are described, and a succinct review of this entity is presented.
2. Gazzaniga AB, Dalen JE. Paradoxical embolism: its pathophysiology and clinical recognition. Ann Surg 1970; 171:137–42.
   Of 117 reported cases of paradoxical embolism, only 7 have been diagnosed during life.
3. Corrin B. Paradoxical embolism. Br Heart J 1964; 26:549–53.
   Two men with postmortem evidence of paradoxical embolism are described.
4. Gill TJ III, Dammin GJ. Paradoxical embolism with renal failure caused by occlusion of the renal arteries. Am J Med 1958; 25:780–7.
   At the time of this report, paradoxical embolism had been reported and proved at autopsy in 100 cases; in 35 of these the kidneys were involved.
5. Padula RT, Camishion RC. Paradoxical embolization. Ann Surg 1968; 167:598–601.
   The case report of a 61-year-old man with a major neurologic event due to paradoxical embolism.
6. Gleysteen JJ, Silver D. Paradoxical arterial embolism: collective review. Am Surg 1970; 36:47–54.
   A complete review of all cases of paradoxical embolism reported in the literature, emphasizing that the vast majority of the intracardiac communications have been a patent foramen ovale.
7. Steiger BW, Libanoff AJ, Springer EB. Myocardial infarction due to paradoxical embolism. Am J Med 1969; 47:995–8.
   A report of a 23-year-old woman with an atrial septal defect and an anterior myocardial infarction presumably due to paradoxical embolism.
8. Banas JS Jr, Meister SG, Gazzaniga AB, O'Connor NE, Haynes FW, Dalen JE. A simple technique for detecting small defects in the atrial septum. Am J Cardiol 1971; 28:467–71.
   A description of the technique for demonstrating right-to-left intracardiac shunting by the indicator dilution method.

MARFAN'S SYNDROME

Marfan's syndrome is one of several inherited disorders of connective tissue. Although it is usually transmitted as an autosomal dominant trait, about 15 percent of cases are sporadic and the result of a new genetic mutation. Paternal age is a contributing factor in cases that appear sporadically, since the fathers

.ch sporadic cases are several years older than the fathers of those with the gularly inherited syndrome.

The clinical manifestations of Marfan's syndrome result from the involvement of four systems. First, most patients with this syndrome have characteristic skeletal features. The tubular bones are excessively long, resulting in arachnodactyly and abnormal body proportions, so that the lower half of the body (pubis to feet) is unusually long in comparison to the upper half (pubis to crown), and the arm span exceeds the height. Excessive longitudinal rib growth may result in sternal deformities (pectus carinatum [pigeon breast] or pectus excavatum [inward displacement]). The patient may have unusually loose joints due to redundant ligaments, tendons, and joint capsules, and recurrent joint dislocation is a common problem. Young female patients with Marfan's syndrome are especially likely to develop kyphoscoliosis.

Second, many patients with Marfan's syndrome have ocular involvement. *Ectopia lentis* (subluxation of the lens or dislocated lens) is the ocular hallmark of this syndrome, and on occasion, the lens is totally dislocated into the anterior chamber. High-grade myopia is usually present, and spontaneous retinal detachment occurs with some frequency.

Third, some patients with Marfan's syndrome have pulmonary cystic disease, leading to recurrent spontaneous pneumothoraces. Fourth, patients with Marfan's syndrome have a weakened aortic media, making them susceptible to the development of both saccular and dissecting aortic aneurysms. As a result of aortic dilatation, aortic regurgitation may develop. In addition to aortic involvement, many patients with this syndrome have enlarged and redundant mitral valve leaflets, so that mitral valve prolapse is particularly common. Occasionally, the resultant mitral regurgitation is substantial, necessitating mitral valve replacement. Whichever left-sided valve is involved by Marfan's syndrome, bacterial endocarditis is always a possibility.

Pathologically, the most striking abnormalities in Marfan's syndrome are present in the aortic media, where the alterations are identical to those of cystic medial necrosis. In the advanced form, one may see a loss of elastic fibers and dilatation of the vasa vasorum. Since Marfan's syndrome is a constellation of clinical findings without a specific biochemical or hematologic abnormality, it can be diagnosed only clinically. In the patient with obvious skeletal, ocular, and cardiovascular involvement, there is little problem in making the diagnosis. However, problems sometimes arise in making the diagnosis in the patient with only a portion of the clinical characteristics. For example, it may be difficult to decide whether the patient with only skeletal abnormalities (without ocular, pulmonary, or cardiovascular involvement) has Marfan's syndrome.

It is important to distinguish Marfan's syndrome from homocystinuria. In brief, homocystinuria is inherited as an autosomal recessive trait. Although arachnodactyly is often present, it is generally less striking than in the patient with Marfan's syndrome. Chest deformities and scoliosis are common in patients with homocystinuria, and ectopia lentis is usually severe. Mental retardation is a frequent clinical characteristic of homocystinuria, whereas it is distinctly uncommon in patients with Marfan's syndrome.

Therapy of patients with Marfan's syndrome should be undertaken if specific organ systems are involved. In young girls who begin to develop scoliosis, estrogen therapy is often initiated in an attempt to terminate upward growth prematurely and to hasten puberty. In all patients with Marfan's syndrome and clinical or radiographic evidence of aortic involvement, propranolol probably is beneficial in reducing morbidity and mortality from aortic dissection. If aortic or mitral regurgitation is present, antibiotic prophylaxis (against endocarditis) is required. If severe aortic or mitral regurgitation is present, digitalis and diuretics are indicated to control congestive heart failure, and valve replacement may even be necessary.

1. Brown OR, DeMots H, Kloster FE, Roberts A, Menashe VD, Beals RK. Aortic root dilatation and mitral valve prolapse in Marfan's syndrome: an echocardiographic study. Circulation 1975; 52:651–7.

   By echocardiography, aortic root dilatation was found in 60% of patients with Marfan's syndrome, and mitral valve prolapse was found in 91%.

2. Murdoch JL, Walker BA, Halpern BL, Kuzma JW, McKusick VA. Life expectancy and causes of death in the Marfan syndrome. N Engl J Med 1972; 286:804–8.

   The cardiac complications of the Marfan syndrome lead to a greatly reduced life expectancy. Of the 72 deceased Marfan's patients described in this report, the average age at death was 32 years.

3. Pyeritz RE, McKusick VA. The Marfan syndrome: diagnosis and management. N Engl J Med 1979; 300:772–7.

   An excellent overview of this syndrome, including its clinical characteristics, diagnosis, and management.

4. Murdoch JL, Walker BA, McKusick VA. Paternal age effects on the occurrence of new mutations for the Marfan syndrome. Ann Hum Genet 1972; 35:331–6.

   In a review of 249 patients with Marfan's syndrome, 23 apparently sporadic cases were found. The fathers of these 23 were an average of 6.8 years older than the fathers of the other 226 patients.

5. Phornphutkul C, Rosenthal A, Nadas AS. Cardiac manifestations of Marfan syndrome in infancy and childhood. Circulation 1973; 47:587–96.

   In a series of children with this syndrome, 61% had cardiac abnormalities, the most common of which was mitral regurgitation.

6. Raghib G, Jue KL, Anderson RC, Edwards JE. Marfan's syndrome with mitral insufficiency. Am J Cardiol 1965; 16:127–32.

   The description of a young girl with Marfan's syndrome and severe mitral regurgitation due to elongation of the chordae tendineae.

7. Boucek RJ, Noble NL, Gunja-Smith Z, Butler WT. The Marfan syndrome: a deficiency in chemically stable collagen cross-links. N Engl J Med 1981; 305:988–91.

   The reduced tensile strength of tissues supporting the ocular lenses, cardiac valves, and aorta in Marfan's syndrome is probably due to a defective organization of collagen. This paper demonstrates that patients with Marfan's syndrome have a reduced number of collagen cross-links.

8. Lababidi Z, Monzon C. Early cardiac manifestations of Marfan's syndrome in the newborn. Am Heart J 1981; 102:943–5.

   The case report of a newborn male with obvious skeletal and vascular evidence of Marfan's syndrome.

9. Come PC, Fortuin NJ, White RI Jr, McKusick VA. Echocardiographic assessment of cardiovascular abnormalities in the Marfan syndrome: Comparison with clinical findings and with roentgenographic estimation of aortic root size. Am J Med 1983; 74:465–74.

   Echocardiography was better than physical exam and chest x-ray in detecting valvular and aortic root abnormalities in this group of 61 patients with the Marfan syndrome.

10. Pyeritz RE, Wappel MA. Mitral valve dysfunction in the Marfan syndrome: clinical and echocardiographic study of prevalence and natural history. Am J Med 1983; 74:797–807.

    Of 166 patients with the Marfan syndrome, 113 (68%) had echocardiographic evidence of mitral valve dysfunction, generally prolapse. By the third decade, serious mitral regurgitation had developed in 1 of every 8 of these patients.

CARDIAC TRANSPLANTATION

The first human heart transplant was performed by Dr. Christian Barnard at Groote Schuur Hospital, Cape Town, South Africa, in 1967. The patient survived only 18 days, then died of pneumonia. From 1968 to 1970, more than 100 transplants were performed by 58 different teams in all parts of the world. Subsequently, however, the consistently low survival rates caused the procedure to be abandoned in all but a few centers. During the 1970s, several teams—those at Stanford University, the University of Cape Town, South Africa, and the Medical College of Virginia—continued to perform transplants. Their success with them gradually improved, so that over the past 3 to 4 years these centers have reported a 1-year survival rate above 60 percent.

Heart transplantation can be performed in one of two ways. With *orthotopic transplantation,* the recipient's heart is removed, and the donor heart is placed in the normal intrathoracic position. Specifically, the atria are transected above the atrioventricular grooves but posterior to the level of the atrial appendages. The donor heart is implanted by opening its left and right atria and anastomosing them to the remnants of the recipient left and right atria. Then, the stumps of the donor aorta and pulmonary artery (transected a few centimeters above the aortic and pulmonary valves) are anastomosed to the recipient ascending aorta and pulmonary artery, respectively. With *heterotopic transplantation,* the recipient's heart is left in situ, and the donor heart is placed adjacent to the recipient's heart in the thoracic cavity. In particular, the donor heart is placed to the right of the recipient heart, and the left and right atria, aorta, and pulmonary artery (with an attached dacron graft) are anastomosed to the respective recipient structures. The advantages of heterotropic transplantation include the following: (1) transplantation is possible despite a markedly increased pulmonary vascular resistance; (2) the recipient heart provides some hemodynamic assistance (which may be small but crucial) in the immediate postoperative period; (3) the transplanted donor heart may be removed if the recipient heart recovers function; and (4) the recipient heart may maintain vital functions during severe rejection. Conversely, the potential disadvantages of heterotopic transplantation are as follows: (1) there may be a possible compromise of pulmonary function; (2) the poorly contracting recipient heart is a potential source of emboli; (3) the recipient heart may be the source of lethal arrhythmias; (4) the patient may still experience angina from the recipient heart; (5) consistent differentiation of donor and recipient electrical activity may be difficult; and (6) signs and symptoms of rejection may be difficult to detect because of the hemodynamic assistance provided by the recipient heart.

The potential recipient of a heart transplant must be chosen carefully. He should have terminal cardiac disease that is not amenable to any other form of cardiac surgery and that assures the patient of a poor prognosis with maximal medical therapy. The patient should be less than 50 years of age, should have normal or reversible function of other organ systems, and should have no evidence of systemic illness that would limit recovery or survival. There are several absolute contraindications to cardiac transplantation: (1) active infection, (2) recent pulmonary infarction, (3) diabetes mellitus requiring insulin therapy, (4) psychosis or mental deficiency, (5) drug addiction, and (6) a pulmonary vascular resistance greater than 8 Wood units unresponsive to vasodilators. This final contraindication need not apply to the patient receiving a heterotopic transplant.

Since irreversible functional and structural changes occur in the normothermic heart after 20 to 30 minutes of anoxia, it is necessary that the heart from the potential donor be removed while it is still beating but after the donor has been certified to have "brain death." However, not all patients with brain death are suitable donors. The potential donor should be screened for any cardiac abnormality, infection, or cancer. A detailed history should be elicited and a physical examination performed. Male donors should preferably be under 35 years of age and female donors under 40 years. In an older potential donor, cardiac catheterization and coronary angiography are recommended. Since brain death is often accompanied by derangements of homeostatic control mechanisms, the maintenance of cardiovascular stability in the potential donor heart may require vigorous fluid replacement, vasodilators, and vasopressors. Prophylactic broad-spectrum antibiotics, vigorous pulmonary care, avoidance of hypothermia, and the administration of vasopressin (for diabetes insipidus) may be necessary. Recently, distant heart procurement, which necessitates the transport and storage of donor hearts for several hours, has proved to be feasible.

The postoperative management of the heart transplant recipient must be performed in an intensive care unit with full reverse isolation for one to several weeks. The patient is extubated as soon as he is awake and cardiovascular status is stable. Immunosuppressive therapy is usually initiated immediately before operation and includes corticosteroids, azathioprine, rabbit antithymocyte globulin (RATG), and (in some centers) cyclosporin A. Azathioprine and RATG are usually given preoperatively. In the immediate postoperative period, methylprednisolone is given intravenously and RATG intramuscularly, and inotropic agents are given as required for cardiovascular support. Once oral intake is possible, prednisone, azathioprine, dipyridamole, and aspirin are instituted and continued long-term. Although the transplanted heart is denervated, the adrenergic receptors are intact and, therefore, are responsive to exogenously administered catecholamines and adrenergic receptor antagonists.

In the post-transplant period, the two most serious complications are *acute transplant rejection* and *infection*. The diagnosis of acute rejection was initially made on symptoms and signs (malaise, weakness, anorexia, and physical findings of right ventricular strain and failure) and electrocardiographic alterations (a decrease in QRS voltage). However, these appear relatively late. Transvenous endomyocardial biopsy and immunologic monitoring techniques allow an earlier and more sensitive detection of impending graft rejection. Indeed, one of the major advances in cardiac transplantation has been the earlier recognition and more successful treatment of acute rejection. Such rejection is treated with RATG, large doses of intravenous and oral corticosteroids, actinomycin D, and intravenous heparin. The incidence of acute rejection decreases markedly after the first 3 months, and subsequent rejection can often be treated with an increase in the dosage of oral prednisone alone.

Infection is the most common cause of death after cardiac transplantation, accounting for 62 percent of all deaths in the first postoperative month and 46 percent of deaths after the first 3 months. The average transplant recipient has three infectious episodes during the post-transplant period. Although nearly every organ system may be involved, pulmonary infections are most common. Bacterial organisms predominate and are followed by viral, fungal, protozoan, and nocardial organisms. *Aspergillus* and the gram-negative bacteria (*Escherichia coli, Klebsiella,* and *Pseudomonas*) are most commonly associated with a fatal outcome. Although the risk of infection is highest in the first 3 months, there is a three-fold increase in the incidence of serious infection when a rejection episode is treated with methylprednisolone and RATG. Prophylactic antibiotics should be administered before transplantation and for 48 hours postoperatively. Meticulous attention should be given to personal hygiene, cross-infection, and the aggressive and early treatment of any infection.

Chronic rejection is manifested as accelerated atherosclerosis of the coronary arteries of the transplanted heart. It may result in painless ischemia or even infarction. In an attempt to prevent this process, the Stanford group recommends (1) anticoagulation with coumadin, (2) dipyridamole, 400 mg per day, (3) weight control with exercise and caloric restriction, and (4) a diet low in saturated fat and cholesterol.

Finally, transplant recipients, like immunosuppressed recipients of other organ grafts, are subject to a higher risk of *malignancy* than the general population. Carcinomas, lymphomas, and leukemias have been reported in this patient population. Factors that appear to be associated with the occurrence of lymphoma include younger age, retransplantation, and treatment with cyclosporin A.

The reported survival rate at Stanford University for cardiac transplant recipients is 65 percent at 1 year and 39 percent at 5 years. There is an inverse relationship between patient age and survival after transplantation: those over age 50 have a 15-percent 3-year survival, those 41 to 50 years of age a 25-percent 3-year survival, and those under age 40 a 55-percent 3-year survival. Infection is the major cause of death in older recipients. Following successful transplantation, most patients are successfully rehabilitated, and more than half return to full-time employment. When the transplanted heart fails, the only viable long-term alternative is retransplantation. Although considerable progress has been made in the development of an artificial heart, even the best device has a limited lifespan (generally less than 1 year) due to material failure, and it requires an external power source.

1. Barnard CN. The operation—a human cardiac transplant: an interim report of a successful operation performed at Groote Schuur Hospital, Cape Town. S Afr Med J 1967; 41:1271–4.
   The original description of the first human heart transplant.
2. Barnard CN, Barnard MS, Cooper DKC, Curchio CA, Hassoulas J, Novitsky D, Wolpowitz A. The present status of heterotopic cardiac transplantation. J Thorac Cardiovasc Surg 1981; 81:433–9.
   A detailed summary of the Cape Town experience with heterotopic heart transplantation.
3. Barnard CN, Wolpowitz A. Heterotopic versus orthotopic heart transplantation. Transplant Proc 1979; 11:309–12.
   A discussion of the advantages and disadvantages of each technique.
4. Baumgartner WA, Reitz BA, Oyer PE, Stinson EB, Shumway NE. Cardiac homotransplantation. Curr Probl Surg 1979; 16(9):6–61.
   An excellent comprehensive report of the Stanford experience. Includes 181 references.
5. Beck W, Barnard CN, Schrire V. Hemodynamic studies in two long-term survivors of heart transplantation. J Thorac Cardiovasc Surg 1971; 62:315–20.
   A detailed hemodynamic study of 2 patients 12 and 18 months after orthotopic heart transplantation.
6. Bieber CP, Reitz BA, Jamieson SW, Oyer PE, Stinson EB. Malignant lymphoma in Cyclosporin A–treated allograft recipients. Lancet 1980; 1:43.
   A brief report of the incidence of lymphomas in cyclosporin A–treated transplant recipients.
7. Cannom DS, Rider AK, Stinson EB, Harrison DC. Electrophysiologic studies in the denervated transplanted human heart. II. Response to norepinephrine, isoproterenol, and propranolol. Am J Cardiol 1975; 36:859–66.

In spite of cardiac denervation, cardiac β-receptors remain responsive to circulating catecholamines.

8. Christopherson LK, Griepp RB, Stinson EB. Rehabilitation after cardiac transplantation. JAMA 1976; 236:2082–4.
   Of 56 patients who survived more than 6 months after cardiac transplantation at Stanford University, 51(91%) were said to be successfully rehabilitated.
9. Clark DA, Stinson EB, Griepp RB, Schroeder JS, Shumway NE, Harrison DC. Cardiac transplantation in man. VI. Prognosis of patients selected for cardiac transplantation. Ann Intern Med 1971; 75:15–21.
   Although a truly randomized study has never been performed, cardiac transplantation appears to prolong life in patients with end-stage cardiac disease.
10. Copeland J, Stinson EB. Human heart transplantation. Curr Probl Cardiol 1979; 4:4–51.
    Another excellent review of the Stanford experience.
11. Griepp RB, Stinson EB, Bieber CP, Reitz BA, Copeland JG, Oyer PE, Shumway NE. Control of graft arteriosclerosis in human heart transplant recipients. Surgery 1977; 81:262–9.
    A review of the Stanford experience with this problem and a proposed course of action to prevent its occurrence.
12. Hastillo A, Hess ML, Richardson DW, Lower RR. Cardiac Transplantation—1980: the Medical College of Virginia Program. South Med J 1980; 73:909–11.
    A summary of the Medical College of Virginia experience.
13. Knox RA. Heart transplants: to pay or not to pay. Science 1980; 209:570–5.
    A detailed consideration of the financial implications of widespread heart transplantation.
14. Kolff WJ, Lawson J. Perspectives for the total artificial heart. Transplant Proc 1979; 11:317–24.
    A review of the status of the total artificial mechanical heart.
15. Oyer PE, Stinson EB, Bieber CP, Reitz BA, Raney AA, Baumgartner WA, Shumway NE. Diagnosis and treatment of acute cardiac allograft rejection. Transplant Proc 1979; 11:296–303.
    A detailed discussion of this problem by the Stanford group.
16. Oyer PE, Stinson EB, Reitz BA, Bieber CP, Jamieson SW, Shumway NE. Cardiac transplantation: 1980. Transplant Proc 1981; 13:199–206.
    An update on the status of human heart transplantation, including its costs.
17. Pope SE, Stinson EB, Daughters GT II, Schroeder JS, Ingels NB Jr, Alderman EL. Exercise response of the denervated heart in long-term cardiac transplant recipients. Am J Cardiol 1980; 46:213–8.
    Increases in cardiac output by the transplanted heart are brought about early in exercise by augmented preload and the Frank-Starling mechanism and later in exercise by chronotropic and inotropic influences due to increased circulating catecholamines.
18. Pennock JL, Oyer PE, Reitz BA, Jamieson SW, Bieber CP, Wallwork J, Stinson EB, Shumway NE. Cardiac transplantation in perspective for the future: survival, complications, rehabilitation, and cost. J Thorac Cardiovasc Surg 1982; 83:168–77.
    This report details the Stanford experience with 227 transplants in 206 patients. Currently, the 5-year survival rate is 39% following transplantation. One hundred and six patients survived at least 1 year after transplantation.
19. Rose AG, Uys CJ, Losman JG, Barnard CN. Evaluation of endomyocardial biopsy in the diagnosis of cardiac rejection: a study using bioptome samples of formalin-fixed tissue. Transplantation 1978; 26:10–13.
    Endomyocardial biopsy is a highly accurate method of diagnosing acute rejection.
20. Thomas FT, Szentpetery SS, Wolfgang TC, Quinn JE, Thomas J, Lower RR. Improved immunosuppression for cardiac transplantation: immune monitoring and individualized modulation of recipient immunity by *in vitro* testing. Ann Thorac Surg 1979; 28:212–23.
    This study shows immune monitoring and individualized modification of recipient immune reactivity with rabbit antithymocyte globulin can improve results with cardiac transplantation.

21. Ad Hoc Committee of the Harvard Medical School to Examine the Definition of Brain Death. A definition of irreversible coma. JAMA 1968; 205:337–40.
    The characteristics of irreversible brain death defined by this committee have been applied to potential transplant donors.

INDEX